Self Assessment and Review
ENT

Ninth Edition

SAKSHI ARORA HANS
Faculty of Leading PG and FMGE Coachings
MBBS "Gold Medalist" (GSVM, Kanpur)
DGO (MLNMC, Allahabad)
India

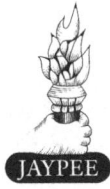

JAYPEE BROTHERS MEDICAL PUBLISHERS
The Health Sciences Publisher
New Delhi | London

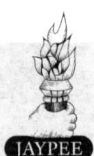

Jaypee Brothers Medical Publishers (P) Ltd

Headquarters
Jaypee Brothers Medical Publishers (P) Ltd
EMCA House, 23/23-B, Ansari Road
Daryaganj, New Delhi 110 002, India
Landline: +91-11-23272143, +91-11-23272703
+91-11-23282021, +91-11-23245672
Email: jaypee@jaypeebrothers.com: www.jaypeebrothers.com

Corporate Office
Jaypee Brothers Medical Publishers (P) Ltd
4838/24, Ansari Road, Daryaganj
New Delhi 110 002, India
Phone: +91-11-43574357
Fax: +91-11-43574314
Email: jaypee@jaypeebrothers.com

Overseas Office
J.P. Medical Ltd
83 Victoria Street, London
SW1H 0HW (UK)
Phone: +44 20 3170 8910
Fax: +44 (0)20 3008 6180
Email: info@jpmedpub.com

Website: www.jaypeebrothers.com
Website: www.jaypeedigital.com

© 2018, Jaypee Brothers Medical Publishers

The views and opinions expressed in this book are solely those of the original contributor(s)/author(s) and do not necessarily represent those of editor(s) of the book.

All rights reserved. No part of this publication may be reproduced, stored or transmitted in any form or by any means, electronic, mechanical, photocopying, recording or otherwise, without the prior permission in writing of the publishers.

All brand names and product names used in this book are trade names, service marks, trademarks or registered trademarks of their respective owners. The publisher is not associated with any product or vendor mentioned in this book.

Medical knowledge and practice change constantly. This book is designed to provide accurate, authoritative information about the subject matter in question. However, readers are advised to check the most current information available on procedures included and check information from the manufacturer of each product to be administered, to verify the recommended dose, formula, method and duration of administration, adverse effects and contraindications. It is the responsibility of the practitioner to take all appropriate safety precautions. Neither the publisher nor the author(s)/editor(s) assume any liability for any injury and/or damage to persons or property arising from or related to use of material in this book.

This book is sold on the understanding that the publisher is not engaged in providing professional medical services. If such advice or services are required, the services of a competent medical professional should be sought.

Every effort has been made where necessary to contact holders of copyright to obtain permission to reproduce copyright material. If any have been inadvertently overlooked, the publisher will be pleased to make the necessary arrangements at the first opportunity. The **CD/DVD-ROM** (if any) provided in the sealed envelope with this book is complimentary and free of cost. **Not meant for sale.**

Inquiries for bulk sales may be solicited at: jaypee@jaypeebrothers.com

Self Assessment and Review: ENT

First Edition: 2010
Second Edition: 2011
Third Edition: 2012
Fourth Edition: 2013
Fifth Edition: 2014
Sixth Edition: 2015
Seventh Edition: 2016
Eighth Edition: 2017
Ninth Edition: 2018, **Reprint:** 2024, **2025**
ISBN: 978-93-5270-430-9
Typeset at JPBMP typesetting unit
Printed at: Samrat Offset Pvt. Ltd.

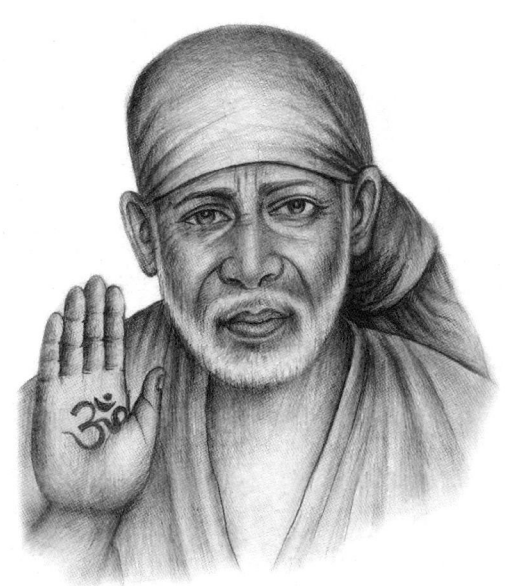

Dedicated to
SAI BABA

Just sitting here reflecting on where I am and where I started, I could not have done it without you Sai Baba.. I praise you and love you for all that you have given me... and thank you for another beautiful day ... to be able to sing and praise you and glorify you .. you are my amazing god

Preface

"It can be very difficult to sculpt the idea that you have in mind. If your idea doesn't match the shape of the stone, your idea may have to change because you have to accept what is available in the rock"

Fevereiro 1999 in Arctic Spirit

Dear Students,

I wish to extend my thanks to all of you for your overwhelming response to all the eight editions of my book. I am extremely delighted by the wonderful response shown by the readers for the 8th edition and proving it again as the bestseller book on the subject. Thanks once again for the innumerable e-mails you have sent in appreciation of the book.

With the experience, which I have gained working as a faculty and being so closely associated with PG Aspirants, **it's not how much you study which matters rather, its how wisely you study which matters the most.**

Since we are not human prodigies (at least I don't consider myself as one and 90% PG Aspirants are somewhat similar), we cannot remember everything about 19 subjects. We need to have a strategic plan to crack AIPG (NEET), which means we have to choose some subjects where we can be sure of not making mistakes.

And believe me friends- ENT is one of those subjects, where if you put efforts, it will not let you down. With the help of this book, I am just helping you to cake walk through the subject.

How to Use This Book

1. *Intern and PG Aspirants:* The scarcity of time which you have and since you have already done ENT in your third year, I would suggest first read all the New Pattern Questions (Marked as N within the theory). See all diagrams, instruments and previously asked questions with answers. Initially do not read the theory, if you are unable to answer the question correctly of some particular topic, then read the theory of that topic from the book. Although, I strongly recommend you to go through anatomy of ear, nose, larynx and pharynx along with their tumors from this book.
2. *Undergraduates and Foreign Graduates:* Read the book cover to cover, do not miss out anything, this book will not only lay a strong foundation for PG Entrance but will also help you in your undergraduate theory and viva exams.

Salient Features of 9th Edition

Important appendices are included:
- Appendix 1: Syndromes in ENT
- Appendix 2: Test in ENT
- Appendix 3: Signs in ENT
- Appendix 4: Named lines and structures

1. *Pretext:* Detailed yet concise pointwise overview of the topic with many flow charts, tables and mnemonics for better understanding and retaining.
2. *New Pattern Questions:* To give students an idea of the new questions which could be formed, over 500 new pattern questions have been added, along side the theory. This will help you to reinforce important points from the topic. These questions are the potential questions for upcoming exams.
3. *Instruments and Diagrams:* All important instruments related to surgery, diagrams, X-rays, CT scans have been given along with the topic. This is to ensure that students do not miss on any important information and can correlate with them.
4. *MCQs:* All MCQs of AIIMS up to November 2017, and state-based MCQs up to November 2017 have been included.
5. *Authentic Explanations:* Explanations from standard and recent edition textbooks have been provided for each answer. Different and controversial MCQs have been explained in details, discussing each option and excluding the incorrect one.

I am thankful to Shri Jitendar P Vij (Group Chairman) for allowing me to use illustrations from eminent ENT Textbooks (like Essentials of ENT by Mohan Bansal, TB of ENT by Mohan Bansal and Diseases of ENT by BS Tuli, 2nd Edition) of Jaypee Brothers Medical Publishers (P) Ltd, New Delhi, India.

Though at most care has been taken to avoid all possible errors, some minor errors might have crept in, inadvertently. I request the readers to kindly point out the same and give their valuable suggestions or feedbacks by e-mail.

I wish you all the very best for your upcoming exams and for your bright future.

New Delhi
March 2018

Dr Sakshi Arora Hans
delhisakshiarora@gmail.com

Acknowledgements

Over the years (even if it is 8-10 years), writing acknowledgement for my books, have become an opportunity for self-reflection.

My Family

- **Dr Pankaj Hans,** my better-half who has always been a mountain of support and who is to a large measure, responsible for what I am today. His calm, consistent approach towards any work, brings some calmness in my hasty, hyperactive, and inconsistent nature.
- **My Father: Shri H.C. Arora,** who has overcome all odds with his discipline, hardwork, and perfection.
- **My Mother: Smt. Sunita Arora,** who has always believed in my abilities and supported me in all my ventures – be it authoring a book or teaching.
- **My in Laws (Hans family):** For happily accepting my maiden surname 'Arora' and taking pride in all achievements.
- **My Brothers: Mr Bhupesh Arora** and **Sachit Arora,** who encouraged me to write books and have always thought (wrong although) their sister is a perfectionist.
- **My Daughter, Shreya Hans** (A priceless gift of God): For accepting my books and work as her siblings (Although now she is showing signs of intense sibling rivalry!!).

My Teachers

- **Dr Manju Verma** (Prof & Head, Gynae & Obs, MLN MC, Allahabad) and **Dr Gauri Ganguli** (Prof & Ex-HEAD, Gynae & Obs, MLNMC, Allahabad) for teaching me to focus on the basic concepts of any subject.

My Colleagues: I am grateful to all my seniors, friends and colleagues of past and present for their moral support.

- Dr Manoj Rawal
- Dr Ruchi Aggrawal
- Dr Parminder Sehgal
- Dr Prakash Khatri
- Dr Pooja Aggrawal
- Dr Shalini Tripathi
- Dr Amit Jain
- Dr Abhishek Singh
- Dr Parul Aggrawal Jain
- Dr Kushant Gupta
- Dr Sonika Lamba Rawal
- Dr Sonia Bhatt

Directors of PG Entrance Coaching, who helped me in realizing my potential as an academician.

- **Dr Vineet Singh:** Director, MIST Coaching
- **Mr Sundar Rao:** Director, SIMS Academy

My Publishers—Jaypee Brothers Medical Publishers (P) Ltd

- **Shri Jitendar P Vij** (Group Chairman) for being the best in the industry.
- **Mr Ankit Vij** (Group President) for having constant faith in me and all my endeavours.
- **Ms Chetna Malhotra Vohra** (Associate Director—Content Strategy) for working hard with the team to achieve the deadlines.
- The entire MCQs team for working laborious hours in designing and typesetting of the book.

Last but not the least

My sincere thanks to all FMGE/UG/PG students, present and past, for their tremendous support, words of appreciation rather I should say e-mails of encouragement and informing me about the corrections, which have helped me in the betterment of the book.

Dr Sakshi Arora Hans
delhisakshiarora@gmail.com

Contents

Appendices .... ix-xv
Color Plates

SECTION 1: EAR

1. Anatomy of Ear 3
2. Physiology of Ear and Hearing 35
3. Hearing Loss 43
4. Assessment of Hearing Loss 54
5. Assessment of Vestibular Function 76
6. Diseases of External Ear 89
7. Diseases of Middle Ear 100
8. Meniere's Disease 136
9. Otosclerosis 144
10. Facial Nerve and its Lesions 154
11. Lesion of Cerebellopontine Angle and Acoustic Neuroma 170
12. Glomus Tumor and Other Tumors of the Ear 178
13. Rehabilitative Methods 184
14. Miscellaneous 192

SECTION 2: NOSE AND PARANASAL SINUSES

15. Anatomy and Physiology of Nose 197
16. Diseases of External Nose and Nasal Septum 210
17. Granulomatous Disorders of Nose, Nasal Polyps and Foreign Body in Nose 223
18. Inflammatory Disorders of Nasal Cavity 237
19. Epistaxis 246
20A. Diseases of Paranasal Sinus—Sinusitis 257
20B. Diseases of Paranasal Sinus—Sinonasal Tumor 277

SECTION 3: ORAL CAVITY

21. Oral Cavity 287

SECTION 4: PHARYNX

22. Anatomy of Pharynx, Tonsils and Adenoids 321
23. Head and Neck Space Inflammation and Thornwaldt's Bursitis 342
24. Lesions of Nasopharynx and Hypopharynx including Tumors of Pharynx 350
25. Pharynx Hot Topics 362

SECTION 5: LARYNX

26. Anatomy of Larynx, Congenital Lesions of Larynx and Stridor 369
27. Acute and Chronic Inflammation of Larynx, Voice and Speech Disorders 386
28. Vocal Cord Paralysis 403
29. Tumors of Larynx 414

SECTION 6: OPERATIVE PROCEDURES

30. Important Operative Procedures 433

Appendices

APPENDIX 1: SYNDROMES IN ENT

Alpert Syndrome
- Progressive sensorineural hearing loss (SNHL)
- Hematuria
- Chronic renal failure
- Anterior lenticonus

Anterior Ethmoidal Syndrome (Sluder's)
- Palm above the superciliary ridge due to pressure on anterior ethmoidal nerve

Behçet Syndrome
- Recurrent aphthous ulcers
- Painful eye ulcers
- Ulcers on genitals

Cogan Syndrome
- SNHL
- Non-syphilitic interstitial keratitis
- Vertigo

Crouzon Syndrome
- Deafness (SN, conductive or mixed HL)
- Shallow orbits
- Proptosis
- Maxillary hypoplasia

Frey Syndrome
- Sweating or flushing of face on parotid or eating food
- Seen after parotidectomy operation

Gradenigo Syndrome
- Pain around the eye
- Otorrhea
- VI nerve palsy causing diplopia
- Facial nerve palsy rarely
- Vestibular Mystagmus

Grisel Syndrome
- Nontraumatic atlantoaxial subluxation due to parapharyngeal infection involving upper cervical region

Lermoyez Syndrome
- Hearing Loss

- Tinnitus
- Vertigo later on
- Loose wire syndrome
- A triad of symptoms after stapedectomy operations that improve with inflation, i.e. auditory acquity, distorted sound, speech discrimination

Melkersson Syndrome

- Recurring attacks of facial palsy
- Swelling of lips
- Congenital furrowing of tongue

Meniere Syndrome

- Episodic vertigo
- Fluctuating deafness
- Tinnitus

Patterson-Kelly-Brown Syndrome/Plummer-Vinson Syndrome

- Iron-deficiency anemia
- Atrophic tongue
- Koilonychia
- Dysphagia
- Esophageal web
- More common in females

Pendred Syndome

- Goiter
- SN deafness

Pierre Robin Syndrome

- Cleft palate, hypoplasia of mandible, glossoptosis
- Club foot
- Mental retardation
- Microcephaly

Ramsay Hunt Sydrome

(Herpes Zoster Oticus)
- Severe in the ear
- Vesicular eruption of pinna or around it
- VII nerve palsy
- Deafness, tinnitus and vertigo may be present

Sjogen's Syndrome

- Xerostomia
- Keratoconjunctivitis sicca
- Swelling of exocrine glands

APPENDIX 2: TEST IN ENT

Named Tests	Used For
• Weber Test • Rinne Test • Bing Test • Gelle Test • Schwabach Test • Absolute Bone Conduction Test	Tuning fork test for hearing loss (Conduction or SNHL)
• Pure Tone Audiometry • Tone Decay	Subjective Audiometry Test
• Speech Audiometry • Impedance Audiometry	Objective Audiometry Test
• Stenger Test • Lombard Test • Stapedial Reflex • BERA	To detect malingering/Nonorganic hearing loss
• Otoacoustic emission • BERA	Initial screening test for hearing loss in infants. IOC for detecting hearing loss in infants
• Caloric Tests • Modified Kobrak Test • Fitzgerald-Hallpike Test	For vestibular function to induce nystagmus
• Galvanic Test • Vestibular Evoked Myogenic Potential	For assessing vestibular function
• Cottle Test	To test the patency of naval value
• Pneumatic otoscopy • Nasopharyngoscopy • Tympanometry • Eustachian Tube Catheterization • Valsalva and Politzer Test • Toynbee Test • Frenzel Maneuver • Sonotubometry	Test for eustachian tube function
• Tobey-Ayer Test • Queckenstedt Test	Lateral sinus/sigmoid sinus thrombophlebitis
• Schimer Test	Method to assess the parasympathetic innervation to lacrimal gland via Greater Superficial Petrosal Nerve in Facial Nerve palsy
• Glycerol Test	Meniere disease
• Frusten berg Test	Encephalocele

APPENDIX 3: SIGNS IN ENT

- **Battle's Sign**
  - It is a post-testicular ecchymosis that occurs due to fracture through the mastoid cortex in cases of head injury or middle cranial fossa fracture.
- **Bierman's Sign**
  - Dark color of anterior pillar of tonsillar fossa in some patients of syphilis.
- **Bocca's Sign**
  - Absence of laryngeal crepitus in postericoid malignancy perichondritis and foreign body cricopharynx.
- **Boyce's Sign**
  - There is gurgling sound on compression of pharyngeal pouch.
- **Brown's Sign**
  - It is seen in glomus tumor. There is blanching of the mass after applying pressure with Siegal's speculum.
- **Charcot's Triad**
  - Consists of nystagmus scanning speech and intentional tremors and triad is a feature of multiple sclerosis.
- **Chvostek's Sign**
  - Facial twitch seen on tapping over the distribution of facial nerve and is seen in hypocalcemia.
- **Crescent Sign**
  - Air shadow in nasopharynx resembles a crescent in the presence of antrochoanal (AC) polyp.
- **Delta Sign**
  - Lateral sinus thrombosis on computerized tomography (CT) or magnetic resonance imaging (MRI) shows enhancement of peripheral angle of dura, whereas there is no enhancement of central pain. It is also called empty triangle sign.
- **Griesinger's Sign**
  - It is seen in lateral sinus thrombosis. There is pitting edema seen over the mastoid process due to thrombosis of mastoid emissary veins.
- **Gutzmann's Test**
  - Frontal pressure on thyroid cartilage lowers the pitch due to counteracting the function of cricothyroid muscle, while lateral pressure has an opposite effect. If the results are abnormal, it suggests cricothyroid paralysis.
- **Halo Sign**
  - Also called **target sign** or **double ring sign** and is seen in traumatic cerebrospinal fluid (CSF) leak due to blood mixed with CSF.
- **Hamman's Sign**
  - When there is air in the mediastinum, there is crepitus present and auscultation with each heartbeat.
- **Hennebert's Sign**
  - It is a false positive fistula test.
- **Hallpike manoeuver** done to rule out benign paroxysm positional of vertigo.
- **Hitselberger's Sign**
  - In this sign, touch sensations of posterosuperior external auditory meatus are found to be absent in cases of vestibular schwannoma.
- **Irwin Moore's Sign**
  - Pressure on anterior pillar, pus comes out from crypto as septic squeeze.
- **Kernig's Sign**
  - This sign is elicited in meningitis. The patient is usually able to touch his chin with his chest.
- **Light House Sign**
  - Pulsatile seen in stage of suppuration of otitis media.
- **Mecca Sign**
  - In malignant lesions of tongue, patient sits with one ear due to referred pain and other hand on mouth for saliva.
- **Paracusis Willisii**
  - Patients of otosclerosis hear better in noisy environment. This is due to good discrimination score and the person has raised his voice.
- **Reservoir Sign**
  - Seen in acute mastoiditis.

- **Rising Sun Sign**
  - There is red vascular hue seen behind the intact tympanic membrane. It is seen in glomus tumor, high jugular bulb and aberrant carotid artery in the floor of middle ear.
- **Spielberg's Sign**
  - Seen in fracture lamina papyracea.
- **Steeple Sign**
  - Narrowing of subglottic on lateral X-ray neck seen in croup.
- **Schwartz's Sign**
  - It is also called flamingo flush. It is seen because of increased vascularity in submucous layer of promontory in otosclerosis.
- **Stellwag's Sign**
  - It is the starting look due to infrequent blinking seen in Grave's disease.
- **Tear Drop Sign**
  - It is defined as a tear drop-shaped opacification seen hanging from the roof of the maxillary sinus on Water's view.
- **Teal's Sign**
  - A feature of acoustic neuroma.
- **Thumb Sign**
  - It is a thumb-like imprssion seen on X-ray in patients with acute epiglottis.
- **Tragus Sign**
  - In acute otitis externa, there is marked tenderness, fragus is pressed against the pinna.
- **Tripod Sign**
  - Seen in acute epiglottitis in children, sitting and forward to have easy breathing.
- **Tullio Phenomenon**
  - Loud sounds may cause vertigo in patients of the disease. It is a variation of Hennebert's sign.
- **Wartenberg's Sign**
  - Intense pruritus of tip of nose and nostril tumor.

APPENDIX 4: NAMED LINES AND STRUCTURES

- Korner's septum : Petrosquamous suture persisting in intrauterine life.
- Shraphell's membrane : Pars flaccida of tympanic membrane
- Canal of Huguier : Exit site of chorda tympani from middle ear
- Jacobson nerve : Tympanic part of glossopharyngeal nerve bounded above by lateral malleolar fold and below by short process of malleus.
- Prussak space : Lies between the neck of malleus and pars flaccida
- Donaldson line : Line extending from lateral semicircular canal and bisecting the posterior semicircular canal. It is the surgical landmark for endolymphatic sac.
- Ohngren's line : Imaginary line extending from medial rectus of eye to the angle of mandible. Used to know the prognosis of PNS tumors
- Lines of Sebileau : Two lines, one line passing through the floor of orbit and other through floor of maxillary antrum used for knowing prognosis of PNS tumor
- Rosenthal canal : Inside the bony spiral lamina, containg 8th nerve ganglion
- Deiters cell
- Claudius cell : Supporting outer hair cells
- Hoarser cell
- Falciform crest : Divides the internal acoustic meatus into superior and inferior parts
- Bells bar : Divides the superior compartment of IAM into anterior and posterior parts

Sinus of Morgagni

It is a large gap between base of skull and upper border of superior constrictor muscle through which pass eustachian tube, levator palatini muscle and ascending palatine artery.

Sinus Tympani

Also called infrapyramidal recess or medial facial recess, it is a triangular space between ponticulus and subiculum process.

Sublingual Space

It is bounded by lingual surface of body of mandible, mucous membrane of floor of mouth and the upper surface of mylohyoid muscle. It contains submandibular, sublingual salivary glands, and lingual and hypoglossal nerves.

Submandibular Space

It is bounded by body of mandible, lower surface of mylohyoid muscle above and the superficial layer of deep cervical fascia below. It contains superficial part of submandibular salivary gland, anterior belly of digastric muscle and submandibular and submental lymph nodes.

Sinodural Angle

It is the angle between tegmen antri and sigmoid sinus.

Simon's Triangle

Anteriorly: It is bounded by recurrent laryngeal nerve (RLN).
Posteriorly: Common carotid artery
At the base: Inferior thyroid artery.

Soft Triangle of Nose

It is the apex of nostril beneath the lobule.
Citelli angle: Sinodural angle

Solid Angle

It is the angle formed by three semicircular canals.

Submental Triangle

- Apex : At the chin
- Base : Body of hyoid
- Floor : Mylohyoid muscle

Macewen's Triangle

- Above : Posterior root of zygoma
- Anterior : Posterosuperior canal wall
- Behind : Imaginary line tangential to posterior canal wall below and cuts the posterior root of zygoma above

Submental Triangle

- Apex : Body of hyoid
- At the chin : Floor
- Base : Mylohyoid muscle

Trautmann's Triangle: Triangular area on medial wall of mastoid antrum

- Posterior : Sigmoid sinus
- Anterior : Bony labyrinth
- Superior : Superior petrosal sinus

It is landmark to approach posterior cranial fossa

Trotter's Triad
- Seen in carcinoma nasopharynx
- Unilateral middle ear effusion (conductive deafness)
- Pain in ear, jaw or tongue

COLOR PLATES

Image Based Questions

PLATE 1

Q N1. Identify the area marked 'X':

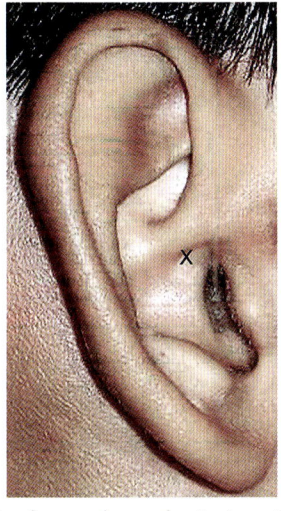

a. Cymba concha   b. Incisura terminalis
c. Scaphoid fossa   d. Ascending crux of helix

Ans. See Chapter 1, Q. N5 for Explanation

PLATE 2

Q N2. Space between pars tensa and anterior malleolar fold is called as:

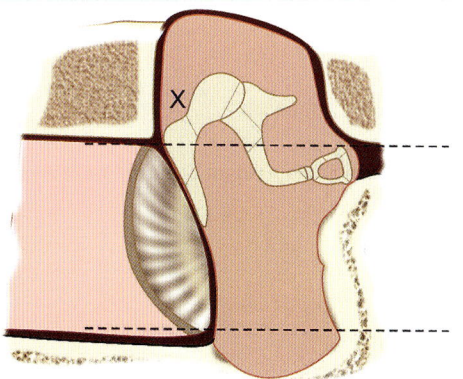

a. Von Troeltsch anterior pouch
b. Facial recess
c. Sinus tympani
d. Prussak's space

Ans. See Chapter 1, Q. N12 for Explanation

PLATE 3

Q N3. Identify the condition shown in the figure:

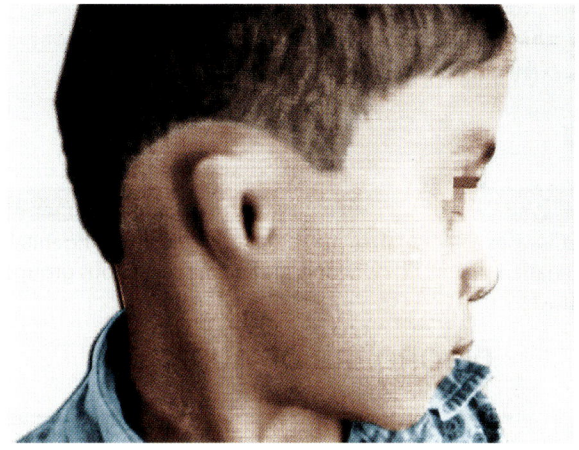

a. Bat ear
b. Microtia
c. Macrotia
d. Crotia

Ans. See Chapter 1, Q. N15 for Explanation

PLATE 4

Q N4. Identify the condition shown in the figure:

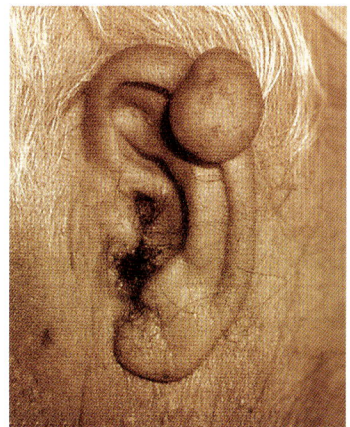

a. Dermoid cyst of pinna
b. Keloid on pinna
c. Cauliflower ear
d. Preauricular sinus

Ans. See Chapter 1, Q. N16 for Explanation

PLATE 5

Q N5. Which of the following is being done in the figure?

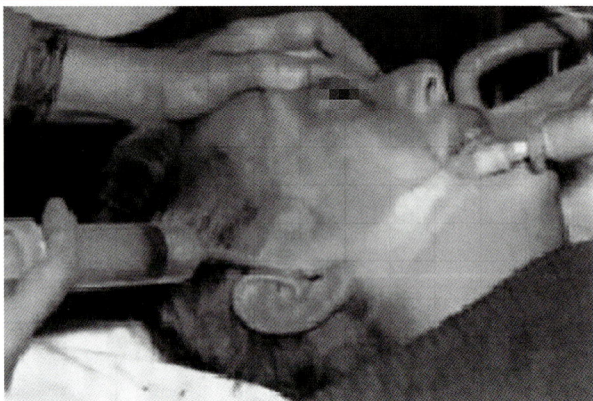

a. Determining Eustachian tube patency
b. Testing vestibulo-ocular reflex by injecting cold water
c. Politzerization
d. Syringe of ear in patient with CSOM and meningitis

Ans. See Chapter 5, Q. N40 for Explanation

PLATE 7

Q N7. Identify the instrument shown in the figure:

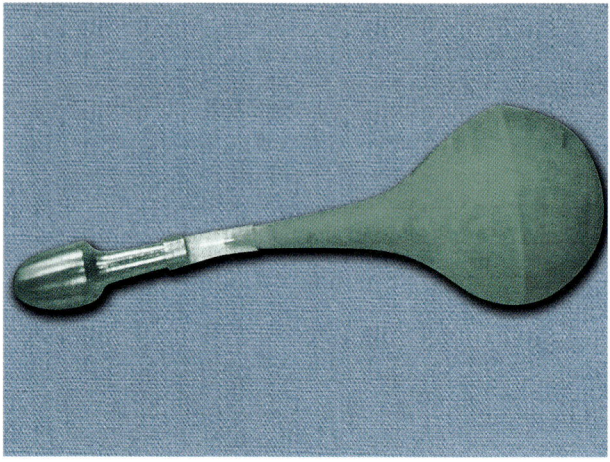

a. Otoendoscope
b. Siegel speculum
c. Politzer bag
d. Otoscope

Ans. See Chapter 5, Q. N10 for Explanation

PLATE 6

Q N6. Identify the procedure being done in the figure:

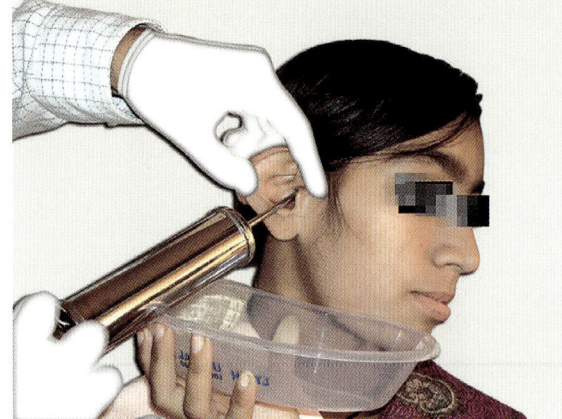

a. Determining Eustachian tube patency
b. Syringing
c. Politzerization
d. Fitzgerald test

Ans. See Chapter 5, Q. N9 for Explanation

PLATE 8

Q N8. An intraoperative photograph of cortical mastoidectomy. Which of the following is the lateral semicircular canal? **[AIIMS Nov 2017]**

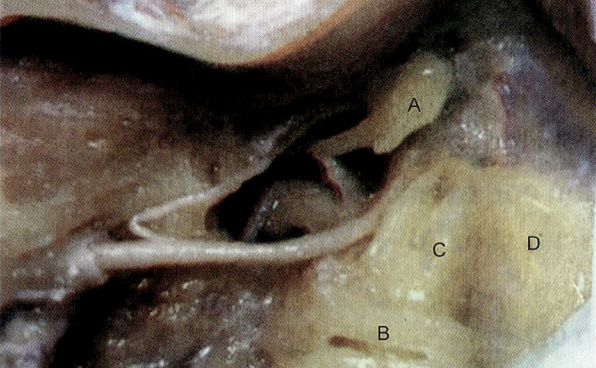

a. A
b. B
c. C
d. D

Ans. See Chapter 7, Q. N110 for Explanation

PLATE 9

Q N9. In the pure tone audiogram shown below, identify the likely cause: [AIIMS May 2017]

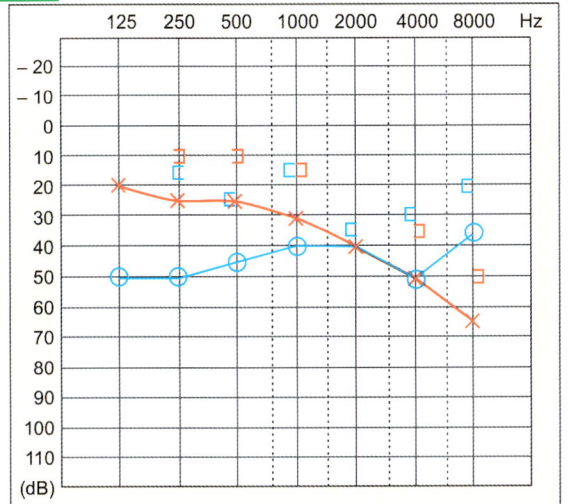

a. Meniere's disease   b. Noise induced hearing loss
c. Otosclerosis   d. Ototoxicity

Ans. See Chapter 9, Q. N18 for Explanation

PLATE 11

Q N11. The figure shows structure seen on posterior rhinoscopy—Identify the structure shown by 'X':

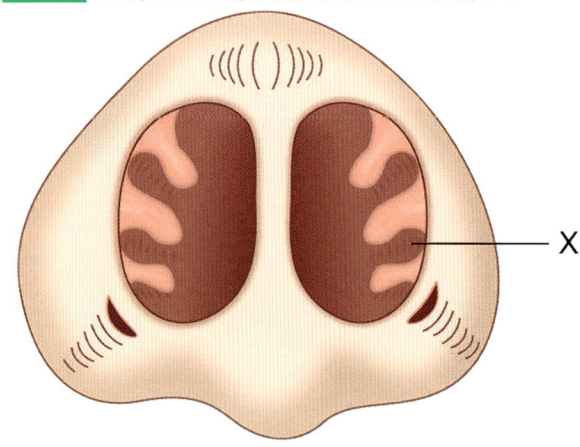

a. Superior meatus
b. Middle meatus
c. Inferior meatus
d. Eustachian tube opening

Ans. See Chapter 15, Q. N24 for Explanation

PLATE 10

Q N10. The plate show an important area of nose—identify it:

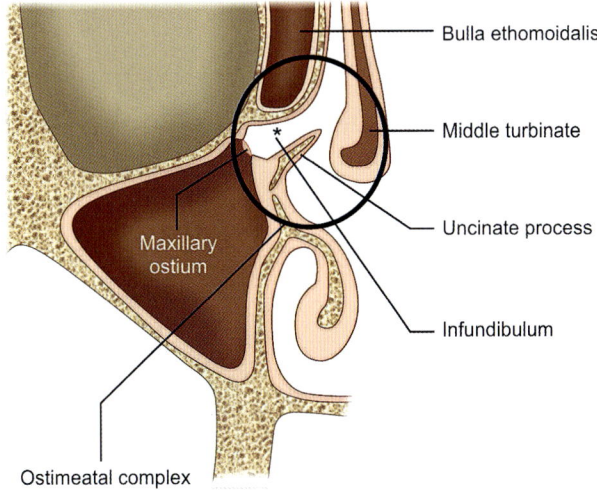

a. Nasal valve   b. Columella
c. Osteomeatal complex   d. Vestibule

Ans. See Chapter 15, Q. N11 for Explanation

PLATE 12

Q N12. Identify the condition of nose shown in plate:

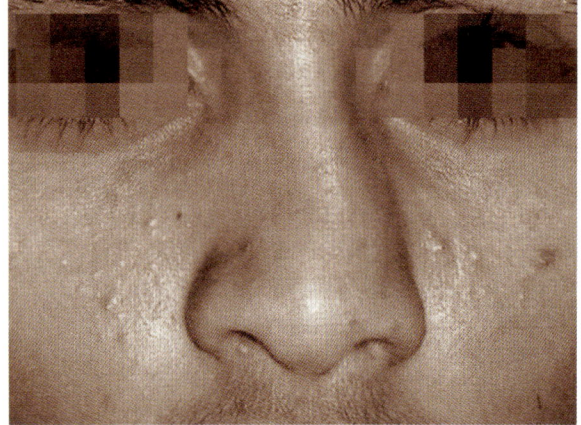

a. Crooked nose
b. Deviated nose
c. Saddle nose
d. Humped nose

Ans. See Chapter 16, Q. N2 for Explanation

PLATE 13
Q N13. Identify the condition of nose shown in plate:

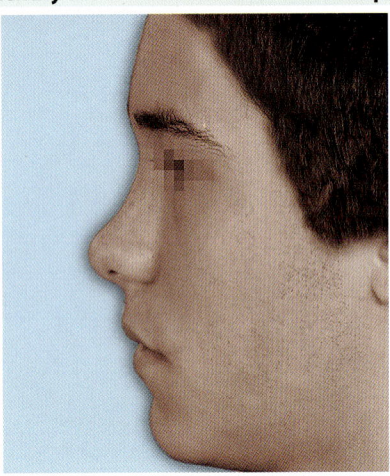

a. Crooked nose
b. Deviated nose
c. Saddle nose
d. Humped nose

Ans. See Chapter 16, Q. N3 for Explanation

PLATE 15
Q N15. Identify the condition shown in the nose in the plate:

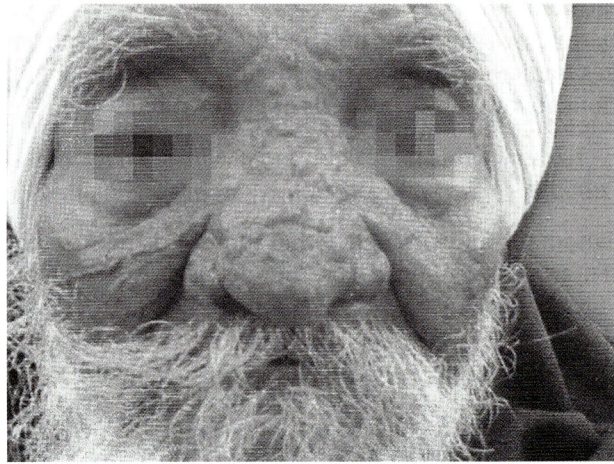

a. Hemangioma of nose
b. Rhinophyma of nose
c. Papilloma of nose
d. Neurofibroma

Ans. See Chapter 16, Q. N15 for Explanation

PLATE 14
Q N14. Identify the incision shown in plate:

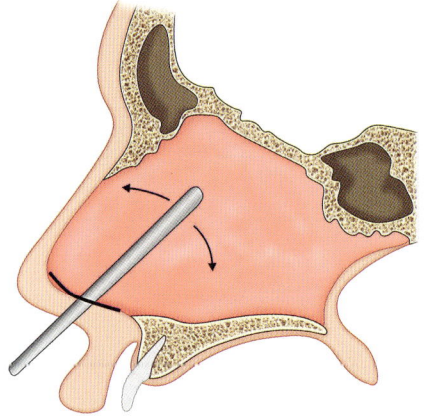

a. Killian's incision
b. Freer's incision
c. Weber-Ferguson incision
d. Schobinger incision

Ans. See Chapter 16, Q. N9 for Explanation

PLATE 16
Q N16. Identify the line marked on face in the picture below:

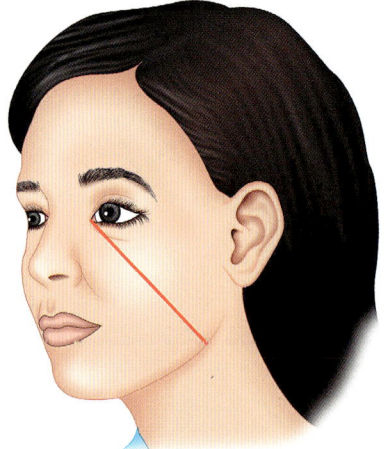

a. Ohngren's line   b. Kasami line
c. Frankfurt's line d. Donaldson line

Ans. See Chapter 20B, Q. N16 for Explanation

PLATE 17

Q N17. The patient came with an ulcer on the side of the nose as shown, which bleeds on itching. What is the diagnosis? [AIIMS Nov 2017]

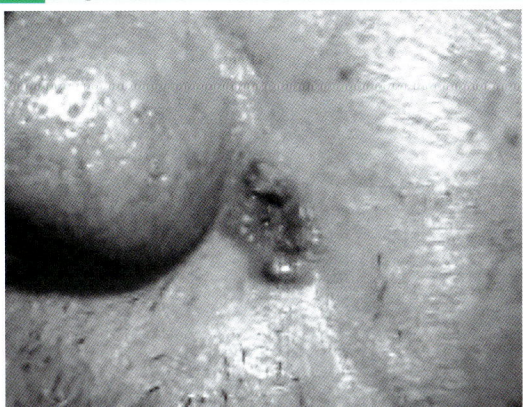

a. Squamous cells carcinoma
b. Basal cell carcinoma
c. Marjolin's ulcer
d. Nevus

Ans. See Chapter 20B, Q. N18 for Explanation

PLATE 19

Q N19. Identify the membrane marked as 'X' in the figure:

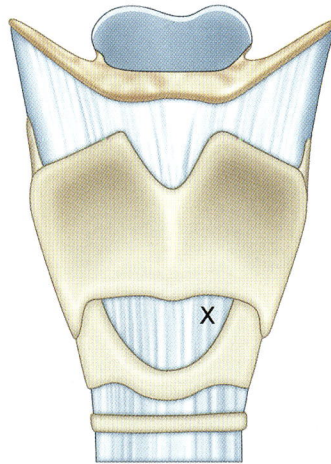

a. Thyrohyoid membrane
b. Cricothyroid membrane
c. Cricotracheal membrane
d. None

Ans. See Chapter 26, Q. N4 for Explanation

PLATE 18

Q N18. Identify the condition of palate shown in the plate:

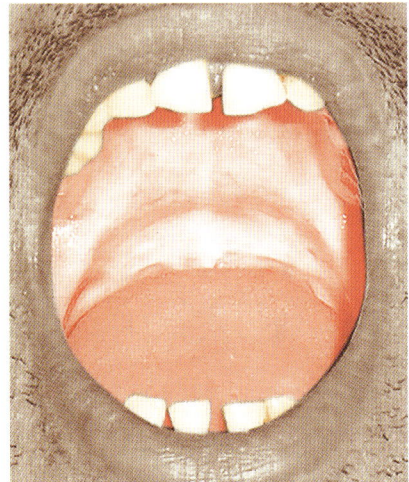

a. Leukoplakia   b. Erythroplakia
c. Submucous fibrosisd. Malignancy of tongue

Ans. See Chapter 21, Q. N28 for Explanation

PLATE 20

Q N12. A 6-year-old girl complaining of high fever, hoarseness of voice and respiratory distress was bought to ENT OPD. The child gets some relief in the position shown in figure. The most probable diagnosis is:

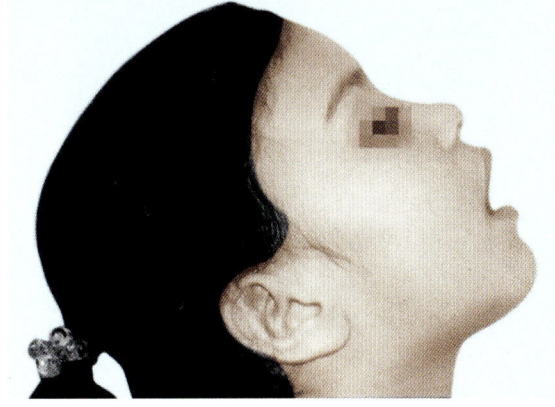

a. Croup   b. Laryngitis
c. Epiglottitis   d. Pseudocroup

Ans. See Chapter 27, Q. N2 for Explanation

PLATE 21

Q N21. Identify the condition shown in plate:

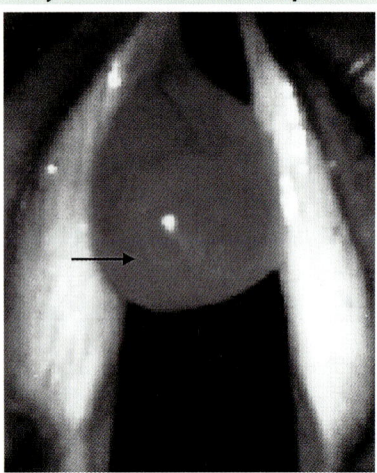

a. Vocal nodule
b. Vocal polyp
c. Leucoplasia of vocal cords
d. Vocal cord cyst

Ans. See Chapter 27, Q. N10 for Explanation

PLATE 22

Q N22. Identify the condition shown in the plate:

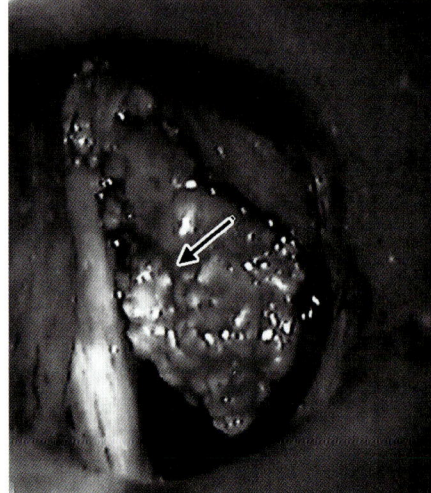

a. Supraglottic CA
b. Glottic CA
c. Subglottic CA
d. None

Ans. See Chapter 29, Q. N6 for Explanation

PLATE 23

Q N23. The patient came with an ulcer on the side of the nose as shown, which bleeds on itching. What is the diagnosis? *[AIIMS Nov 2017]*

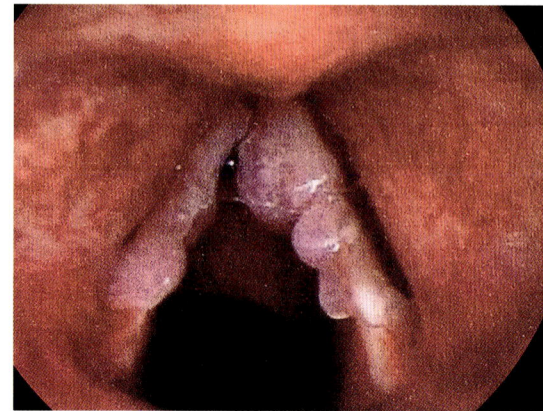

a. Vocal nodule
b. Acute epiglottis
c. Respiratory papillomatosis
d. Carcinoma larynx

Ans. See Chapter 29, Q. N33 for Explanation

PLATE 24

Q N24. A construction worker met with an accident and presented to the trauma centre when a heavy concrete block fell over his face. He was found to have severe maxillofacial and laryngeal injury. He was not able to open his mouth and, on examination, he is found to have multiple fractures and obstruction in nasopharynx as well as oropharynx. In order to maintain a patent airway, the following procedure was done for him. Which of the following options correct define the procedure? *[AIIMS 2016]*

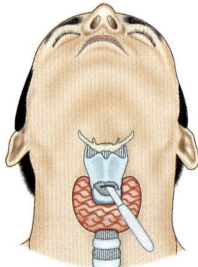

a. Submental endotracheal intubation
b. Emergency tracheostomy
c. Cricothyroidotomy
d. Subcutaneous tracheostomy

Ans. See Chapter 30, Q. N32 for Explanation

IMPORTANT PICTURES FOR PICTORIAL QUESTIONS
EAR

1. **Auricular cartilage: external features**

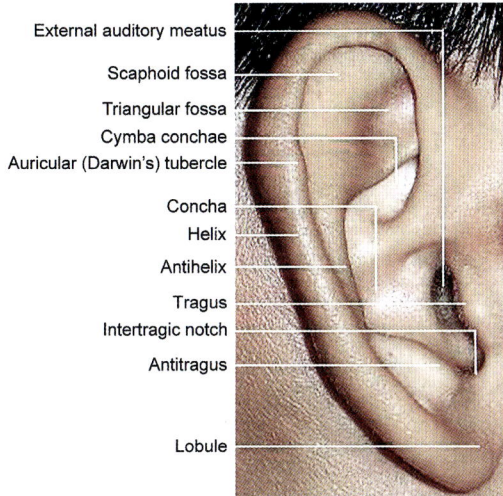

2. **Nerve supply of Pinna**

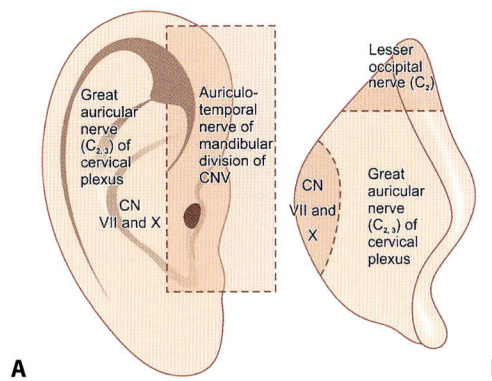

A. Lateral surface   B. Medial surface

3. **Tympanic membrane as seen on otoscopy**

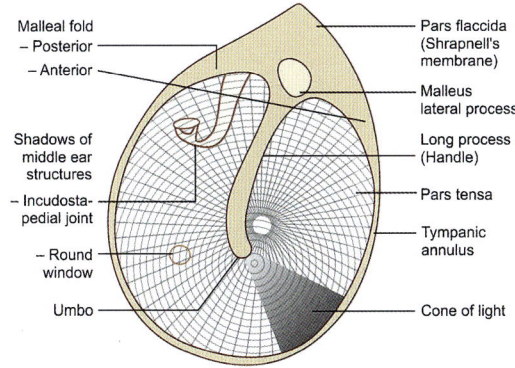

4. **Parts of middle ear cleft**

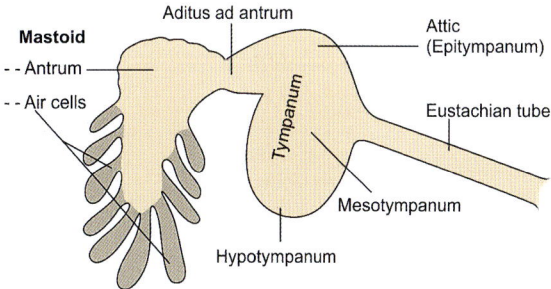

5. **Parts of middle ear as in seen on coronal section**

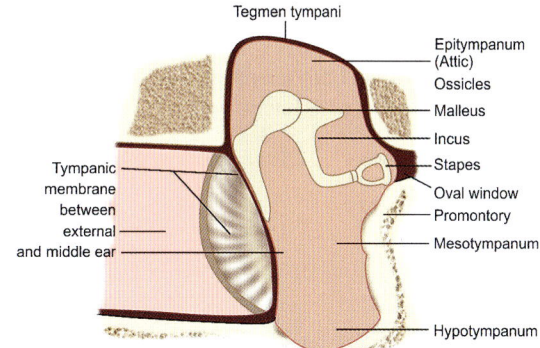

6. **Mc-Ewan triangle: Surface landmark for mastoid antrum**

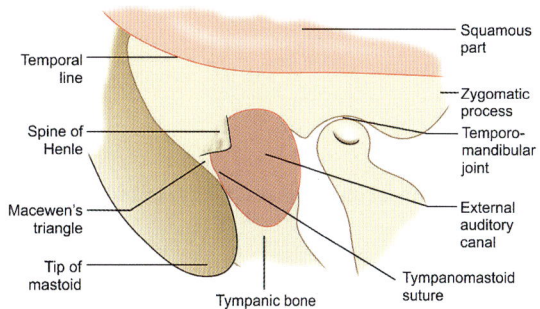

7. **Middle ear ossicles**

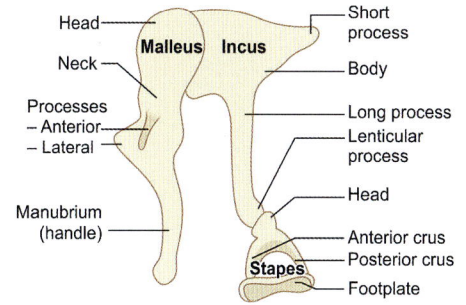

8. **Cochlea: Peri and endolymphatic systems: relation**

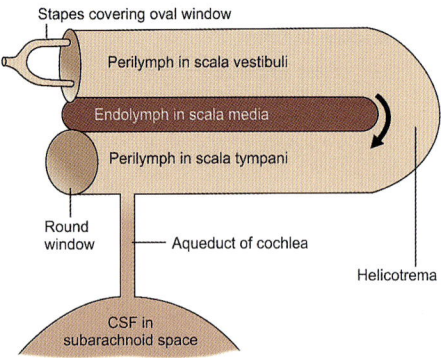

11. **Structure of Organ of Corti**

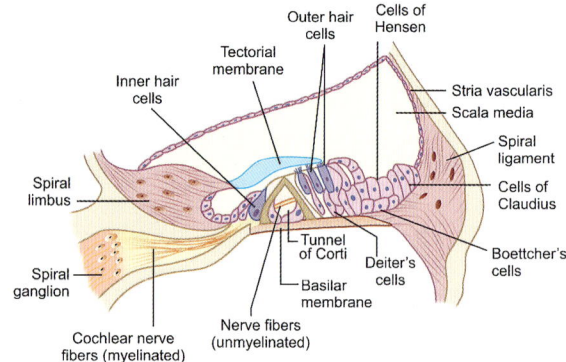

12. **Central auditory pathway**

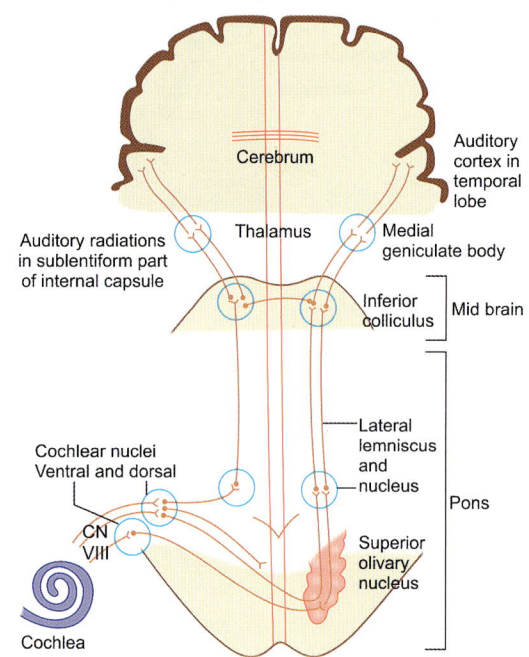

9. **Medial wall of left bony labyrinth seen from lateral side after the removal of its lateral wall**

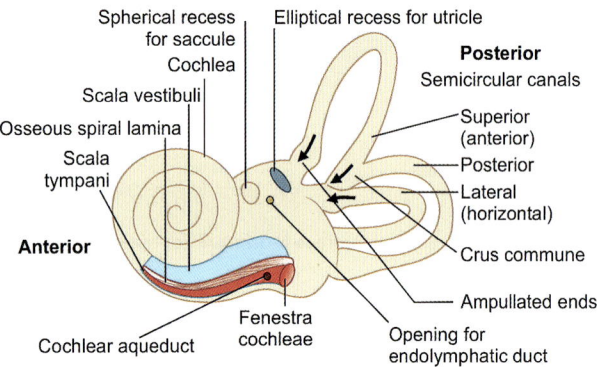

10. **Structure of cochlear canal after its cut section**

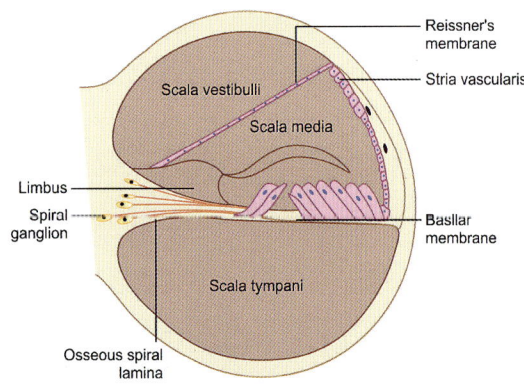

13. **Vestibular pathway**

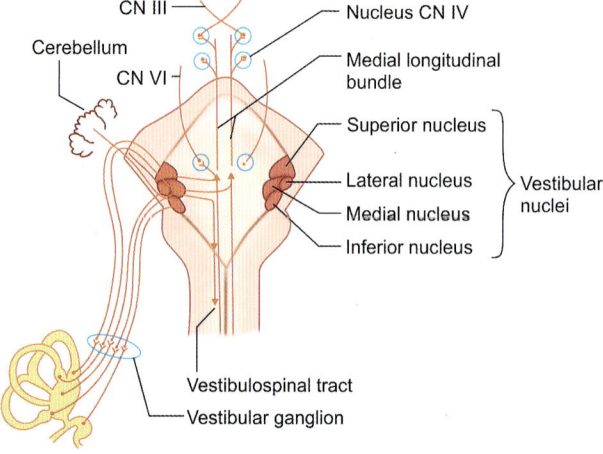

14. Acoustic reflex pathway

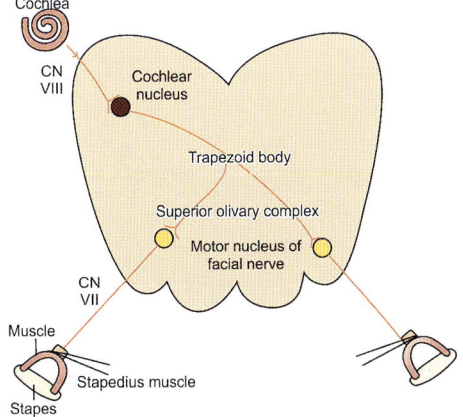

15. BERA

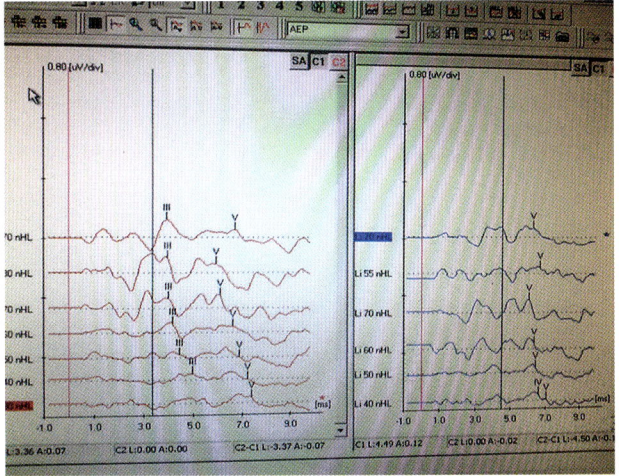

A. Normal with normal latency

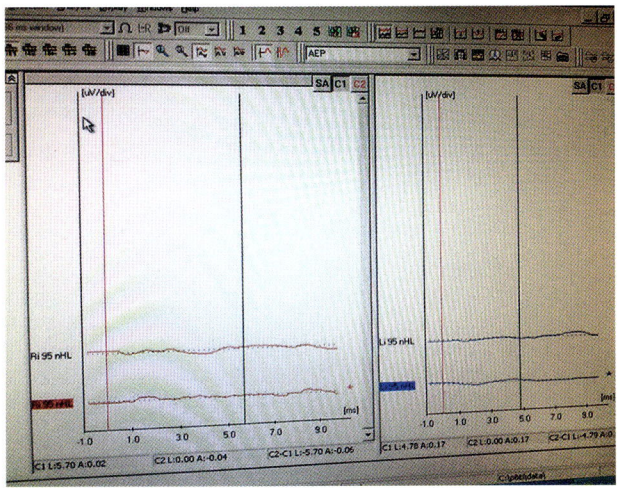

B. BERA in severe hearing less. Note: No peaks seen

16. Symbols used in audiogram charting

Modality	Ear	
	Right	Left
AC unmasked	O	X
AC masked	△	□
BC unmasked	<	>
BC masked	[	]
No response	⌕	⤫

17. Audiogram of left normal ear

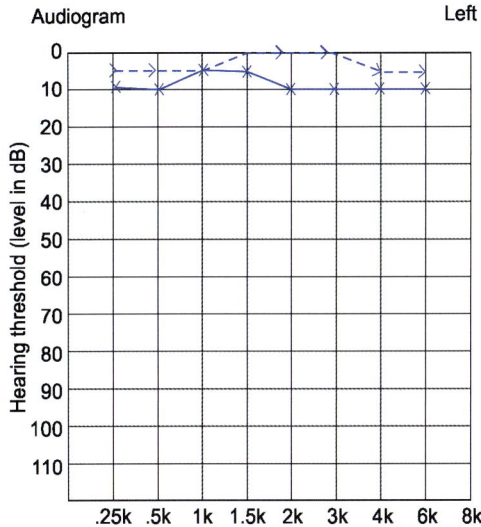

In normal persons, hearing threshold values with both air and bone remain between 0 and 10 dB

18. Audiogram of left ear with conductive hearing loss

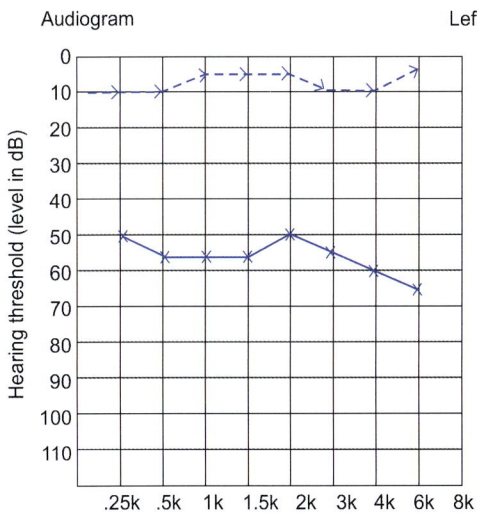

In this graph, bone-air gap is seen which means a patient can hear by bone under 10-20 dB, while with air hearing is much below, depending on the severity, indicating conductive hearing loss.

19. **Audiogram of left ear with SNHL**

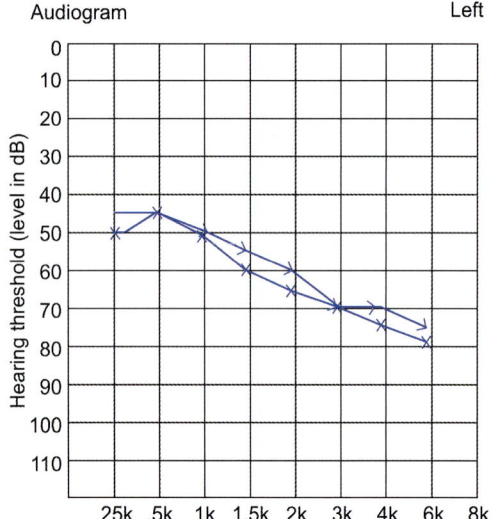

In SNHL, both bone and air conduction values are decreased and may even overlap each other.

20. **Audiogram in Early case of noise-induced hearing loss.**

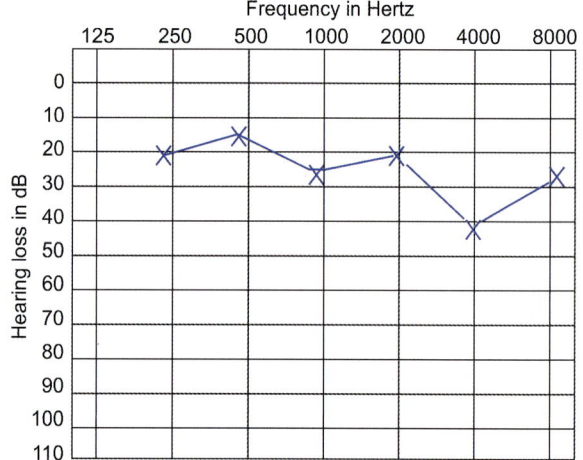

In acoustic trauma, there is a sudden dip at 4000 Hz both in air and bone conduction values

21. **Alternate binaural loudness balance test**

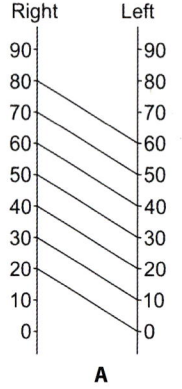
A

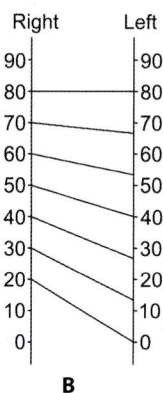
B

(A) Nonrecruiting ear. The initial difference of 20 dB between the right and left ear is maintained at all intensity levels.
(B) Recruiting ear right side. At 80 dB loudness perceived by right ear is as good as left ear though there was difference of 30 dB initially

22. Types of Tympanogram: Impedene Audiometry Curves:

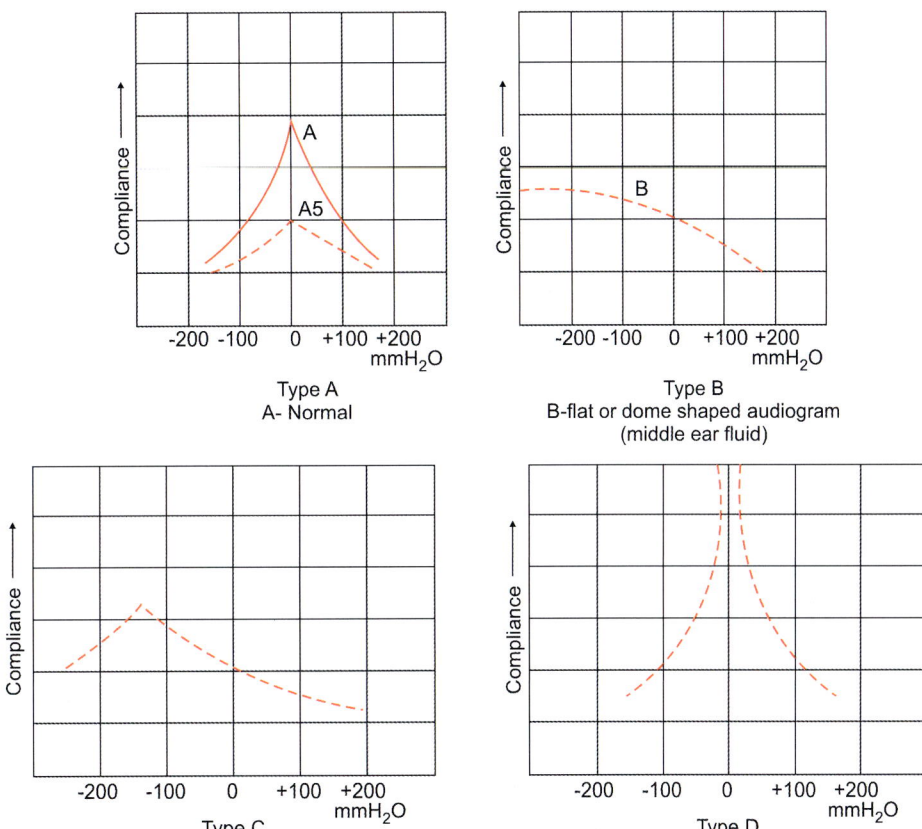

Type A
A- Normal

Type B
B-flat or dome shaped audiogram
(middle ear fluid)

Type C

Type D

Types of curve	Conditions seen in
A curve (Normal peak height and pressure	Normal Eustachian tube obstruction
As curve[Q] (It is also a variant of normal tympanogram but may be shallow	Otosclerosis[Q] Tumors of middle ear Fixed malleus syndrome Tympanosclerosis
Ad curve (Variant of normal with high peak)	Ossicular discontinuity Post stapedectomy Monometric ear drum
B curve (Flat or dome-shaped curve)[Q] Indicating lack of compliance	Fluid on middle ear[Q] Secretory otitis media[Q] Tym+anic membrane perforation[Q] Grommet in ear[Q]
C curve (negataive peak pressure)	Retracted tympanic membrane Faulty function of Eustachian tube/ Eustachian tube obstruction

23. **Incisions for myringotomy**

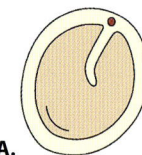
A.
In case of Acute Suppurative Otitis Media (ASOM)

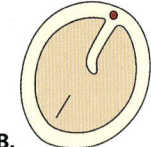
B.
In case of Serous Otitis Media ± grommet insertion

24. **Different view of X-ray for diseases of the ear**

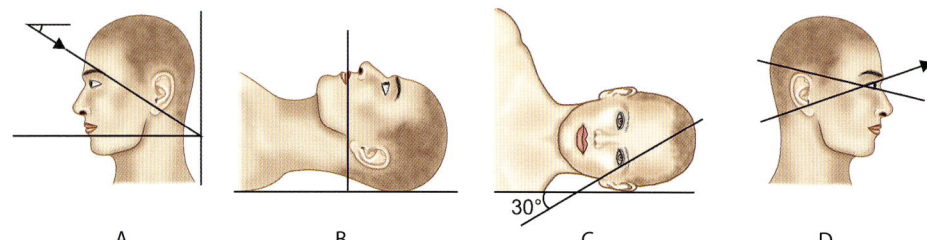

A.   B.   C.   D.

(A) Towne's (Fronto-occipital): (B) Submento-vertical view, (C) Stockholm-B view (Lateral-oblique): (D) Stenvers view (Oblique-posterior anterior)

NOSE

1. **Openings of paranasal sinus as in lateral wall of nose after removal of turbinates**

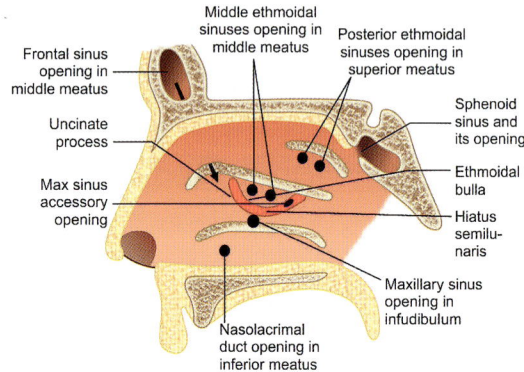

2. **Blood supply of nasal septum**

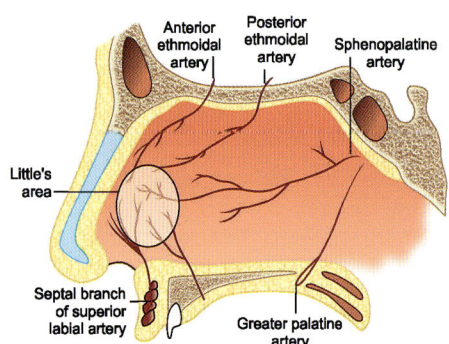

3. **Tripod fracture**

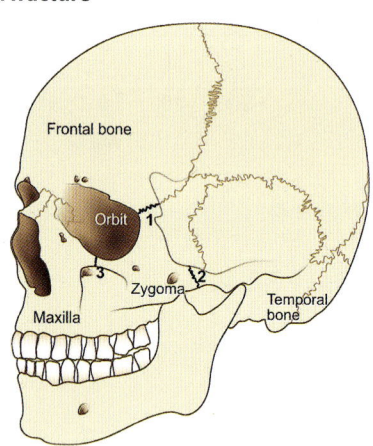

Left zygoma (tripod) fracture showing three sites of fracture.
(1) Zygomaticofrontal: (2) Zygomaticotemporal; (3) Infraorbital

4. **Le fort classification of fracture of nasomaxillary complex**

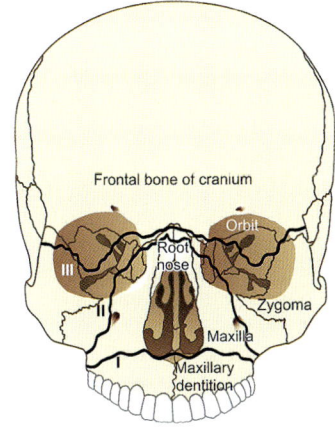

Le Fort classification of fractures of nasomaxillary complex crossing nasal septum and pterygoid plates. (I) Transverse (separating maxillary dentition); (II) Pyramidal (fracture of root of nose, medial wall and floor of orbit and maxilla), (III) Craniofacial disjunction (separating face from the cranium)

5. **Ohngrens classification for malignant neoplasm of PNS**

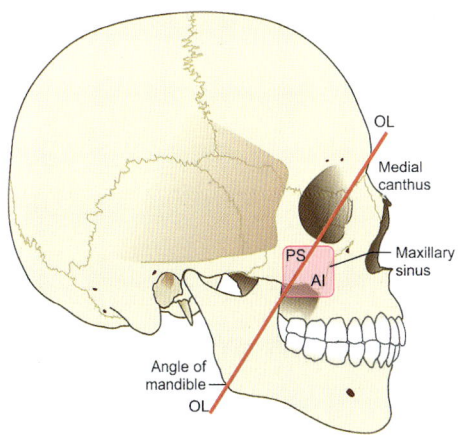

Ohngren's classification: Ohngren's line is an imaginary line (OL), which extends between medial canthus and the angle of mandible, divides the maxilla into two regions anteroinferior (AI) and posterosuperior (PA). AI growths are easy to manage and have better prognosis than PS tumors

6. **Structures seen an posterior rhinoscopy**

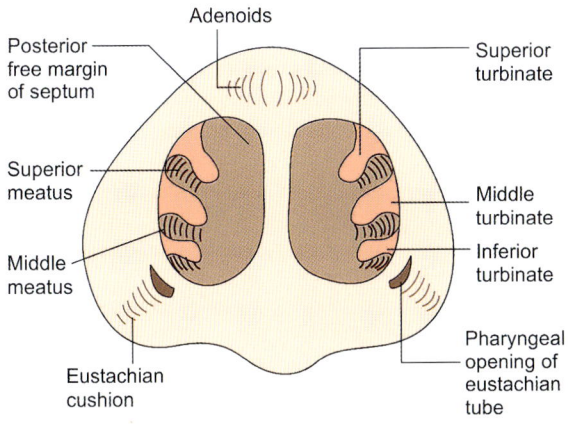

7. **A radiopaque foreign body in the nose of a child**

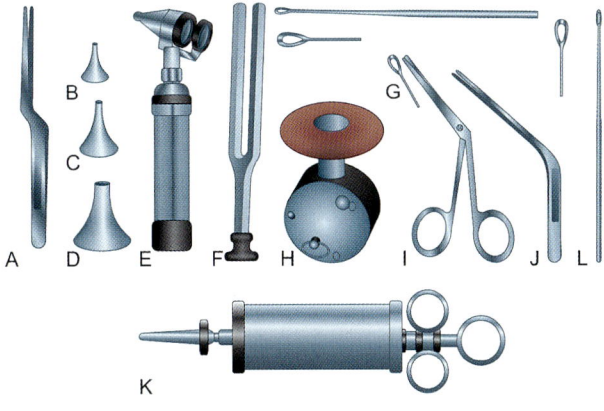

8. **X-ray: PNS, Water's view**

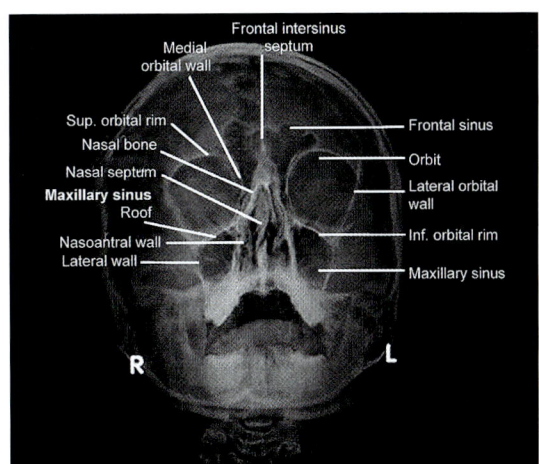

9. **View for the paranasal sinuses**

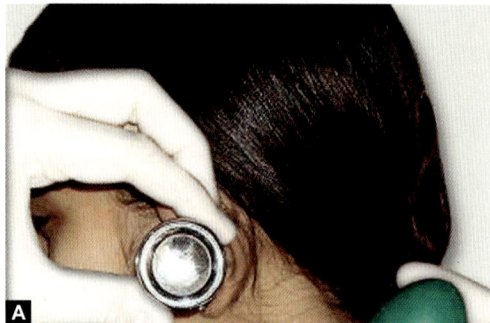

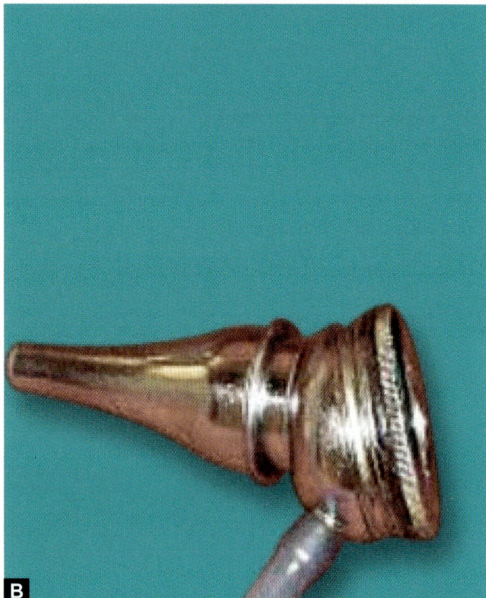

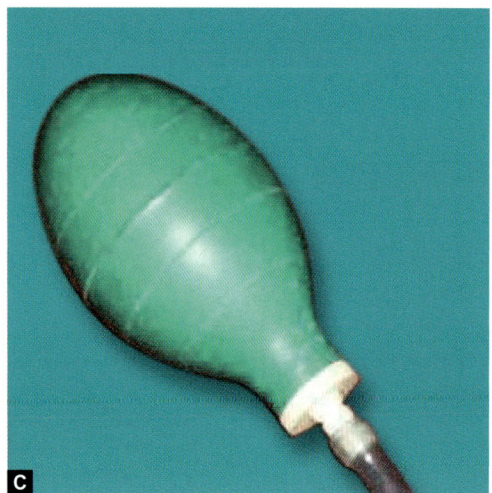

Radiology of nasal structures: (A) Occipitomental view: (B) Occipitofrontal view: (C) Submentovertical view

It is difficult to examine all the paranasal sinuses on one projection, so the examination of individual sinus requires many views. The few standard views that are taken, which give an adequate idea about the condition of paranasal sinuses are as follow:

- **Occipitomental view (Waters view):** The X-ray is taken in the nose-chin position with an open mouth. The film demonstrates mainly the maxillary sinuses, nasal cavity, septum, frontal sinuses and few cells of the ethmoids. The view taken in the standing position may show fluid level in the antrum (Fig. A)
- **Occipitofrontal view (Caldwell view):** The patient's forehead and tip of the nose are kept in contact with the film. This view is particularly useful for fontal sinuses. A portion of the maxillary antrum and nasal cavity are also shown (Fig. B)
- **X-ray, the base of the skull (Submentovertical view):** The neck and head are fully extended so that vertex faces the film and the rays are directed beneath the mandible. The view is useful for demonstrating sphenoid sinuses, ethmoids, nasopharynx, petrous apex, posterior wall of the maxillary sinus and fracture of the zygomatic arch (Fig. C)
- **Lateral view:** The patient's head is placed in a lateral position against the film and the ray is directed behind the outer canthus of the eye towards the film.

The maxillary, ethmoidal and frontal sinuses superimpose each other but this film is useful for the following purposes:
   - To demonstrate the extent of pneumatization of the sphenoid and frontal sinuses.
   - To demonstrate the position of a radiopaque foreign body in the nasal cavity or nasopharynx.
   - To demonstrate the thickness of soft tissues of the nasopharynx which should not normally be more than 5 mm.
   - To show the nasopharyngeal airway.
   - To demonstrate the adenoid mass or a tumor in the nasopharynx.
- **Lateral oblique view for ethmoids:** If the disease involves the ethmoids, a special lateral oblique view provides an idea about the ethmoidal air cells, being relatively free of superimposition by other structures.

On plain radiography, the normal sinuses appear as air filled translucent cavities. Opacity of the sinuses can be caused by fluid, thickened mucosa or tumors. Bony erosion can occur because of tumors, osteomyelitis or mucoceles.

PHARYNX

1. **Waldeyers ring**

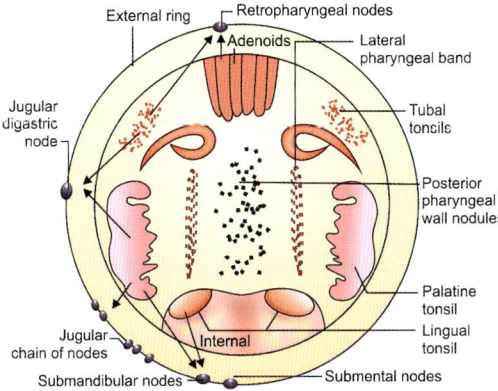

2. **Blood supply of tonsil**

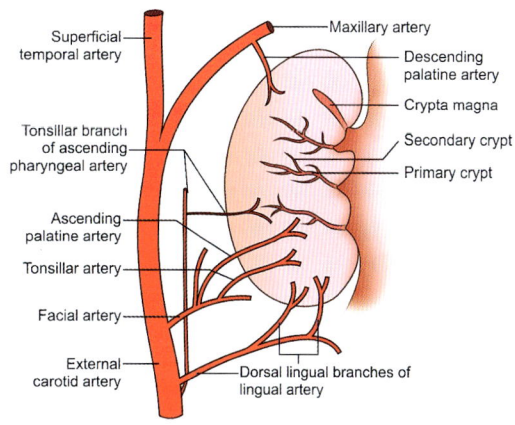

IMPORTANT INCISIONS AND POSITION IN ENT SURGERY

1. **Abbe estander flap**

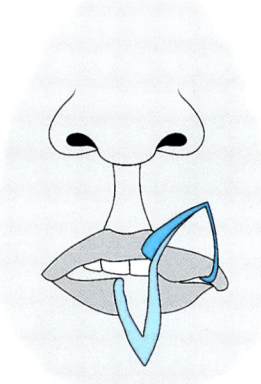

Used for lip reconstruction

2. **Rose Position**

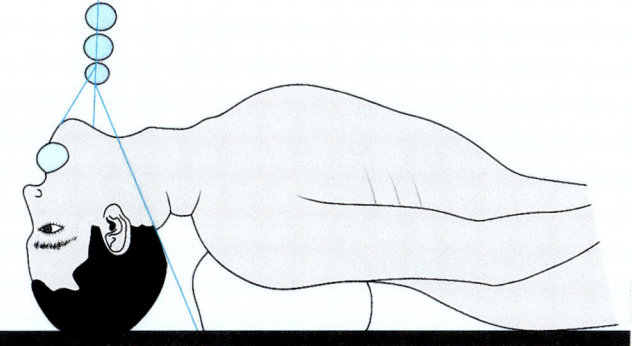

Used during I. Tonsillectomy II. Abenoidectomy III. Tracheostomy

INSTRUMENTS

1. Head mirror

2. Head light

3. Aural speculum

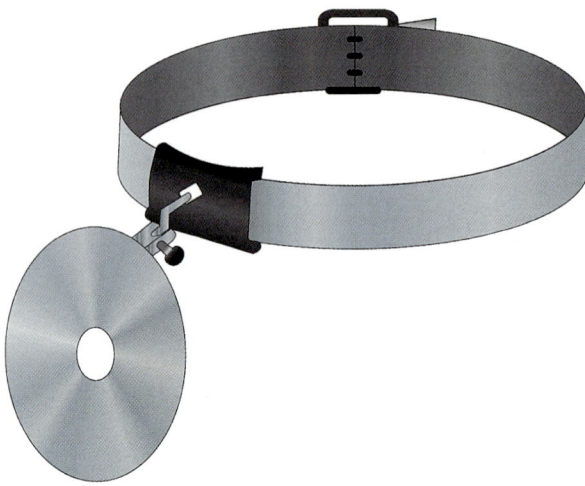
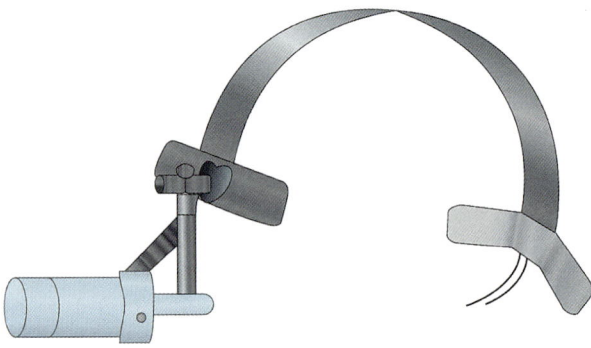
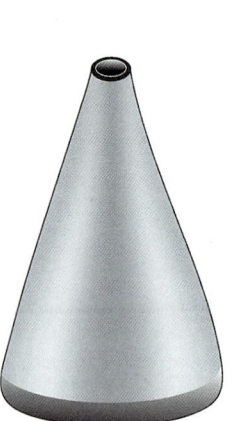
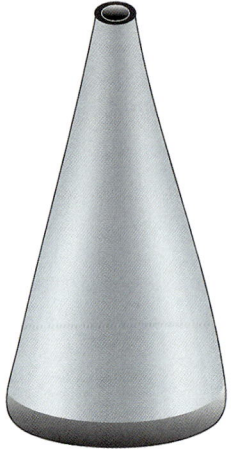

4. Electrical otoscope

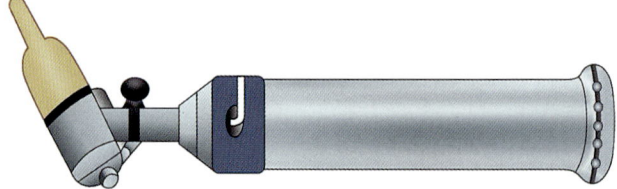

5. Jobson's aural probe

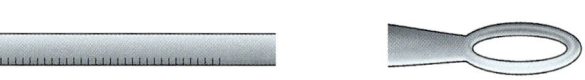
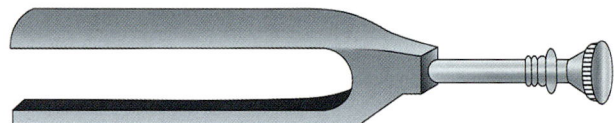

6. Tuning fork

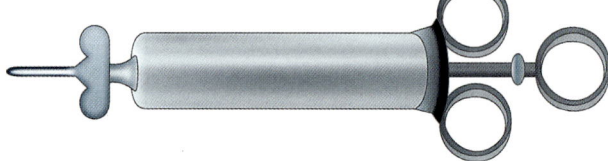

7. Aural syringe

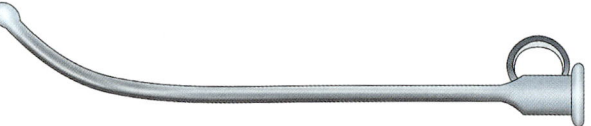

8. Eustachian catheter

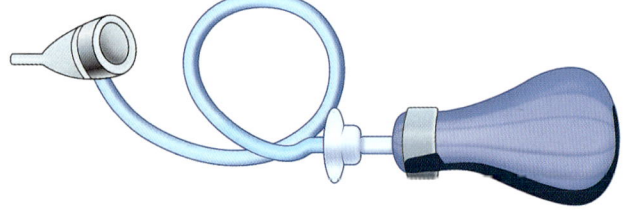

9. Siegel's pneumatic speculum

10. Politzer bag

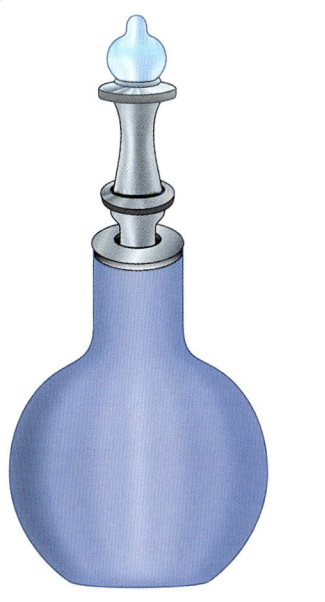

11. Myringotome

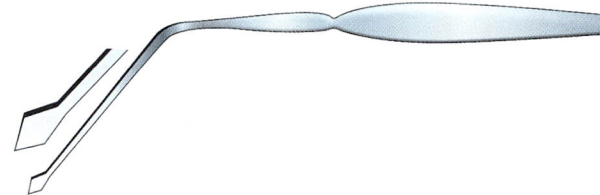

12. Mastoid retractor

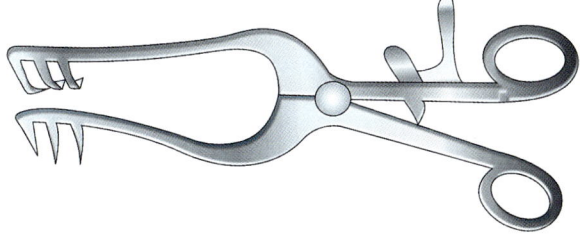

13. Mastoid gouge

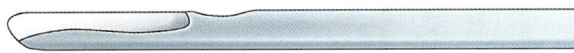

14. Mallet

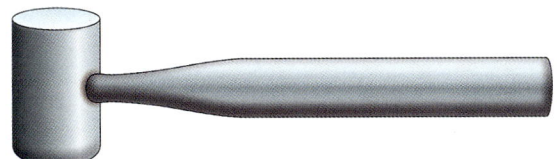

15. Mastoid cell seeker with scoop

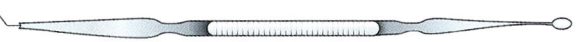

16. Thudicum's nasal speculum

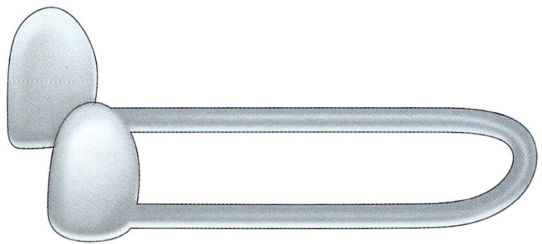

17. Correct method of holding Thudicum's nasal speculum

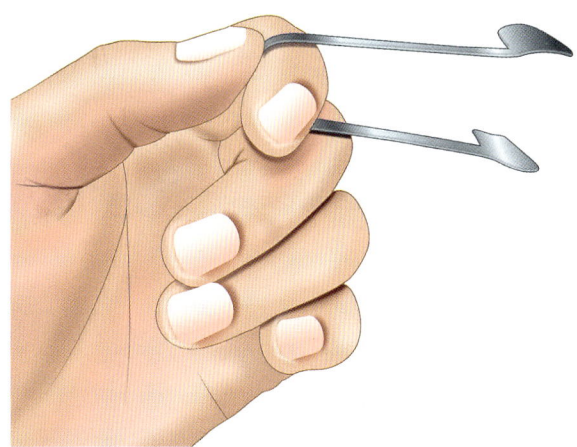

18. St Clair-Thompson's nasal speculum

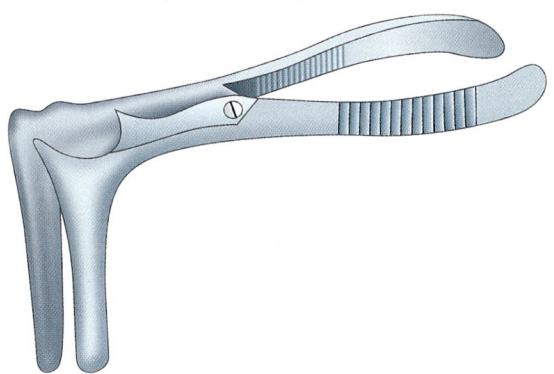

19. Posterior rhinoscopy mirror

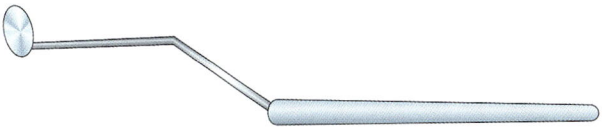

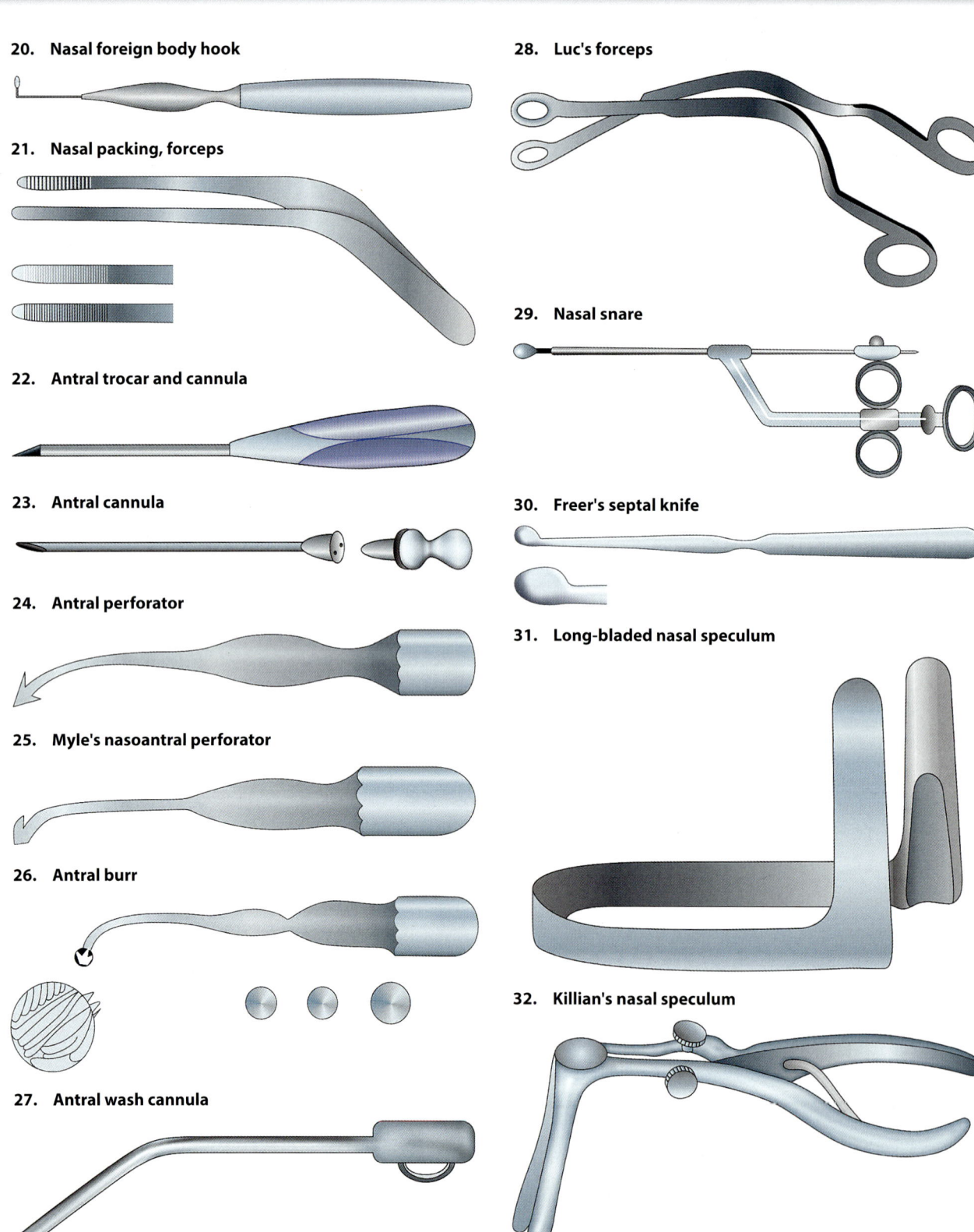

33. Ballinger's swivel knife

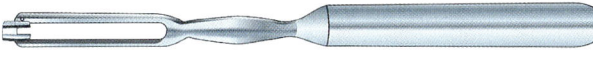

34. Bayonet-shaped gouge

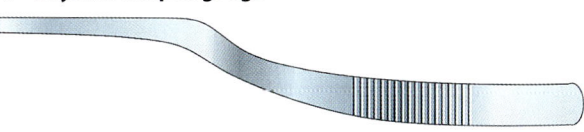

35. Walsham's forceps

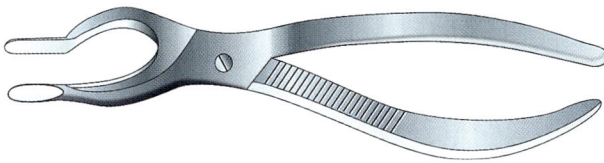

36. Lackj's spatula

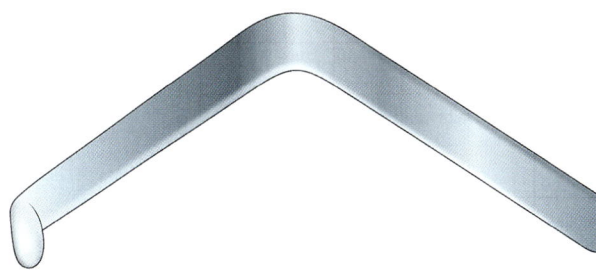

37. Laryngeal mirror

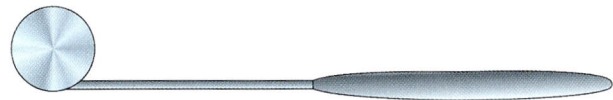

38. Direct laryngoscope

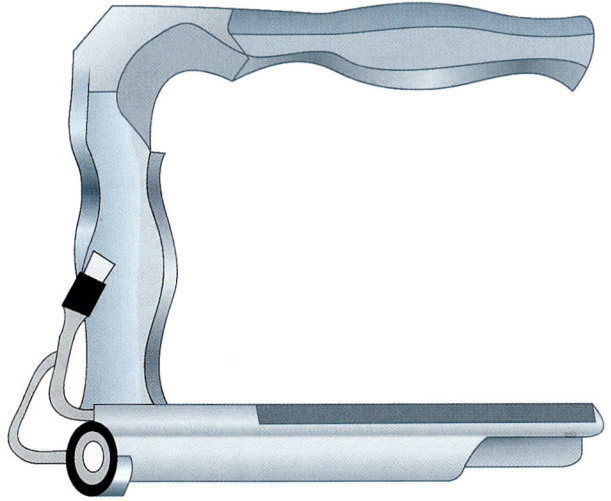

39. Chevalier-Jackson laryngoscope with removable slide

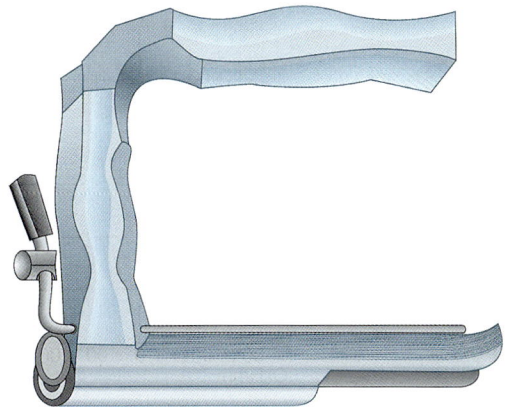

40. Distal light arrangement

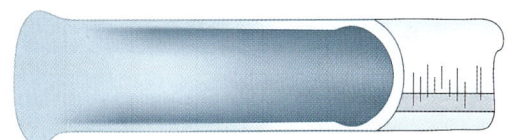

41. Anterior commissure larynogoscope

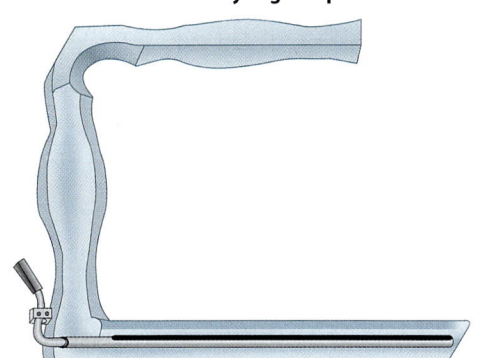

42. Negus bronchoscope

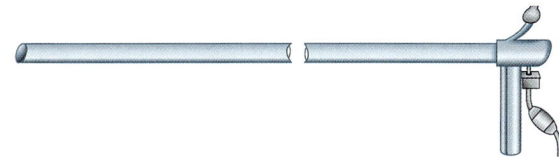

43. Chevalier-Jackson bronchoscope

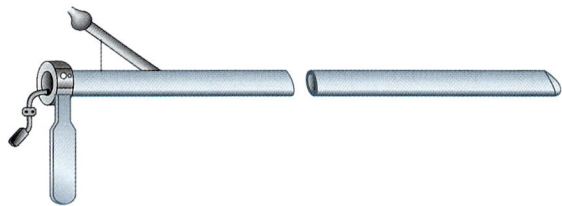

44. Chevalier-Jackson esophagoscope

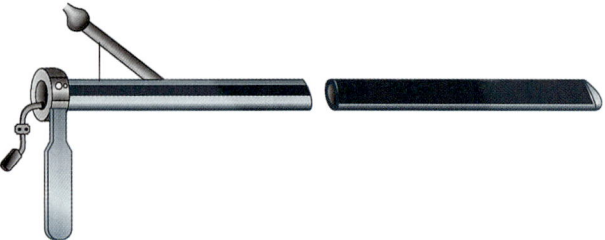

45. Negus esophagoscope

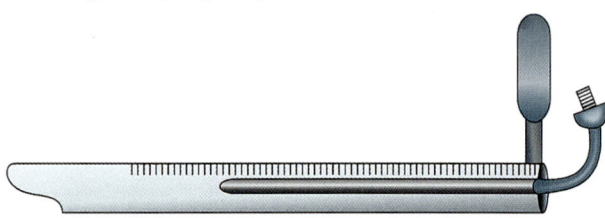

46. Esophageal speculum

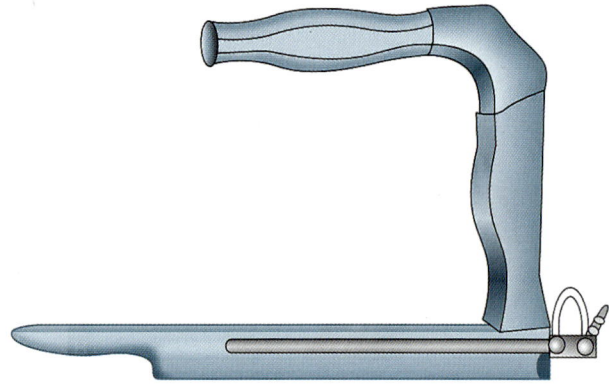

47. Laryneal forceps

48. Crocodile punch biopsy foreps

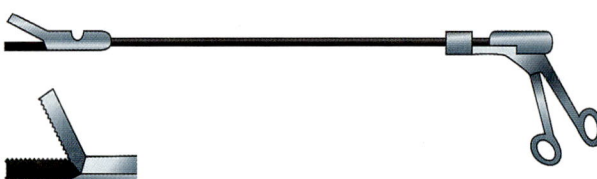

49. Boyle-Davis mouth gag

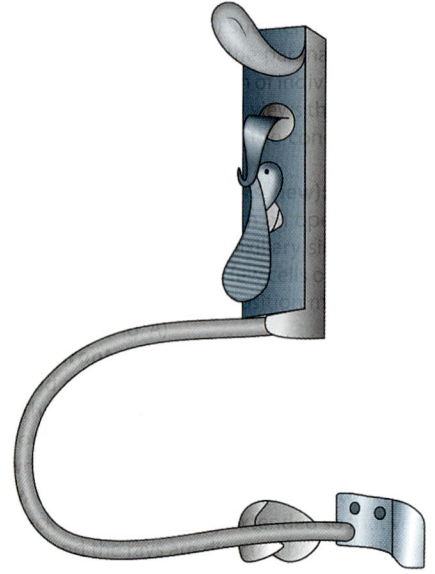

50. Tongue plate with throat suction

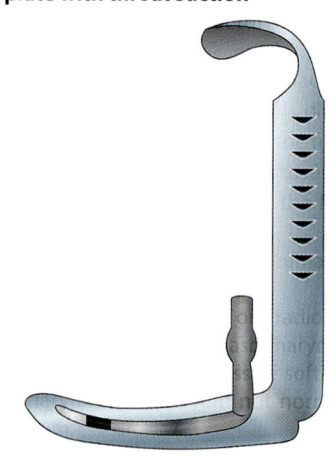

51. Tonsil holding forceps

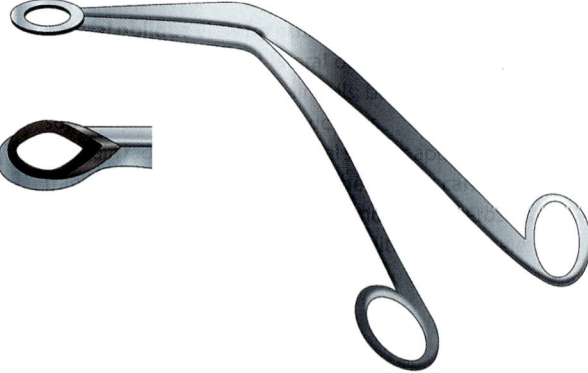

52. **Tonsillar suction**

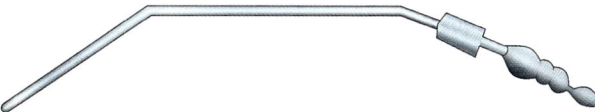

53. **Tonsil pillar retractor and dissector**

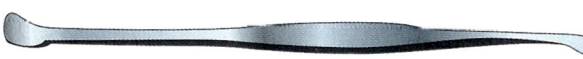

54. **Tonsillar snare**

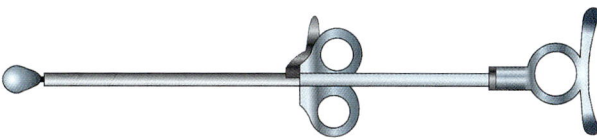

55. **Guillotine**

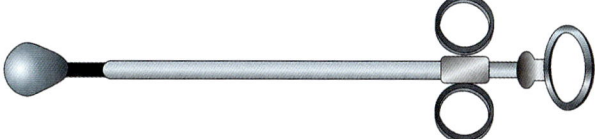

56. **Adenoid curette with cage**

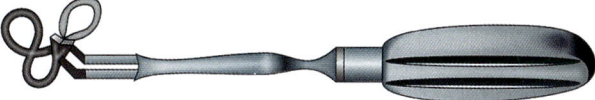

57. **Peritonsillar abscess drainage forceps**

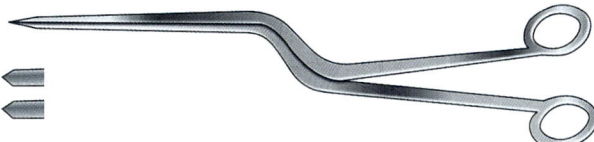

58. **Fuller's tracheostomy tube**

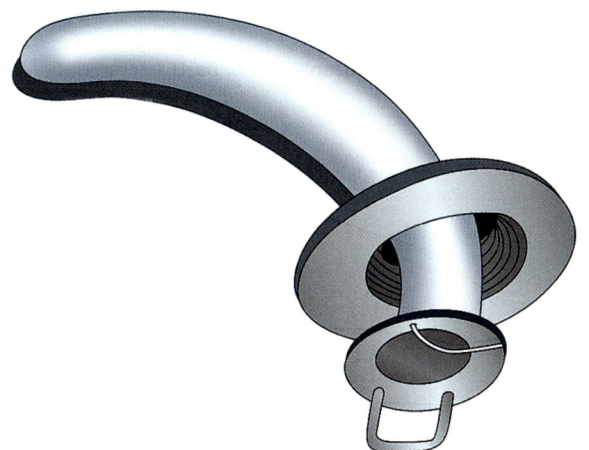

59. Jackson's tracheostomy tube

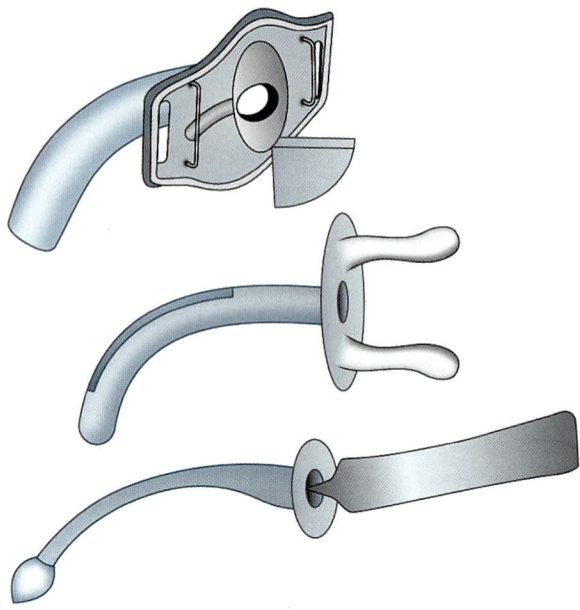

61. Sharp tracheal hook

62. Draffin bipod stand with plate

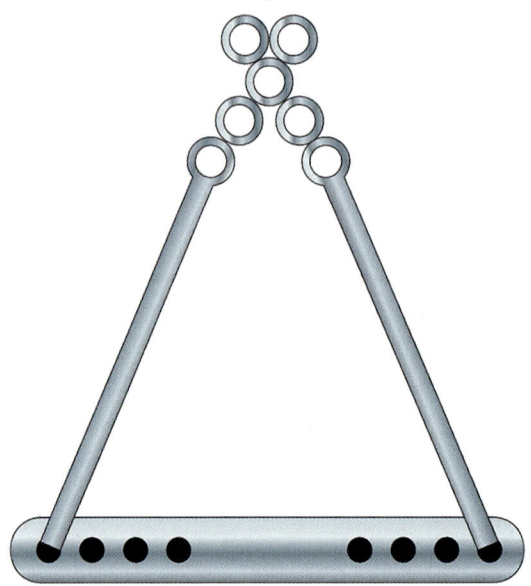

60. Blunt tracheal hook

SECTION 1

Ear

Section Outline

1. Anatomy of Ear
2. Physiology of Ear and Hearing
3. Hearing Loss
4. Assessment of Hearing Loss
5. Assessment of Vestibular Function
6. Diseases of External Ear
7. Diseases of Middle Ear
8. Meniere's Disease
9. Otosclerosis
10. Facial Nerve and its Lesions
11. Lesion of Cerebellopontine Angle and Acoustic Neuroma
12. Glomus Tumor and Other Tumors of the Ear
13. Rehabilitative Methods
14. Miscellaneous

CHAPTER 1

Anatomy of Ear

Ear can be divided into three parts:
I. External ear
II. Middle ear
III. Inner ear (situated in petrous part of temporal bone).

EXTERNAL EAR

- It consists of (A) Pinna (B) External auditory canal and (C) Tympanic membrane.

PINNA/AURICLE (FIG. 1.1)

- It is made of single yellow elastic cartilage except at the lobule, where it is absent.

> Its lateral surface has characteristic prominences and depressions (as shown in figure) which are different in every individual even among identical twins. This unique pattern is comparable to fingerprints and can allow for identification of persons.

- The cartilage of pinna is continuous with the cartilage of external auditory canal.
- The cartilage is covered with skin which is closely attached on lateral surface and slightly loose on medial surface.^{Q}
- The cartilage itself is **avascular** and derives its supply of nutrients from the perichondrium covering it.
- **Clinical importance**-stripping of the perichondrium from the cartilage as occurs following injuries that cause hematoma can lead to cartilage necrosis and so-called 'boxers ear'.
- **Various landmarks on the pinna (Fig. 1.1)**
  - **Cymba concha** is the area lying between crest of helix and antihelix.

> **Applied Anatomy:**
> ➢ The cymba conchae is an important landmark for mastoid antrum

  - Another important landmark for mastoid antrum is **Mc Ewen's triangle or suprameatal triangle.** Mastoid antrum lies 1 cm deep to it. **McEwen's triangle** can be felt under cymba concha (*Discussed later*).
  - **Incisura terminalis:** Area between the ascending crus of the helix and tragus. It is devoid of cartilage.

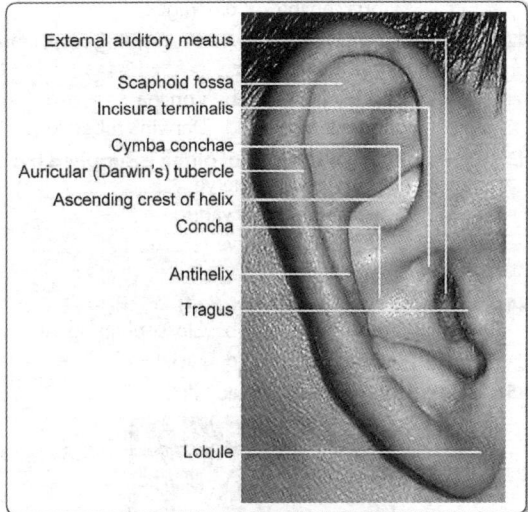

Fig. 1.1: External features of auricle
Courtesy: Textbook of Diseases of Ear, Nose and Throat, Mohan Bansal, Jaypee Brothers Medical Publishers Pvt. Ltd., p 3

Clinical importance: An incision made in this area does not cut through the cartilage and is used for endaural approach in surgery.

- Pinna has **3 extrinsic muscle:** 1. Auricularis anterior, 2. Auricularis superior and 3. Auricularis posterior. These are all attached to epicranial aponeurosis and supplied by the **facial nerve**
- **Intrinsic muscles** are 6 in number and are small, inconsistent and without any useful information
- ^{Q}**Innervation of the pinna:**

Lateral surface	Medial surface
1. **Auriculotemporal nerve**	1. **Lesser occipital nerve**—supplies upper part
2. **Greater auricular nerve**	2. Most of the medial surface is supplied by **great auricular nerve**
3. **Auricular branch of vagus** also called as Arnold nerve	3. Auricular branch of vagus
4. **Facial nerve (VII)**	4. Facial nerve

- **Lymphatic Drainage:**
  - From posterior surface – lymph node at mastoid tip
  - From tragus and upper part of anterior surface – Pre-auricular nodes
  - Rest of auricle → upper deep cervical nodes

Section 1: Ear

- **Clinical Correlation:**
  - *Grafts in rhinoplasty:* Conchal cartilage is used to correct depressed nasal bridge.
  - *Graft in tympanoplasty:* Tragal and conchal cartilage and perichondrium are used during tympanoplasty.

NEW PATTERN QUESTIONS

Q N1. Part of pinna which lies behind the external auditory meatus is:
a. Scaphoid fossa b. Concha
c. Cymba concha d. Tragus

Q N2. Part of pinna lying between ascending crest of helix and tragus is called as:
a. Scaphoid fossa b. Concha
c. Incisura terminalis d. Darwin's tubercle

Q N3. Major part of the skin of pinna is supplied by:
a. Auriculotemporal nerve
b. Auricular branch of vagus
c. Lesser occipital nerve
d. Greater auricular nerve

Q N4. Arnolds nerve is a branch of:
a. Vagus b. Glossopharyngeal
c. Auditory d. Facial

Q N5. Identify the area marked 'X':

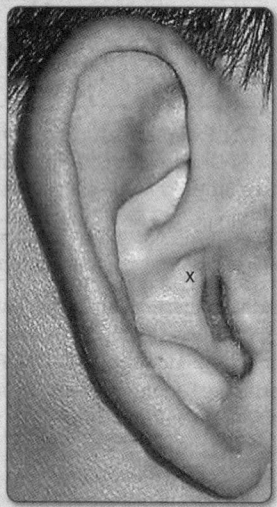

See Color Plate 1

a. Cymba concha b. Incisura terminalis
c. Scaphoid fossa d. Ascending crux of helix

EXTERNAL AUDITORY CANAL/EXTERNAL ACOUSTIC MEATUS

Length	:	24–25 mm^Q	
Parts	:	Lateral/outer 1/3 (8 mm) :	Cartilaginous^Q
		Medial/inner 2/3 :	Osseous^Q
Shape	:	'S'- shaped curve	

External Auditory Canal develops from = First brachial cleft/groove^Q

Cartilaginous Part

Forms the outer/lateral 1/3 (8 mm) of external auditory canal.

Has a fissure/deficiency — in the anterior part called as **Fissures of Santorini^Q** through which parotid or superficial mastoid infection can appear in the canal and like vice versa.

- Skin covering is thick and has ceruminous glands *(modified apocrine sweat glands^Q)*, pilosebaceous glands and hair.
- Ceruminous and pilosebaceous glands secrete wax (mixture of cerumen, sebum and desquamated cells is wax).
- Since hair is confined to cartilaginous part – furuncles are seen only in the outer third of canal.^{Q}

Bony Part

- It forms inner two-thirds (16 mm)^Q of external auditory canal.
- Skin lining the bony canal is thin and is devoid of hair and ceruminous glands.^{Q}
- 5 mm lateral to tympanic membrane, bony meatus is narrow and called *Isthmus* (**Applied** – Foreign bodies get lodged in it and are difficult to remove). Beyond the narrow isthmus, lies a dilatation called as **Anterior meatal recess**. Any discharge of middle ear collects in the recess.

- **Foramen of Huschke^Q** is a deficiency present in anteroinferior part of bony canal in children up to 4 years of age, permitting infection to and from the temporomandibular joint.

Blood supply: It is also supplied by **External carotid artery**.
Lymphatic drainage—follows the auricle
Relationship of external auditory canal (Flowchart 1.1)

Flowchart 1.1: Relations of middle external auditory canal

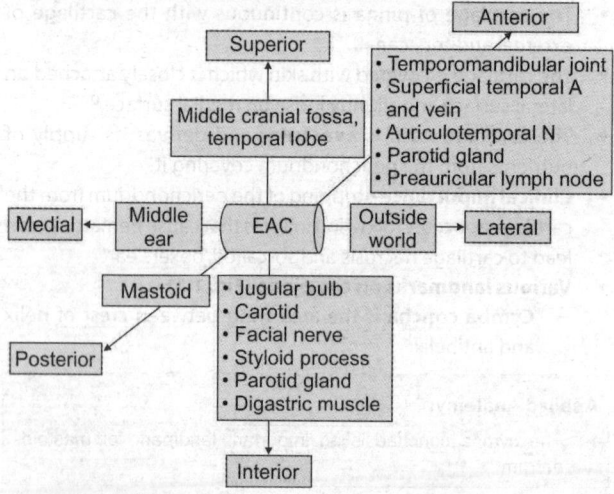

- ^{Q}**Nerve supply:**
  - Anterior wall and roof: **Auriculotemporal nerve**
  - Floor and posterior wall: *Vagus* (Arnold nerve)
  - Posterior wall also receives innervation from: *Facial nerve* (Importance–Hypoesthesia of the posterior meatal wall is seen in case of facial nerve injury, **known as Hitzelberger's sign**).

Chapter 1: Anatomy of Ear

NEW PATTERN QUESTIONS

Q N6. Which of the following statement is correct with respect to EAC of newborn?
   a. In newborn, cartilaginous part of EAC is absent
   b. In newborn, bony part of EAC is absent
   c. Both bony and cartilaginous part are present but EAC is short
   d. Both bony and cartilaginous part are present and EAC of newborn and adults are of same size

Q N7. All of the following are seen in bony part of EAC except:
   a. Foramen of Huschke   b. Fissure of Santorini
   c. Isthmus   d. Anterior meatal recess

Q N8. The cough response caused while cleaning the ear canal is mediated by stimulation of:
   a. The V cranial nerve
   b. Innervation of external ear canal by C_1, C_2
   c. The X cranial nerve
   d. Branches of the VII cranial nerve

TYMPANIC MEMBRANE (FIG. 1.2)

- It is the partition between external acoustic meatus and middle ear, i.e. it lies at medial end of external auditory meatus.
- Tympanic membrane is 9–10 mm tall, 8–9 mm wide and 0.1 mm thick and is positioned at angle of 55° to external auditory canal.
- Area of adult tympanic membrane is 90 mm² of which only 55 mm² is functional.
- It is shiny and pearly gray^Q in color.
- Normal tympanic membrane is mobile with maximum mobility being in the peripheral part.^{Q}

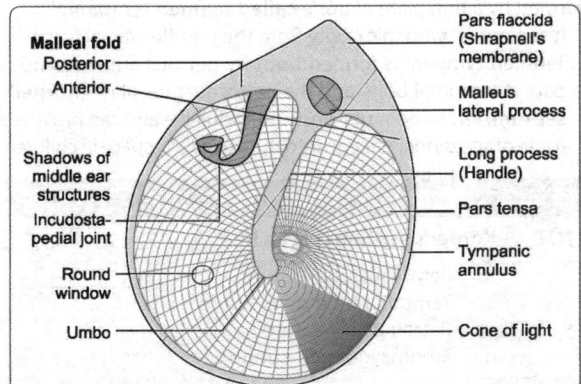

Fig. 1.2: Tympanic membrane showing attic, malleus handle, umbo, cone of light and structures of middle ear seen through it on otoscopy

Courtesy: Textbook of Diseases of Ear, Nose and Throat, Mohan Bansal, Jaypee Brothers Medical Publishers Pvt. Ltd., p 5

It has 2 parts:

Pars tensa	Pars flaccida/Shrapnell's membrane
It forms most of tympanic membrane	Situated above the lateral process of malleus between the notch of Rivinus and the anterior and posterior malleal folds
Periphery is thickened to form a fibrocartilaginous ring called **the annulus tympanicus**	It is more mobile and flaccid
This ring is deficient above in the form of a notch called **the notch of Rivinus**	**Prussak's space** is a shallow recess within the posterior part of pars flaccida
The central part is tented inward at the level of tip of malleus & is called as **umbo**	**Note:** Negative pressure in middle ear due to blockage of Eustachian tube leads to formation of retraction pocket and primary cholesteatoma in pars flaccida as PF is more flaccid.
Cone of light is seen radiating from tip of malleus to the periphery in the anteroinferior quadrant.^{Q}	

Layers of Tympanic Membrane
- Outer – Epithelial
- Middle – Fibrous
- Inter – Mucosal continuous – the middle ear mucosa

 Note: When a tympanic membrane perforation heals spontaneously, it heals in two layers as it is often closed by squamous epithelium before fibrous elements develop.

Arterial supply: Vessels are present only in connective tissue layer of the lamina propria.

Arteries supplying tympanic membrane are:

Mnemonic

M = Maxillary artery
A = Postauricular artery
M = Middle meningeal branch artery

Nerve supply of tympanic membrane
- **Lateral/outer surface**
   - Anterior half: **Auriculotemporal nerve**
   - Posterior half: **Vagus nerve (Arnold nerve)**
- **Medial/inner surface**
   - **Tympanic branch of glossopharyngeal nerve (k/a Jacobson's nerve)**

➤ *Auriculotemporal nerve (CN V3):* It is a branch of mandibular division of trigeminal nerve and supplies anterior half of lateral surface of TM.
➤ *CN X (vagus nerve):* Its auricular branch (**Arnold's nerve**) supplies to posterior half of lateral surface of TM.
➤ *CN IX (glossopharyngeal nerve):* Its tympanic branch (**Jacobson's nerve**) supplies to medial surface of tympanic membrane.

	NEW PATTERN QUESTION
Q N9	True about tympanic membrane:
	a. Attached to oval window
	b. Forms an angle of 55° with external auditory canal
	c. Chorda tympani nerve passes through pars tensa
	d. Cone of light forms on arteriosuperior quadrant

MIDDLE EAR CLEFT (FIG. 1.3)

Ear cleft in the temporal bone, consists of tympanic cavity (middle ear), Eustachian tube and mastoid air cell system.

TYMPANIC CAVITY (MIDDLE EAR CAVITY) (FIG. 1.4)

It is divided into:
- Mesotympanum (Opposite pars tensa)
- Epitympanum (widest part) (above pars tensa)
- Hypotympanum (below pars tensa)

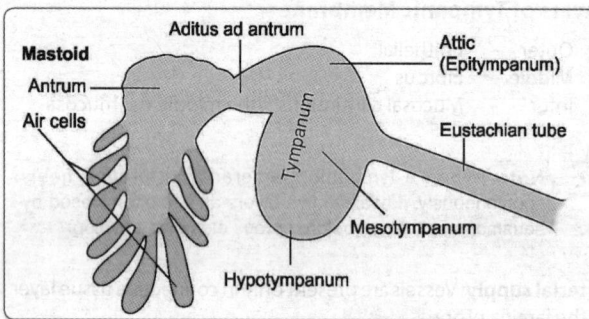

Fig. 1.3: Parts of middle ear cleft
Courtesy: Textbook of Diseases of Ear, Nose and Throat, Mohan Bansal, Jaypee Brothers Medical Publishers Pvt. Ltd., p 6

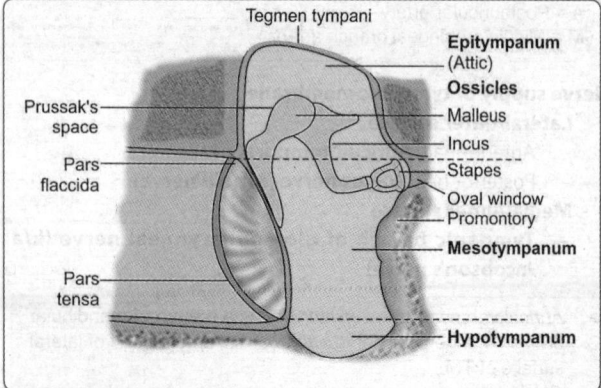

Fig. 1.4: Parts of middle ear seen on coronal section
Courtesy: Textbook of Diseases of Ear, Nose and Throat, Mohan Bansal, Jaypee Brothers Medical Publishers Pvt. Ltd., p 6

Note:
- Sometimes the portion of middle ear around the tympanic orifice of the Eustachian tube is called as *protympanum*.
- Narrowest part of middle ear: mesotympanum
- Widest part of middle ear: epitympanum

Epitympanum	Mesotymparum	Hypotymparum
• Part which lies above the level of Pars tensa	• Part which lies at the level of Pars tensa	• Part which lies below the level of Pars tensa
• Widest part (6 mm)	• Transverse diameter: 2 mm	• Transverse diameter: 4 mm
• Contains Malleus – Head – Neck – Anterior process – Lateral process	• Contains: – Malleus: Handle – Incus long process – Whole of stapes – Incudosta- pedial joint	• Contains nothing.
• Incus: – Body – Short process		
• Incudomalleolar joint		
• Chorda tympani		

Prussak's Space

- Also called **superior recess** of Tympanic membrane. It lies between neck of malleus (medially) and pars flaccida (laterally in the epitympanum. It is bounded above the fibers of lateral malleolar fold and below by lateral process of malleus.
- *Importance of this space:* It is most common site of cholesteatoma. The cholesteatoma may extend to posterior mesotympanum infection here does not drain easily and causes attic pathology.

Boundaries of Middle Ear

- **Middle ear** is like a six sided box with a: roof, floor, medial wall, lateral wall, anterior wall, and posterior wall

Roof

Is formed by a thin plate of bone **called tegmen tympani.**^Q
- It separates tympanic cavity from the middle cranial fossa.^Q
- Tegmen tympani is formed both by petrous and squamous part of temporal bone and the petrosquamous line **(Korner's septum)** Which does not close until adult life and can provide a route of access for infection into the extradural space in children.

	NEW PATTERN QUESTIONS
Q N10	Korner's septum is seen in:
	a. Petrosquamous suture
	b. Temporal squamous suture
	c. Petromastoid suture
	d. Frontozygomatic suture
Q N11.	Space between pars flaccida and neck of malleus is called as:
	a. Von Troeltsch anterior pouch
	b. Facial recess
	c. Sinus tympani
	d. Prussak's space

Chapter 1: Anatomy of Ear

Q N12. Space between pars tensa and anterior malleolar fold is called as:
a. Von Troeltsch anterior pouch
b. Facial recess
c. Sinus tympani
d. Prussak's space

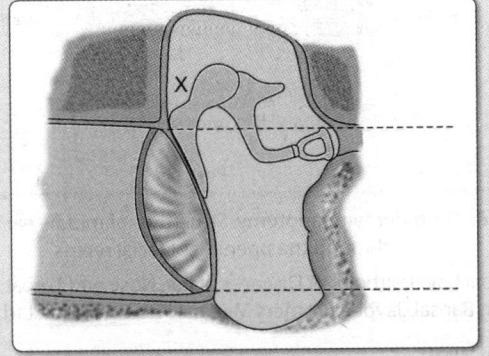

See Color Plate 2

Q N13. Identify the space marked as 'X' in above figure:
a. Epitympanum
b. Mesotympanum
c. Hypotympanum
d. Prussak's space

Q N14. Portion of middle ear around the tympanic orifice of Eustachian tube is:
a. Mesotympanum   b. Epitympanum
c. Hypotympanum   d. Protympanum

Q N15. Stenvers view is used for:
a. Mastoid air cells   b. Temporal bone
c. Paranasal sinuses   d. Tonsils

Floor or Jugular Wall

It is a thin plate of bone which separates tympanic cavity from the jugular bulb.^{Q}
- In the floor close to the medial wall lies a small opening which allows entry of tympanic branch of glossopharyngeal nerve (**Jacobson nerve**) into the middle ear.

Anterior Wall or Carotid Wall (Figs. 1.5 and 1.6)

- It is a thin plate of bone which separates the cavity from internal carotid artery.
- From above downwards features seen on anterior wall are
  - **Canal for tensor tympani (canal containing tensor tympani muscle** which extends to the medial wall to form a pulley called as processus cochleariformis). The cochleariformis process, serves a useful landmark and denotes the location of anterior most part of horizontal segment of facial nerve.
  - Opening for **Eustachian tube.**
  - **Internal carotid artery (carotid canal)**

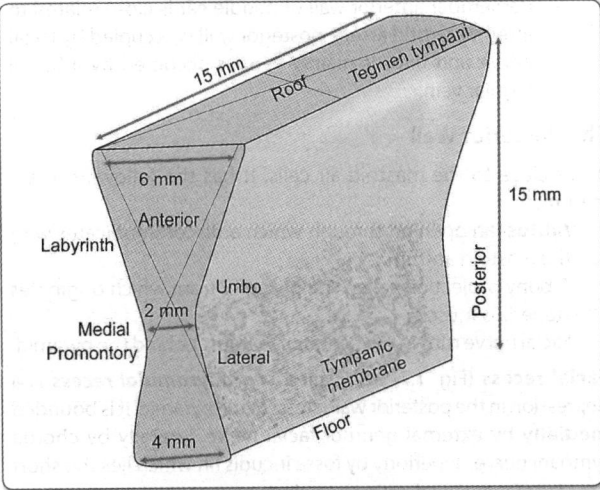

Fig. 1.5: Dimensions of tympanum
Courtesy: Textbook of Diseases of Ear, Nose and Throat, Mohan Bansal, Jaypee Brothers Medical Publishers Pvt. Ltd., p 6

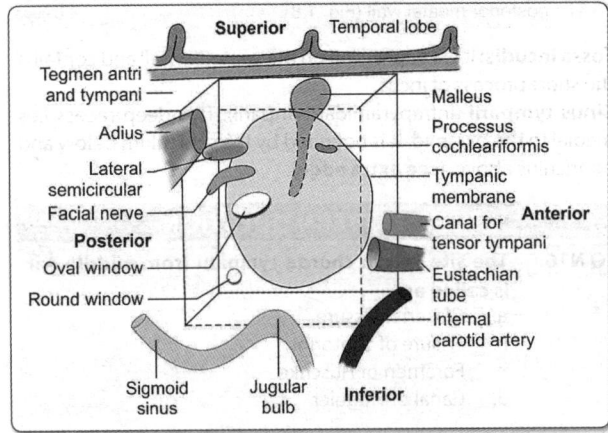

Fig. 1.6: Six boundaries of tympanum. Medial wall is seen through the tympanic membrane
Courtesy: Textbook of Diseases of Ear, Nose and Throat, Mohan Bansal, Jaypee Brothers Medical Publishers Pvt. Ltd., p 7

- **Canal of Huguier** for passage of chorda tympani nerve out of temporal bone anteriorly through the medial end of petrotympanic fissure to join the lingual nerve in the infratemporal fossa. It carries taste from anterior two-thirds of tongue and secretomotor fibers to submaxillary and sublingual gland.
- **Glaserian fissure** below canal of Huguier transmits tympanic artery and anterior ligament of malleus.

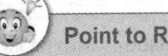

Point to Remember

Anterior wall of middle ear is close related to internal carotid artery; posterior wall is occupied by facial nerve and floor is mainly venous occupied by internal jugular vein.

– Remember anterior wall of middle ear is close related to internal carotid artery; posterior wall is occupied by facial nerve and floor is mainly venous occupied by internal jugular vein.

The Posterior Wall

It lies close to the mastoid air cells. It has the following main features:
- **Aditus**–an opening through which attic communicates with the mastoid antrum.
- A bony projection called **the pyramid** from which originates stapedius muscle.
- Facial nerve runs in the posterior wall just behind the pyramid.

Facial recess (Fig. 1.7) also called *suprapyramidal recess* is a depression in the posterior wall lateral to the pyramid. It is bounded **medially** by external genu of facial nerve, laterally by chorda tympani nerve, superiorly by fossa incudis (in which lies the short process of incus) and anterolaterally by tympanic membrane.

 Note: In the intact canal wall mastoidectomy, middle ear is approached (posterior tympanotomy or facial recess approach) through the facial recess without disturbing posterior meatal wall (Fig. 1.8).

Fossa Incudis: It is a depression on the posterior wall and contains the short process of incus.

Sinus tympani (Infrapyramidal tympani): This deep recess lies medial to the pyramid. It is bounded by the subiculum below and ponticulus above. **(see extra edge).**

NEW PATTERN QUESTION

Q N16. The site exit of chorda tympani from middle ear is called as:
a. Glaserian fissure
b. Fissure of Santorini
c. Foramen of Huschke
d. Canal of Huguier

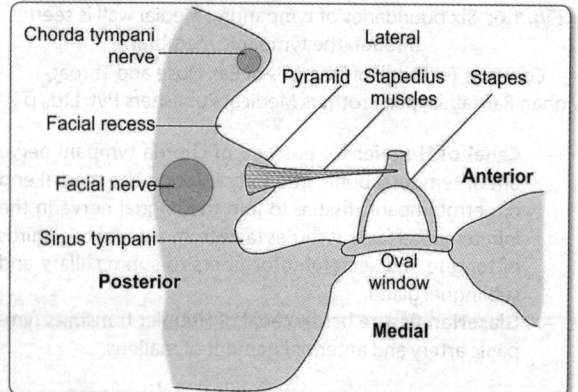

Fig. 1.7: Facial recess and sinus tympani relations with facial nerve and pyramidal eminence

Courtesy: Textbook of Diseases of Ear, Nose and Throat, Mohan Bansal, Jaypee Brothers Medical Publishers Pvt. Ltd., p 7

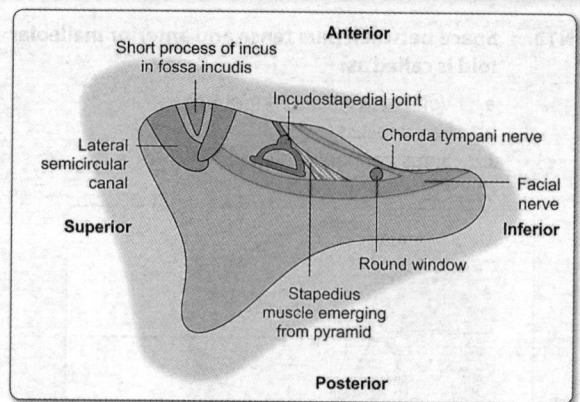

Fig. 1.8: Posterior tympanotomy. Structures of middle ear seen through the opening of facial recess

Courtesy: Textbook of Diseases of Ear, Nose and Throat, Mohan Bansal, Jaypee Brothers Medical Publishers Pvt. Ltd., p 7

Medial Wall

It separates the tympanic cavity from internal ear. It is formed by labyrinth. The main features on medial wall are (Fig. 1.9):
- A bulge called as **promontory formed** by basal turn of cochlea.^{Q}
- **Fenestra vestibuli (oval window** ^{Q}**)** lies posterosuperior (behind and above) to the promontory and opens into scala vestibuli. It is occupied by foot plate of stapes fixed by annular ligament. Its size on average is 3.25 mm long and 1.75 mm wide.
- **Fenestra cochleae (round window)** lies posteroinferior to the promontory and opens into scala tympani of cochlea. It is closed by **secondary tympanic membrane**. The round window is closest to ampulla of posterior semicircular canal. Round window is a triangular opening.
- Prominence of facial nerve canal (k/a Fallopian canal) lies above the fenestra vestibuli curving downward into posterior wall of middle ear.

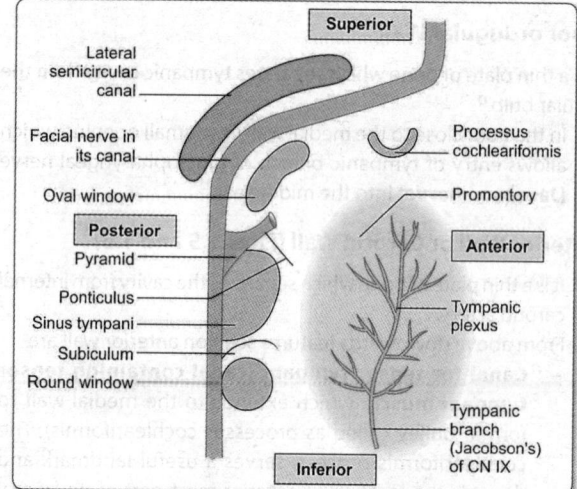

Fig. 1.9: Medial wall of middle ear

Courtesy: Textbook of Diseases of Ear, Nose and Throat, Mohan Bansal, Jaypee Brothers Medical Publishers Pvt. Ltd., p 8

- Anterior to oval window lies a hook-like projection called the **processus cochleariformis**[Q] for tendon of tensor tympani[Q].
- The cochleariform process marks the level of the genu of the facial nerve which is an important landmark for surgery of the facial nerve.

Lateral Wall
- The lateral wall of middle ear is formed by Tympanic membrane and a small bone '*scutum*'.
- The scutum is the bone above pars flaccida lateral to the attic.

NEW PATTERN QUESTION
Q N17. Scutum is:
- a. Bony part of outer attic wall
- b. Bony part of inner attic wall
- c. Cartilaginous part of outer attic wall
- d. Cartilaginous part of inner attic wall

Extra Edge
- The round window opening is separated from the oval window opening by a bony ridge called the **subiculum**.
- The **ponticulus** – is another bony ridge below oval window.
- Medial to the pyramid is a deep recess called as **sinus tympani** (infrapyramidal recess or medial facial recess) which is bounded below by **subiculum** and above by ponticulus. **It is the most inaccessible site in the middle ear and mastoid. Its importance is that cholesteatoma which has extended up to it, is difficult to eradicate.**
- Facial recess is superficial to sinus tympani and is separated from it by descending part of facial N.

Nerve supply of middle ear
Is by Tympanic Plexus
- *Tympanic plexus is formed by:*
  - Tympanic branch of IX nerve (Jacobson nerve)
  - The sympathetic plexus
- They form a plexus on the promontory and provide branches to the tympanic cavity, Eustachian tube and mastoid antrum and air cells.

Blood supply
- Arteries supplying the walls and contents of the tympanic cavity arise from both the internal and external carotid system. Arteries involved are:
(i) Anterior tympanic artery, (ii) Inferior tympanic artery, (iii) Stylomastoid artery.

Lymphatic drainage
Middle ear: Retropharyngeal and Parotid nodes
Eustachian tube: Retropharyngeal group

Point to Remember
Contents of Tympanic Cavity:
- The tympanic cavity contains the
- Ossicles
- Muscles viz:
  - Tensor tympani and stapedius
- Chorda tympani
- Tympanic plexus

AUDITORY OSSICLES (FIG. 1.10)
- These are malleus, incus and stapes (MIS)

Malleus
- It is shaped like a mallet
- It is placed most laterally
- It is 7.5–9 mm long
- It comprises of head, neck, anterior process, lateral process, manubrium and umbo

Incus
- It is shaped like an anvil
- It is the largest of the three ossicles
- It is placed medially to malleus
- It has body, short process, long process and lenticular process

Stapes
- It is the shortest bone of the body
- It is shaped like a stirrup
- It is placed most medially
- **Stapes consists of a capitulum, two crura and foot plate**
- The average dimensions of footplate are 3 mm long and 1.4 mm wide
- Footplate of stapes is held on the oval window by annular ligament

Also know
Lenticular process is sometimes called as the fourth ossicle as it is a sesamoid bone

Development of Ossicles
- Maleus and incus develop mainly from first brachial arch (Meckels cartilage)
- Stapes develops mainly from second brachial arch except the footplate which along with annular ligament is derived from the otic capsule.
- **Ossicles ossify by fourth month of intrauterine life (first bones in the body to do so).**

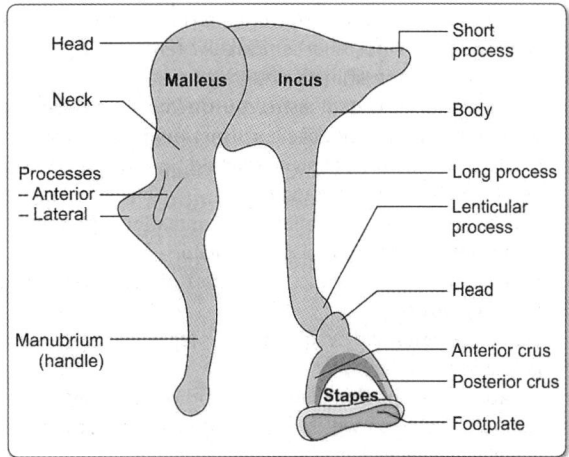

Fig. 1.10: Middle ear ossicles
Courtesy: Textbook of Diseases of Ear, Nose and Throat, Mohan Bansal, Jaypee Brothers Medical Publishers Pvt. Ltd., p 8

> **Joints of the Ossicles**
> a. The incudomalleolar joint
>   – Saddle joint
> b. Incudostapedial joint
>   – Ball and socket joint
> Both of them are synovial joints.

Function of Ossicle

- Ossicles conduct sound energy from the tympanic membrane to oval window and then to inner ear fluid.

Muscles of Tympanic Cavity: *Tympanic Cavity has Two Muscles*

Tensor tympani develops from 1st arch
  Origin: Cartilaginous pharyngotympanic tube, greater wing of sphenoid, its own bony canal
  Insertion: Upper part of handle of malleus
  Nerve supply: Mandibular nerve (anterior or motor branch)
  Function: Contraction pulls handle of malleus medially, tensing tympanic membrane to reduce the force of vibrations in response to loud noise

Stapedius develops from 2nd Arch
  Origin: Attached to inside of pyramidal eminence
  Insertion: Neck of stapes
  Innervation: *Branch of facial nerve*
  Function: Contraction usually in response to loud noises, pulls the stapes posteriorly and prevents excessive osscillation.

MASTOID ANTRUM

Mastoid bone is a **cancellous or spongy bone**
- It has numerous air cells. The largest of which is **mastoid antrum**.

  Types → Pneumatic (80%)
          → Sclerotic (20%)
          → Diploic (mixed)

- It is an air sinus in the petrous temporal bone.
- Its upper anterior wall has the opening of aditus, while medial wall is related to posterior semicircular canal (SCC).
- Posteriorly lies the sigmoid sinus.
- The posterior belly of digastric muscle forms a groove in the base of mastoid bone. The corresponding ridge inside the mastoid lies lateral not only to sigmoid sinus but also to facial nerve and is a useful landmark.
- The roof is formed by tegmen antri separating it from middle cranial fossa and temporal lobe of brain.^{Q}
- Anteroinferior is the descending part of facial nerve canal (or Fallopian canal).
- Lateral wall is formed by squamous temporal bone and is easily palpable behind the pinna.
- Mastoid develops from squamous and petrous part bone of temporal between which lies petrosquamous suture which usually disappears.

The mastoid antrum unlike the other air sinuses are well developed at birth and almost adult in size. Pneumatization begins in the first year and is complete by 4 to 6 years of age.

Korner's septum: Korner's septum is persistence of petrosquamous suture in the form of a bony plate which separates superficial squamous cells from the deep petrosal cells. Korner's septum is surgically important as it may cause difficulty in locating the antrum and the deeper cells, and thus lead to incomplete removal of disease at mastoidectomy. Mastoid antrum cannot be reached unless the Korner's septum has been removed.

Landmark for Mastoid Antrun

Macewen's Triangle (Fig. 1.11)

The mastoid antrum lies 1.25 cm deep to Macewen triangle.
It is bounded by:

- Above by temporal line
- Anteroinferiorly by posterosuperior segment of bony external auditory canal.
- Posteriorly by a line drawn as a tangent to the external canal.

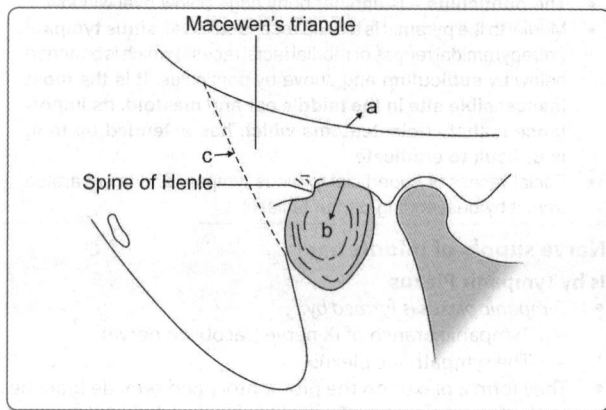

Fig. 1.11: a. Supramastoid crest or temporal line, b. Posterosuperior segment of EAC, c. Tangent drawn to external canal

 Note: Anterior to Macewen's triangle on the mastoid bone, a projection can be seen. This is called **spine of Henle**. It is also an important landmark for mastoid antrum.

Extra Edge

Master Antrum: In an adult, it lies 12–15 mm deep to suprameatal triangle. But at the time of birth, it just lies 2 mm deep to suprameatal triangle. The thickness of the bone increase up to puberty at the rate of 1 mm per year.

NEW PATTERN QUESTION

Q N18. Which of the following is not a pneumatic bone?
  a. Ethmoid   b. Sphenoid
  c. Maxillary d. Mastoid

Chapter 1: Anatomy of Ear

EUSTACHIAN TUBE

It is a channel connecting the tympanic cavity with the nasopharynx. (Fig. 1.12) It is also called **pharyngotympanic tube**. It is lined by Ciliated columnar epithelium.

- It helps to equalize pressure on both sides of tympanic membrane.
- Length of Eustachian tube is 36 mm (reached by the age of 7 years) and 3 mm wide.
- Lateral third (i.e. 12 mm) is bony.
- Medial 2/3 (i.e. 24 mm) is fibrocartilaginous.
- In adults it is placed at **an angle of 45°** with saggital plane, while in infants, it is short (length 13–18 mm), wide and placed horizontally.
  So in infants infections of middle ear are more common.
- **Muscles of Eustachian tube:**
  - Levator veli palatini (innervated by the vagus N)
  - Salpingopharyngeus (innervated by vagus N)
  - Tensor tympani (innervated by mandibular N of CN V)
  - Tensor veli palatini (innervated by mandibular N of CN V)
- Arterial supply is through branches from ascending pharyngeal artery, middle meningeal artery and artery of pterygoid canal (both branches of maxillary artery).
- Venous drainage is to the pterygoid venous plexus.
- Nerve supply is by tympanic plexus.

NEW PATTERN QUESTIONS

Q N19. Length of Eustachian tube is:
- a. 24 mm
- b. 36 mm
- c. 46 mm
- d. 26 mm

Q N20. Patulous Eustachian tube is seen in:
- a. Pregnancy
- b. Cleft lip
- c. Down syndrome
- d. Turner's syndrome

Q N21. Eustachian tube is opened if pressure difference is more than:
- a. 15 mm of Hg
- b. 30 mm of Hg
- c. 50 mm of Hg
- d. 90 mm of Hg

Q N22. Schuller's view is for:
- a. Sphenoid sinus
- b. Mastoid air cells
- c. Round window
- d. Carotid canal

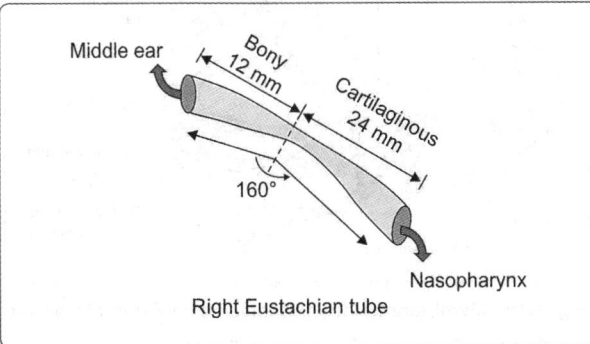

Fig. 1.12: Right Eustachian tube

INNER EAR (ALSO CALLED LABYRINTH)

- It consists of a bony labyrinth (contained within the petrous temporal bone) along with the membranous labyrinth.
- It serves the most important function of hearing and equilibrium.
- The inner ear is connected to posterior cranial fossa by an opening in petrous temporal bone called as internal acoustic meatus.
- **Parts:** A. Bony labyrinth, B. Membranous labyrinth.

BONY LABYRINTH (FIG. 1.13)

- It lies in the temporal bone
- It consists of *vestibule, the semicircular canals* and *the cochlea which are filled with perilymph*^{Q}, which resembles CSF but is rich in Na$^+$ and poor in K$^+$.
- **Fallopius in 1561 described cochlea and labyrinth.**

Vestibule

- Central portion of the bony labyrinth around the utricle and saccule.
- **Posterosuperior wall:** Has '5' openings of the semicircular canals.
- **Medial wall** of vestibule has:

❏ Spherical recess	❏ Elliptical recess	❏ Opening of aqueduct of vestibule
For the saccule	For the utricle	Carries endolymphatic duct

- **In the lateral wall** lies the oval window (Fenestra vestibule).

Semicircular Canals (SCC)

They are three in number, the **lateral, posterior and superior** and lie at right angles (90°) to each other. The area of bony labyrinth which lies in between 3 SCC is called **solid angle.**^{Q}

- *Ampulla:* One end of each canal dilates to form the ampulla, which contains the vestibular sensory epithelium and opens independently in vestibule. Ideally there should be 6 openings of 3 SCC but the non ampullated ends of posterior and superior SCC fuse together to form a common crus called as **'crus commune'** (4 mm length) which then opens into the vestibule, So the 3 semicircular canals open in vestibule by "5" openings.

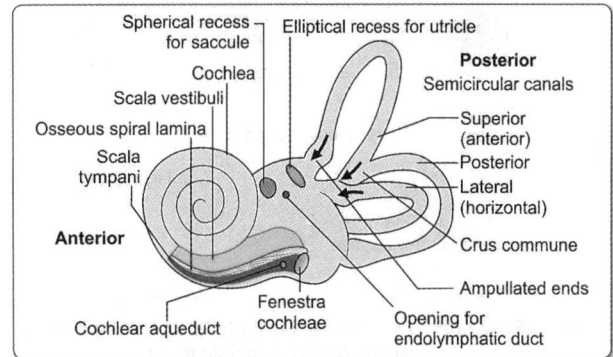

Fig. 1.13: Bony labyrinth of left side. External features seen from lateral side

Cochlea (Bony Cochlea)

- Has approximately two- and- one half turns.^Q
- Coils turn about a central bone called *modiolus*.^Q
- The cochlear tube is 30 mm long.
- Cochlea converts mechanical sound waves to electrical signal which can be transmitted to brain. This function is primarily performed by cochlea hair cells.
- The modiolus houses spiral ganglion cells destined to innervate cochlea hair cells, in an area **called as Rosenthal canal**.
- Arising from the modiolus is a thin shelf of bone which spirals upward within the lumen of the cochlea as the **bony spiral lamina**.
  - Spira lamina divides the cochlear canal into **upper scala vestibuli and lower scale tympani**. The scala vestibuli and tympani scala are continuous with each other through **helicotrema at the** apex of cochlea (Fig. 1.14)
  - Scala vestibuli is closed by the footplate of stapes, which separates it from the air-filled middle ear.
  - The scala tympani is closed by secondary tympanic membrane.
  - **Aqueduct of cochlea connects the** scala tympani with the subarachnoid space.
  - Spiral lamina gives attachment to the basilar membrane.

Point to Remember

> The bony labyrinth (bony cochlea) has 3 openings
> - The **oval window (fenestra vestibule)** present in scala vestibule and closed by footplate of stapes.
> - **Round window (fenestra cochleae)** present in scala tympani and covered by secondary tympanic membrane.
> - **Cochlear canaliculus** which transmits a small vein to inferior petrosal sinus
>
> The bony labyrinth communicates with subarachnoid space via **cochlear aqueduct**. Thus, infection of labyrinth can lead to meningitis and vice versa.

■ MEMBRANOUS LABYRINTH (FIG. 1.15)

- It lies within the osseus/bony labyrinth and is filled with endolymphatic fluid.^Q
- It is separated from the bony labyrinth by perilymphatic fluid.^Q
- It consists of cochlear duct, utricle, saccule, semicircular ducts, endolymphatic duct and sac.

Semicircular Ducts

- They are three in number and correspond exactly to the three bony canals.
- They open in **the utricle**. The ampullated end of each duct contains a thickened ridge of neuroepithelium called **crista ampullaris**^Q which responds **to angular acceleration**.^Q

Utricle and Saccule

- The utricle lies in the posterior part of bony vestibule.
- **It receives the five openings of the three semicircular ducts.**
- It is connected to the saccule through **utriculosaccular ducts**.^Q
- The sensory epithelium of the utricle is **called the *macula*** and is concerned with linear acceleration^Q and deceleration.^Q
- The **saccule** also lies in the bony vestibule.
- Its sensory epithelium is also called **the *macula*.**^Q Its exact function is not known. It probably also responds to linear acceleration^Q and deceleration.^Q

Endolymphatic Duct and Sac

Endolymphatic duct is formed by the union of two ducts, one each from the saccule and the utricle.^Q i.e. utriculosaccular ducts. Its terminal part is dilated to form **endolymphatic sac** which lies under the dura on the posterior surface of the petrous bone. Thus, endolymphatic duct connects utriculosaccular duct to brain. The endolymphatic sac is responsible for absorption of endolymph (fluid which fills whole of membranous labyrinth).

> **Donaldson's line:** This line is a surgical landmark for endolymphatic sac. It passes through horizontal bisecting the posterior semicircular canal. The endolymphatic sac that appears as thickening of the posterior cranial fossa dura is situated inferior to Donaldson's line.

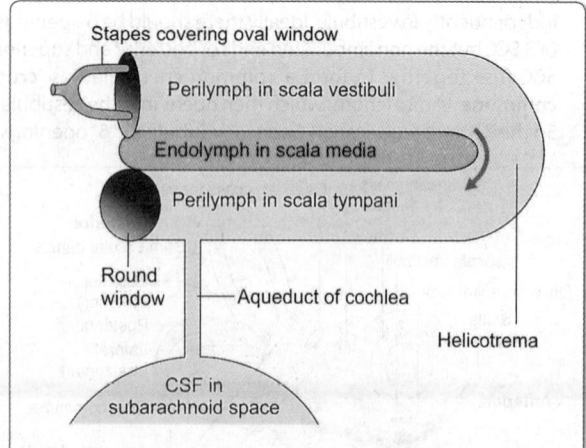

Fig. 1.14: Cochlea: Peri- and endolymphatic systems relations with cerebrospinal fluid (CSF)

Courtesy: Textbook of Diseases of Ear, Nose and Throat, Mohan Bansal, Jaypee Brothers Medical Publishers Pvt. Ltd., p 14

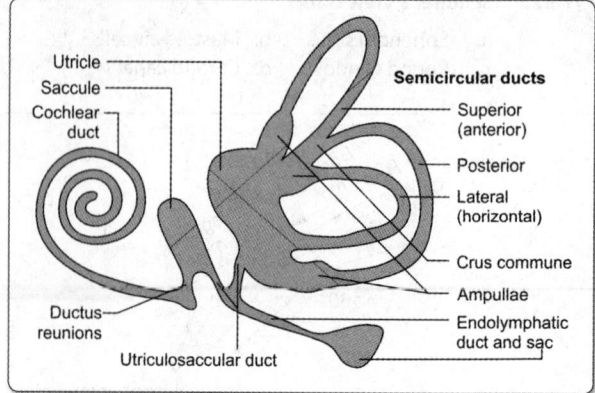

Fig. 1.15: Membranous labyrinth of left side: External features

Courtesy: Textbook of Diseases of Ear, Nose and Throat, Mohan Bansal, Jaypee Brothers Medical Publishers Pvt. Ltd., p 15

Cochlear Duct (Membranous Cochlea)

- Also called *membranous cochlea*[Q] or the scala media.[Q] It is a blind coiled tube, Which takes $2^{1}/_{2} - 2^{3}/_{4}$ turns around a bony axis called '**modulus**'.
- It appears triangular on cross section and has three walls formed by:
    - The basilar membrane, which supports the organ of Corti[Q]
    - The Reissner's membrane which separates it from the scala vestibuli[Q] (Fig. 1.16)
    - The stria vascularis, which contains vascular epithelium and is concerned with secretion of endolymph.[Q]
- Cochlear duct is connected to the saccule by ductus reunions.[Q]

> The basal coil of cochlea responds to higher frequency sounds whereas the apical turns respond to low frequency sounds.

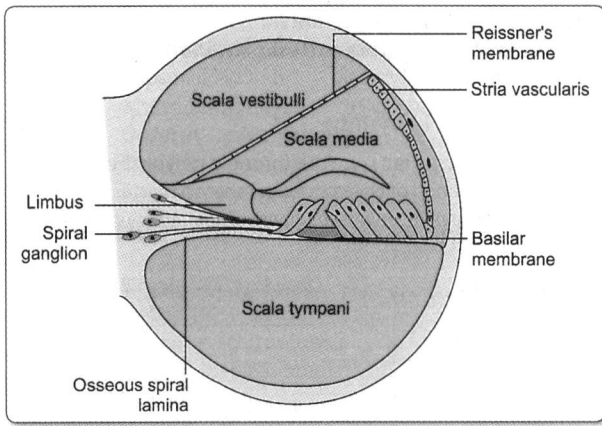

Fig. 1.16: Structure of cochlear canal after its cut section
Courtesy: Textbook of Diseases of Ear, Nose and Throat, Mohan Bansal, Jaypee Brothers Medical Publishers Pvt. Ltd., p 15

NEW PATTERN QUESTIONS

Q N23. Not included in bony labyrinth:
   a. Cochlea
   b. Semicircular canal
   c. Organ of Corti
   d. Vestibule

Q N24. The bony cochlea is a coiled tube making...turns around a bony pyramid called:
   a. 2, 1/4 modiolus
   b. 2, 1/2 helicotrema
   c. 2, 3/4 modiolus
   d. 2, 3/4 helicotrema

Q N25. Sense organ for hearing:
   a. Organ of Corti
   b. Cristae
   c. Macula
   d. None

Q N26. Where is electrode kept in cochlear implant?
   a. Round window
   b. Oval window
   c. Scala vestibuli
   d. Scala tympani

Q N27. Surgical landmark for endolymphatic sac during surgery is:
   a. Solid angle
   b. Trautman triangle
   c. Utelli's angle
   d. Donaldson line

Q N28. Cochlea endolymph has potential of:
   a. + 80 mV
   b. – 80 mV
   c. + 60 mV
   d. – 60 mV

Q N29. The bony labyrinth has following *except*:
   a. Oral window
   b. Round window
   c. Endolymphatic sac
   d. Cochlear aqueduct

Q N30. Inner ear communicates with cranium by:
   a. Cochlear aqueduct
   b. Internal acoustic meatus
   c. Both
   d. None

Inner Ear Fluids and their Circulation

- There are two main fluids in the inner ear, perilymph and endolymph.
- **Perilymph** resembles extracellular fluid and is rich in Na ions[Q]. It fills the space between the bony[Q] and the membranous labyrinth.[Q] It communicates with CSF through the aqueduct of cochlea[Q] which opens into the scala tympani near the round window.
- **Endolymph** fills the entire membranous labyrinth[Q] and resembles intracellular fluid[Q], being rich in K ions[Q]. It is secreted by the secretory cells of the stria vascularis[Q] of the cochlea and by the dark cells (present in the utricle and near the ampullated ends of semicircular ducts).

NEW PATTERN QUESTIONS

Q N31. Function of structure marked with 'X' is:

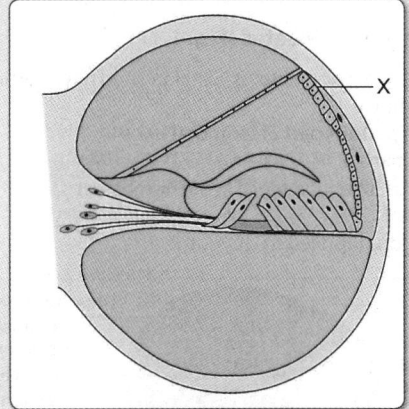

   a. Perilymph secretion
   b. Endolymph secretion
   c. Both perilymph and endolymph secretion
   d. CSF secretion

Q N32. Endolymph is present in:
a. Scala media b. Scala vestibulae
c. Scala tympani d. Cochlear aqueduct

Blood Supply of Labyrinth

- Blood supply of labyrinth is through labyrinthine artery[Q] which is a branch of anteroinferior cerebellar artery[Q] but may sometimes arise from basilar artery.
- It divides in the labyrinth – as

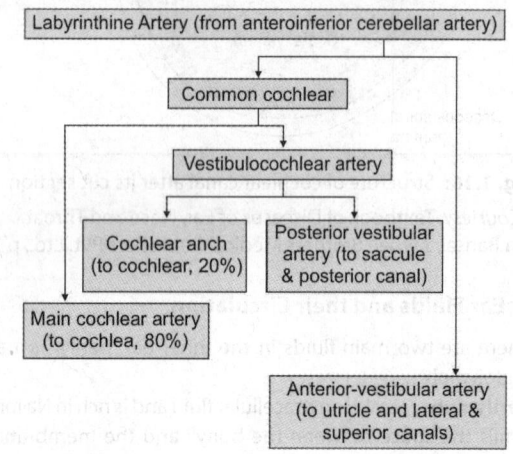

Venous Drainage

- It is through three veins namely internal auditory, vein of cochlear aqueduct and vein of vestibular aqueduct which ultimately drain into inferior petrosal sinus and lateral venous sinus.

Note:
- Blood supply to the inner ear is independant of blood supply to middle ear and bony otic capsule, and there is no cross circulation between the two.
- Blood supply to cochlea and vestibular labyrinth is segmental, therefore, independent ischemic damage can occur to these organs causing either cochlear or vestibular symptoms.

Internal Acoustic Meatus (Fig. 1.17)

- Internal acoustic meatus is 1 cm long and has a vertical length of 2–8 mm
- It lies in petrous part of temporal bone
- It has 3 parts:
  - Perus (inlet of interval acoustic meatus)
  - Canal
  - Fundus (applied to labyrinth)

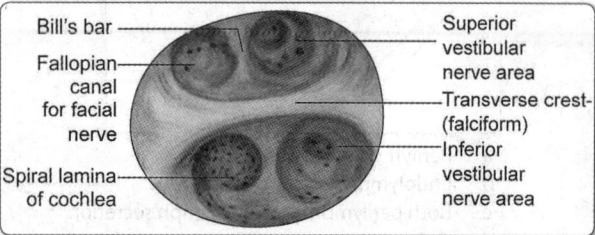

Fig. 1.17: Fundus of internal acoustic meatus

- **Bills bar** is a vertical crest of bone, which divides superior compartment of canal into anterior compartment for facial N and posterior compartment for superior vestibular N.
- It is divided into superior and inferior compartment by Falciform (Transverse) crest.
- Structures which pass through internal acoustic meatus to cranium and vice versa.

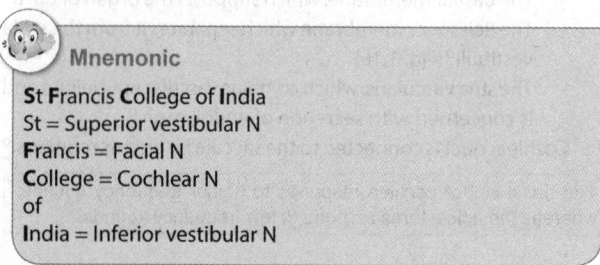

Mnemonic

St Francis **C**ollege **of I**ndia
St = Superior vestibular N
Francis = Facial N
College = Cochlear N
of
India = Inferior vestibular N

Sensory end Organs of Balance

The sensory organs or balance are:

Cristae:
- Present in semicircular canal
- Responsible for sensing rotational and angular movements.

Maculae:
- Present in utricle and saccule
- Responsible for sensing linear acceleration, head tilt and gravity.

■ DEVELOPEMENT OF EAR

Pinna

- In the sixth week of embryonic life, six tubercles (**Hillocks of His**) (Fig 1.18) appear around the first and second branchial arch. They progressively grow and coalesce and form the auricle.
- Tragus develops from the first branchial arch. The remaining pinna develops from second arch.
- By the 20th week, pinna attains adult shape.

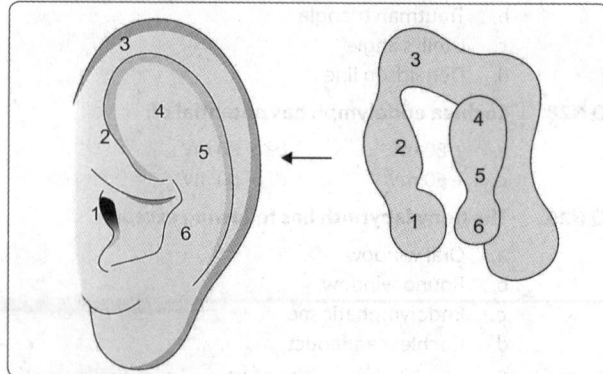

Fig. 1.18: Development of pinna (A) from six hillocks of His (B) around the first branchial cleft (1 from first and 2–6 from second branchial arch)

Courtesy: Textbook of Diseases of Ear, Nose and Throat, Mohan Bansal, Jaypee Brothers Medical Publishers Pvt. Ltd., p 19

Chapter 1: Anatomy of Ear

Point to Remember

Applied Anatomy:
- **Preauricular sinus:** Results due to defective fusion between 1st and 2nd arch, hence it is situated between tragus and rest of pinna
  Opening of the sinus is found in front of the ascending limb of the helix.
- **Anotia** is complete absence of pinna and usually forms a part of the first arch syndrome
- **Microtia:** It is developmental anomaly where size of pinna is small.
- The surgical reconstruction of pinna is done after 6 years of age using costal cartilage. This is because pinna attains adult size by that time.

NEW PATTERN QUESTIONS

Q N33. Pinna attains adult size by:
  a. 6 hours after birth
  b. 8–9 years after birth
  c. 6–8 months after birth
  d. 2–4 years after birth

Q N34. A new born presents with bilateral microtia and external auditory canal atresia. Corrective surgery is usually performed at:
  a. < 1 year of age
  b. 5–7 years of age
  c. Puberty
  d. Adulthood

Q N35. Identify the condition shown in the figure:

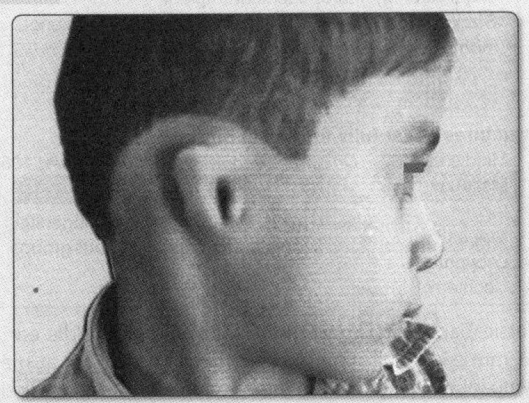

See Color Plate 3

  a. Bat ear
  b. Microtia
  c. Macrotia
  d. Crotia

External Auditory Canal

- External auditory canal (EAC) develops from the first branchial cleft.
- At birth external canal is cartilaginous, the bony part develops later.
- At the time of birth, the tympanic membrane is nearly horizontal in orientation Tympanic membrane becomes more vertical (50–60 from horizontal) during 3rd year of life.

Point to Remember

Applied Anatomy:
Atresia of canal: The recanalization of meatal plug, which begins from the deeper part near the tympanic membrane and progresses outwards, forms the epithelial lining of the bony meatus. This is the reason why deeper meatus is sometimes developed while there is atresia of canal in the outer part.

Tympanic Membrane

It develops from all the three germinal layers:
- **Ectoderm:** Outer epithelial layer is formed by the ectoderm.
  – of 1st brachial cleft
- **Mesoderm:** The middle fibrous layer develops from the mesoderm.
  – of 1st pharyngeal pouch (tubo tympanic recess)
- **Endoderm:** Inner mucosal layer is formed by the endoderm.

NEW PATTERN QUESTIONS

Q N36. External auditory canal is formed by:
  a. 1st branchial groove
  b. 1st visceral pouch
  c. 2nd branchial groove
  d. 2nd visceral pouch

Q N37. Call Aural fistula is:
  a. 1st branchial cleft anomaly
  b. 2nd branchial cleft anomaly
  c. 1st branchial pouch anomaly
  d. 2nd branchial pouch anomaly

Middle Ear

- **Endoderm of Tubotympanic Recess:** The Eustachian tube, tympanic cavity, attic, antrum and mastoid air cells are derived from the endoderm of **tubotympanic recess** which arises from the first and partly from the second pharyngeal pouches. The distal part of tubotympanic recess forms tympanic cavity and proximal part becomes Eustachian tube.
- **First Branchial Arch:** Malleus and incus develop from mesoderm of the first arch.
- **Second Branchial Arch:** The stapes suprastructures (i.e. head, neck and the 2 crura) develops. from the second arch. Whereas the stapes footplate and annular ligament are derived from the otic capsule.
- The ossicles attain their adult configuration by 20 weeks.

Inner Ear

- Development of the inner ear, which begins in third week of fetal life, is complete by the 16th week.
- **Auditory Placode (Otic placode):** The auditory placode, which is thickened ectoderm of hind brain, gets invaginated and forms auditory vesicle (otocyst).

- **Auditory Vesicle:** The auditory vesicle differentiates into endolymphatic duct and sac, utricle, semicircular ducts, saccule and cochlea, i.e. **membranous labyrinth develops from ectoderm.**
- Development of pars superior (semicircular canals and utricle) takes place earlier than pars inferior (saccule and cochlea). The pars superior is phylogenetically older part of labyrinth.
- **Bony labyrinth develops from mesoderm.**
- The cochlea develops by 20 weeks of gestation and the fetus can hear in the womb of the mother. The great Indian epic of Mahabharata, which was written thousands of years ago, mentions that Abhimanyu son of great warrior Arjun while in his mother's womb heard conversation (regarding the art of battle ground) of his mother and father.

NEW PATTERN QUESTIONS

Q N38. Which of the following is derived from otic placode?
  a. Mastoid
  b. Tympanic antrum
  c. Ear ossicles
  d. Cochlea

Q N39. Which of the following is a derivative of otic capsule?
  a. Membranous labyrinth
  b. Perilymphatic labyrinth
  c. Bony labyrinth
  d. Ossicles

Q N40. Identify the condition shown in the figure:

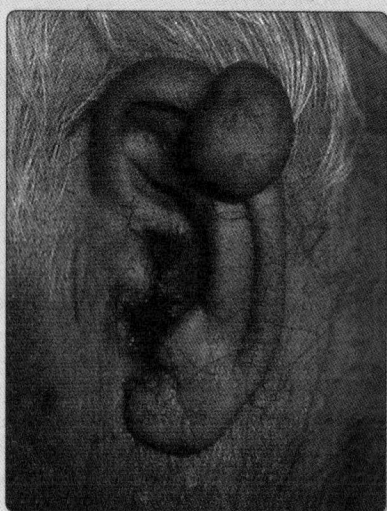

See Color Plate 4

  a. Dermoid cyst of pinna
  b. Keloid on pinna
  c. Cauliflower ear
  d. Preauricular sinus

Q N41. Identify the ear instrument shown in figure:

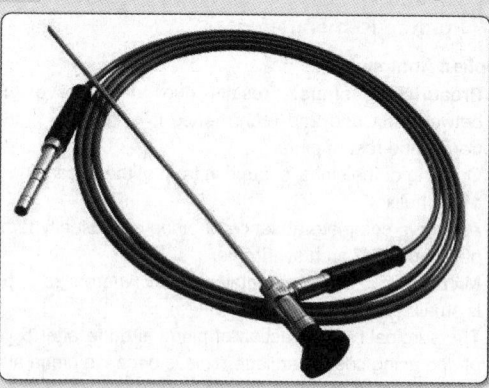

  a. Ear speculum   b. Otoendoscope
  c. Siegel speculum d. Politzer bag

Point to Remember

Applied Anatomy:
Dysplasias of Inner Ear (Dhingra 6/e, p 115)
- **Mondini dysplasia:** The cochlea takes only 1.5 turns instead of $2\frac{1}{4}$ to $2\frac{3}{4}$ turns. Cochlear implants are useful in this condition
- **Scheibe dysplacia:** M/C inner ear malformation. The bony labyrinth is normal. Involves dysplasia of cochlea and saccule (hence also called cochleosaccular dysplasia). Inherited as Autosomal Recessive trait.
- **Alexandar dysplasia:** Affects the basal turn of cochlea. Thus high frequencies are only affected. Hearing aids are beneficial in this condition.
- **Michel aplasia:** Complete absence of bony and membranous labyrinth. These patients are not benefited with either hearing and/or cochlear implant.
- **Bing Siebenmann dysplasia:** Complete absence of membranous labyrinth.

Extra Edge

- **Structures of ear fully formed at birth:**
  - Middle ear[Q]   *Dhingra 4/e, p 403; 5/e, p 462; point 106*
  - Malleus[Q]
  - Incus[Q]
  - Stapes[Q]
  - Labyrinth[Q]
  - Cochlea[Q]

- Vertical and anteroposterior dimensions of middle ear are 15 mm each while transverse dimension is 2 mm at mesotympanum, 6 mm above at the epitympanum and 4 mm below in the hypotympanum. Thus, middle ear is the narrowest between the umbo and promontory.
- Boundaries of **facial recess** are facial nerve medially, chorda tympanic (laterally) and fossa incudis (above).
- Eddy currents[Q] in the external auditory meatus do not allow water to reach TM while swimming.
- Organ of Corti is filled with cortilymph.
- The electrodes in cochlear implant are placed in the scala tympani via round window.

Chapter 1: Anatomy of Ear

Explanations and References to New Pattern Questions

N1. Ans. is b i.e. Concha

For this, refer to Figure 1.1—Concha is the part which is lying behind the external auditory meatus.

N2. Ans. is c i.e. Incisura terminalis

For this, refer to Figure 1.1—The part of pinna lying between ascending crest of helix and tragus is incisura terminalis.

N3. Ans. is d i.e. Greater auricular nerve. *Ref. Dhingra 6/e, p 4*

Major part of pinna is supplied by greater auricular nerve ($C_{2,3}$)

N4. Ans. is a i.e. Vagus *Ref. Dhingra 6/e, p 4*

Auricular branch of vagus (CNX) is called as Arnold nerve.

N5. Ans. is b i.e. Incisura terminalis

See the text for explanation

N6. Ans. is b i.e. In newborn, bony part of EAC is absent *Ref. Tuli 2/e, p 6*

In newborns, bony part of EAC is absent cartilaginous part is present and EAC is short 20 mm

N7. Ans. is b i.e. Fissure of Santorini *Ref. Dhingra 6/e, p 2*

Fissures of Santorini are seen in cartilaginous part of external auditory canal and not bony part. Rest all are seen in bony part.

N8. Ans. is c i.e. The X- cranial nerve *Ref. BDC 4/e, p Vol. 3, p 185*

"Irritation of the auricular branches of the vagus in the external ear (by ear wax, syringe, etc.) may reflexly cause cough, vomiting, or even death due to sudden cardiac inhibition."

Auricular branch of the vagus nerve is also known as **Arnold's nerve or Alderman's nerve**.

Also Know

Similarly irritation of recurrent laryngeal nerve by enlarged lymph nodes in children may also produce a persistent cough.

N9. Ans. is b i.e. Forms an angle of 55° with external auditory canal

See the text for explanation

N10. Ans. is a i.e. Petrosquamous suture *Ref. Dhingra 6/e, p7*

The petrosquamous suture may persist as a bony plate - the Korner's septum.

N11. Ans. is d i.e. Prussak's space

Prussak's space: It is bounded by pars flaccida (laterally), neck of malleus (medially), lateral process of malleus (inferiorly), and lateral malleal ligament (superiorly). Posteriorly, it opens into epitympanum.

N12. Ans. is a i.e. Von Troeltsch anterior pouch

Von Troeltsch anterior pouch: It is situated between the pars tensa and anterior malleolar fold.

N13. Ans. is d i.e. Prussak's space

See the text for explanation

N14. Ans. is d i.e. Protympanum

The part of middle ear around tympanic orifice of the Eustachian tube is called as protympanum.

N15. Ans. is b i.e. Temporal bone

Stenvers view is for imaging of temporal bone.

N16. Ans. is d i.e. Canal of Huguier *Ref. Essential of Mohan Bansal p 11*

See the text for explanation

N17. Ans. is a i.e. Bony part of outer attic wall

Scutum is a bone above pars flaccida in the lateral wall of middle ear, i.e. outer attic wall.

N18. Ans. is d i.e. Mastoid *Ref. Read below*

Mastoid is a spongy bone. Maxilla, frontal, sphenoid and ethmoid.

N19. Ans. is b i.e. 36 mm

See the text for explanation

N20. Ans. is a i.e. Pregnancy *Ref. Internet Search*

Patulous Eustachian tube is seen in pregnancy.

N21. Ans. is a i.e. 15 mm of Hg

The closed tube can be opened against a pressure difference of 10–15 mm of Hg. However, when the difference in pressure between the middle ear and atmosphere is 90 mm of Hg or more, the Eustachian tube can no longer be opened by swallowing.

N22. Ans. is b i.e. Mastoid air cells

N23. Ans. is c i.e. Organ of Corti *Ref. Dhingra 6/e, p 10*

Organ of Corti is a part of membranous labyrinth, not bony labyrinth.

N24. Ans. is c i.e. 2¾ modiolus *Ref. Dhingra 6/e, p 9*

"The bony cochlea is a called tube making 2.5 to 2.75 turns around a central pyramid of bone called modulus"

N25. Ans. is a i.e. Organ of Corti *Ref. Dhingra 6/e, p 13*

"Organ of Corti is the sense organ of hearing and is situated on the basilar membrane"

N26. Ans. is d i.e. Scala tympani *Ref. Dhingra 6/e, p 125*

The electrodes of cochlear implant are placed into the scala tympani by passing through round window.

N27. Ans. is d i.e. Donaldson line *Ref. Essential of Mohan Bansal p 12*

Donaldson line—Details given in text

Also Know:
- **Citelli's angle (sinodural angle):** It lies between the sigmoid sinus and middle fossa dura mater.
- **Bill's island:** This thin plate of bone left on sigmoid sinus during mastoidectomy helps in retracting the sigmoid sinus. It should not be confused with Bill's bar, which lies in the fundus of internal auditory canal.
- **Solid angle:** This area of bony labyrinth lies between the three semicircular canals.
- **Trautmann's triangle:** This area is bounded by the bony labyrinth anteriorly, sigmoid sinus posteriorly and the superior petrol sinus superiorly. Any infection in the posterior canal fossa can spread through this triangle and can be approached by removing the bone in between the triangle.

N28. Ans. is a i.e. +80 mV

Endocochlear potential is the positive voltage of 80–100 mV seen in the endolymph.

N29. Ans. is c i.e. Endolymphatic sac *Ref. Dhingra 6/e, p 10*

Endolymphatic sac is present in the membranous labyrinth and not bony labyrinth.

Read the text for explanation.

N30. Ans. is c i.e. Both

> As discussed in the text—cochlear aqueduct connects bony labyrinth to subarachnoid space. Internal acoustic meatus lies in petrous part of temporal bone, also connects inner ear to cranium

N31. Ans. is b i.e. Endolymph secretion

> The structure shown in the figure is stria vascularis which secretes endolymph:
> There are two theories for the origin of perilymph
> 1. It is a futrate of blood serum from the capillaries of spiral ligament
> 2. CSF reaching labyrinth via aqueduct of cochlea.

N32. Ans. is a i.e. Scala media

> See the text for explanation

N33. Ans. is b i.e. 8–9 years after birth

> Tympanic membrane attains adult size by 8–9 years of age

N34. Ans. is b i.e. 5–7 years of age

> Read the preceding text for explanation

N35 Ans. is b i.e. Microtia

> The condition in the figure shows a small sized pinna, i.e. microtia.

N36. Ans. is a i.e. 1st branchial groove *Ref. Dhingra 6/e, p 11*

> External auditory canal develops from the first branchial cleft.

N37. Ans. is a i.e. 1st branchial cleft anomaly *Ref. Dhingra 6/e, p 50*

> **Collaural fistula:** This is an abnormality of the first branchial cleft. The fistula has two openings: one situated in the neck just below and behind the angle of mandible and the other in the external canal. The track of the fistula passes through the parotid in close relation to the facial nerve. Treatment is excision of the tract.

N38. Ans. is d i.e. Cochlea

> The inner ear is derived from a pair of otic placodes that appear during 4th week and lie behind second pharyngeal arch. It forms a fluid filled otocyst which finally gives rise to cochlea and semicircular canals.

N39. Ans. is d i.e. Ossicles

> Otic placode forms the inner ear along with semicircular canal and utricles
> In:
> Ossicles—malleus and incus are derived from first arch and stapes from second arch.
> Only the stapes footplate and annular ligament are derived from otic capsule

N40. Ans. is b i.e. Keloid of pinna

N41. Ans. is b i.e. Otoendoscope

QUESTIONS

1. **Ceruminous glands present in the ear are:**
   [AIIMS May 05]
   a. Modified eccrine glands
   b. Modified apocrine glands
   c. Mucous gland
   d. Modified holocrine glands

2. **Nerve supply for external ear are all except:** [MAHE 07]
   a. Greater occipital nerve
   b. Greater auricular nerve
   c. Auriculotemporal nerve
   d. Lesser occipital nerve

3. **All of the following nerves supply auricle and external meatus except:** [TN 03]
   a. Trigeminal nerve
   b. Glossopharyngeal nerve
   c. Facial nerve
   d. Vagus nerve

4. **Which of the following nerves has no sensory supply to the auricle?** [AI 12]
   a. Lesser occipital nerve
   b. Greater auricular nerve
   c. Auricular branch of vagus nerve
   d. Tympanic branch of glossopharyngeal nerve

5. **Sensory supply of external auditory meatus is by:**
   a. Pterygomandibular ganglion [PGI June 07]
   b. Geniculate ganglion
   c. Facial nerve
   d. Auriculotemporal nerve

6. **Skin over pinna is fixed:** [JIPMER 95]
   a. Firmly on both sides
   b. Loosely on medial side
   c. Loosely on lateral side
   d. Loosely on both side

7. **Dehiscence of anterior wall of the external auditory canal cause infection in the parotid gland via:**
   a. Fissure of Santorini
   b. Notch of ramus
   c. Petrous fissure
   d. Retropharyngeal fissure

8. **What is the color of the normal tympanic membrane?**
   a. Pearly white
   b. Gray [CUPGEE 96]
   c. Yellow
   d. Red

9. **The most mobile part of the tympanic membrane:**
   a. Central
   b. Peripheral [TN 98]
   c. Both
   d. None of the above

10. **Pars flaccida of the tympanic membrane is also called:**
    a. Reissner's membrane [MP 07]
    b. Shrapnell's membrane
    c. Basilar membrane
    d. Secondary tympanic membrane

11. **Anterior wall of tympanic cavity contains:** [PGI May 11]
    a. Promontory
    b. Bony part of pharyngotympanic tube
    c. Processus cochleariformis
    d. Pyramid
    e. Tensor tympani muscle

12. **The distance between tympanic membrane and medial wall of middle ear at the level of center is:** [PGI]
    a. 3 mm
    b. 4 mm
    c. 6 mm
    d. 2 mm

13. **Distance of promontory from tympanic membrane:**
    a. 2 mm
    b. 5 mm [Delhi 05]
    c. 6 mm
    d. 7 mm

14. **Narrowest part of middle ear is:** [PGI 97]
    a. Hypotympanum
    b. Epitympanum
    c. Attic
    d. Mesotympanum

15. **Surface area of tympanic membrane:** [Manipal 06]
    a. 55 mm^2
    b. 70 mm^2
    c. 80 mm^2
    d. 90 mm^2

16. **The effective diameter of the tympanic membrane:** [UP 05]
    a. 25 mm^2
    b. 30 mm^2
    c. 40 mm^2
    d. 45 mm^2

17. **Lever ratio of tympanic membrane is:** [UP 01]
    a. 1.4:1
    b. 1.3:1
    c. 18.2:1
    d. 1.5:1

18. **"Cone of light" is due to:** [AIIMS 96]
    a. Malleolar fold
    b. Handle of malleus
    c. Anterior inferior quadrant
    d. Stapes

19. **In otoscopy, the most reliable sign is:** [AIIMS 92]
    a. Lateral process of malleus
    b. Handle of malleus
    c. Umbo
    d. Cone of light

20. **Nerve supply of the tympanic membrane is by:** [AI 95]
    a. Auriculotemporal
    b. Lesser occipital
    c. Greater occipital
    d. Parasympathetic ganglion

21. **Nerve supply of tympanic membrane:** [PGI Dec 02]
    a. Auriculotemporal
    b. Auricular branch of vagus
    c. Occipital NV
    d. Great auricular NV
    e. Glossopharyngeal NV

22. **Which of the following is false about tympanic membrane?** [Delhi 08]
    a. Cone of light is anteroinferior
    b. Shrapnell's membrane is also known as pars flaccida
    c. Healed perforation has three layers
    d. Anterior malleolar fold is longer than posterior

23. **Sensory nerve supply of middle ear cavity is provided by:** [AI 95]
    a. Facial
    b. Glossopharyngeal
    c. Vagus
    d. Trigeminal

24. **In carcinoma base of tongue pain is referred to the ear through:** [Kerala 94]
    a. Hypoglossal nerve
    b. Vagus nerve
    c. Glossopharyngeal nerve
    d. Lingual nerve

25. **Which of the following pain is not referred to ear?**
    a. Pharynx
    b. Tongue [Rj 2008]
    c. TM joint
    d. Vestibule of nose

26. **Stapedius is supplied by:** [JIPMER 92]
    a. Maxillary nerve
    b. Facial nerve
    c. Auditory nerve
    d. Mandibular disease
27. **Regarding stapedial reflex, which of the following is true?** [AI 00]
    a. It helps to enhance the sound conduction in middle ear
    b. It is a protective reflex against loud sounds
    c. It helps in masking the sound waves
    d. It is unilateral reflex
28. **Tensor tympani is supplied by:** [JIPMER 2002]
    a. Anterior part of V nerve
    b. Posterior part of V nerve
    c. IX nerve
    d. VII nerve
29. **Nerve of the pterygoid canal is also known as:** [PGI]
    a. Arnold's nerve
    b. Vidian nerve
    c. Nerve of Kuntz
    d. Criminal nerve of Grassi
30. **All are components of epitympanum except:** [AI 02]
    a. Body of incus
    b. Head of malleus
    c. Chorda tympani
    d. Footplate of stapes
31. **Prussak's space is situated in:** [MAHE 02]
    a. Epitympanum
    b. Mesotympanum
    c. Hypotympanum
    d. Ear canal
32. **Tegmen seperates middle ear from the middle cranial fossa containing temporal lobe of brain by:** [Karn. 06]
    a. Medical wall of middle ear
    b. Lateral wall of middle ear
    c. Roof of middle ear
    d. Anterior wall of middle ear
33. **Facial recess or the posterior sinus is bounded by:**
    a. Medially by the vertical part of VII nerve [TN 2003]
    b. Laterally by the chorda tympani
    c. Above by the fossa incudis
    d. All of the above
34. **While doing posterior tympanotomy through the facial recess there are chances of injury to the following except:** [AIIMS 2013, AI 2007]
    a. Facial nerve horizontal part
    b. Chorda tympani
    c. Dislodgement of short process of incus from fossa incudis
    d. Vertical descending part of facial nerve
35. **All are true about facial recess except:** [JIPMER 2006]
    a. Suprapyramical recess
    b. Medially it is bounded by chorda tympani and laterally by facial nerve
    c. Important in cochlear implant
    d. Middle ear can be approached through it
36. **Floor of middle ear cavity is in relation with:** [AI 2001]
    a. Internal carotid artery
    b. Bulb of the internal jugular vein
    c. Sigmoid sinus
    d. Round window
37. **Promontory seen in the middle ear is:** [PGI June 98]
    a. Jugular bulge
    b. Basal turn of cochlea
    c. Semicircular canal
    d. Head of incus
38. **Process cochleariformis attaches to:** [JIPMER 95]
    a. Tendon of tensor tympani
    b. Basal turns of helix
    c. Handle of malleus
    d. Incus
39. **Macewen's triangle is the landmark for:** [MP98]
    a. Maxillary sinus
    b. Mastoid antrum
    c. Frontal sinus
    d. None
40. **The suprameatal triangle overlies:** [JIPMER 91]
    a. Mastoid antrum
    b. Mastoid air cells
    c. Antrum
    d. Facial nerve
41. **Anatomical landmark indicating position of mastoid antrum:** [CUPGEE 96]
    a. Suprameatal triangle
    b. Spine of Henle
    c. Tip of the mastoid process
    d. None
42. **All of the following form the boundary of Macewen's triangle except:** [Delhi 2008]
    a. Temporal line
    b. Posterosuperior segment of bony external auditory canal
    c. Promontory
    d. Tangent drawn to the external auditory meatus
43. **What is the type of joint between the ossicles of ear?** [AI 08]
    a. Fibrous joint
    b. Primary cartilaginous
    c. Secondary cartilaginous
    d. Synovial joint
44. **Eustachian tube opens into middle ear cavity at:**
    a. Anterior wall
    b. Medial wall [UP 2000]
    c. Lateral wall
    d. Posterior wall
45. **The length of Eustachian tube is:** [AP99; TN 06]
    a. 16 mm
    b. 24 mm
    c. 36 mm
    d. 40 mm
46. **True about Eustachian tube are:** [PGI June 02]
    a. 24 mm in length
    b. Outer 1/3rd is cartilaginous
    c. Inner 2/3rd is bony
    d. Inner 2/3rd is cartilaginous
    e. Opens during swallowing
47. **True about Eustachian tube is/are:** [PGI June 01]
    a. Size is 3.75 cm
    b. Cartilaginous 1/3 and 2/3rd bony
    c. Opens during swallowing
    d. Nasopharyngeal opening is narrowest
    e. Tensor palati helps to open it
48. **Which of the following causes opening of Eustachian tube?** [Maharashtra 2010]
    a. Salpingopharyngeus
    b. Levator veli palatine
    c. Tensor veli palatini
    d. None of the above
49. **True about Eustachian tube:** [PGI Nov 10]
    a. Length is 36 mm in adults and 1.6 to 3 mm in children
    b. Higher elastin content in adults
    c. Ventilatory function of ear better developed in infants
    d. More horizontal in adults
    e. Angulated in infants

50. **Inner ear is present in which bone:** [PGI 97]
    a. Parietal bone
    b. Petrous part of temporal bone
    c. Occipital bone
    d. Petrous part of squamous bone
51. **Inner ear bony labyrinth is:** [Karn. 06]
    a. Strongest bone in the body
    b. Cancellous bone
    c. Cartilaginous bone
    d. Membranous bone
52. **Cochlear aqueduct:** [PGI June 98]
    a. Connects internal ear with subarachnoid space
    b. Connects cochlea with vestibule
    c. Contains endolymph
    d. Same as S media
53. **Infection of CNS spread in inner ear through:**
    [AIIMS May 10, May 11]
    a. Cochlear aqueduct   b. Endolymphatic sac
    c. Vestibular aqueduct d. Hyrtl fissure
54. **Which of the following is not a route of spread of infection from middle ear?** [AI 12]
    a. Directly through openings such as round window and oval window
    b. By bony invasion
    c. Osteothrombotic route
    d. Lymphatics
55. **Crus commune is a part of:** [Jharkhand 06]
    a. Cochlea
    b. Middle ear
    c. Semicircular canal
    d. Vestibule
56. **Stapes footplate covers:** [AIIMS May 03]
    a. Round window   b. Oval window
    c. Inferior sinus tympani d. Pyramid
57. **Organ of Corti is situated in:** [Kerala 98]
    a. Scala media   b. Sinus tympani
    c. Sinus vestibuli d. Saccule
58. **Movement of stapes causes vibration in:** [DNB 03]
    a. Scala media   b. Scala tympani
    c. Scala vestibuli d. Semicircular canal
59. **Lateral wall of middle ear formed by:** [FMGE 13]
    a. Tegmen tympani
    b. Mastoid process
    c. Promontory
    d. Tympanic membrane
60. **Bone which is pneumatic:** [PGI June 07]
    a. Maxillary   b. Parietal
    c. Temporal   d. Frontal
    e. Ethmoidal
61. **Spine of Henle is a:** [MH 2003]
    a. Cortical bone
    b. Cancellous bone
    c. Sclerotic bone
    d. Long bone with Haversian system
62. **Labyrinthine artery is a branch of:** [AIIMS 91]
    a. Internal carotid artery
    b. Basilar artery
    c. Posterior cerebellar artery
    d. Anteroinferior cerebellar artery
63. **Endolymphatic duct connects which structure:**
    a. Scala media to subdural space [Delhi 05]
    b. Scala vestibule to aqueduct of cochlea
    c. Scala tympani to aqueduct of cochlea
    d. Scala tympani to subdural space
64. **Site where endolymph is seen:** [Kerala 97]
    a. Scala vestibuli   b. Scala media
    c. Helicotrema   d. Organ of Corti
65. **Endolymph in inner ear:** [AIIMS May 10]
    a. Is a filtrate of blood serum
    b. Is secreted by striae vascularis
    c. Is secreted by basilar membrane
    d. Is secreted by hair cells
66. **The function of stria vascularis is:** [AI 2002]
    a. To produce perilymph
    b. To absorb perilymph
    c. To maintain electric milieu of endolymph
    d. To maintain electric milieu of perilymph
67. **Pinna develops from:** [MH 02]
    a. 1st pharyngeal arch
    b. 1st and 3rd pharyngeal arch
    c. 1st and 2nd pharyngeal arch
    d. 2nd pharyngeal arch
68. **The following structure represents all the 3 components of the embryonic disc:** [TN 98]
    a. Tympanic membrane   b. Retina
    c. Meninges   d. None of the above
69. **Vertical crest at the internal auditory canal is:**
    [AIIMS May 11]
    a. Bill's bar   b. Ponticulus
    c. Cog   d. Falciform crest
70. **Eustachian tube develops from:** [PGI 97]
    a. 2nd and 3rd pharyngeal pouch
    b. 1st pharyngeal pouch
    c. 2nd pharyngeal pouch
    d. 3rd pharyngeal pouch
71. **All of the following are of adult size at birth except?**
    a. Mastoid antrum   b. Ear ossicles [AIIMS 2009]
    c. Tympanic cavity   d. Maxillary antrum
72. **Which of the following attain adult size before birth?**
    a. Ear ossicles   b. Maxilla [AIIMS Nov 2010]
    c. Mastoid   d. Parietal bone
73. **True regarding "Preauricular sinus" is:** [MAHE 07]
    a. Improper fusion of auricular tubercles
    b. Persistent opening of first branchial arch
    c. Autosomal recessive pattern
74. **Stapes develop from:** [AI 2009]
    a. 1st arch   b. 2nd arch
    c. 3rd arch   d. 4th arch

75. **True regarding development of the ear:** *[PGI 2007]*
    a. Eustachian tube develops from 1st cleft
    b. Eustachian tube opens behind the level of inferior turbinate
    c. Pinna develops from 1st pouch
    d. Growth of organ of Corti is completed by 5th month
    e. Ossicles are adult size at birth
76. **Fetus starts hearing by what time in intrauterine life:**
    a. 14 weeks
    b. 20 weeks *[DNB 2011]*
    c. 32 weeks
    d. 33 weeks
77. **The commonest genetic defect of inner ear causing deafness is:** *[AIIMS 2010]*
    a. Michel aplasia
    b. Mondini aplasia
    c. Scheibe dysplasia
    d. Alexander aplasia
78. **Feature(s) of Scheibe's syndrome is/are:** *[PGI May 2016]*
    a. Semicircular canal fistula
    b. Abnormality in bony labyrinth
    c. Dysplasia of cochlea
    d. Middle ear anaomaly
79. **What are the boundaries of Trauttmann's triangle?**
    a. Bony labyrinth anteriorly *[PGI Nov 2012]*
    b. Bony labyrinth posteriorly
    c. Sigmoid sinus posteriorly
    d. Sigmoid sinus anteriorly
    e. Superior petrosal sinus superiorly
80. **Not correctly matched pair is:** *[TN 2007]*
    a. Utricle and sacule –Semicircular canal
    b. Oval window –Footplate of staps
    c. Aditus ad antrum –Macewen's triangle
    d. Scala vestibule –Reissner's membrane
81. **Which is the most common type of congenital ossicular dysfunction?** *[AIIMS Nov 2015]*
    a. Isolated stapes defect
    b. Stapes defect with fixation of footplate and lenticular process involvement
    c. Defective lenticular process of incus
    d. None of the above
82. **True about development of Cochlea:** *[PGI May 17]*
    a. Cochlea start developing from 3rd week of gestation
    b. Semicircular canals develop after cochlea
    c. Cochlea development completes by 20-week of gestation
    d. Cochlea development completes at 2-year of age

Explanations and References

1. **Ans. is b i.e. Modified apocrine glands** *Ref. IB Singh Histology 6/e, p 214-215*

   Sweat glands are of 2 types:

Eccrine / typical sweat glands	Apocrine / Atypical sweat glands
• Distributed all over the body • Innervated by cholinergic nerves • They open on the skin surface	• Confined to some parts of body • Innervated by adrenergic nerves • They open into the hair follicle • **Located on:** Axilla, Mons pubis, Circumanal area, Areola, Nipple Ceruminous glands of external acoustic meatus and ciliary glands of eyelids are modified apocrine glands.

2. **Ans. is a i.e Greater occipital nerve** *Ref. Dhingra 5/e, p 5; 6/e, p 4 Scott Brown 7/e, Vol. III p 3106–3107*
3. **Ans. is b i.e. Glossopharyngeal nerve**
4. **Ans. is d i.e. Tympanic branch of glossopharyngeal nerve**
5. **Ans. is d i.e. Auriculotemporal nerve** *Ref. Dhingra 6/e, p 4; 5/e, p 5; BDC 4/e, Vol. III p 254*

Nerve Supply of Ear

External ear Auricle/pinna	External acoustic meatus	Tympanic membrane	Middle ear Cavity	Muscles
Lateral surface	• **Anterior wall and roof** by auriculotemporal nerve	*Lateral surface*	Tympanic plexus formed by:	**Tensor tympani** by mandibular nerve:
1. Upper 1/3 by **auriculotemporal nerve** 2. Lower 2/3 by **greater auricular nerve**	• Posterior wall and floor by **auricular branch of vagus nerve (Arnold N)** • **Posterior wall of auditory canal also receives** innervations by facial nerve through auricular branch of vagus	1. Anteroinferior part by **auriculo-temporal nerve** 2. Posteriosuperior part by **auricular branch of vagus nerve**	1. Tympanic branch of **glossopharyngeal** nerve. 2. Superior and inferior Carotympanic nerves (Sympathetic plexus around internal carotid)	**Stapedius** by facial nerve
Medial surface 1. Upper 1/3 by **lesser occipital nerve** 2. Lower 2/3 by **greater auricular nerve** 3. Root of auricle by **auricular branch of vagus nerve (Arnold nerve)**		*Medial surface* • Tympanic branch of **glossopharyngeal nerve (Jacobson nerve)**		

 Note: Auriculotemporal nerve is a branch of mandibular nerve (branch of trigeminal nerve)

> **Remember**
>
> **Pinna is supplied mainly by 4 nerves:**
> Greater auricular N
> Lesser occipital nerve
> Auricular br of Vagus (Arnold N)
> Auriculotemporal N
> • The Glossopharyngeal nerve does not supply external ear and external acoustic meatus. It gives sensory supply to middle ear.

6. **Ans. is b i.e. Loosely on medial side** *Ref. Dhingra 6/e, p 2, 5/e, p3*
   Skin over the pinna is closely adherent to the perichondrium on the lateral surface while it is loosely attached on the medial surface.
7. **Ans. is a i.e. Fissure of Santorini** *Ref. Dhingra 6/e, p 2, 5/e, p4*
   - The cartilaginous part of external auditory canal—the **"fissures of Santorini"** through which infections can pass from external ear to parotid and vice versa.
   - The deficiency present in bony part is "Foramen of Huschke" seen in children up to the age of 4. Through this infections of ear can also pass to parotid gland.
8. **Ans. is a i.e. Pearly white** *Ref. Dhingra 5/e, p 61; Maqbool 11/e, p 33; Turner 10/e, p 240*
   Such a simple appearing question can also confuse us with its options. Most of the texts say that tympanic membrane is pearly gray in color.
   "Normal tympanic membrane is shiny and pearly gray in color." *Ref. Dhingra 6/e p55; 5/e, p 61*
   "Tympanic membrane appears as a grayish white translucent membrane." *Ref. Maqbool 11/e, p 33*
   "In health, the drum head presents a highly gray surface." *Ref. Turner 10/e, p 240*
   So, neither **option "a"** i.e. pearly white nor **option "b"** i.e. gray is fully correct but from ages the answer is taken as pearly white, so I am in also taking **option "a"** i.e. pearly white as the correct option.
9. **Ans. is b i.e. Peripheral** *Ref. Dhingra 5/e, p 18*
   "Movements of tympanic membrane are more at the periphery than at the center where malleus handle is attached."
10. **Ans. is b i.e. Shrapnell's membrane** *Ref. Dhingra 6/e, p 2, 5/e, p 4*
    Pars flaccida /Shrapnell's membrane
    Situated above the lateral process of malleus between the notch of Rivinus and the anterior and posterior malleal folds.

    > **Also know**
    > - **Reissner's membrane** – Separates scala media from scala vestibuli in the inner ear *(Dhingra 6/e p10, 5/e, p12)*
    > - **Basilar membrane** – Seen in scala media and supports the organ of Corti *(Dhingra 6/e, p10, 5/e p12)*
    > - **Secondary tympanic membrane** – Closes the scala tympani at the site of round window *(Dhingra 5/e, p11)*

11. **Ans. is e i.e. Tensor tympani muscle** *Ref. Dhingra 6/e, p 7-8, 5/e, p 6*
    The anterior wall has a thin plate of bone which separates the cavity from internal carotid. It also has two openings; the lower one for Eustachian tube and the upper one for the canal of tensor tympani muscle.
12. **Ans. is d i.e. 2 mm**
13. **Ans. is a i.e. 2 mm**
14. **Ans. is d i.e. Mesotympanum** *Ref. BDC Vol. III 4/e, p 258; Dhingra 6/e, p 450; p 129*
    "**When seen in coronal section, the cavity of the middle ear is biconcave, as the medial and lateral walls are closest to each other in the center.**"
    The distances separating them are:
    - Near the roof 6 mm → Epitympanum (Attic)
    - In the center 2 mm → Mesotympanum (between promontory and umbo)
    - Near the floor 4 mm → Hypotympanum
15. **Ans. is d i.e. 90 mm^2** *Ref. Maqbool 11/e, p 19; Dhingra 6/e, p 446; point 8, 5/e, p 457; point 8*
16. **Ans. is d i.e. 45 mm^2**
    - Area of tympanic membrane is 90 mm^2.
    - Effective area is 55 mm^2 (approximately 2/3rd of the total area).
    - Significance of large area of tympanic membrane – The area of tympanic is much larger than area of stapes footplate, which helps in converting sound of greater amplitude but lesser force to that of lesser amplitude and great force.
17. **Ans. is b i.e. 1.3:1** *Ref. Dhingra 6/e, p 14, 5/e, p 18*

    Lever-Action of Ossicles
    Handle of malleus is 1.3 times longer than process of the incus which constitutes for the lever-action.
    Area Ratio: The area ratio of tympanic membrane is 14:1
    Lever ratio = 1.3 : 1
    = Their product is 18:1, i.e. the pressure exerted at oval window.
    This helps in the transformer action of the middle ear (impedance matching mechanism), i.e. converting sound of greater amplitude and less force to that of lesser amplitude but greater force.
18. **Ans. is b i.e. Handle of malleus** *Ref. Logan and Turner 10/e, p 240*
    Cone of Light
    - Seen in anteroinferior quadrant of the tympanic membrane is actually the reflection of the light projected into the ear canal to examine it.

- This part reflects it because it is the only part of tympanic membrane that is approximately at right angles to the meatus.
- This difference in different parts of the tympanic membrane is due to the handle of malleus which pulls the tympanic membrane and causes it to tent inside.

Thus, the handle of malleus causes tenting and because of tenting the anteroinferior quadrant is at right angles to the meatus and thus reflects the light (leading to cone light).

19. **Ans. is a i.e. Lateral process of malleus** *Ref. Maqbool 11/e, p 33*

Otoscopy

- Helps to view the inside of external auditory canal.
- For proper view: Pinna is pulled
  - Backward and upward in adults.^{Q}
  - Downward and outward in infants.^{Q}
- The tympanic membrane appears as a grayish white, translucent membrane set obliquely inside the canal.

The important landmarks on membrane are:

Landmark	Importance
• The short process: (Lateral process of malleus)	It is the most important landmark as it is least obliterated in disease
• Anterior and posterior malleolar folds	Separates pars tensa from pars flaccida
• Handle of malleus: It is directed downward and backward; ending at the umbo	Cone of light radiates from it. Pars tensa is arbitrarily divided into four quadrants by a vertical line passing along the handle of malleus and horizontal line intersecting it at umbo

Since, short process/lateral process of malleus is least obliterated by diseases so I think it is the most reliable sign in otoscopy.

20. **Ans. is a i.e Auricultemporal nerve**
21. **Ans. is a, b and e i.e. Auriculotemporal nerve; Auricular branch of vagus nerve and Glossopharyngeal nerve**
22. **Ans. is c i.e. Healed perforation has three layers** *Ref. Dhingra 6/e, p 2, 3, 5/e, p 4,79*

    Let's see Each option one by one

    Option a – Cone of light is anteroinferior

    This is correct – *"A bright cone of light can be seen radiating from the tip of malleus to the periphery in the anteroinferior quadrant"*
    Ref. Dhingra 5/e, p 4

    Option b – Shrapnell's membrane is also called as pars flaccida. This is absolutely correct *Ref. Dhingra 6/e, p 2, 5/e, p 4*

    Option c – Healed perforation has 3 layers

    This is incorrect

    - When perforation of tympanic membrane heals, it heals in two layers and not in three layers. *Ref. Dhingra 6/e, p 55-56)*
    - "Healed chronic otitis media is the condition when tympanic membrane has healed (usually by two layers) is atrophic and easily retracted if there is negative pressure in the middle ear" *Ref. Dhingra 5/e p79*

    Option d – Anterior malleal fold is longer than posterior fold. Well! it is not given anywhere that anterior fold is longer than posterior, but we have to eliminate one option and that definitely is option 'c'.

23. **Ans. is b i.e. Glossopharyngeal nerve** *Ref. Dhingra 6/e, p 8, 5/e, p 10*
    - The nerve supply of middle ear is derived from tympanic plexus which lies over the promontory.
    - The inferior ganglion of the glossopharyngeal nerve gives off the tympanic nerve which enters the middle ear through the tympanic canaliculus and takes part in formation of the tympanic plexus on the medial wall of middle ear.
    - This distributes it fibers to the middle ear, and also to the auditory tube, aditus ad atrum mastoideum (aditus to mastoid antrum).

    Glossopharyngeal nerve → Tympanic nerve/tympanic plexus → Middle ear / Auditory tube / Mastoid antrum

Chapter 1: Anatomy of Ear

24. **Ans. is c i.e. Glossopharyngeal nerve** *Ref. Dhingra 6/e, p 228, 5/e, p 241*

    Note: Pain in the base of tongue is referred to ear via glossopharyngeal N.

25. **Ans. is d i.e. Vestibule of nose** *Ref. Read below*
   Lets analyze each option separately.
   - Pain from pharynx is referred to ear because it is supplied by vagus and Glossopharyngeal nerves (via pharyngeal plexus), both of which supply ear also. Hence any pain in pharynx can be referred to ear.
   - Tongue as explained previously can cause referred pain to ear
   - Pain from TM joint is also referred to ear because it is the Auriculotemporal N which also supplies the ear.
   - Pain from vestibule of nose is not referred to ear because it is supplied by maxillary nerve which does not supply the ear.
26. **Ans. is b i.e. Facial nerve** *Ref. Dhingra 6/e, p 5, 5/e, p 10*
27. **Ans. is b i.e. It is a protective reflex against loud sounds** *Ref. Dhingra 5/e, p 9-10, 30*
   Stapedius muscle helps to dampen very loud sound and thus prevents noise trauma to the inner ear. It is supplied by VII nerve *(facial nerve)*. Lesions of facial nerve lead to loss of stapedial reflex and hyperacusis or phonophobia, i.e. intolerance to loud sounds. For more details see chapter – physiology of hearing and assessment of hearing loss of the guide.

    Note: Stapedial reflex = Acoustic reflex

28. **Ans. is a i.e. Anterior part of V nerve**
   The tensor tympani is supplied by 1st anterior branch of mandibular (nerve of 1st arch).
29. **Ans. is b i.e. Vidian nerve** *Ref. Dhingra 5/e, p 154; Tuli 1/e, p 84*
   - Greater superficial petrosal nerve joins the deep petrosal nerve to form the nerve of pterygoid canal or also called as *Vidian nerve*.
   - Vidian nerve reaches pterygopalatine ganglion to supply the lacrimal gland and mucus glands of nose, palate and pharynx.
   Arnold nerve: It is a branch of cranial nerve X which carries fibers that supply sensory innervation to the ear canal
   Jacobson nerve: It is a branch of cranial nerve IX that runs along the promontory of the middle ear supplying sensation and parasympathetic fibers to the parotid gland.
30. **Ans. is d i.e. Footplates of stapes** *Ref. Dhingra 6/e, p 5 Fig. 1.8, 5/e, p Fig. 1.4*
   See text for explanation
31. **Ans. is a i.e. Epitympanum** *Ref. Dhingra 6/e p449; point 149, 5/e p461; point 90; Maqbool 11/e p13*
   Prussak's space is the space between pars flaccida, and the neck of malleus in the Epitympanum (see Fig. 1.4)
   - It is the M/C site for primary cholesteatoma.
32. **Ans. is c i.e. Roof of middle ear** *Ref. Dhingra 4/e, p 5, 5/e, p 5, 6/e, p 5*
   - The roof of middle ear is formed by a thin plate of bone called **tegmen tympani**. It separates tympanic cavity from middle cranial fossa.
   - Tegmen tympani is formed by squamous and petrous part of temporal bone.^Q
33. **Ans. is d i.e. All of the above** *Ref. Dhingra 6th/e, p 5, 5/e, p 6*

   Facial recess or Posterior sinus – It is a depression in the posterior wall of the middle ear.
   It is bounded by:
   Medially – Vertical part of VIII nerve
   Laterally – Chorda tympani
   Above – Fossa incudis
   Importance – This recess is important surgically, as direct access can be made through this into the middle ear without disturbing posterior canal wall. (Posterior tympanotomy approach)

34. **Ans. is a i.e. Facial nerve horizontal part**
35. **Ans. is b i.e. Medially it is bounded by chorda tympani and laterally by facial nerve**
   As discussed in the above question, all are boundaries of facial recess except horizontal part of VII nerve, so it cannot be damaged (Ans 34).
36. **Ans. is b i.e. Bulb of the internal jugular vein** *Ref. Dhingra 6/e, p 5, 5/e, p 6; Scott Brown 7/e, Vol. III p 3110*
   Read the text for explanation.

37. **Ans. is b i.e. Basal turn of cochlea** *Ref. Dhingra 6/e, p 5, 5/e, p 6*
Promontory is seen in the medial wall of middle ear and is due to basal coil of cochlea.

38. **Ans. is a i.e. Tendon of tensor tympani** *Ref. Dhingra 6/e, p 5, 5/e, p 6*
- Anterior to oval window lies a hook-like projection called the processus cochleariformis[Q] for tendon of tensor tympani[Q].
The **cochleariform process** marks the **level of the Genu** of the facial nerve which is an important landmark for surgery of the facial nerve.

39. **Ans. is b i.e. Mastoid antrum**

40. **Ans. is a i.e. Mastoid antrum**

41. **Ans. is a i.e. Suprameatal triangle**

42. **Ans. is c i.e. Promontory** *Ref. Dhingra 6/e, p 5, 5/e, p 7*
Mastoid antrum is marked externally on the surface by suprameatal (Macewen's) triangle.
For details on Macewen's triangle read the preceding text.

43. **Ans. is d i.e. Synovial joint** *Ref. Grays 38/e, p 485, 617 and 1275*

> **Joints of the ossicles are synovial joints**
>
> - The incudomalleolar joint is a saddle joint (variety of synovial joint)
> - Incudostapedial joint is a ball and socket joint (type of synovial joint)

44. **Ans. is a i.e. Anterior wall** *Ref. Dhingra 6/e, p 5, 5/e, p 6; Scott Brown 7/e, Vol. III p 3114 Fig. 225.13*
- The **tympanic end** of the eustachian tube is bony and is situated in the **anterior wall of middle ear**. The **pharyngeal end** of the tube is slit like and is situated in the lateral wall of the nasopharynx, 1–1.25 cm behind the posterior end of **inferior tubinate**.[Q]

45. **Ans. is c i.e. 36 mm**

46. **Ans. is d and e i.e. Inner 2/3rd is Cartilaginous; and Opens during swallowing**
Ref. Logan and Turner 10/e, p 227; Dhingra 6/e, p 57, 5/e, p 63

47. **Ans. is a, c and e i.e. Size is 3.7 cm; Opens during swallowing; and Tensor palati helps to open it**

48. **Ans. is c i.e. Tensor veli palatini** *Ref. Dhingra 6/e, p 57, 5/e, p 63*
- The Eustachian tube/auditory tube in the adult is 36 mm in length. **(Range 32–38 mm)** From its **tympanic** end, it runs downward forward and medially joining an angle of 45° with horizontal.
- In infants, the tube is shorter, wider and is more horizontal.
- It has two parts—a pharyngeal cartilaginous part which forms 2/3rd (24 mm) of its length (i.e. inner or medial part) and a tympanic bony part which forms remaining 1/3rd (outer or lateral part) (12 mm). This is just reverse of external auditory canal

> **Remember**
> Mnemonic **ICE 2/3**: **I**nner part **C**artilaginous in **E**ustachian tube and forms **2/3** part.

- The two parts meet at **isthmus** which is the **narrowest part of tube**.
- The fibers of origin of **tensor palati** muscles are attached to lateral wall of the tube. **Contraction of this muscle during swallowing, yawning and sneezing opens the tube** and this helps in maintaining equality of air pressure on both sides of tympanic membrane. Contraction of levator palati muscles which runs below the floor of cartilaginous part also helps in opening the tube.
- It is lined by pseudostratified columnar ciliated epithelium (cartilaginous part contains numerous mucus glands).

49. **Ans. is b i.e. Higher elastin content in adults** *Ref. Dhingra 6/e, p 57, 5/e, p 65*
The Developing Humans: Kleith 8/e, p 431-32, Langman's Embryology 10/e, p 317-323
"Eustachian tube serves to ventilate the middle ear and exchange nasopharyngeal air in the middle ear. In children, ET is relatively narrow. It is prone to obstruction[Q] when mucosa swell in response to infection or allergic challenge and it results in middle ear effusion"

Ref. Gray's 40/e, p 626

Chapter 1: Anatomy of Ear

Table: Differences between infant and adult Eustachian tube

	Infant	Adult
Length	13–18 mm birth (about half as long as in adult)	36 mm (31–38 mm)
Direction	More horizontal°, At birth it forms an angle of 10° with the horizontal at age 7 and later it is 45°	Forms an angle of 45° with the horizontal
Angulation at isthmus	No angulation	Angulation persent
Bony versus cartilaginous	Bony part is slightly longer than 1/3 of the total length of the tube and is relatively wider	Bony part 1/3; cartilaginous part 3/2/3
Tubal cartilaginous part	Flaccid. Retrograde reflux of nasopharyngeal Secretion can occur	Comparatively rigid, Remains closed and protects middle ear from reflux.
Density of elastin at the hinge	Less dense; tube does not efficiently close by recoil	Density of elastin more and helps to keep the tube closed by recoil of cartilage
Ostmann's pad of fat	Less in volume	Large and helps to keep the tube closed

50. **Ans. is b i.e. Petrous part temporal bone** *Ref. Turner 10/e, p 228; BDC 4/e, Vol. III p 264*
    Inner ear lies within the petrous part of temporal bone.
51. **Ans. is c i.e. Cartilaginous bone**
    Bony labyrinth is an example of cartilaginous bone.
52. **Ans. is a i.e. Connects internal ear with subarachnoid space** *Ref. Dhingra 6/e, p 9*
    Cochlear aqueduct connects scala tympani with the subarachnoid space. This is the reason why otitis media can lead to meningitis

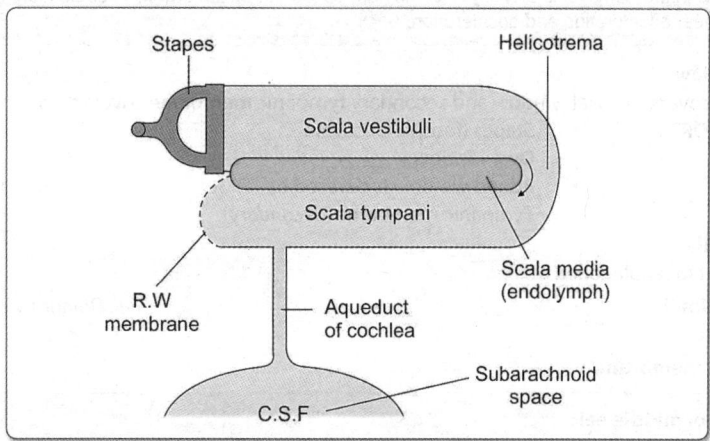

53. **Ans. is a i.e. Cochlear aqueduct**
    Ref. Grey 40/e p635; Dhingra 5/e p112; http://Journalsleww.com/Otology, Pediatric audiology: Diagnosis, Technology and Management by Jane R. Madell, Carol Flexer 2008, p28
    - As we know that cochlear aqueduct (Aqueduct of Cochlea) is a connection between scala tympani (containing perilymph) and the subarachnoid space (containing CSF). On occasions, particularly in young children, the Cochlear aqueduct is large and open.
    - Infection can spread to the inner ear from the infected CSF or vice versa, via the cochlear aqueduct resulting in severe profound hearing loss (meningitic labyrinthitis).
54. **Ans. is d i.e. Lymphatics** *Ref. ENT, PL Dhingra 5/e, p 84*
    Pathways of spread of infection from middle ear

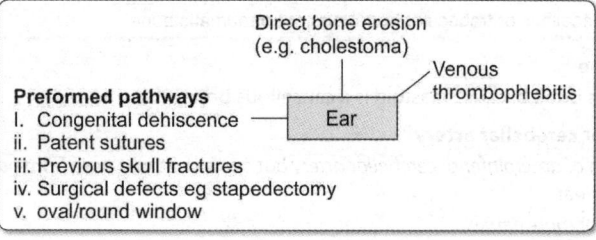

55. **Ans. is c i.e. Semicircular canal** *Ref. Dhingra 6/e, p 10 , 5/e, p 11*

Semicircular Canals
- There are 3 semicircular canals – the lateral, posterior and superior which lie in a plane of right angles to one another
- Each canal has an ampullated end which opens independently into the vestibule and a nonampullated end
- The non-ampullated ends of posterior and superior canals unite to form a common channel called the **crus commune**.

So the three canals open into the vestibule by 5 openings.

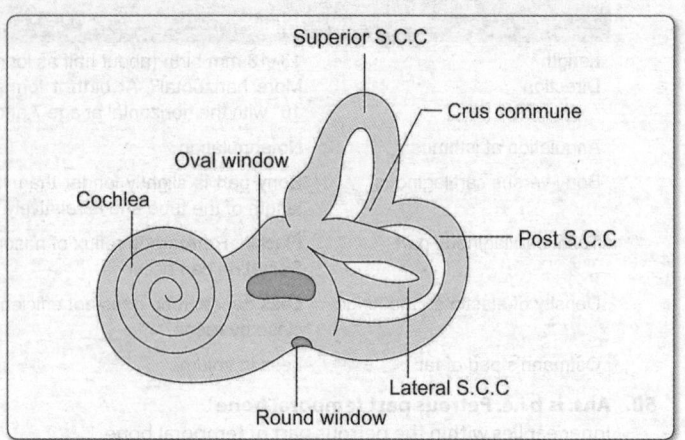

> **Also Remember**
> - Crista ampullaris: It is located in the ampullated end of the three semicircular duct and is a receptor which responds to angular acceleration.
> - Utricle and saccule lie in the bony vestibule, together they are called the otolith organ. Their sensory epithelium is called as Macula which responds to linear acceleration and deceleration.

56. **Ans. is b i.e. Oval window** *Ref. BDC 4/e, Vol. 3, p 258*
    - Footplate of stapes covers the oval window and secondary tympanic membrane covers the round window.
    - *Mnemonic:* **SORT:**
      - **S**tapes (footplate) covers
      - **O**val window
      - **R**ound window is covered by
      - **T**ympanic membrane *(Secondary)*

57. **Ans. is a i.e. Scala media**
    Read the preceding text for explanation.

58. **Ans. is c i.e. Scala vestibuli** *Ref. Dhingra 5/e, p 11 & 18, 6/e, 9, Tuli 1/e, p 18*
    Read the preceding text

59. **Ans. is d i.e. Tympanic membrane** *Ref. Dhingra 6/e, p 5*

> **Important Relations of middle ear:**
> - Roof – Thin plate called as tegmen tympani
> - Floor – Jugular bulb
> - Anterior wall – Internal carotid artery
> - Posterior wall – Lies close to mastoid air cells
> - Medial wall – Labyrinth
> - Lateral wall – Tympanic membrane

60. **Ans. is a, d and e i.e. Maxillary; Frontal and Ethmoidal** *Ref. BDC Handbook of General Anatomy 4/e, p 32*
    Pneumatic bones are one which contain large air spaces lined by epithelium, e.g.: maxilla, sphenoid, ethmoid, frontal, etc. They make the skull light in weight, help in resonance of voice, and act as air conditioning chambers for the inspired air.

    > **Remember**
    > Mastoid is a spongy bone (cancellous or trabecular bone) and not pneumatic bone.

61. **Ans. is b i.e. Cancellous bone**
    Spine of Henle is a cancellous bone because mastoid is a cancellous bone.

62. **Ans. is d i.e. Anteriorinterior cerebellar artery** *Ref. Dhingra 6/e, p 11; 5/e, p 13*
    Labyrinthine artery is a branch of anteroinferior cerebellar artery but can sometimes arise from basilar artery.
    It supplies whole of the inner ear.
    Kindly see the preceding text for more details.

Chapter 1: Anatomy of Ear

63. **Ans. is a i.e. Scala media to subdural space** *Ref. Dhingra 6/e, p9, 5/e, p 12*
    Endolymphatic duct – It is a part of membranous labyrinth (Scala media)
    - It is formed by union of saccule and utricle
    - It connects scala media to subdural space
    - Its terminal part is dilated to form the endolymphatic sac
    - Endolymphatic sac lies between the two layers of dura on the posterior surface of petrous bone
    - Surgical importance – Endolymphatic sac is exposed for drainage or shunt operation in Meniere's disease

    ALSO KNOW
    - Ductus reuniens – connects cochlear duct to saccule
    - Aqueduct of cochlea – connects scala tympani to subarachnoid space

64. **Ans. is b i.e. Scala media** *Ref. Dhingra 6/e, p 10, 5/e, p 12*
65. **Ans. is b i.e. secreted by striae vascularis**
66. **Ans. is c i.e. To maintain electric mileu of endolymph**
    Scala vestibuli and scala tympani are filled with perilymph, whereas scala media/membranous cochlea is filled with endolymph.
    Origin and absorption of inner ear fluids.

Origin	Absorption

• Perilymph (It resembles ECF and is rich in Na$^+$ ions)
  – From CSF
  – Direct blood filtrate from the vessels of spiral ligament
	• Through aqueduct of cochlea to subarachnoid space

• Endolymph (It resembles ICF and is rich in K$^+$ ions)
  – Secreted by stria vascularis or by the adjacent tissues of outer sulcus
  – Derived from perilymph across Reissner's membrane
	• Endolymphatic sac
	• Stria vascularis

67. **Ans. is c i.e. 1st and 2nd pharyngeal arch** *Ref. Dhingra 6/e, p 11, 5/e, p 14*

    Pinna
    - It develops from both 1st and 2nd brachial arches
    - Period of development starts from 4–6 weeks and adult configuration is attained by 20th week
    - From the
1st arch	2nd arch
• Tragus • Crus of helix • Adjacent helix	Rest of the pinna
    - The tissue condensations of the mesoderm of the 1st and 2nd brachial arch form 6 hillocks of His, which fuse to form the pinna

    Also know
    - External auditory canal – develops from the 1st brachial cleft/groove^Q
    - Tympanic membrane – develops from all 3 germ layers (Ecoderm, mesoderm and endoderm)^Q

68. **Ans. is a i.e. Tympanic membrane** *Ref. Dhingra 6/e, p 12, 5/e, p 14*
    See the text for explanation

69. **Ans. is a i.e. Bill's bar** *Ref. Tuli 2/e, p 6*
    See the text for explanation

70. **Ans. is b i.e. First pharyngeal pouch and c i.e. 2nd pharyngeal pouch** *Ref. IB Singh Embryology 8/e, p 110*
    The **Eustachian tube, tympanic cavity, attic, antrum and mastoid develops** from endoderm of tubotympanic recess which arises from **the first and partly from the second pharyngeal pouch**. Since this question is of PGI – we are taking both 1st and 2nd pouch as correct answer but if single option is to be marked, it will be 1st pharyngeal pouch.

71. **Ans. is d i.e. Maxillary antrum** *Ref Scotts Brown 7/e, Vol. III p 3118*
    "Mastoid antrum is an air-filled sinus within the petrous part of temporal bone. It communicates with the middle ear by way of the aditus and has mastoid air cells arising from its walls. The antrum, but not the air cells is well developed at birth"
    Ref. Scott Brown 7/e, Vol. 3 p 3118
    "Development of the mastoid air cell system does not occur until afterbirth, with about 90% of air cell formation being completed by the age of six with the remaining 10% taking place up to age of 18" *Ref. Scotts Brown 7/e, Vol. 3 p 3122*

> **Structures of adult size in newborn**
> - Tympanic cavity
> - Tympanic membrane
> - Ear ossicles
> - Mastoid antrum
> - Internal ear—cochlea, vestibule semicircular canals.

72. **Ans. is a i.e. Ear ossicles** *Ref. Pediatric Neuroradiology, edited by Paolo Tortori Donati 1/e, p 1362*

> - The ossicles begins to form during 4th week of gestation from the mesenchymal tissue.
> - They originate as cartilaginous models that reach adult size by the 18th week of gestation. Ossification of malleus begins at 15th week gestation, while stapes begins to ossify at 18th week of gestation. At birth, the ossicles are of nearly adult size.

ALSO KNOW

> **Structures which are not adult size at birth**
> - Mastoid process
> - External ear
> - Ext auditory canal
> - Tegmen tympani
> - Eustachian tube

73. **Ans. is a i.e. Improper fusion of auricular tubercles** *Ref. Dhingra 6/e, p 11, 49; 5/e, p 54*
    - Failure of fusion of 1st and 2nd arch leads to the formation of preauricular sinus.
    - It is commonly seen at the root of helix
    - It is a blind track lined by squamous epithelium
    - It may get repeatedly infected causing purulent discharge
    - Abscess may also form
    - Treatment is surgical excision of the track if the sinus gets repeatedly infected.

ALSO KNOW

> **Collaural Fistula** It is an anomaly of first brachial cleft:
> - Treatment is excision of tract

74. **Ans. is b i.e. 2nd arch** *Ref. Dhingra 6/e, p 12*
    Malleus and incus are derived from mesoderm of 1st arch. Stapes develops from second arch except its footplate and annular ligament which are derived from the otic capsule.

75. **Ans. is b, d and e i.e. Eustachian tubes open behind the level of inferior turbinates, growth of organ of Corti is complete by 5th month and ossicles are adult size at birth.** *Ref. Dhingra 6/e, p 12, 57*

    > Refer text for explanation.

76. **Ans. is b i.e. 20 weeks** *Ref. Dhingra 6/e, p 12*
    Formation of cochlea is complete by 20 weeks & a fetus can hear by 20 weeks.

77. **Ans. is c i.e. Scheibe dysplasia** *Ref. Dhingra 6/e, p 115*
    'Scheibe dysplasia. It is the most common inner ear anomaly.'

78. **Ans. is c i.e. Dysplasia of cochlea** *Ref. Dhingra 6/e, p 115*
    Scheibe dysplasia: It is the most common inner ear anomaly. Bony labyrinth is normal. Superior part of membranes labyrinth (utricle and semicircular ducts) is also normal. Dysplasia is seen in cochlea and saccula hence also called **cochleo saccular dysplasia**. It is inherited as Autosomal Recessive trait.

79. **Ans. is a, c and e, i.e. a. Bony labyrinth anteriorly; c. Sigmoid sinus posteriorly; e. Superior petrosal sinus superiorly**
    Ref. Dhingra 6/e, p 450 point 122
    "Trautmann's triangle is bounded by the bony labyrinth anteriorly, sigmoid sinus posteriorly and the dura or superior petrosal sinus superiorly" *Ref. PL Dhingra 6/, p 450 point 122*

Chapter 1: Anatomy of Ear

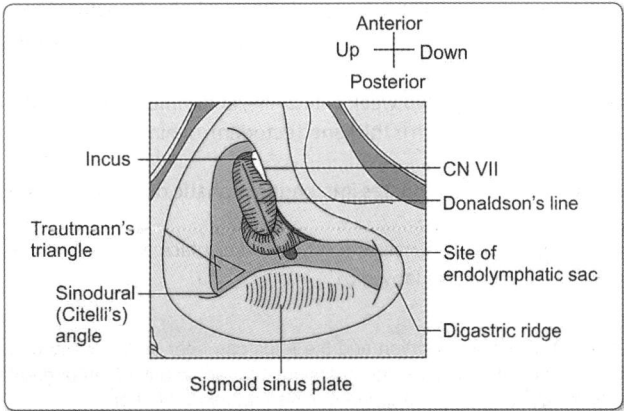

80. Ans. is c i.e. Aditus ad antrum – Macewen's triangle *Ref. Scott Brown 7/e, Vol. 3 p 3120*

Let's analyze each option separately.

Option a:
- Utricle and saccule – Semicircular canal
- Utricle lies bony vestibule and receives the five openings of the three semicircular ducts/semicircular canals
- Saccule also lies in the bony vestibule, anterior to the utricle and together both of these are called otolith organs.
- Hence, this pair is correct

Option b:
- Oval window – footplate of stapes
- Oval window is closed by the footplate of stapes.
- Hence, this pair is also related to each other

Option c:
- Aditus ad antrum – Macewen's triangle
- Aditus ad antrum is an opening through which the attic communicates with the antrum.
- Mastoid antrum and not the aditus is marked externally on by Macewen's triangle
- Hence, this pair is not correctly matched.

Option d:
- Scala vestibule – Reissner's membrane
- Reissner's membrane separates scala vestibule from scala media
- Hence, this pair is also related to each other.

81. Ans. is b. i.e. Stapes defect with fixation of footplate and lenticular process involvement.
Ref. Nelson Textbook of Pediatrics 20/e p3071

Congenital Stapes Anomalies with Normal Eardrum

 Point to Remember

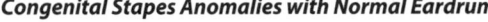

➢ Incus and stapes anomalies > isolated stapes anomalies > anomalies in all 3 ossicles.

- Among ossicular anomalies, stapes anomaly is the most common.
- Footplate fixation(Stapes super-structure) is the most common anomaly, mostly with involvement of long apophysis/ lenticular process of incus.
- Among stapes anomalies: Stapes footplate fixation only > Mobile stapes footplate with other anomalies > Stapes footplate fixation with other anomalies > Isolated stapes defect.

Teunissen and Cremers' Classification of Congenital Malformations of Ear

Class	Malformations	%
1	Ankylosis or isolated congenital fixation of the stapes(Footplate or Superstructure fixation)	30.6%
2	Stapes ankylosis associated with other malformations of ossicular chain like: deformities of incus and/or malleus, or aplasia of long apophysis of the incus or bone fixation of malleus and/or incus	38.1%
3	Congenital anomalies of the ossicular chain with mobile stapes footplate like: disruption of ossicular chain, epitympanic or tympanic fixation	21.6%
4	Congenital aplasia or severe dysplasia of oval and round windows	9.7%

82. **Ans. is a. i.e. Cochlea start developing from 3rd week of gestation** and **c i.e. Cochlea development completes by 20-week of gestation**
    (Ref: Essentials of ENT, Mohan Bansal, page 19-20)

    Inner Ear:
    - Development of inner ear, which begins in third week of fetal life, is complete by the 16th weak.
    - **Auditory placode:** The auditory placode, which is thickened ectoderm of hind brain, gets invaginated and forms auditory vesicle (otocyst).
    - **Auditory vesicle:** The auditory vesicle differentiates into endolymphatic duct and sac, utricle, semicircular ducts, saccule, and cochlea.
    - Development of pars superior (semicircular canals and utricle) takes place earlier than pars inferior (saccule and cochlea). The pars superior is phylogenetically older part of labyrinth.

    Note: The cochlea develops by 20 weeks of gestation and the fetus can hear in the womb of the mother. The great Indian epic of Mahabharata, which was written thousands of years ago, mentions that Abhimanyu (son of great warrior Arjun) while in his mother's womb heard conversation (regarding the art of battle ground) of his mother and father.

CHAPTER 2

Physiology of Ear and Hearing

PHYSIOLOGY OF HEARING

The pinna collects sound signal from the environment. Sound waves pass through external auditory canal (EAC) and vibrates the tympanic membrane (Fig. 2.1) Vibrations of the tympanic membrane are transmitted to the stapes footplate through the chain of ossicles. Vibrations of stapes footplate are transmitted to the oval window → scala vestibuli → helicotrema → scala tympani. This leads to movement of basilar membrane which has organ of Corti. Organ of Corti has hair cells. The hair cells of cochlea act as transducers and convert the mechanical energy into electrical impulses which travel along the auditory nerve.

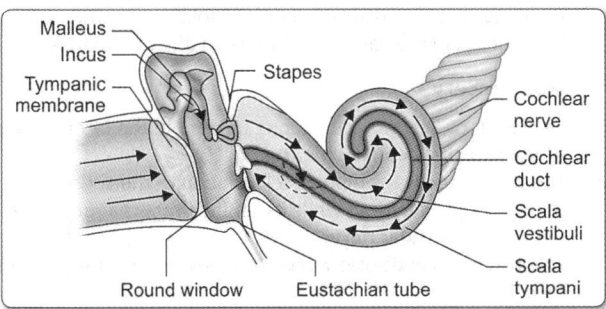

Fig. 2.1: Physiology of hearing. Arrows show sound waves
Source: Essentials of Mohan Bansal, Jaypee Brothers Medical Publishers Pvt. Ltd.

AUDITORY PATHWAY

Inner hair cells → **afferent nerves which from** cochlear nerve → spinal ganglion (present in Rosenthal canal) → Fibres exit through internal acoustic meatus → Dorsal cochlear nucleus + Ventral cochlear nucleus (Pons) → All fibres of from dorsal and ventral cochlear nucleus synapse to form trapezoid body → Fibres now pass to opposite and same side Superior olivary nucleus → Lateral lemniscus → Inferior colliculus → Medial geniculate body → Auditory cortex **(Brodmann area 41)**

Mnemonic

ECOLIMA
Mnemonic for auditory pathway
- E – **E**ighth nerve
- C – **C**ochlear nuclei
- O – **S**uperior **o**livary nucleus
- L – **L**ateral lemniscus
- I – **I**nferior colliculus
- M – **M**edial geniculate body
- A – **A**uditory cortex.

The auditory fibers travel via the ipsilateral and contralateral routes and have multiple decussation points of which 3 are main.

(a) At the trapezoid body (b) In the commissure between the 2 nuclei of lateral lemniscus (c) In the commissure connecting the two inferior colliculi. Thus, each ear is represented in both cerebral hemispheres.

> The area of cortex, concerned with hearing is situated in the transverse temporal gyrus (Brodmann's area 41).

 Point to Remember
> Higher auditory centres are concerned with sound localisation.

Organ of Corti

It is the sense organ of hearing and is situated on the basilar membrane in scala media.

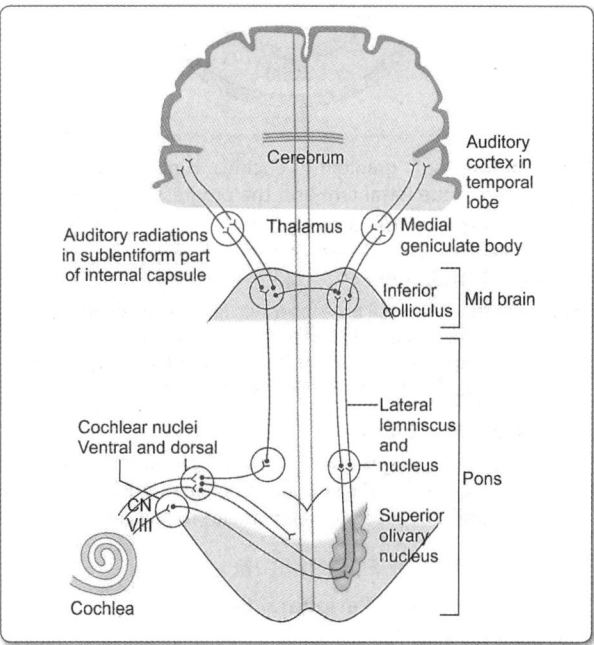

Fig. 2.2: Central auditory pathways
Courtesy: Textbook of Diseases of Ear, Nose and Throat, Mohan Bansal, Jaypee Brothers Medical Publishers Pvt. Ltd., p 21

Important components of the organ of Corti are:
1. Tunnel of Corti, which is formed by the inner and outer rods. It contains a fluid called *cortilymph*.
2. Cells:

Sensory hair cells		Supporting cells
Inner hair cell	**Outer hair cell**	• **P**illar cells
• Nerve supply primarily afferent	• Nerve supply mainly efferent	• **H**ensen's cells
• Resistant to noise and ototoxicity drugs	• Susceptible to ototoxic drugs and noise	• **D**eiter's cells (PHD).
• Function: To transmit auditory stimulus	• Function: To modulate the function of inner hair cells and to generate otoacoustic emission.	

Point to Remember
In cochlea-higher frequencies are represented in the basal turn and progressively lower tones towards the apex of cochlea.

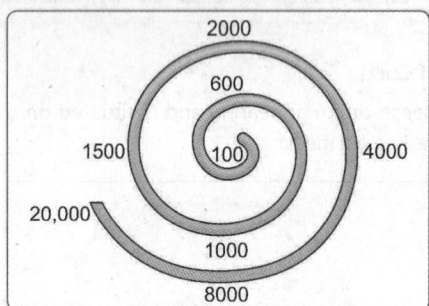

Fig. 2.3: Tonotopic gradient in cochlea. Higher frequency are represented in the basal turn and the progressively lower tones towards the apex of the cochlea

Clinical Correlation
With age, hair cells at base are lost more than at the apex. Significance—so hearing loss is more for higher frequencies than lower with aging. Whereas in Meniere's disease dilatation begins from the apex, hence lower frequencies affected first.

3. **Tectorial Membrane**
It consists of gelatinous matrix with delicate fibers. It overlies the organ of Corti. The shearing force between the hair cells and tectorial membrane produces the stimulus to hair cells.

■ PHYSIOLOGY OF EQUILIBRIUM
Vestibular System—Peripheral Receptors
They are two types:
- **Cristae:** They are located in the ampullated ends of the three semicircular canals.ᵩ These receptors respond to **angular**ᵩ **acceleration and deceleration.**ᵩ
- **Maculae:** They are located in otolith organs (i.e. utricle and saccule).ᵩ Macula of the utricle lies in its floor in a horizontal plane. Macula of saccule lies in its medial wall in a vertical plane. They sense position of head in response **to gravity and linear acceleration.**ᵩ

Structure of a Crista
It has 2 types of hair cells which project into a gelatinous matrix called as **'cupula'**.
- **Type 1:** Cells are flask-shaped with a single large cup-like nerve terminal, contains bipolar cells.
- **Type 2:** Cell are cylindrical with multiple nerve terminals. From the upper surface of each cell, project a single hair, **the kinocilium** and a number of other cilia.

Structure of Macula
A macula consists mainly of two parts:
a. A sensory neuroepithelium, made up of type I and type II cells, similar to those in the crista.
b. An otolithic membrane, which is made up of a gelatinous mass and on the top, the crystals of calcium carbonateᵩ called *otoliths* or *otoconia*.ᵩ The linear, gravitational and head tilt movements cause displacement of otolithic membrane and thus stimulate the hair cells which lie in different planes.

Vestibular Nerve
- Vestibular or Scarpa's ganglion is situated in the **lateral part of the internal acoustic meatus.**
- The distal process of bipolar cells innervate the sensory epithelium of the labyrinth while its central process aggregate to form the **vestibular nerve**.
- **The inferior vestibular nerve** supplies the maculae in the saccule.
- A branch of inferior vestibular nerve called as **singular nerve** supplies the hair cells of cristae in the posterior semicircular canal.
- The superior vestibular nerve supplies the hair cells of cristae in the superior and lateral semicircular canal and maculae in the utricle.

Central Vestibular Connections
- The fibers of vestibular nerve end in vestibular nuclei and some go to the cerebellum directly.

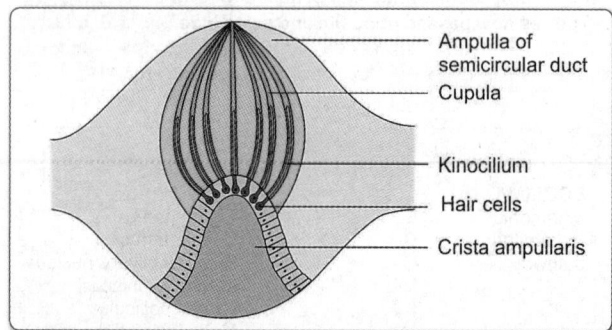

Fig. 2.4: Structure of ampullary end of semicircular duct

Chapter 2: Physiology of Ear and Hearing

NEW PATTERN QUESTIONS

Q N1. Impedance matching occurs due to:
a. Difference of surface are of tympanic membrane and foot plate
b. Semicircular canal fluid
c. Utricle and saccule
d. None of the above

Q N2. Primary receptor cells of hearing:
a. Supporting cell
b. Tectorial membrane
c. Tunnel of corti
d. Hair cells

Q N3. Otolith organs are concerned with function of:
a. Hearing
b. Rotatory nystagmus
c. Linear acceleration
d. Angular acceleration

Q N4. Appreciation of sound occurs in:
a. Organ of Corti
b. Basilar membrane
c. Cochlear nuclei
d. Transverse temporal gyrus

Q N5. Trapezoid body is associated with:
a. Auditory pathway
b. Visual pathway
c. Extrapyramidal system
d. Pyramidal system

Q N6. Best discrimination of pitch occurs at _____ frequency:
a. 100-400 Hz
b. 100-1000 Hz
c. 1000-4000 Hz
d. 20-20000 Hz

Q N7. Threshold of hearing in a young normal adult is:
a. 0 dB
b. 10 dB
c. 20 dB
d. 30 dB

Q N8. All of the following are true for organ of Corti *except*:
a. Hensen cell
b. Hensen node
c. Deiters cell
d. Pillar cell

Explanations and References to New Pattern Questions

N1. Ans. is a i.e. Difference of surface area of tympanic membrane and foot plate *Ref. Dhingra 6/e, p 14*
The area of tympanic membrane is much larger than area of stapes footplate, the average ratio being 21:1. As the effective vibratory area of tympanic membrane is only two thirds, the effectives area ratio is reducted to 14:1 which helps in impedance matching/transformer action.

N2. Ans. is d i.e. Hair cells *Ref. Dhingra 6/e, p 13*
Hair cells are important receptor cells of hearing and transduce sound energy into electrical energy.

N3. Ans. is c i.e. Linear acceleration *Ref. Dhingra 6/e, p 16*
Otolith organs (present in maculae) are concerned with linear acceleration, gravity and head tilt movements and they also help to maintain static equilibrium.

N4. Ans. is d i.e. Transverse temporal gyrus
Sound localisation and appreciation is a function of higher centres, i.e. auditory cortex located in transverse temporal gyrus (Broadman area 411)

N5. Ans. is a i.e. Auditory pathway *Ref. Dhingra 6/e, p 14, Fig. 2.2*
Trapezoid body is an integral part of auditory pathway.

N6. Ans. is c i.e. 1000-4000 Hz
Human ear can detect sounds ranging in frequency from 20 to 20,000 Hz. Pitch discrimination is best between 1000 to 3000 Hz.

N7. Ans. is a i.e. 0 dB
The hearing threshold is defined as the lowest threshold of acoustic pressure sensation possible to perceive by an organism. It is 0 dB for normal young person.

N8. Ans. is b i.e. Hensen node
See the text for explanation

Chapter 2: Physiology of Ear and Hearing

QUESTIONS

1. **Hair cell of organ of Corti supported by:** [PGI Nov 09]
   a. Onodi cells
   b. Deiter cell
   c. Hensen cell
   d. Bullar cell
   e. Heller cell

2. **The centre of stapedial reflex is:** [AIIMS Nov 2016]
   a. Superior olivary complex
   b. Medial geniculate body
   c. Superior colliculus
   d. Lateral lemniscus

3. **Stapedial reflex is mediated by:** [JIPMER 92]
   a. V and VII nerves
   b. V and VIII nerves
   c. VII and VI nerves
   d. VII and VIII nerves

4. **Perilymph contains:**
   a. Na^+
   b. K^+
   c. Mg^{++}
   d. Cl^-

5. **Endolymph in the inner ear:** [AIIMS May 09]
   a. Is a filtrate of blood serum
   b. Is secreted by stria vascularis
   c. Is secreted by basilar membrane
   d. Is secreted by hair cells

6. **All of the following are concerned with auditory pathway except:** [AI 95]
   a. Trapezoid body
   b. Medial geniculate body
   c. Genu of internal capsule
   d. Lateral lemniscus

7. **Higher auditory center determine:** [AIIMS May 09]
   a. Sound frequency
   b. Loudness
   c. Speech discrimination
   d. Sound localization

8. **Bones of middle ear are responsible for which of the following?** [MH 03]
   a. Amplification of sound intensity
   b. Reduction of sound intensity
   c. Protecting the inner ear
   d. Reduction of impedance to sound transmission

9. **Semicircular canals are stimulated by:** [MP 2000]
   a. Gravity
   b. Linear acceleration
   c. Rotation
   d. Sound

10. **Horizontal semicircular canal responds to:** [UP 2005]
    a. Horizontal acceleration
    b. Rotational acceleration
    c. Gravity
    d. Anteroposterior acceleration

11. **Angular movements are sensed by:** [JIPMER 93]
    a. Cochlea
    b. Saccule
    c. Utricle
    d. Semicircular canals

12. **All are correctly matched except:** [TN 07]
    a. Otolith—Made up of uric acid crystals
    b. Position of otolith—Changes with head position
    c. Otoliths—Stretch receptors
    d. Otolith organs—Stimulated by gravity and linear acceleration

13. **Singular nerve is a:** [AP 2007]
    a. Superior vestibular nerve supplying posterior semicircular canal
    b. Interior vestibular nerve supplying posterior semicircular canal
    c. Superior vestibular nerve supplying anterior semicircular canal
    d. Interior vestibular nerve supplying anterior semicircular canal

14. **Endocochlear potential is:** [AIIMS Nov 2016]
    a. +45 mv
    b. −45 mv
    c. +60 mv
    d. +85 mv

Section 1: Ear

Explanations and References

1. **Ans. is b, and c i.e. Deiter cell and Hensen cell**
   Ref. PL Dhingra 5/e, p 16; Logan and Turner 10/e, p 231, 32; Maqbool 11/e, p 18

   Supporting cells in organ of corti are PHD i.e. **P**illar cells, **H**ensen cells and **D**ecten cells.

   Hellar cells are ethmoidal air cell that extend along the medial roof of the maxillary sinus. They may exist as a discrete cells or the may open into maxillary sinus or infundibulum.^{Q}
   – Cummings Otolaryngology 4/e, p1162

   "Onodi cells are posterior and lateral extension of posterior ethmoidal cells. These cells can surround the optic nerve tract^Q and put the nerve at risk during surgery"
   – Cummings Otolaryngology 4/e, p1162

2. **Ans. is a i.e. Superior olivary complex**

3. **Ans. is d i.e. VII and VIII nerves** *Ref. Dhingra 5/e, p 30; 6/e, p 24, 25; Current Otolaryngology 2/e, p 602.*

Acoustic Reflex/Stapedial Reflex

It is based on the fact that a loud sound of 70–100 dB above the threshold of hearing of particular ear, causes bilateral contraction of the stapedial muscle which can be detected by tympanometry. This can be seen both in the stimulating ear (ipsilateral ear) and in the non stimulating ear (contralateral ear).

Note: I/L = Ipsilateral   C/L = Contralateral

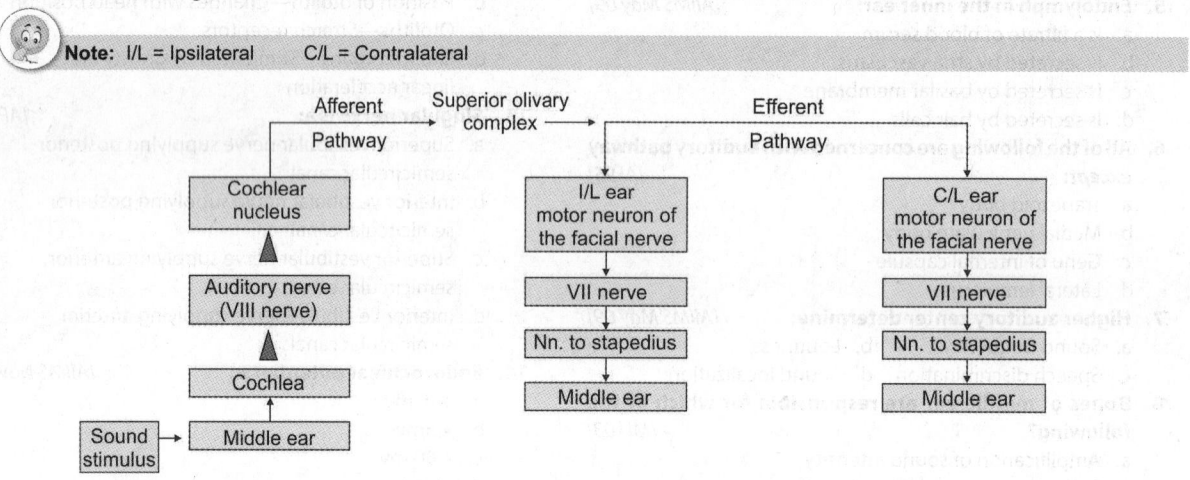

Also know

Stapedial reflex can be used
- As an objective method to test hearing in infants and young children
- To detect malingers – as stapedial reflex is positive in people faking hearing loss
- To detect

Lesion	Test response
a. Cochlear pathology	Presence of stapedial reflex at lower intensities, i.e. 40–60 dB means recruitment is positive, i.e. cochlear pathology
b. VIII nerve lesion	It eliminates both the contralateral and ipsilateral acoustic reflex when the affected ear is stimulated. But contralateral and ipsilateral reflex are present, if normal side is stimulated
c. VII nerve lesion	Absence of stapedial reflex in presence of normal hearing indicates lesion of VIIth nerve proximal to the nerve of stapedius
d. Brainstem lesion	If ipsilateral reflex is present but contralateral reflex is absent, it indicates lesion in the area of crossed pathway in the brainstem

4. **Ans. is a i.e. Na$^+$** *Ref. Dhingra 5/e, p12; 6/e, p 10; Current Otolaryngology 2/e, p 583*

Chapter 2: Physiology of Ear and Hearing

5. **Ans. is b. i.e. is secreted by stria vascularis** *Ref. Dhingra 5/e, p 12*

   There are 2 main fluids in the inner ear.

Perilymph	Endolymph
• Fills the space between the bony and membranous labyrinth, i.e. it is found in scala vestibuli and scala tympani	• Fills the entire membranous labyrinth, i.e. found in scala media
• Resembles extracellular fluid /CSF	• Resembles intracellular fluid
• Rich in Na$^+$ ions	• Rich in K$^+$ ions.

6. **Ans. is c i.e. Genu of internal capsule** *Ref. Guyton Physiology 11/e, p 657, 658; Dhingra 5/e, p 17; 6/e, p 13*

   Genu of internal capsule is not a part of auditory pathway. The fibres from medial geniculate body, pass through the posterior limb of internal capsule to reach auditory cortex.

7. **Ans. is d i.e. Sound localization** *Ref. Scott Brown 7/e, Vol. 3, p 3144; Ganong 23/e, p 213*

   Auditory cortex—main function is sound localization^Q
   "Sound localization is markedly disrupted by lesions of the auditory cortex." — *Ganong 23/e, p. 213*

8. **Ans. is d i.e. Reduction of impedance to sound transmission**
   Ref. Scott Brown 7/e, Vol. 3, p 3181; Dhingra 5/e, p 18; 6/e, p 14-16

   Broadly hearing mechanism can be divided into:
   - Mechanical conduction of sound (done by middle ear).
   - Transduction of mechanical energy into electrical impulses (done by sensory system of cochlea)
   - Conduction of electrical impulse to brain (i.e. auditory pathway)

   Detailed Information

   i. **Conduction of sound:**
      It is done mainly by middle ear and discussed earlier. Middle ear not just simply conducts the sound but converts sound of great amplitude and less force to that of less amplitude and greater force. This function of the middle ear is called as **impedance matching mechanism or the transformer action**.
      - This function of middle ear is accomplished by

   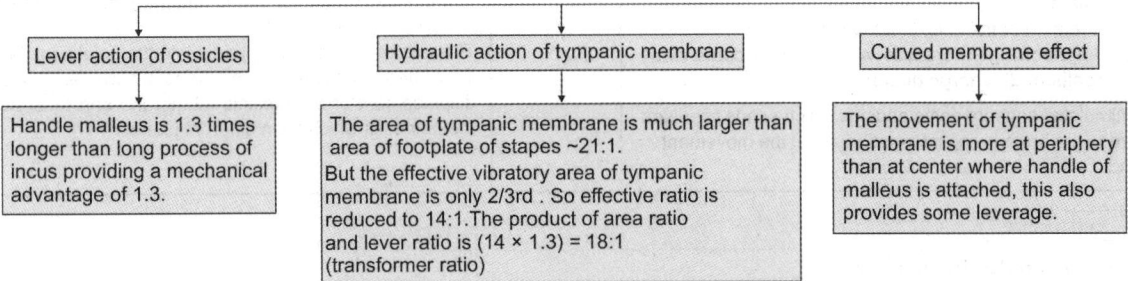

Lever action of ossicles	Hydraulic action of tympanic membrane	Curved membrane effect
Handle malleus is 1.3 times longer than long process of incus providing a mechanical advantage of 1.3.	The area of tympanic membrane is much larger than area of footplate of stapes ~21:1. But the effective vibratory area of tympanic membrane is only 2/3rd. So effective ratio is reduced to 14:1. The product of area ratio and lever ratio is (14 × 1.3) = 18:1 (transformer ratio)	The movement of tympanic membrane is more at periphery than at center where handle of malleus is attached, this also provides some leverage.

   ii. **Transduction of mechanical energy to electrical impulse:**
       Movements of the stapes footplate causes vibrations in scala vestibuli followed by scala tympani and is transmitted to the cochlear fluids which brings about movement of the basilar membrane. This sets up shearing force between the tectorial membrane and the hair cells. The distortion of hair cells gives rise to **electrical nerve impulse**.

       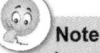**Note:**
       - A sound wave, depending on its frequency, reaches maximum amplitude on a particular place on the basilar membrane, and stimulates that segment (traveling wave theory of von Bekesy). Higher frequencies are represented in the basal turn of cochlea and the progressively lower one toward the apex.

   iii. **Neural pathway/Auditory pathway:**
       - Hair cells get innervation from bipolar cells of spiral ganglion. Central axons of these cells collect to form the cochlear nerve. (Cochlear division of VIII nerve) and end in the cochlear nuclei (the dorsal and ventral on each side of medulla).
       - From cochlear nuclei crossed and uncrossed fibers pass via superior olivary nucleus complex → nucleus of lateral lemniscus → inferior colliculus → Medial geniculate body and finally reach the auditory cortex of the temporal lobe.

9. **Ans. is c i.e. Rotation**
10. **Ans. is b i.e. Rotational acceleration**
11. **Ans. is d i.e. Semicircular canals** *Ref. Scott Brown 7/e, Vol. 3, p 3211; Dhingra 5/e, p 21; 6/e, p 17, 18*

Vestibular systems includes

	Semicircular canals/ducts	Peripheral receptors	Utricle and saccule (otolith organ)
	↓ Cristae		↓ Macula
	Located in the ampullated end of the semicircular ducts ↓		
	Angular/Rotational acceleration and deceleration	Respond to	Linear acceleration/gravity/change in position of head
	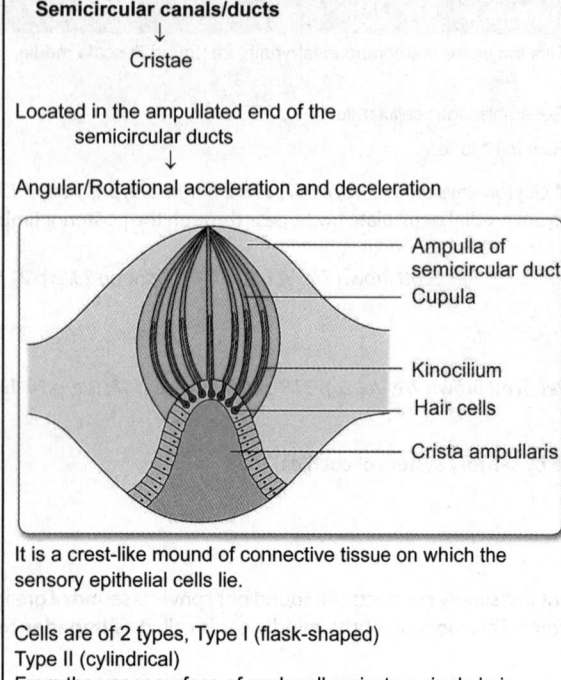	Structure	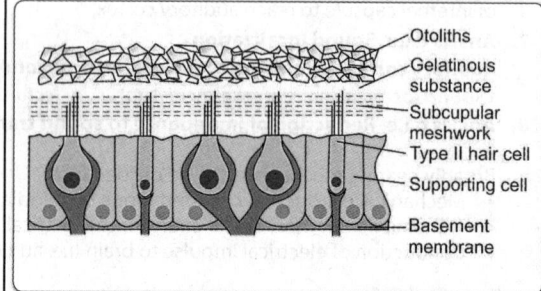
	It is a crest-like mound of connective tissue on which the sensory epithelial cells lie. Cells are of 2 types, Type I (flask-shaped) Type II (cylindrical) From the upper surface of each cell projects a single hair **k/a kinocilium.** When movement of the endolymph occurs toward **kinocilium discharge increases, and when it occurs away from kinocilium discharge decreases** This stimulates sensory nerve endings which sends impulses upward to the brain giving information about the movement of head		It has 2 parts: • A sensory neuroepithelium made of Type I and Type II cells (similar to crista) • **An otolithic membrane which is** made of gelatinous mass and on the top has crystals of calcium carbonate called as otolith.º The cilia of the hair cells project into the gelatinous layer The linear, gravitation and head tilt movement causes displacement of the otolithic membrane and thus stimulate the hair cells which lie in different planes.

Extra Edge

Between the utricle and saccule:
Utricle	Senses horizontal linear acceleration
Saccule	Senses vertical linear acceleration
Utricle + saccule	Both sense gravity and position of head in space

- **Coriolis effect**: It is a specific type of angular acceleration (i.e. sensed by semicircular ducts) that causes motion sickness in space craft due to rotation of earth.
- Type I cells correspond to the inner hair cells of organ of Corti and Type II cells correspond to the outer hair cells.

12. **Ans. is a i.e. Otolith—Made up of uric acid crystals** *Ref. Dhingra 5/e, p 20-22; 6/e, p 16; Tuli 1/e, p 23,24*

    As discussed in text: Otolith is made of crystals of calcium carbonate and not uric acid. Rest all options are correct.

13. **Ans. b i.e. Interior vestibular nerve supplying posterior semicircular canal** *Ref: 5/e, 7/e, Vol 3, p 3120*

    As discussed in the preceding text, singular nerve is a branch of inferior vestibular nerve which supplies the posterior semicircular canal.

14. **Ans. is d i.e. +85 mv** *Ref. Scott Brown Vol 3, pg 3136-3187*

    Endocochlear potential is +85 mv- it is the resting potential recorded from scala media. It is generated from stria vascularis by Na^+/K^+AT Pase pump. Endolymph has high K^+ concentration. It acts as a battery and helps in driving the current through the hair cells when they move after exposure to any sound stimulus.

Chapter 3

Hearing Loss

Deafness can be of two types **based on its etiology** viz:
- Congenital
- Acquired

Deafness can also be classified as conductive type/sensorineural type **based on the site of lesion** given as follows:

- **Conductive hearing loss:** Any disease process which interferes with the conduction of sound to reach cochlea causes conductive hearing loss. The lesion may **lie in the external ear tympanic membrane, middle ear or ossicles up to stapediovestibullar joint**.
- **Sensorineural hearing loss:** Results from **lesions of the cochlea, VIIIth nerve or central auditory pathways**. It may be present at birth (congenital) or start later in life (acquired).

Table 3.1: Congenital causes of conductive hearing loss
- Meatal atresia
- Fixation of stapes footplate
- Fixation of malleus head
- Ossicular discontinuity
- Congenital cholesteatoma

Table 3.2: Acquired causes of conductive hearing loss

External ear	Any obstruction in the ear canal, e.g. wax, foreign body, furuncle, acute inflammatory swelling, benign or malignant tumor or atresia of canal.
Middle ear	• Perforation of tympanic membrane, traumatic or infective • Fluid in the middle ear, e.g. acute otitis media, serous otitis media ear, e.g. benign or malignant tumor • Mass in middle ear, e.g. benign or malignant tumor • Disruption of ossicles, e.g. trauma to ossicular chain, chronic suppurative otitis media, cholesteatoma • Fixation of ossicles, e.g. otosclerosis, tympanosclerosis, adhesive otitis media • Eustachian tube blockage, e.g. retracted tympanic membrane, serous otitis media

Sensorineural Hearing Loss

Congenital Causes

Etiology
It is present at birth and is the result of anomalies of the inner ear or damage to the hearing apparatus by prenatal or perinatal factors.

Acquired Causes
- Infections of labyrinth—viral, bacterial or spirochaetal
- Trauma to labyrinth or VIII nerve, e.g. fractures of temporal bone or concussion of the labyrinth or the ear surgery
- Noise-induced hearing loss
- Ototoxic drugs
- Presbycusis
- Meniere's disease
- Acoustic neuroma
- Sudden hearing loss
- Familial progressive SNHL
- Systemic disorders, e.g. diabetes, hypothyroidism, kidney disease, autoimmune disorders, multiple sclerosis, blood dyscrasias.

NEW PATTERN QUESTIONS

Q N1. Conductive hearing loss occurs in:
a. Travelling in an aeroplane
b. Trauma to labyrinth
c. Stapes abnormal at oval window
d. High noise

Q N2. All are causes of sensorineural deafness *except*:
a. Old age
b. Cochlear otosclerosis
c. Loud sound
d. Rupture of tympanic membrane

Q N3. Resonance of tympanic membrane is:
a. 800 Hz
b. 800-1600 Hz
c. 3000 Hz
d. None of the above

Q N4. TM and ear ossicles efficiently transmit sound of frequency:
a. 3000-5000 Hz   b. 300-500 Hz
c. 500-2000 Hz   d. 5000-20000 Hz

Q N5. Virus causing acute SNHL:
a. Corona virus   b. Mumps virus
c. Adenovirus   d. Rotavirus

Table 3.3: WHO Classification of hearing loss

Grade of Impairment*	Corresponding Audiometric ISO Value**	Performance	Recommendations
0-No impairment	25 dB or better (better ear)	No or very slight hearing problems, able to hear whispers.	
1-Slight impairment	26-40 dB (better ear)	Able to hear and repeat word spoken in normal voice at 1 meter	Counselling hearing aids may be needed
2-Moderate impairment	41-60 dB (better ear)	Able to hear repeat words spoken in raised voice at 1 meter	Hearing aids usually recommended
3-Severe impairment	60-80 dB (better ear)	Able to hear words when shouted into better wear	Hearing aids needed. If no hearing aids available, lip-reading and signing should be taught
4-Profound impairment including deafness	81 dB or greater (better ear)	Unable to hear and understand even a shouted voice	Hearing aids may help understanding words. Additional rehabilitation needed. Lip-reading and sometimes signing essentials.

*Grades 2,3, and 4 are classified as disabling hearing impairment (for children, it starts at 31 dB)
**The audiometric ISO values are averages of values at 500, 1000, 2000, 4000 Hz

Table 3.4: Average Hearing Loss seen in Different Lesions of Conductive Apparatus

Condition	Average hearing loss
Closure of oval window	60 dB
Ossicular interruption with intact TM	54 dB
Ossicular interruption with perforation	38 dB
Complete obstruction of ear canal	30 dB
TM perforation	10-40 dB
Occlusion of EAC	30-40 dB

Common Terminology

- **Hearing loss:** It is an impairment of hearing, and its severity may vary from mild to severe or profound.
- **Deafness:** It is used when there is little or no hearing at all.

WHO Definition of 'Deaf'

- The term deaf should be applied only to those individual whose hearing impairment is so severe that they are unable to benefit from any type of amplification.
- **According to the Ministry of social welfare, Govt. of India:**
  - **Deaf** are those in whom the sense of hearing is non functional for ordinary purposes of life.
  - They do not, hear/understand sounds at all even with amplified speech.
  - The cases included in this category are those who have either loss more than 90 dB hearing loss in better ear or total hearing loss in both ears.
- **Partially hearing** are those falling under any one of the following categories:

Category	Hearing
Mild impairment	Between 30 and 45 dB in better ear
Serious impairment	Between 45-60 dB in better ear
Severe impairment	Between 60-90 dB in better ear

Table 3.5: WHO classification of degree of hearing loss and Difficulty in Hearing Speech
Ref. Essential of Mohan Bansal, p 66

Hearing threshold in better ear (average of 500, 1000, 2000 Hz)	Degree of impairment (WHO classification)	Ability to understand speech
0-25	Not significant	Can hear faint speech
26-40	Mild	Difficulty with faint speech
41-55	Moderate	Frequent difficulty with normal speech
56-70	Moderately severe	Difficulty even with loud speech
71-90	Severe	Can understand only shouted or amplified speech
Above 91	Profound	Cannot understand even amplified speech

Hearing loss causes as impairment, which leads to disability and handicap.

The simplest way to find it out in a person is to do **pure tone audiometry test** of both ears and calculate the average of 3 speech frequencies: 500, 1000 and 2000 Hz.

Suppose the result is:

Right ear = 55 dB

Left ear = 35 dB

As per WHO, classification, there is no disability upto 25 dB, so it will be Right ear = 55-25 = 30 dB

Left ear = 35-25 = 10 dB

Now multiply it with 1.5:

Right ear 30 × 1.5 = 45%

Left ear = 10 × 1.5 = 15%

Percentage of handicap of the person will be:

> Better hearing ear × 5 + percentage of bad ear divided by 6.
> So, in above case = 15 × 5 + 45 ÷ 6 = 20%

Thus total disability is 20%.

Chapter 3: Hearing Loss

NEW PATTERN QUESTIONS

Q N6. Threshold for moderate hearing loss is:
- a. 26-40 dB
- b. 0-25 dB
- c. 41-55 dB
- d. More than 91 dB

Q N7. A person has frequent difficulty in understanding normal speech. The approximate hearing loss in the person is:
- a. 26-40 dB
- b. 41-55 dB
- c. 56-70 dB
- d. 71-90 dB

ALSO KNOW

Another important thing to remember in this chapter is that SNHL can be of cochlear or retrocochlear variety

Table 3.6: Differences between Cochlear and Retrocochlear SNHL

Cochlear SNHL	Retrocochlear SNHL
Hair cells are damaged mainly	Lesion is of VIII nerve or its central connections
Recruitment is present	Recruitment absent
NO significant tone decay	Tone decay is significant
SISI is positive	SISI is negative
Bekesy shows no gap between I and C tracings (Type II)	Bekesy shows wide gap between I and C tracings (type III)
Speech discrimination is not highly impaired (SDS) is low) and roll over phenomenon is not present	Speech discrimination is highly impaired (SDS very poor) and roll over phenomenon is present
Subjective feeling of diplacusis, hyperacusis or fullness in the ear	No such sensation or feeling

Contd...

NEW PATTERN QUESTIONS

Q N8. All of the following are true regarding retrocochlear SNHL *except*:
- a. Recruitment present
- b. Tone decay significant
- c. Speech discrimination is highly impaired
- d. Rollover phenomenon present

Q N9. Impairment of hearing due to noise starts at:
- a. 1000 Hz
- b. 2000 Hz
- c. 3000 Hz
- d. 4000 Hz

Q N10. Delayed speech in a 5-year-old child with normal motor and adaptive development, is most likely due to:
- a. Mental retardation
- b. Cerebral palsy
- c. Kernicterus
- d. Deafness

Explanations and References to New Pattern Questions

N1. Ans. is c i.e. Stapes abnormal at oval window *Ref. Dhingra 6/e, p 29, 30*
As discussed in previous chapter.
Noise induced hearing loss and trauma to labyrinth leads to SNHL.
Travelling in air plane, leads to ear ache and temporary conductive hearing loss.
Stapes abnormal at oval window will lead to conductive hearing loss.

N2. Ans. is d i.e. Rupture of tympanic membrane *Ref. Dhingra 6/e, p 29, 30*
Read the text for explanation.

N3. Ans. is b i.e. 800-1600 Hz

N4. Ans. is c i.e. 500-2000 Hz
Friends these are 2 facts which you need to memorize.

N5. Ans. is b i.e. Mumps virus
SNHL can be due to viral infections: mumps, measles. It is also due to syphilis. SNHL can also be due to drugs like
- Aminoglycoside - M/c cause - e.g. tobramycin
- Loop diuretics, e.g. furosemide
- Antimetabolites, e.g. methotrexate
- Salicylates, e.g. aspirin

N6. Ans. is c i.e. 41-55 dB *Ref. Dhingra 6/e, p 38*
See Table in preceeding text for explanation.

N7. Ans. is b i.e. 41-55 dB *Ref. Essentials of ENT, Mohan Bansal, p 66.*
If a person faces frequent difficulty in understanding normal speech the approximate hearing loss is 41-55 dB.
See Table 3.5 in the text.

N8. Ans. is a i.e. Recruitment present
Recruitment is present in cochlear variety of SNHL not retrocochlear. See Table 3.6 for details.

N9. Ans. is d i.e. 4000 Hz
Noise trauma can be divided into two types:
1. *Acoustic trauma* — It is caused by a single brief exposure to very intense sound which may damage outer hair cells, disrupt Organ of Corti and rupture the Reissner membrane. A severe blast may rupture tympanic membrane and disrupt ossicular chain.
2. *Noise-induced hearing loss*—It is caused by chronic exposure to less intense sound.
   a. **Temporary threshold shift**—The hearing is impaired immediately after exposure to noise but recovers after an interval of a few minutes to a few hours.
   b. **Permanent threshold shift**—Hearing impairment is permanent.
      A noise of 90 dB, 8 hours a day for 5 days per week is the maximum safe limit.
      The audiogram of NIHL shows a typical notch at 4000 Hz. NIHL causes damage to hair cells, starting in the basal turn of cochlea. Outer hair cells are affected before the inner hair cells.

N10. Ans. is d i.e. Deafness

Chapter 3: Hearing Loss

QUESTIONS

1. According to WHO definition of hearing loss, what is the value to clarify as profound hearing loss: [AIIMS Nov 2016]
   a. 61-71dB
   b. >81 dB
   c. >91 dB
   d. >101 dB
2. According to WHO classification, for severe degree of impairment of hearing is at: [TN 2004]
   a. 26-40 dB
   b. 41-60 dB
   c. 61-80 dB
   d. > 81 dB
3. At which level sound is painful: [Jharkhand 2004]
   a. 100-120 dB
   b. 80-85 dB
   c. 60-65 dB
   d. 20-25 dB
4. Ear sensitive to: [Jharkhand 2003]
   a. 500-3500 Hz
   b. 1000-3000 Hz
   c. 300-5000 Hz
   d. 5000-8000 Hz
5. After rupture of tympanic membrane the hearing loss is: [PGI June 99]
   a. 10-40 dB
   b. 5-15 dB
   c. 20 dB
   d. 300 dB
6. Which of the following conditions causes maximum hearing loss?
   a. Ossicular disruption with intact tympanic membrane
   b. Disruption of malleus and incus with intact tympanic membrane
   c. Partial fixation of the stapes footplate
   d. Otitis media with effusion
7. In a patient audiogram shows hearing loss of 54 dB. Most probably it is due to:
   a. Ossicular disruption with intact TM
   b. Ossicular disruption with TM perforation
   c. Complete fixation of stapes footplate
   d. Otitis media with effusion
8. Commonest cause of hearing loss in children is: [AIIMS Dec. 95]
   a. CSOM
   b. ASOM
   c. Acoustic - neuroma
   d. Chronic secretory otitis media
9. Commonest cause of hearing loss in children is: [CUPGEE 95]
   a. Microtia with atresia of external auditory meatus
   b. Trauma
   c. Otitis media with effusion
   d. Bony canal
10. Commonest cause of deafness is: [AP 97]
    a. Trauma
    b. Wax
    c. Acute mastoiditis
    d. Meniere's disease
11. All of the following can cause hearing loss except: [UP 2001]
    a. Measles
    b. Mumps
    c. Chickenpox
    d. Rubella
12. Hyperacusis is defined is: [PGI Dec. 97]
    a. Hearing of only loud sound
    b. Normal sounds heard as loud and painful
    c. Completely deaf
    d. Ability to hear in noisy surroundings
13. Conductive hearing loss is seen in all of the following except: [AI 12]
    a. Otosclerosis
    b. Otitis media with effusion
    c. Endolymphatic hydrops
    d. Suppurative otitis media
14. A patient has bilateral conductive deafness, tinnitus with positive family history. The diagnosis is: [AIIMS Nov. 93]
    a. Otospongiosis
    b. Tympanosclerosis
    c. Meniere's disease
    d. B/L otitis media
15. Conductive deafness occurs in: [UP 07]
    a. Travelling in aeroplane or ship
    b. Trauma to labyrinth
    c. Stapes abnormal at oval window
    d. High noise
16. A 55-year-old female presents with tinnitus, dizziness and h/o progressive deafness. Differential diagnosis includes all except: [AIIMS Nov. 01]
    a. Acoustic neuroma
    b. Endolymphatic hydrops
    c. Meningioma
    d. Histiocytosis-X
17. True about conductive hearing loss: [PGI May'15]
    a. Presbycusis
    b. Cholesteatoma
    c. Acoustic neuroma
    d. Perforation of tympanic membrane
    e. Serous otitis media
18. All are ototoxic drugs except: [RJ 2000]
    a. Streptomycin
    b. Quinine
    c. Diuretics
    d. Propranolol
19. Post head injury, the patient had conductive deafness and on examination, tympanic membrane was normal and mobile. Likely diagnosis is:
    a. Distortion of ossicular chain
    b. Hemotympanum
    c. EAC sclerosis
    d. Otosclerosis
20. All are causes of sensorineural deafness except: [2001]
    a. Old age
    b. Cochlear otosclerosis

c. Loud sound
d. Rupture of tympanic membrane

21. **Virus causing acute onset sensorineural deafness:**
    [PGI Dec. 04]
    a. Corona virus
    b. Rubella measles
    c. Mumps
    d. Adenovirus
    e. Rota virus

22. **Sensorineural deafness may be feature of all, *except*:**
    a. Nail-patella syndrome
    b. Distal renal tubular acidosis
    c. Bartter syndrome
    d. Alport syndrome

23. **Sensorineural deafness is seen in:** [PGI June 02]
    a. Alport's syndrome
    b. Pendred's syndrome
    c. Treacher Collins syndrome
    d. Crouzon's disease
    e. Michel's aplasia

24. **Fluctuating recurring variable sensorineural deafness is seen in:** [APPGI 06]
    a. Serous otitis media
    b. Hebimotympanum
    c. Perilabyrinthine fistula
    d. Labirinthine concussion

25. **True about presbycusis:** [PGI May 2014]
    a. Degeneration of outer Hair cell of organ of Corti in sensory type
    b. High frequency is affected first in sensory type
    c. Can be treated with hearing aids
    d. Usually unilateral hearing loss occurs

26. **Prolonged exposure to noise levels greater than the following can impair hearing permanently:** [Karnat 96]
    a. 40 decibels
    b. 85 decibels
    c. 100 decibels
    d. 140 decibels

27. **A steel factory worker is suffering from noise induced hearing loss. Which of the following is most likely to be affected?** [AIIMS Nov 2017]
    a. Inner hair cells
    b. Macula
    c. Crista ampullaris
    d. Saccule

Chapter 3: Hearing Loss

Explanations and References

1. **Ans. is b i.e >81dB**

2. **Ans. is c i.e. 61-80 dB** *Ref. Dhingra, 6/e, p 38 (Table 5.9)*

   WHO Classification of hearing loss

Grade of Impairment	Corresponding Audiometric ISO Value	Performance
0-No impairment	25 dB or better (better ear)	No or very slight hearing problems, able to hear whispers.
1-Slight impairment	26-40 dB (better ear)	Able to hear and repeat word spoken in normal voice at 1 meter
2-Moderate impairment	41-60 dB (better ear)	Able to hear repeat words spoken in raised voice at 1 meter
3-Severe impairment	60-80 dB (better ear)	Able to hear words when shouted into better wear
4-Profound impairment including deafness	81 dB or greater (better ear)	Unable to hear and understand even a shouted voice

3. **Ans. is a i.e. 100-120 dB** *Ref. Dhingra, 6/e, p 19*

   Intensity

Whisper	30 dB
Normal conversation	60 dB
Shout	90 dB
Discomfort of ear	120 dB
Pain in ear	130 dB

   Since the highest intensity given in the question is 100-120 dB, hence we are taking it as our correct answer.

4. **Ans. is a i.e. 500-3500 HZ** *Ref. Guyton 11/e, p 657*

   Ear best perceives sound in the frequency of 500-5000 HZ.

5. **Ans. is a i.e. 10-40 dB**

6. **Ans. is a i.e. Ossicular disruption with intact tympanic membrane** *Ref. Dhingra, 6/e, p 29*

7. **Ans. is a i.e. Ossicular disruption with intact TM**

   Average hearing loss seen in different lesions of conductive apparatus:

Condition	Average hearing loss
Closure of oval window	60 dB
Ossicular interruption with intact TM	54 dB
Ossicular interruption with perforation	38 dB
Complete obstruction of ear canal	30 dB
TM perforation	10-40 dB

   Ans. 5 and 7 are straight forward:

   Coming on to **Ans 6:**
   - Hearing loss in otitis media with effusion:
     - Mean = 20-30 dB. ... *Internet search*
   - Hearing loss in ossicular fixation:
     - Malleus fixation = 10-25 dB – *Dhingra, 6th/ed, p 29*
     - Stapes fixation = upto 50 dB ... *Internet search*

   So it is clear - ossicular disruption with intact tympanic membrane causes maximum hearing loss. **Option 'b'** (of Ans 5) can give rise to some confusion but option b is disruption of malleus and incus *(with stapes intact)* whereas in **option 'a' of ans 5,** malleus, incus and stapes are all disrupted which definitely will lead to more hearing loss.

8. **Ans. is d i.e. Chronic secretory otitis media** *Ref. Ghai 6/e, p 334; Ghai 7/e, p 333; Current Otolaryngology 2/e, p 658*
9. **Ans. is c i.e. Otitis media with effusion**

    "The most common cause of conductive deafness in children is otitis media with effusion, which is typically of mild to moderate severity." ... *Ref. Ghai 6/e, p 334; Ghai 7/e, p 333*

    Otitis media with effusion/glue ear/chronic serous or secretory otitis media -

    "It is the most common cause of hearing loss in children in the developed world and has peak incidence at 2 and 5 years of age" *Ref. Current otolaryngology 2/e, p 658*

    For more details on Secretory otitis media or Otitis media with effusion, see Chapter: Diseases of middle ear in this book.
10. **Ans. is b i.e. Wax** *Ref. Dhingra 3/e, p 68*

    Searching.
11. **Ans. is c i.e. Chickenpox** *Ref. OP Ghai 7/e, p 333*

    "The most common postnatal cause of acquired SNHL is meningitis, while the most common prenatal cause is intrauterine infection (eg TORCH infections, syphilis, mumps, measles)". *Ref. OP Ghai 7/e, p 333*
12. **Ans. is b i.e. Normal sounds heard as loud and painful** *Ref. Turner 10/, p 237; Maqbool 11/e, p 31*

Hyperacusis	Sensation of discomfort or pain on exposure to normal sounds. Seen in injury to nerve to stapedius and in case of congenital syphilis (Hennebert sign).
Diplacusis	Condition where same tone is heard as notes of different pitch in either ear.
Paracusis Willisii	Condition where patient hears a sound better in presence of background noise. Seen in case of otosclerosis.

Also Know

Tullio phenomenon condition where the subject gets attacks of vertigo/dizziness by loud sounds. It occurs in patients with labyrinthine fistula or those who have undergone fenestration operation.

13. **Ans. c i.e. Endolymphatic hydrops** *Ref. 6/e, p 30 (Tables 5.1 and 5.2)*

    Endolymphatic hydrops, i.e. Menier's disease leads to SNHL and not conductive hearing loss. All the rest can lead to conductive hearing loss.
14. **Ans. is a i.e. Otospongiosis** *Ref. Dhingra 6/e, p 30, 87*

    Conductive deafness means the disease process leading to deafness is limited to external ear tympanic membrane, middle ear including the footplate of stapes.

    Bilateral conductive deafness rules out Meniere's disease (as it presents with SNHL).

    Amongst the remaining three options, positive family history is seen mainly in case of otosclerosis (Otospongiosis), so it is our answer.
15. **Ans. is a, c and d i.e. Travelling in aeroplane or ship; Stapes abnormal at oval window; and High noise**

    Ref. Dhingra, 6/e, p 66, 30, 33, 35

    Otitic Barotrauma or **travelling in aeroplane/ship** leads to conductive hearing loss but sensorineural type of loss may also be seen. *Ref. Dhingra 6/e, p 66*
    - Trauma to labyrinth leads to SNHL. *Ref. Dhingra 6/e, p 33*
    - Abnormal attachment of stapes at oval window *(otosclerosis)* will lead to conductive deafness. *Ref. Dhingra 6/e, p 30*

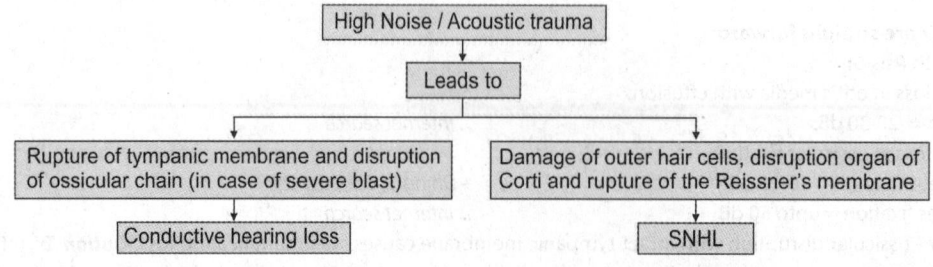

Ref. Dhingra, 6/e, p 34

Chapter 3: Hearing Loss

16. **Ans. is d i.e. Histiocytosis-X** *Ref. Dhingra 5th/ed, p 38; Harrison 17th/ed, p 2603*

    Acoustic neuroma and endolymphatic hydrops **(Meniere's disease)** can lead to SNHL and tinnitus *(Dhingra 5/e, p 38)*. Meningioma can cause deafness, and tinnitus as a part of Neurofibromatosis type 2 syndrome *(Harrison 17th/ed, p 2603)* and its peak incidence occurs in middle age.

    No where it is mentioned histiocytosis X causes deafness and tinnitus. Another point which goes against it is the age of patient (55 years) as histiocytosis occurs mainly in children.

17. **Ans. is b, d and e i.e. cholesteatoma, tympanic membrane perforation and serous otitis media.**
    See the text for explanation.

18. **Ans. is d i.e. Propranolol** *Ref. Scott's Brown 7/e, Vol 3 p 3568 (Table 238 d.1)*

    Ototoxic Drugs

Class	Examples	Predominant ototoxic effects
1. Antimalarial	Quinine	Temporary hearing loss, tinnitus
2. Analgesia, Antipyretics	Aspirin	Temporary hearing loss, tinnitus
3. Aminoglycoside	Amikacin, gentamicin, kanamycin, streptomycin, Neomycin, netilmicin, tobramycin, isepamicin	Permanent hearing loss and /or vestibular injury
4. Antineoplastics	Cisplatin/Carboplatin	Permanent hearing loss and /or vestibular injury
5. Diuretics	Ethacrynic acid, furosemide	Temporary hearing loss
6. Industrial solvents	Toluene benzene	Permanent hearing loss in animals, inconclusive evidence in man.
7. Polypeptide antibiotics	Viomycin, vancomycin	Permanent vestibular injury and / or hearing loss
8. Macrolide antibiotics	Erythromycin, azithromycin clarithromycin	Temporary hearing loss

    Agents for which there have been isolated reports of ototoxicity are:
    Arsenals, Bromides, chloramphenicol, chlorhexidine, erythromycin, Mercury, polymyxin B, Tetracycline, vinblastine and Vincristine

19. **Ans. is a i.e. Distortion of ossicular chain** *Ref. Turner 10/e, p 347*

    In post head injury, the conductive deafness may occur due to:
    - Fracture temporal bone *(more commonly longitudinal)* extending to external canal: tympanic membrane is frequently torn and inner ear is spared.
    - Blood or CSF in external and middle ear.
    - Damage to ossicle *(most frequent being incudostapedial joint)* resulting in more severe and permanent conductive deafness.
    - Aseptic necrosis of long process of incus can lead to late conductive deafness.

    In the Question it is given:

    Tympanic membrane is normal and mobile: In hemotympanum - tympanic membrane will appear red/blue (due to presence of blood pigments) so it is ruled out. *Ref. Turner 10/e, p 441*
    Otosclerosis and EAC sclerosis do not occur in case of head injury and hence they are ruled out.

    ALSO KNOW

    Causes of SNHL in case of head injury:
    - Labyrinthine concussion
    - Vestibular damage.

20. **Ans. is d i.e. Rupture of tympanic membrane** *Ref. Dhingra, 6/e, p 32*
    See proceeding text for explanation.

21. **Ans. is b and c i.e. Rubella measles; and Mumps** *Ref. Scott Brown 7/e, p 3579; OP Ghai 7/e, p 333*

    "The most common postnatal cause of acquired SNHL is meningitis, while the most common prenatal cause is intrauterine infection (eg TORCH infections, syphilis, mumps, measles)". *Ref. OP Ghai 7/e, p 333*
    According to Scotts Browth 7/e, p 3579 – Specific viruses like mumps and syphilis and encephalitis can cause sudden sensorineural hearing loss.

22. **Ans. is None** *Ref. Harrison 16/e, p 1692;17/e, p 1794; Dhingra 6/e, p 30, 116; Maqbool 11/e, p 116*

Section 1: Ear

23. Ans is a, b, c and e i.e. Alport's syndrome; Pendred's syndrome; Treacher-Collins syndrome and Michel's aplasia.

Causes of Congenital Deafness

Conductive hearing loss
- Meatal atresia
- Fixation of stapes footplate
- Fixation of malleus head
- Congential cholesteatoma
- Ossicular discontinuity
- Crouzon syndrome
- Apert syndrome.

Mnemonic

Sensorineural Hearing Loss

Assistant	:	**A**plasia
Branch	:	**B**artter's syndrome
Manager	:	**M**ELAS
W	:	**W**aardenburg syndrome/Wildervanck syndrome
A	:	**A**lport syndrome (SNHL develops by the age of 30 years)
R	:	**R**efsum syndrome
K	:	**K**lippel-feil syndrome
U	:	**U**shers syndrome
T	:	**T**reacher Collins syndrome
Just	:	**J**ervell and Lange-Neilson syndrome
Loves	:	**L**eopard syndrome
To	:	**T**risomy 13, 15, 21
Have	:	**H**yper pigmentation
Pineapple	:	**P**endred syndrome
And	:	**A**lbinism
Orange	:	**O**nychodystrophy
Raita	:	**R**enal tubular acidosis (Distal/Type I)

Note: Stickler syndrome, Treacher Collins syndrome (Current Otolaryngology 2/e p 700), van der Hoeve syndrome, Pierre Robin syndrome can lead to both SNHL or conductive hearing loss.

24. Ans. is c i.e. Perilabyrinthine fistula *Ref. Dhingra 4/e, p 46, 5/e, p 52*

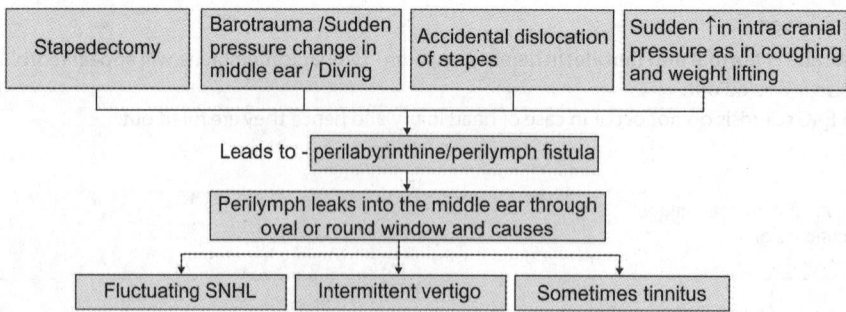

25. Ans. is a, b and c i.e. degeneration of outer hair cell of organ of Corti in sensory type, high frequency is affected first in sensory type and can be treated with hearing aid *Ref. Dhingra 6/e, pgs37; Logan Turner 10/e, pgs324*

Presbycusis
- Sensorineural hearing loss associated with physiological ageing process in the ear is called presbycusis
- For pathological types can be identified–Sensory, neural, strial or metabolic & cochlear conductive
- Sensory **type:** This is **characterized by degeneration of organ** of **Corti**, starting at the basal coil & progressing gradually to the apex **(remember-basal coil is concerned with higher frequencies of sound, whereas apical coils** are **concerned with lower frequencies).** Higher frequency are affected but speech discrimination remains good

- Patients have great difficulty in hearing in the presence of background noise though they may hear well in **quiet surroundings**
- Patients of presbycusis can be helped by a hearing aid
- It is a bilateral condition.

26. **Ans. is c i.e. 100 decibels**   *Ref. Park 19/e, p 599*
"Repeated or continuous exposure to noise around 100 decibels may result in a permanent hearing loss."   *Ref. Park 19th/ed p 599*
"A noise of 90 dB SPL, 8 hours a day for 5 days per week is the maximum safe limit as recommended by ministry of labour, govt. of India rules under factories act."   *Ref. Dhingra 4/e, p 35; 5/e, p 40*

Note: Impulse noise (single time exposure) of more than 140 dB is not permitted.

27. **Ans. is a i.e. Inner hair cells**   *Ref. Mohan Bansal, Essentials of ENT, p 63)*
Noise induced hearing loss is a major preventable cause of SNHL.
Noise level of 90 dB, 8 hours a day for 5 days per week is highest safe limit in factories.
Exposure of more than 115 dB is not permitted. Impulse noise which is greater than 140 dB is not permitted.
Pathology: NIHL damages hair cells, which begins at the basal turn of cochlea. Outer hair cells are affected earlier than the inner hair cells.

Chapter 4

Assessment of Hearing Loss

FUNCTIONAL ASSESSMENT OF HEARING

TUNING FORK TESTS

They are:
- Qualitative test (as they indicate the type of hearing loss)
- Most common used tuning fork = 512 Hz. because of – Longer tone decay and distinct sound.

- Air conduction (AC) is tested by—placing tuning fork 1/2–1 inch in front of external acoustic meatus. (It indicates integrity of tympano-ossicular chain).
- Bone conduction (BC) is tested by—placing tuning fork on mastoid bone or on forehead. (It indicates integrity of inner ear).

NEW PATTERN QUESTION

Q N1. Frequency of tuning fork mostly used in most commonly ENT is:
- a. 256 Hz
- b. 512 Hz
- c. 1024 Hz
- d. 2048 Hz

Rinne Test

In this test, AC is compared with BC of the patient. Tuning fork is struck and placed in front of external auditory meatus. When the patient stops hearing, move it on to the mastoid bone and ask the patient if he/she still hears and then reverses the process. The object is to find out whether the patient hears longer by air or by bone conduction. **Rinne test will be negative in conductive deafness of more than 15 dB.**^{Q}

Interpretation is as follows

- Normally, AC is 2 times better than BC– positive Rinne^Q
- In conductive deafness – BC > AC → Negative Rinne^Q
- In SNHL – AC > BC → Low positive Rinne^Q
- In severe SNHL–BC>AC → False negative Rinne (Due to transcranial transmission of sounds to the normal ear)^Q

 Note: A negative Rinne with 256, 512 and 1024 Hz shows air bone gap of ≈ 15, 30, 45 dB respectively.

NEW PATTERN QUESTIONS

Q N2. Positive Rinne test indicates:
- a. AC > BC
- b. BC > AC
- c. BC = AC
- d. None of the above

Q N3. A negative Rinne's test indicates the presence of:
- a. Profound SNHL
- b. Conductive hearing loss
- c. Recruitment
- d. None

Weber's Test

In this test vibrating tuning fork is placed in the middle of forehead and the patient is asked about the lateralization of sound to left or right ear or in which the sound is heard better. It is a very sensitive test^Q and even less than 5 dB difference in 2 ears hearing level will be indicated by this test.

In Conductive Deafness
- The sound is lateralized to the deaf ear^Q and in bilateral conductive loss, sound is lateralized to the more deaf ear or it is centrally heard if both ears are equally deaf.

In Sensorineural Hearing Loss (SNHL):
- The sound is lateralized to better hearing ear or is heard centrally if both ears are equally bad.

In Normal Ear
- No lateralization of sound occurs.
- Weber test is quite sensitive as difference of only 3-5 dB hearing level can result in lateralization. Weber test readily detects false Rinne negative.

Test	Normal	Conductive deafness	SN deafness
Rinne	AC>BC (Rinne test positive)	BC>AC (Rinne test negative)	AC> BC (Rinne test positive)
Weber	Not lateralized	Lateralized to poorer ear	Lateralized to better ear
ABC	Same as examiner	Same as examiner	Reduced
Schwabach	Equal	Lengthened	Shortened

Chapter 4: Assessment of Hearing Loss

Point to Remember

- Ideal tuning fork for testing hearing - 512 Hz.
- Gelle's test - Test for bone conduction.
  - Positive in normal persons and sensorineural deafness.
  - Negative in otosclerosis.
- Stenger's test/Chimani-Moos test/Lombard's test/Teel's test—They are tuning fork test for detecting non-organic deafness (malingering).
- Most sensitive TFT – Weber's test (5 dB difference needed to lateralize).
- Least sensitive TFT – Schwabach's test.
  (TFT = Tuning fork test)

NEW PATTERN QUESTIONS

Q N4. In conductive deafness, Weber's test is lateralized to:
- a. Deaf ear
- b. Normal ear
- c. Both ears
- d. Any of the above

Q N5. In a patient, Rinne test positive in both ears, Weber's lateralizes to the right. This implies:
- a. Right sensorineural deafness
- b. Left sensorineural deafness
- c. Right conductive deafness
- d. Left conductive deafness

Absolute Bone Conduction Test

In this test, bone conduction of the patient is tested after occluding the external auditory meatus and compared with the BC of the examiner if he has a normal hearing.

The test detects sensorineural hearing loss.

Conclusion

- If both the patient and examiner hear equally either hearing is normal in patient or there is conductive deafness.
- If patient ceases to hear before examiner (i.e. ABC is reduced)– it indicates SNHL

Schwabach's Test

Bone conduction of the patient and examiner is compared, but meatus is not occluded.

Conclusion

- **Sch**wabach is **sho**rtened in **SNHL (Remember 3S)**.
- Schwabach is lengthened in conductive hearing loss.

Gelle's Test

It is also a test of bone conduction and examines the effect of *increased air pressure* in ear canal on the hearing. Normally, when air pressure is increased in the ear canal by Siegel's speculum, it pushes the tympanic membrane and ossicles inwards, raises the intralabyrinthine pressure and causes immobility of basilar membrane and decreased hearing, but no change in hearing is observed when ossicular chain is fixed or disconnected. Gelle's test is performed by placing a vibrating fork on the mastoid while changes in air pressure in the ear canal are brought about by Siegel's speculum.

Gelle's test is positive in normal persons and in those with sensorineural hearing loss. It is negative when ossicular chain is fixed or disconnected. It was a popular test to find out stapes fixation in otosclerosis but has now been superceded by tympanometry.

Point to Remember

Tuning fork tests are not 100% reliable, but are a useful screening test. They should be correlated with an audiogram.

Point to Remember

Other Tuning Fork Tests
- Bing test
- Stenger's test^Q
- Teel's test^Q
- Lombard's test^Q
- These tests are done for those patients who feign deafness but actually are normal subjects.

NEW PATTERN QUESTION

Q N6. In Bing test on alternately compressing and relaxing the tragus the sound increases and decreases. This indicates:
- a. Sensorineural deafness
- b. Adhesive otitis media
- c. Otosclerosis
- d. CSOM

AUDIOMETRY

Pure Tone Audiometry

- This *non-invasive subjective test is* a graphic recording of hearing level both quantitatively and qualitatively done with the help of *audiometer*. An audiometer is an electronic device this generates pure tones. The intensity of these tones are either increased or decreased in 5 dB steps. The audiometer is so calibrated that the hearing of a normal person is at zero dB level.
- The air conduction thresholds are measured usually for tones of 250, 500, 1,000, 2,000, 4,000 and 8,000 Hz. The bone conduction thresholds are measured usually for 250, 500, 1,000, 2,000 and 4,000 Hz. The speech frequencies range from 500-2,000 Hz.

Method

- Audiometry is done in a soundproof room (ideal) or a quiet room. First air conduction and then bone conduction is recorded separately for each ear. The pure tones are presented to the ears by headphone (for air conduction) and vibrator (for bone conduction). The graph on which these thresholds are charted is called an **audiogram**.

Indications—PTA is an Accurate Measure to know

- ***Degree of hearing loss:*** Hearing loss may be mild, moderate, severe or profound.

- **Type of hearing loss:** Hearing loss may be conductive, sensory, neural or mixed.
- **Progress of the disease:** Hearing loss can be fluctuating progressive and stationary.
- **Response to the treatment:** It is important to know whether the hearing loss is improving or not with the therapy.
- **Hearing aids:** The type and necessary setting of hearing aids can be determined.
- **Degree of handicap:** It is needed for compensation and certain benefits.

Hearing Loss

Degree of Hearing Loss

As discussed in Chapter 3:
- In normal persons, normal hearing threshold values with air and bone remain between 0 to 10 dB.
- Hearing threshold up to 25 dB is considered as normal. Further hearing loss is classified as:

WHO classification of hearing loss.

Hearing loss	dB
Mild	26-40
Moderate	41-55
Moderately severe	56-70
Severe	71-91
Profound	> 91

The result of PTA are plotted on audiograph. **The symbols used in audiogram**

- Blue line for left ear
- Red line for right ear (Remember R-R)
- Continuous line for air conduction
- Broken line for Bone conduction (Remember B-B)

	Left ear	Right ear
Air conduction - Unmasked - Masked	X ▨	○ △
Bone conduction - Unmasked - Masked	> ⏌	< ⌊
No response		
Air conduction - Unmasked - Masked	X ⟲	○ △
Bone conduction - Unmasked - Masked	⌐ ⌐	⌐ ⌐

Fig. 4.1: Symbols used in audiogram

Masking

- One of the most important yet confusing aspect of hearing test is to ensure that the auditory function of each ear is measured independently.
- When a sound is given to one ear, via air conduction it gets transmitted to the other ear also.
- Here it should be remembered, that during this process, there is a loss of 40 dB to the other ear for eg if a sound of 70 dB is presented to left ear, it will be heard as 30 dB in right ear.
- This is troublesome because if a person has hearing loss in one ear, lets say right, then a sound projected to right ear would be heard by the left ear via air conduction. This can create confusions.
- Thus masking is done by a noise presented to the non test ear to prevent it from responding to a signal presented to test ear.
- Masking is required for air conduction whenever the difference between healthy and deaf ear is at least 40 dB. In all such cases better ear should be masked.
- For BC testing, masking should be done in all conditions as crossover may occur even at 0 dB difference between the two ears.

Now lets study the graphs obtained in PTA in various situations.

A. Normal hearing (Fig. 4.2)

- This is the PTA graph seen in normal persons.
- In normal persons, hearing threshold values with both air and bone remain between 0 and 10 dB

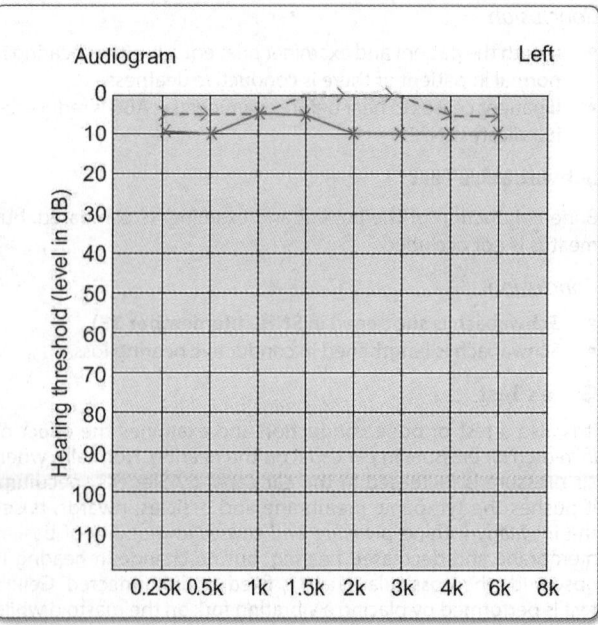

Fig. 4.2: Graph in normal person

Chapter 4: Assessment of Hearing Loss

Note in Audiogram:

On vertical axis: Intensity is measured in decibels. The top line at 0 dB represents a very soft sound. Intensity increases as we move further down.
Remember: 0 dB does not mean that there is no sound at all. Rather, it is the softest sound that a person with normal hearing ability would be able to detect at least 50% of the time. Audiologist considers 0-15 dB to be 'N' hearing in children. 0-25 dB to be 'N' hearing in adults.

This means if a graph does not start from top—the person cannot hear soft sounds (Fig. 4.3).

On horizontal axis: Frequency is measured in Hertz. The frequencies are low on left side and then gradually become higher on right side (Fig. 4.4).

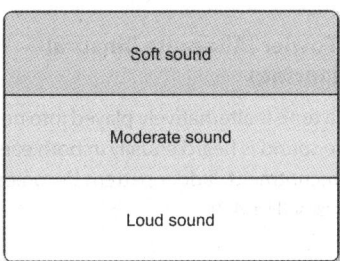

Fig. 4.3

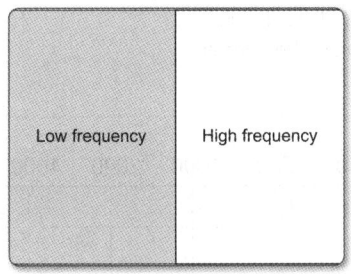

Fig. 4.4

B. Conductive hearing loss: (Fig. 4.5)

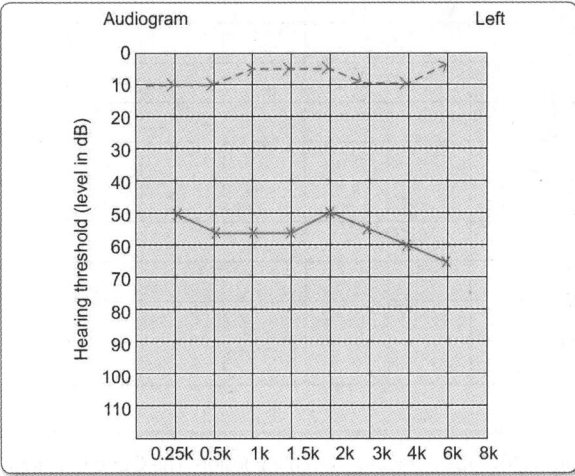

Fig. 4.5: Graph in conductive hearing loss

- In this graph, air-bone gap is seen which means a patient can hear by bone under 10-20 dB, while with air hearing is much below, depending on the severity indicating conductive hearing loss.

 Note: In this audiogram, an **air-bone gap** is seen, i.e. a gap between AC and BC curves of more than 15-20 dB. Remember in conductive hearing loss air-bone gap is seen.

C. Sensorineural hearing loss: (Fig. 4.6)

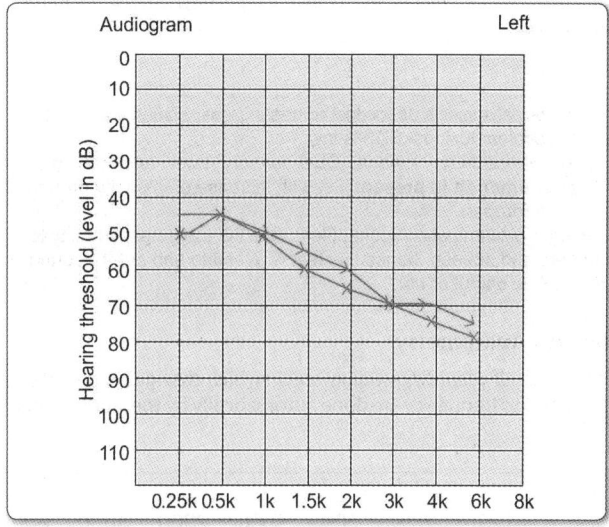

Fig. 4.6: Graph in SNHL

In SNHL, both bone and air conduction value are decreased and may even overlap each other.

 Note: In this graph air-bone is not seen. Thus in sensorineural hearing loss, air-bone gap is never more than 15-20 dB.

NEW PATTERN QUESTIONS	
Q N7.	**Advantages of PTA ever tuning force tests are all *except*:**
	a. It confirms the type of hearing loss
	b. It confirms the degree of hearing loss
	c. It can tell response to the treatment
	d. It can be used in neonates
Q N8.	**U-shaped curve in audiometry is seen in:**
	a. Congenital SNHL b. Otitis media with effusion
	c. Otosclerosis d. Meniere's disease
Q N9.	**A down sloping audiogram is characteristic of:**
	a. Meniere's disease b. Otosclerosis
	c. Presbycusis d. Congenital hearing loss

Speech Audiometry

In this audiometry, recorded spondee words are presented to the ear at various sound pressures. The patient is asked to write the words, which are then cross-checked with the list.

Speech Reception Threshold (SRT)

SRT of a person is the minimum intensity level (in dB) at which 50% of the spondee words can be repeated correctly.

Speech Discrimination Score (SDS) or Optimum Discrimination Score (ODS)

It is the maximum percentage of correct score when phonetically balanced single syllable words such as pin, day, bus, fun, and rum are used.

Results

- In normal subjects or conductive hearing loss, SDS is 95 – 100%.
- In cochlear lesions, SDS is low.
- In retrocochlear lesions, SDS is very poor and **roll over phenomenon is present,** i.e. with increase of intensity ground, score drops.

As poor discrimination score of less than 80% affects the ability to understand speech, hence this test is useful to find out if hearing aid will be useful or not.

Bekesy Audiometry

- It is a self-recording audiometer in which changes in the intensity and frequency are done automatically by the audiometer.
- It is outdated these days.
- Various graphs recorded in Bekesy audiometer are given in Figures 4.7A to D.

■ TEST FOR RECRUITMENT

- Recruitment is an abnormally rapid increase in loudness with increasing sound intensity. Ear which does not hear low intensity sounds will hear greater intensity sounds as loud or even louder than normal ear.[Q]
- **This phenomenon of recruitment is seen in cochlear type of SNHL, e.g.** Meniere's disease[Q] and presbycusis[Q]. In normal persons and conductive hearing loss, the test is negative.

ABLB Test of Fowler (Alternate Binaural Loudness Balancing)

- In this test, a tone is alternatively played into normal and deaf ear, until the sound is heard equally in both ears
- In positive recruitment, ladder pattern becomes horizontal at higher intensity (Fig. 4.8).

Disadvantage

- Difference between the hearing thresholds of the two ears should be at least 25 dB.
- One ear should be normal.

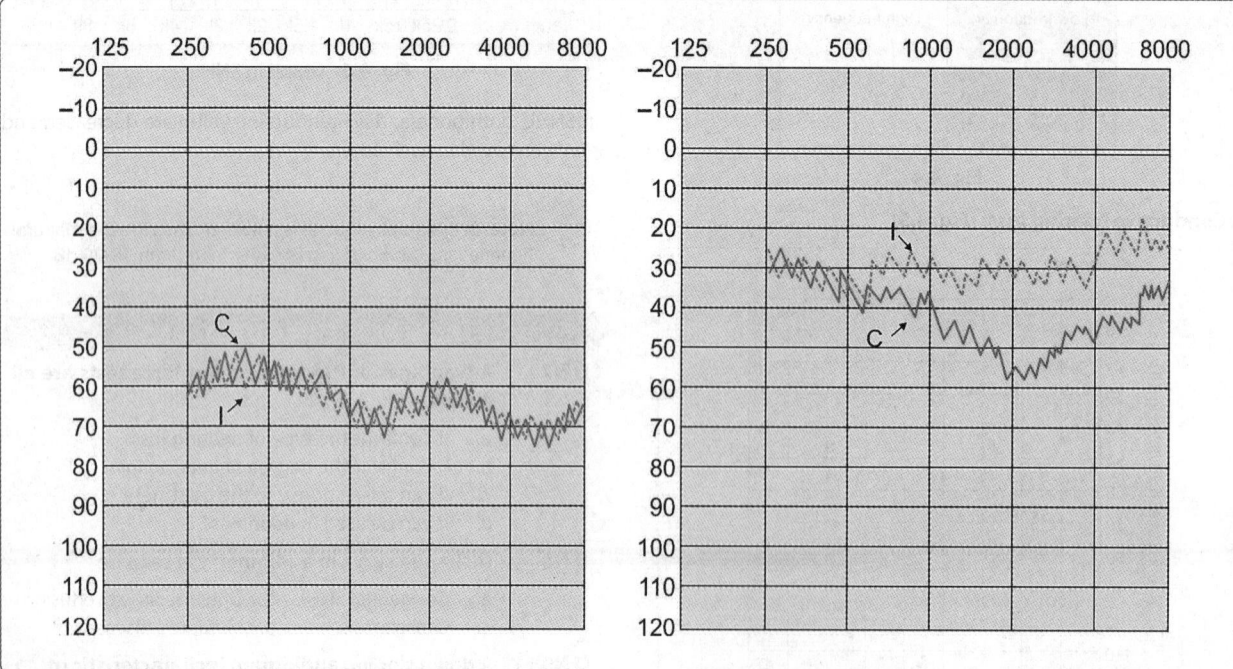

Fig. 4.7A: Type I tracing – Normal person or conducting hearing loss. The C and I tracings overlap in all frequencies

Fig. 4.7B: Type II tracing – Cochlear lesion. The C and I tracings overlaps till 1000 Hz after which C tracing drops by 15–20 dB

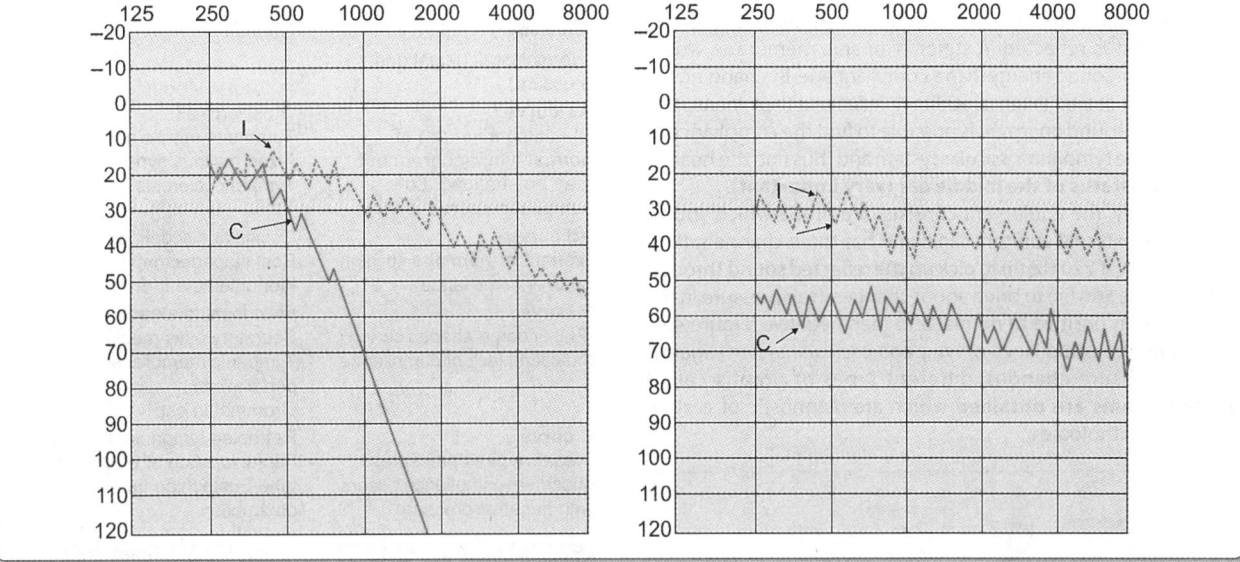

Fig. 4.7C: Type III tracing – retrocochlear lesion/neural lesion. The C tracing drops to > 20 dB below Type I tracing

Fig. 4.7D: Type IV tracing – in acoustic nerve lesion or non-organic hearing loss. The C and I tracings never overlaps

- In nerve fatigue, he stops hearing earlier.
- A decay of more than 25 dB is diagnostic of retrocochlear lesions.

OBJECTIVE TEST FOR HEARING LOSS

Impedance Audiometry

It is an objective test for hearing as compared to tuning fork tests and PTA which are subjective tests.
- *Principle:* It measures the change in the impedance of the middle ear system at the level of the tympanic membrane as a result of changes in the air pressure in the external auditory canal.

Uses

- To differentiate between conductive and sensorineural hearing loss.
- Differential diagnosis of conductive hearing loss.
- Measurement of middle ear pressure and evaluation of Eustachian tube function.
- To differentiate between cochlear and retrocochlear type of sensorineural hearing loss.
- To identify the site of lesion in facial paralysis.

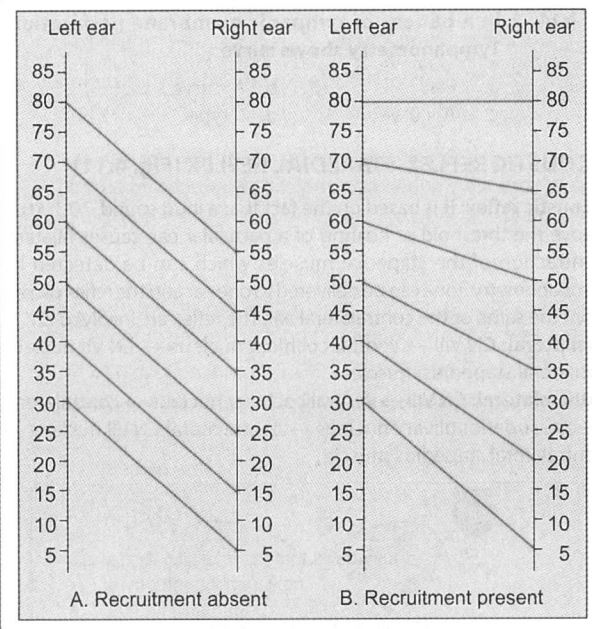

Fig. 4.8: Recruitment phenomenon

Tone Decay Test (or Nerve Fatigue Test)

- Measure of nerve fatigue[Q] and is used to detect retrocochlear lesions.[Q]
- Normally, a person can hear a tone continuously for 60 seconds.

It has two components, i.e. tympanometry and acoustic reflex measurement.
- **Tympanometry:** It is the measure of change in the impedance of the middle ear system at the plane of tympanic membrane – in response to pressure changes in the external auditory canal.
- **Acoustic reflex:** It is the measure of change in the impedance of the middle ear system in response to loud stimulus.

Tympanometry: It is based on a simple principle, i.e. when a sound strikes tympanic membrane, some of the sound energy is absorbed while the rest is reflected. A stiffer tympanic membrane would reflect more of sound energy than a compliant one. By changing the pressures in a sealed external auditory canal and then measuring the reflected sound energy, it is possible to find the compliance or stiffness of the tympano-ossicular system and thus find the healthy or **diseased status of the middle ear (very important)**.

Essentially, the equipment consists of a probe which snugly fits into the external auditory canal and has three channels: (i) to deliver a tone of 220 Hz, (ii) to pick up the reflected sound through a microphone and (iii) to bring about changes in air pressure in the ear canal from positive to normal and then negative (Figure 4.9). By charting the compliance of tympano-ossicular system against various pressure changes, different types of graphs called **tympanograms are obtained** which are diagnostic of certain middle ear pathologies.

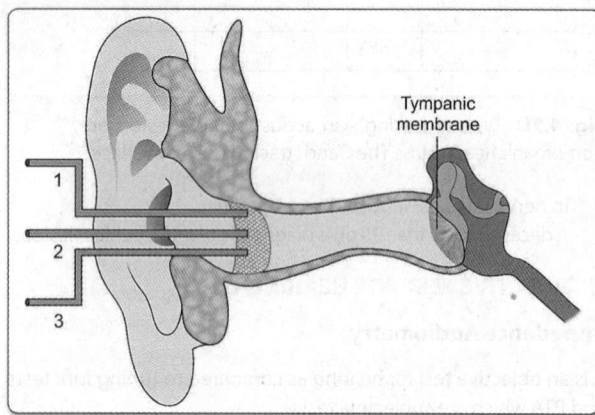

Fig 4.9: Principle of impedance audiometry. **1.** Oscillator to produce a tone of 220 Hz. **2.** Air pump to increase or decrease air pressure in the air canal. **3.** Microphone to pick up and measure sound pressure level reflected from the tympanic membrane.

Types of Tympanogram (Fig. 4.10)

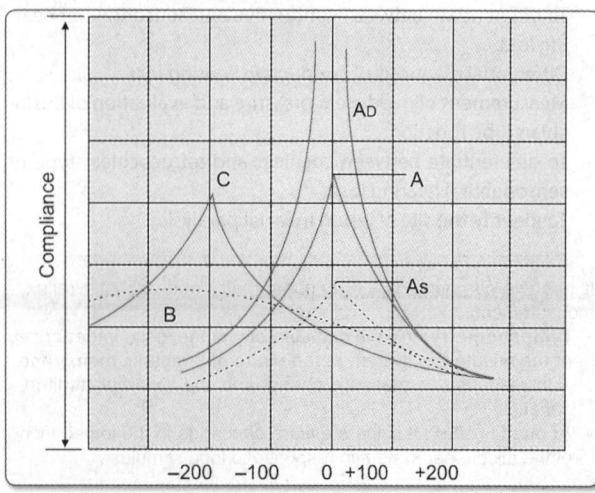

Fig. 4.10: Curves of impedance audiometry

Type of curve	Condition
A curve (Normal peak height and pressure).	– Normal
As curve[Q] (It is also a variant of normal tympanogram but may be shallow). Low compliance curve	– Otosclerosis[Q] – Tumors of middle ear – Fixed malleus syndrome – Tympanosclerosis
Ad curve (Variant of normal with high peak or compliance)	– Ossicular discontinuity – Post stapedectomy – Monometric ear drum
B curve (Flat or dome-shaped curve)[Q] Indicating lack of compliance	– Fluid in middle ear[Q] – Secretory otitis media[Q] – Tympanic membrane perforation[Q] – Grommet in ear[Q]
C curve (negative peak pressure) Maximum compliance occurs with negative pressure	– Retracted tympanic membrane – Faulty function of Eustachian tube/Eustachian tube obstruction

NEW PATTERN QUESTIONS

Q N10. Impedance audiometry is for pathology of:
 a. External ear   b. Middle ear
 c. Mastoid air cell   d. Inner cell

Q N11. In a patient of tympanic membrane perforation Tympanometry shows curve:
 a. Flat   b. A_s curve
 c. A_d curve   d. C type

ACOUSTIC REFLEX/STAPEDIAL REFLEX (Fig. 4.11)

Acoustic reflex: It is based on the fact that a loud sound, 70-100 dB above the threshold of hearing of a particular ear, causes bilateral contraction of the stapedial muscles which can be detected by tympanometry. Tone can be delivered to one ear and the reflex picked from the same or the contralateral ear. The reflex arc involved is:

Ipsilateral: CN VIII → ventral cochlear nucleus → CN VII nucleus ipsilateral stapedius muscle.

Contralateral: CN VIII → ventral cochlear nucleus → contralateral medial superior olivary nucleus → contralateral CN VII nucleus → contralateral stapedius muscle.

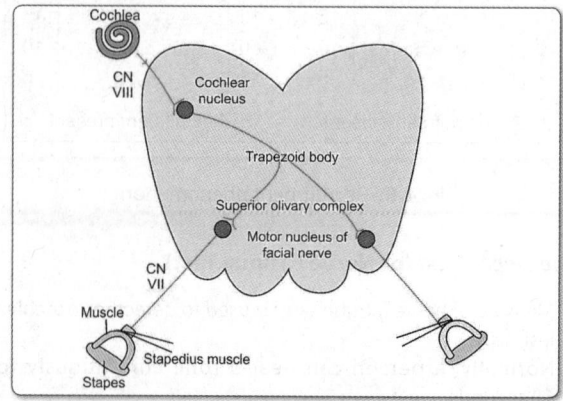

Fig. 4.11: Acoustic reflex pathways

Causes of Absent Stapedial Reflex

Afferent pathway	Efferent pathway

• Middle ear diseases
   – Otosclerosis
   – Ossicular discontinuity
   – Atelectasis
• Colchlea/VIII nerve/ superior olivary complex lesion
   – Severe SNHL
   – Acoustic neuroma
   – Multiple sclerosis
	• VII nerve diseases
	   – Facial palsy
	   – Ramsay Hunt syndrome
	
	• Stapedius muscle involvement
	   – Poststapedectomy
	   – Myasthenia gravis

NEW PATTERN QUESTIONS

Q N12. Stapedial reflex is absent in:
   a. VI nerve lesion   b. X nerve lesion
   c. VIII nerve lesion   d. V nerve lesion

Q N13. In facial nerve palsy of right side, Stapedial reflex will be absent on:
   a. Right side   b. Left side
   c. Both sides   d. Not absent

■ SPECIAL TESTS OF HEARING

BERA: (Brainstem Evoked Response Audiometry)/ ABR (Auditory Brainstem Response)/Indications

- It is the IOC for detection of deafness in difficult to test cases like infants^Q, mentally retarted or malingers.
- For assessment of the nature of deafness (conductive or sensorineural)^Q
- For identification of the site of lesion in retrocochlear pathologies^Q
- To study the maturity of the CNS in newborns, objective assessment of brain-death.
- For assessing prognosis in a comatosed patients.
- To diagnose brainstem pathology example multiple sclerosis or pontine tumor
- Unlike pure tone audiometry, BERA does not require subjective patient response.

Principle

It is noninvasive technique to find the integrity of central auditory pathway through the VIII nerve, pons and midbrain.

Sound in the Cochlea → is converted into → Electrical impulse (Various wave forms) → Passes from → Cochlea → Produces → Auditory cortex

These waves are studied for latency, amplitude and morphology. Out of the following waves generated the 1st, 3rd and 5th waves are most stable and the ones which are studies.

According to *Dhingra 4th/ed p29 and Scott Browns 7th ed p3283*

- Wave I = E = Distal part of eight nerve
- Wave II = E = Proximal part of eight nerve
- Wave III = C = Cochlear nucleus/Lower pons
- Wave IV = O = Superior olivary complex
- Wave V = L = Lateral leminiscus—Upper pons
- Wave VI-VII = Inferior colliculus

NEW PATTERN QUESTIONS

Q N14. In monaural diplacusis the lesion is in the:
   a. Cochlea   b. Auditory nerve
   c. Brainstem   d. Cerebrum

Q N15. 40 dB compared to 20 dB is:
   a. Double   b. 10 times
   c. 100 times   d. 1000 times

Otoacoustic Emissions

Otoacoustic emissions (OAE) are low-intensity sounds, which are produced by movements of the outer hair cells of the cochlea. They are produced spontaneously and in response to the acoustic stimuli.

- The spontaneous OAE are present in only 50% of normal hearing people
- The evoked OAE are produced in response to a sound stimulus and are seen in all normal hearing individuals.

Hence we test for evoked OAE. If Evoked OAE are also absent it indicates damage to outer hair cell. (i.e. cochlear pathology).

This non-invasive objective test can diagnose damage to the outer hair cells due to acoustic trauma and ototoxic drugs. It aids in the assessment of hearing in infants.

Note: Sedation does not interfere with OAE.

The OAE travels through basilar membrane, perilymph, oval window, ossicles, tympanic membrane and ear canal. OAE are present in nerve hearing loss as the outer hair cells are normal.

Uses

- Screening test of hearing in neonates, uncooperative or mentally challenged patients. In neonates if OAE are absent then confirm citory test BERA is done.
- Distinguish between cochlear (acoustic trauma and ototoxic drugs) and retrocochlear hearing losses (auditory neuropathy).
- Early detection of noise induced hairing loss on hearing loss due to ototoxic drugs.

Point to Remember
➢ Screening test for detecting hearing loss in infant is Oto acoustic emission
➢ Diagnostic test-BERA/ABR

Concepts of Acoustic

Frequency: The number of cycles or vibrations per second. It is described in Hertz (Hz) after the name of a German scientist, *Heinrich Rudolf Hertz*.
➢ Pure tone is a sound of a single frequency such as 250, 500 Hz or 1 kHz to 8 kHz

Amplitude: The intensity of the sound, hence the cloudness.
Pitch: Determined by frequency of sound waves, higher the frequency, higher the pitch.
Loudness: Depends upon intensity of sound waves.
Intensity: Denoted in decibels (dB) (1/10 of a Bel). Bel a log of the ratio of intensity of that sound and standard sound.

(Alexander Graham Bell) 1 Bel = Log of $\dfrac{\text{Intensity of sound}}{\text{Intensity of standard sound}}$

Explanations and References to New Pattern Questions

N1. Ans. is b i.e. 512 Hz *Ref. Essentials of Mohan Bansal, p 41*
See the text for explanation.

N2. Ans. is a i.e. AC > BC *Ref. Dhingra 6/e, p 22*
Rinne's positive means AC > BC; it is seen in normal persons or those having SNHL.

N3. Ans. is b i.e. Conductive hearing loss
See the text for explanation

N4. Ans. is a i.e. Deaf ear
See the text for explanation

N5. Ans. is b i.e. Left sensorineural deafness *Ref. Read below*
- Rinne test positive in both ears indicates either hearing is normal or there is SNHL.
- Weber lateralizes to the right means that the left ear has SNHL. This cannot be conductive hearing loss of any side as rinne is positive.

N6. Ans. is a i.e. Sensorineural deafness *Ref. Dhingra 6/e, p 22*
Bing Test *Ref. Dhingra 6/e, p 22*
It is a test of bone conduction and examines the effect of occlusion of ear canal on the hearing. A vibrating tuning fork is placed on the mastoid while the examiner alternately closes and opens the ear canal by pressing on the tragus inward.
- Positive in normal and SNHL i.e. person hears louder when ear canal is occluded and softer when ear canal is open.
- Negative in conductive hearing loss – i.e. no change.

N7. Ans. is d i.e It can be used in neonates *Ref. Essentials of ENT, Mohan Bansal, p 44*

PTA has all the advantages as discussed in the question over tuning fork tests, except that it can be used in neonates. This is because in neonates/infants only objective tests are used, not subjective tests.

N8. Ans. is a i.e. Congenital SNHL

N9. Ans. is c i.e. Presbycusis

In Audiograms of SNHL specific characteristic signify Specific Disease	
Characteristic on Audiogram	Disease condition
Down sloping audiogram (meaning higher frequencies affected more) as on right side higher frequencies are indicated 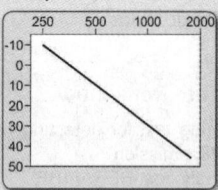	1. Presbycusis 2. Noise induced hearing loss 3. Ototoxicity
Upsloping audiogram (i.e. lower frequencies affected more) 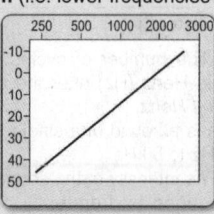	1. Meniere Disease (Early stages)
U-shaped	Congenital SNHL
Carhart's notch (dip at 2000 Hz)	Oto sclerosis

Also Know
Types of audiograms in conductive hearing loss.
- **Left sloping** – loss in lower frequencies is seen in otospongiosis
- **Right sloping** – loss in higher frequencies is seen in secretory otitis media

Chapter 4: Assessment of Hearing Loss

N10. Ans. is b i.e. Middle ear *Ref. Dhingra 6/e, p 24*

Impedance audiometry is used to find the health or diseased status of middle ear.

N11. Ans. is a i.e. Flat

In perforation of tympanic membrane, tympanometry cannot be done. So a flat curve is obtained on tympanometry.

N12. Ans. is c i.e. VIII nerve lesion *Ref. Dhingra 6/e, p 47*

See the text for explanation.

N13. Ans. is a i.e. Right side

Facial nerve forms the efferent of stapedial reflex, so in facial nerve palsy of right side, the stapedial reflex is absent on right side only.

> **Remember**
> VIII N forms the afferent of the reflex ∴ in VIII N lesions, stapedial reflex is absent in both ipsilateral and contralateral ears.

N14. Ans. is a i.e. Cochlea *Ref. Tuli 1/e, p 114*

Subjective feeling of diplacusis, hyperacusis or fullness in the ear occurs in cochear pathology or cohlear, sensorineural hearing loss (SNHL).

Differences between Cochlear and Retrocochlear SNHL

Cochlear SNHL	Retrocochlear SNHL
Hair cells are damaged mainly	Lesion is of VIIth nerve or its central connections
Recruitment is present	Recruitment is absent
No significant tone decay	Tone decay is significant
Short increment sensitivity index (SISI) is positive	SISI is negative
Bekesy shows no gap between I and C tracing (Type II)	Bekesy shows wide gap between I and C tracings (Type III)
Speech discrimination is not highly impaired (SDS is low) and roll over phenomenon is not present	Speech discrimination is highly impaired (SDS very poor) and roll over phenomenon is present
Subjective feeling of diplacusis, hyperacusis or fullness in the ear	No such sensation or feeling

 Note: SDS = Speech Discrimination Score

It is the maximum percentage of correct score when phonetically balanced single syllable words such as pin, day, bus are used.

Results

- In normal subject or conductive hearing loss, SDS is 95–100%
- In cochlear lesions SDS is low

In retrocochlear lesions, SDS is very poor and roll over phenomenon is present (which means with increase of intensity, drop of score occurs)

N15. Ans. is b i.e 10 times *Ref. Dhingra 6/e, p 19; Essential's of Mohan Bansal, p 39*

As discussed in the text:	**Remember:**
I Bel = Log of $\dfrac{\text{Intensity of sound being described (S1)}}{\text{Intensity of standard sound (So)}}$	Log 1 = 0
Or it can also be expressed as:	Log 10 = 1
= 20 Log $\dfrac{\text{SPL of S1}}{\text{SPL of So}}$	Log 100 (10^2) = 2
SPL = Sound pressure level	Log 1000 (10^3) = 3
If a sound has an SPL of 1000 i.e (10^3) times, the reference of sound, it is expressed as	Log 10000 (10^4) = 4
20 × log 1000 = 20 × 3 = 60 dB (as log 1000 = 3)	Log 100,000 (10^5) = 5
Now in the Q sound is 20 dB, that means to get 20 as the answer, 20 has to be multiplied by 1, i.e the SPL of this sound is 10 (because log 10 is 1).	
Now it is being compared with 40 dB	
To get 40 dB as the answer.	
20 has to be multiplied by 2 which means log of x = 2, therefore x = 100	
So it means this sound should have SPL = 100	
Now see = 20 dB = SPL 10	
40 dB = SPL 100	
i.e. 40 dB is 10 times of 20 dB	

QUESTIONS

1. All are tunning fork test except: [UP 02/DNB 02]
   a. Schwaback test
   b. Grant's test
   c. Rinne's test
   d. Weber's test
2. Tuning fork of 512 FPS is used to test the hearing because it is: [Karn. 06]
   a. Better heard
   b. Better felt
   c. Produces over tones
   d. Not heard
3. Gelle's test is done in: [JIPMER 98]
   a. Senile deafness
   b. Traumatic deafness
   c. Osteosclerosis
   d. Serous otitis media
4. Which one of the following test is used to detect malingering? [TN 07]
   a. Stenger's test
   b. Bunge's test
   c. Weber's test
   d. Rinne's test
5. Rinne's test is negative in: [AIIMS Nov 94]
   a. Sensorineural deafness
   b. Acoustic neuroma
   c. Tympanosclerosis
   d. Meniere's disease
6. Rinne's test negative is seen in: [JIPMER 92]
   a. Presbycusis
   b. CSOM
   c. Labyrinthitis
   d. Meniere's disease
7. Rinne's test is negative if minimum deafness is: [SRMC 02]
   a. 15–20 dB
   b. 25–30 dB
   c. 35–40 dB
   d. 15–50 dB
8. Positive Rinne test is seen in: [JIPMER 91]
   a. Otosclerosis
   b. CSOM
   c. Wax impacted ear
   d. Presbycusis
9. Rinne's test is positive in: [AIIMS 91]
   a. Chronic suppurative otitis media
   b. Normal individual
   c. Wax in ear
   d. Otomycosis
10. Weber test is best elicited by: [AI 02]
    a. Placing the tuning fork on the mastoid process and comparing the bone conduction of the patient with that of the examiner
    b. Placing the tuning fork on the vertex of the skull and determining the effect of gently occluding the auditory canal on the threshold of low frequencies
    c. Placing the tuning fork on the mastoid process and comparing the bone conduction in the patient
    d. Placing the tuning fork on the forehead and asking him to report in which ear he hears it better.
11. In the right middle ear pathology, Weber's test will be: [AI 04]
    a. Normal
    b. Centralized
    c. Lateralized to right side
    d. Lateralized to left side
12. Weber's test in conductive deafness: [CUPGEE 96]
    a. Sound louder in normal ear
    b. Sound louder in diseased ear
    c. Heard with equal intensity in both ears
    d. Inconclusive test
13. What should be the least hearing loss for Weber test to lateralize? [Rj 2004]
    a. 5 dB
    b. 10 dB
    c. 15 dB
    d. 20 dB
14. A 38-year-old gentleman reports of decreased hearing in the right ear for the last two years. On testing with a 512Hz tuning fork the Rinne's test without masking is negative on the right ear and positive on the left ear. With the Weber's test the tone is perceived as louder in the left ear. The most likely patient has: [AIIMS Nov 02]
    a. Right conductive hearing loss
    b. Right sensorineural hearing loss
    c. Left sensorineural hearing loss
    d. Left conductive hearing loss
15. A middle-aged women presented with right sided hearing loss, Rinne's test shows positive result on left side and negative result on right side Weber's test showed lateralization to left side, diagnosis is: [AIIMS June 00]
    a. Right sided conductive deafness
    b. Right sided sensorineural deafness
    c. Left sided sensorineural deafness
    d. Left sided conductive deafness
16. One man had 30 dB deafness in left ear with Weber test showing more sound in left ear and BC (Bone conduction) more on left side and normal hearing in right ear, his test can be summarized as:
    a. Weber's test—left lateralized; Rinne test—right positive, BC>AC on left side
    b. Weber's test—right lateralized; Rinne test—left positive, AC>BC on right side
    c. Weber's test—left lateralized; Rinne test—false positive on right side, BC>AC on left side
    d. Weber's left lateralized; Rinne test—equivocal, BC>AC on right side
17. A patient presents to your clinic for evaluation of defective hearing. Rinne's test shows air conduction greater than the bone conduction on both sides with Weber test lateralized to right ear. What is the next logical step? [AIIMS Nov 2015]
    a. Normal test
    b. Schwabach's test
    c. Repeat Rinnie's test on right side
    d. Wax removal
18. A 38-year-old male presented with a suspected diagnosis of suppurate labyrinthitis. A positive Rinne's test and positive fistula test was recorded on initial examination. The patient refused treatment, and returned to the emergency department after 2 weeks complaining of deafness in the affected ear. On examination, fistula test was observed be negative. What is the likely expected finding on repeating the Rinne test? [AI 09]
    a. True positive Rinne's test
    b. False positive Rinne's test

c. True negative Rinne's test
d. False negative Rinne's test
19. In pure tone audiogram the symbol X is used to mark: [JIPMER 02]
    a. Air conduction in right ear
    b. Air conduction in left ear
    c. Bone conduction in right ear
    d. No change in air conduction in right ear
20. The 'O' sign in a pure tone audiogram indicates: [AP 2005]
    a. Air conduction of right ear
    b. Air conduction of left ear
    c. Bone conduction of right ear
    d. Bone conduction of left ear
21. Tone decay test is done for: [Manipal 01]
    a. Cochlear deafness   b. Neural deafness
    c. Middle ear problem   d. Otosclerosis
22. All are subjective tests for audiometry except:
    a. Tone decay   b. Impedance audiometry
    c. Speech audiometry   d. Pure tone audiometry
23. Impedance audiometry is for pathology of: [UP 04]
    a. External ear   b. Middle ear
    c. Mastoid air cell   d. Inner ear
24. Impedance audiometry is done using frequency probe of: [Delhi 07]
    a. 220 Hz   b. 550 Hz
    c. 440 Hz   d. 1000 Hz
25. Which of the following test assesses resistance in middle ear? [MAHE 2000]
    a. Pure tone audiometry
    b. Impendence audiometry
    c. Caloric test
    d. Brainstem evoked response audiometry (BERA)
26. True about pure tone audiometry: [PGI May 2014]
    a. The frequency tested is 2000-9000Hz
    b. Done in silent room
    c. Air conduction for right ear is represented on audiogram by symbol 'X'
    d. Air conduction for left ear is represented on audiogram by symbol 'O'
27. High frequency audiometry is used in:
    a. Otosclerosis   [AIIMS May 09; Nov 12]
    b. Ototoxicity
    c. Nonorganic hearing loss
    d. Meniere's disease
28. A lady has B/L hearing loss since 4 years which worsened during pregnancy. Type of impedance audiometry graph will be: [AIIMS May 07; Nov 06]
    a. Ad   b. As
    c. B   d. C
29. Flat tympanogram is seen in: [PGI 00]
    a. ASOM   b. Otosclerosis
    c. Serous otitis media   d. Ossicular chain disruption
30. B-type tympanogram is seen in: [Bihar 04]
    a. Serous otitis media   b. Ossicular discontinuity
    c. Otosclerosis   d. All of the above
31. Flat and dome-shaped graph in tympanogram is found in: [RJ 03]
    a. Otosclerosis
    b. Ossicular discontinuity
    c. TM perforation   d. Middle ear fluid
32. In osteogenesis imperfecta, the tympanogram is: [DNB 03]
    a. Flat   b. Noncompliance
    c. High-compliance   d. Low-compliance
33. A young man presents with an accident leading to loss of hearing in right ear. On otoscopic examination, the tympanic membrane was intact pure tone audiometry that shows an air-bone gap of 55 dB in the right with normal cochlear reserve. Which of the following will be the like tympanometry finding: [AI 09]
    a. As type tympanogram   b. Ad type tympanogram
    c. B type tympanogram   d. C type tympanogram
34. Which is the best test for screening of the auditory function of neonates? [AIIMS May 14, Nov 12]
    a. Pure tone audiometry
    b. Stapedial reflex
    c. Otoacoustic emissions (OAE)
    d. Brainstem evoked auditory response
35. Which is the investigation of choice in assessing hearing loss in neonates? [AIIMS May 11]
    a. Impedance audiometry
    b. Brainstem evoked response audiometry (BERA)
    c. Free field audiometry
    d. Behavioral audiometry
36. Which of the following tests is recommended for neonatal screening of hearing? [AIIMS Nov 2015]
    a. Automated auditory brainstem response
    b. Spontaneous OAE
    c. Evoked OAE
    d. Distorted product OAE
37. True about Otoacoustic emissions: [PGI June 2009]
    a. Are by product of outer hair cell
    b. Are by product of inner hair cell
    c. Used as a screening test of hearing in newborn infant
    d. Useful in ototoxicity monitoring
    e. Disappear in 8th nerve pathology
38. To distinguish between cochlear and post cochlear damage test done is: [PGI Dec 97]
    a. Brainsterm evoked response audiometry
    b. Impedance audiometry
    c. Pure tone audiometry
    d. Auditory cochlear potential
39. In normal adult wave v is generated from: [AIIMS May 14, J and K 05, Delhi 08]
    a. Cochlear nucleus
    b. Superior olivary complex
    c. Lateral lemniscus
    d. Inferior colliculus
40. Test of detecting damage to cochlea [MH PGM CET Jan 05; MH 00]
    a. Caloric test   b. Weber test
    c. Rinne's test   d. ABC test

41. **Threshold for bone conduction is normal and that for air conduction is increased in disease of:** [AP 96]
    a. Middle ear
    b. Inner ear
    c. Cochlear nerve
    d. Temporal lobe
42. **Stapedial reflex is mediated by:**
    a. V and VII nerves
    b. V and VIII nerves
    c. VII and VI nerves
    d. VII and VIII nerves
43. **Vestibular evoked myogenic potential (VEMP) detects lesion of:** [AIIMS May 2012]
    a. Cochlear nerve
    b. Superior vestibular nerve
    c. Inferior vestibular nerve
    d. Inflammatory myopathy
44. **In electrocochleography:** [AIIMS May 2012]
    a. It measures middle ear latency
    b. Outer hair cells are mainly responsible for cochlear microphonics and summation potential
    c. Summation potential is a compound of synchronus auditory nerve potential
    d. Total AP represents endocochlear receptor potential to an external auditory stimulus
45. **Electrocochleography is** [DNB 2012]
    a. Probe, stimulation of outer hair cells only
    b. Summation of microphonics
    c. AP of cochlear nerve
    d. Evoked potential generated in cochlea and auditory nerve
46. **Which one of the following test is used to detect malingering?** [TN 2007]
    a. Stenger test
    b. Bing test
    c. Weber test
    d. Rinne test
47. **Which of the following does not show negative Rinne test in the right ear?** [AIIMS May 2014]
    a. Sensorineural hearing loss of 45 dB in left ear and normal right ear
    b. Profound hearing loss
    c. Conductive hearing loss of 40 dB in both ears
    d. Conductive hearing loss of 40 dB in right ear and left ear normal
48. **A 35 years old pregnant female complaining of hearing loss, which aggravated during pregnancy, was sent for tympanometry. Which of the following graph will be seen?** [AIIMS Nov 2013]
    a. As
    b. Ad
    c. B
    d. C

Chapter 4: Assessment of Hearing Loss

Explanations and References
---

1. **Ans. is b i.e. Grant's test**   *Ref. Dhingra 6/e, p 22,23*
   Tuning Fork tests include.
   - **Rinne's test** – Compares air conduction of the ear with bone conduction
   - **Weber test**
   - **Absolute bone conduction test** – Here bone conduction of the patient is tested after occluding the meatus and then compared with BC of the examiner
   - **Schwabach test** – Here also BC of the patient is compared with the BC of a normal hearing person but meatus is not occluded.
   - **Bing test** – It is a test of BC and examines the effect of occlusion of ear canal on hearing (i.e. external meatus is occluded and released alternatively)
   - **Gelle's test** – It is also a test of BC and examines the effect of increased air pressure in ear canal on hearing.

   Other Tuning Fork Tests
   - Stenger test ⎤
   - Teel's test   ⎬   For detecting malingering
   - Lombard's test ⎦

2. **Ans. is a i.e. Better heard**   *Ref. Tuli 1/e, p 28*
   Tuning fork tests can be done with tuning forks of different frequencies like 128, 256, 512, 1024, 2018 and 4096 Hz but most commonly used is 512 Hz because
   - *"Tests are done with various tuning forks, but 512 Hz is the most commonly used as it has longer tone decay and sound is quite distinct from ambient noise."*
   - Forks of lower frequencies produce a sense of bone vibration while those of higher frequency have a shorter decay time and therefore not commonly used

3. **Ans. is c i.e. Osteosclerosis**   *Ref. Dhingra, 6/e, p 22*
   Gelle's test was once a popular test to find out stapes fixation in otosclerosis, but now it has been superseded by tympanometry.
   In this test, bone conduction is tested and at the same time Siegel's speculum compresses the air in the meatus.

   Principle

   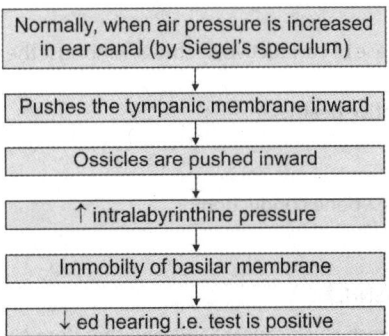

   But if ossicular chain is fixed or disrupted, no such phenomenon occurs i.e. **test is negative**.

   > **Gelle's test is positive:** In normal individuals, SNHL.
   > **Gelle's test is negative:** In case of fixed ossicular chain (otosclerosis) or if ossicular chain is disconnected.

4. **Ans. is a i.e. Stenger's test**   *Ref. Dhingra 6/e, p 37; Tuli 1/e, p31*
   Malingering/Nonorganic hearing loss (also called pseudohypacusis)
   - Ocassionally patients wilfully or subconsciously exaggerate their hearing loss.
   - This is functional hearing loss or pseudohypacusis or malingering
     – The signs in the test behavior that suggest functional component include:
        a. Inconsistent responses
        b. Significant differences between the threshold obtained using ascending and descending administration of test stimuli
        c. A discrepancy of > 8 dB between the SRT (speech reception threshold) and the pure tone average of 500–2000 Hz
        d. Positive Stenger test

Stenger Test
- It is used to identify unilateral or asymmetrical functional hearing loss. It is based on the concept that when both ears are stimulated simultaneously by a tone equal in frequency and phase, the auditory percept is lateralized to the ear with better hearing.
- If speech stimulus is used in Stenger test it is k/a Speech Stenger test or modified Stenger test.
- Other objective tests which can diagnose functional involvement are:
  - **Acoustic reflexes:** Patient saying hearing loss but normal acoustic reflex indicates NOHL
  - Auditory brainstem response
  - Otoacoustic emission

> **Also Know**
> Other tuning fork tests which can be used to detect malingering but are now outdated are:
> - Teel's test
> - Lombard's test
> - Chamini-Moos test
> - Gault test

5. **Ans. is c i.e. Tympanosclerosis**
6. **Ans. is b i.e. CSOM**
7. **Ans. is a i.e. 15 – 20 dB**

Ref. Dhingra, 6/e, p 22

As discussed in the text in Rinne's test—air conduction of the ear is compared with its bone conduction. Hence there is **false negative Rinne test** (BC > AC).

Result	Inference	Seen in
Positive	Air conduction > Bone conduction	• Normal individuals • SNHL
Negative False negative	Bone conduction > Air conduction	• Conductive deafness • Severe SNHL

 Note: A negative Rinne test indicates a minimum air bone gap of 15–20 dB (Ans 7)

Now lets see Qs 5 and 6
Q.5 says Rinne's test is negative in –
We know negative Rinne test is seen in case of conductive deafness. Amongst the options given, only tympanosclerosis is a cause for conductive deafness.
Again in Q.6 – only CSOM causes conductive deafness.

8. **Ans. is d i.e. Presbycusis**
9. **Ans. is b i.e. Normal individual**

Ref. Dhingra 6/e, p 22

Rinne's test is positive, i.e. air conduction > bone conduction
It is seen in:
a. Normal individuals (Ans 9)
b. In case of sensorineural hearing loss (SNHL)

Amongst the options given in Q.8 only presbycusis causes SNHL and therefore gives positive Rinne test

> **Presbycusis:** It is sensorineural hearing loss associated with physiological aging process in the ear. It manifests at 65 years of age.

10. **Ans. is d i.e. Placing the tuning fork on the forehead and asking him to report in which ear he hears it better**

Ref. Dhingra, 6/e, p 22

Test	Method of testing
Rinne's test	Placing the tuning fork on mastoid process and bringing it beside the meatus when patient stops hearing it on mastoid
Weber's test	Placing the tuning fork on forehead and asking him to report in which ear he hears better
Absolute bone conduction	Placing the tuning fork on mastoid process and comparing the bone conduction of the patient with that of examiner after occluding the meatus
Schwabach's test	Test same as absolute bone conduction but meatus is not occluded

Chapter 4: Assessment of Hearing Loss

11. Ans. is c i.e. Lateralized to right side   *Ref. Dhingra 5/e, p 26*

12. Ans. is b i.e. Sound louder in diseased ear

13. Ans. is a i.e. 5 dB

As discussed in the text in Weber's Test
- In normal Individuals – No lateralization of sound occurs as Bone conduction of both ears in normal and equal.
- In conductive deafness – Lateralization of sound occurs to the diseased ear (Ans 12)
- In SNHL – Lateralization of sound occurs to the better ear.

> **Mnemonic**
> M = Maxillary artery
> A = Postauricular artery
> M = Middle meningeal branch artery

Weber's is a very sensitive test and even less than 5 dB difference in 2 ears hearing level can be indicated.

14. Ans. is b i.e. Right sensorineural hearing loss

15. Ans. is b i.e. Right-sided sensorineural deafness   *Ref. Dhingra 6/e, p 22, Table 4.1*

Rinne's Test

Negative on right side means either there is:
- Conductive deafness of Right side or
- Severe SNHL on right side (leading to false negative Rinne test)

To differentiate between the 2 conditions: Let us see the result of Weber's test:
- Patient is complaining of decreased hearing in right ear and Weber's test is lateralized to left ear (as stated in the question) i.e. to the better ear.
- As discussed in the text: Weber's test is lateralized to the better ear in case of SNHL.

So, diagnosis is right sided severe SNHL.

> **Remember**
> If Rinne's test is negative and Weber's test shows lateralization toward healthy side, it indicates **severe SNHL**

16. Ans. is a i.e. Weber's test—left lateralized; Rinne's test—right positive; BC > AC on left side   *Ref. Dhingra, 6/e, p 22*

Let us analyze each information provided in the question.
- This man has deafness of 30 dB in left ear.
- Weber's test is lateralized to left ear i.e. deaf ear which means deafness is conductive type. (As in conductive deafness - Weber's test is lateralized to poorer ear).

This means Rinne test should be negative on left side (as in conductive deafness - Rinne test is negative). Ruling out **options "b" and "d"**.

In the question it is given hearing is normal on right side, so Rinne test will be positive on right side (because in case of normal hearing - Rinne test is positive).

In the question itself it is given, bone conduction is more on left side.

So **option "a"** is correct i.e.:

Weber's test - left lateralized, Rinne test - right positive and BC>AC on left side.

17. Ans. is b i.e. Schwabach's test   *Ref. Dhingra's 6/e p25-27*

Lateralization of Weber's test to right means either right-sided conductive deafness or left-sided sensorineural deafness. In right side conductive deafness BC should be better than AC on Rinne's test, whereas Rinne result shows AC > BC, hence the patient probably has sensorineural deafness involving the left ear.

In such a case, Schwabach's test should be performed to see the absolute bone conduction and confirm the findings.

Tuning Fork Tests and their Interpretation

Test	Normal	Conductive deafness	SN deafness
Rinnie	AC > BC (Rinnie positive)	BC > AC (Rinnie negative)	AC > BC
Weber	Not lateralized	Lateralized to poorer ear	Lateralized to better ear
ABC	Same as examiner's	Same as examiner's	Reduced
Schwabach	Equal	Lengthened	Shortened

Section 1: Ear

18. Ans. is d i.e. False negative Rinne's test *Ref. Dhingra, 6/e, p22*

In the above question: Patient was suffering from suppurative labyrinthitis which was not treated and led to total loss of hearing, i.e. severe SNHL.

In severe SNHL: Rinne's test is false negative and because labyrinth is dead. Fistula test is negative.

False negative Rinne test as explained earlier occurs in case of severe SNHL because patient does not perceive any sound of tuning fork by air conduction but responds to bone conduction due to intracranial transmission of sound from opposite healthy ear.

Fistula Test

The basis of this test is to induce nystagmus by producing pressure changes in the external canal which are then transmitted to the labyrinth. Stimulation of the labyrinth results in nystagmus and vertigo. Normally the test is negative because the pressure changes in the EAC cannot be transmitted to the labyrinth.

Positive Fistula Test is seen in:
- Erosion of horizontal semicircular canal (Cholesteatoma or fenestration operation)
- Abnormal opening in oval window (post stapedectomy fistula) or round window (rupture of round window).

> **A positive fistula test also implies that the labyrinth is still functioning.**
> - False-negative fistula test: Dead labyrinth, cholesteatoma covering site of fistula.
> - False-positive fistula test (Positive fistula test without Fistula): Congenital syphilis, 25% cases of Meniere's disease (Hennebert's sign.)

19. Ans. is b i.e. Air conduction in left ear *Ref. Dhingra 6/e, p 30, 51; Current Otolaryngology 2/e, p 597*

20. Ans. is a i.e. Air conduction of right ear.
For symbols used in audiometry—*See the preceding text*

21. Ans. is b i.e. Neural deafness *Ref. Dhingra 4/e, p 28, 5/e, p31*

> **Tone decay test is** a measure of nerve fatigue *(i.e. neural deafness)* and is used to detect retrocochlear lesions. A decay of more than 25 dB is diagnostic of retro cochlear lesion.
> **Method of doing the test and principle:** A continuous tone of 5 dB above threshold in 500 Hz and 2000 Hz is given to the ear and person should be able to hear it for 60 sec. The result is expressed as dB by which intensity has to be increased so that the patient car – hear the sound for 60 sec. If tone decay of >25 dB is present, it indicates retrocochlear leison, e.g.—acoustic neuroma.

22. Ans. is b. i.e. Impedance audiometry *Ref. Dhingra 6th/ed, p24; Tuli 1st/ed, p31-35*

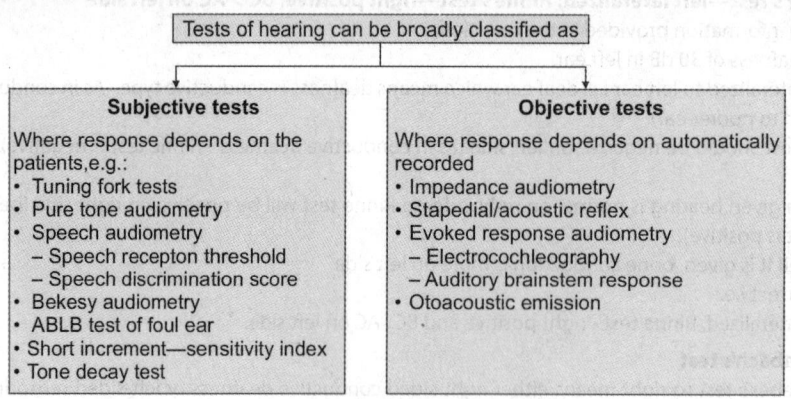

23. Ans. is b i.e. Middle ear

24. Ans. is a i.e. 220 Hz

25. Ans. is b i.e. Impedance audiometry. *Ref. Dhingra 6/e, p 24; Current Otolaryngology 2/e, p 601*

Impedance Audiotmetry

1. It is an objective test for hearing^Q
2. It is very useful in children for assessing the hearing loss.^Q
3. It consists of tympanometry and acoustic reflex

Tympanometry is a measure of the condition of the middle ear at the level of tympanic membrane.

Chapter 4: Assessment of Hearing Loss

Note:
- For infants and neonates, tympanograms obtained using a 220 Hz probe may erroneously appear normal.
  ∴ a higher frequency probe tone (660 or 1000 Hz) must be used.
  Ref. Current Otolaryngology 2nd/ed p601

26. **Ans. is b. i.e. Done in silent room** *Ref. P.L.Dhingra 6/e,pgs23; Logan Turner 10/e,pgs248-49; Textbook of ENT by Maqbool 11/e,pgs134-36*
    Pure Tone Audiometry
    - Usually air conduction thresholds are measured for tones of 125, 250, 1000, 2000, 4000 & 8000 Hz & bone conduction thresholds for 250, 500, 1000, 2000, 4000 Hz (i.e. option a is correct)
    - In a soundproof room, the patient's ability to hear pure tones in the frequency range of about 125 to 8000 Hz is measured
    - **Symbols on audiogram**: Red "0" represents air conduction for the right ear while blue "X" represents air conduction for the left ear. The symbol of > is for bone conduction of the right ear and symbol < for bone conduction of the left ear.

27. **Ans. is b i.e. Ototoxicity** *Ref. Scott Brown 7/e Vol. 3, p 3572; Audiology by Ross J. Roeser, Michael Valente, Holly Hosford-Dunn 2/e, p 242; Ototoxicity by Peter S. Roland, John A. Rutka, p 154*

    High frequency audiometry

    Conventional audiometry tests frequencies between 0.25 kHz - 8 kHz, whereas high frequency audiometry tests in the region of **8 kHz-20 kHz**. Some environmental factors, such as ototoxic medication like aminoglycosides and noise exposure, appear to be more detrimental to high frequency sensitivity than to that of mid or low frequencies. Therefore, high frequency audiometry is an effective method of monitoring losses that are suspected to have been caused by these factors. It is also effective in detecting the auditory sensitivity changes that occur with aging

Note: Ototoxic drugs like aminoglycosides typically affecting higher-frequency hearing first and progressing to lower frequencies.

Remember
- Otoacoustic emissions (OAE) are more sensitive at detecting auditory dysfunction than high-frequency pure tone audiometry. OAEs also have the added advantage of being practical at bedside and do not require a soundproof room.
- Distortion product OAEs are more sensitive than transient evoked OAEs for the detection of early signs of ototoxicity.

28. **Ans. is b i.e. As** *Ref. Dhingra 6/e, p 87*

    Bilateral hearing loss
    +
    Occurring in a female
    +
    25 years of age
    +
    Accentuation of hearing loss during pregnancy
    } → All these features indicate toward **otosclerosis** as the cause of deafness

    Inotosclerosis as type of curve is seen.

29. **Ans. is a and c i.e. ASOM; and Serous otitis media**
30. **Ans. is a i.e. Serous otitis media**
31. **Ans is d i.e. Middle ear fluid** *Ref. Dhingra 6/e, p 24*
    - **Flat (or dome-shaped)** tympanogram is type B curve of tympanogram which is seen in case of fluid in middle ear.
    - **Fluid (i.e. pus)** is seen in case of ASOM and sterile non purulent effusion is seen in case of serous otitis media. So, in both these conditions flat tympanogram/type B tympanogram will be seen.

32. **Ans. is d i.e. Low compliance** *Ref. Scott Brown 7/e Vol. 3, p 3458, Dhingra 6/e, p 87*
    This is a very interesting question – They are testing our knowledge as well as application ability.
    Osteogenesis imperfecta is associated with otosclerosis.
    Van der Hoeve syndrome is a triad of:

    Otosclerosis
       △
    Osteogenesis   Blue
    imperfecta   sclera

Hence – indirectly they are seen asking the type of tympanogram in otosclerosis.

Types of Tympanogram	
Type A	Normal tympanogram
Type AS	Low-compliance tympanogram—Seen in case of fixation of ossicles, i.e. otosclerosis or malleus fixation
Type Ad	High-compliance tympanogram—seen in case of ossicular discontinuityy or laxed tympanic membrane
Type B	Flat/Dome-shaped tympanogram—seen in case of middle ear fluid or tympanic membrane perforation
Type C	Negative compliance tympanogram—seen in case of retracted tympanic membrane

33. **Ans. is b i.e. Ad type tympanogram** *Ref. Dhingra 5/e, p 27, 30 and 34*

This is also a very interesting question:
- The question says. Pure tone audiometry shows an air bone gap of 55 dB in the right ear with normal cochlear reserve.
- The air-bone gap in pure tone audiometry is a measure of total conductive deafness.
- Hence – it means there is a conductive deafness of 55 dB in the right ear.
- Next the question says – Patient has intact tympanic membrane so we have to look for a cause of this 55 dB conductive deafness.

Average hearing loss seen in different lesions of conductive apparatus	*Ref. Dhingra 5th/ed p34*
1. Complete obstruction of ear canal	30 dB
2. Perforation of tympanic membrane	10–40 dB
3. Ossicular interruption with intact drum	54 dB
4. Ossicular interruption with perforation	10–25 dB
5. Closure of oval window	60 dB

As is clear from above table – with tympanic membrane intact and a hearing loss of 55 dB is seen if ossicular chain is disrupted.
Hence– it is a case of ossicular discontinuity.
Tympanogram seen in ossicular discontinuity is a high compliance tympanogram i.e. Ad tympanogram.

34. **Ans. is c i.e. Otoacoustic emissions (OAE)**

35. **Ans. is b i.e. Brainstem evoked response audiometry (BERA)** *Ref. Logan and Turner's 10/e, p 251, 410-415;*
Anirban Biswas Clinical Audio Vestibulometry 3/e, p 68, 99; Dhingra 4/e, p 117; 5/e, p 32, 132

36. **Ans. is c i.e. Evoked OAE**

Remember in children and infants:
- **Best screening test for detecting hearing loss-Otoacoustic emission**
- **Best confirmatory test is BERA.**
- OAE is considered as best screening test as it is less time consuming, easy to perform, child does not need to be sedated and results are available immediately
- Absent OAE indicates cochlear lesion.
- If OAE are absent child is taken up for BERA which is confirmatory.

Extra Edge

Types of Otoacoustic Emissions		
Spontaneous OAE (SOAEs)	Sounds emitted without an acoustic stimulus (spontaneously)	SOAEs are seen in 25–80% of neonates with normal hearing and absence of SOAEs is not necessarily abnormal
Transient evoked OAE (TEOAEs)	Sounds emitted in response to an acoustic stimuli of very short duration; usually clicks but can be tone-bursts	TOAEs commonly are used to screen infant hearing to validate behavioral or electrophysiologic auditory thresholds, and to assess cochlear function
Distortion product OAE (DPOAEs)	Sounds emitted in response to 2 simultaneous tones of different frequencies	Particularly useful for early detection of cochlear damage as they are for ototoxicity and noise-induced damage.
Sustained frequency OAE (SFOAEs)	Sounds emitted in response to a continuous tone	SFOAEs are responses recorded to a continuous tone

37. **Ans. is a, c and d i.e. Are by product of outer hair call, used as a screening test of hearing in newborn infant and useful in ototoxicity monitoring.**
Read the text for explanation

Chapter 4: Assessment of Hearing Loss

38. **Ans. is a i.e. Brainstem evoked response audiometry** *Ref. Dhingra 6/e, p 26*
    BERA is very useful in distinguishing between cochlear pathology and retrocochlear pathology for SNHL
    Impedance audiometry and PTA tests the middle ear pathology.

39. **Ans. is c i.e. Lateral lemniscus** *Ref. Dhingra 6/e, p 27, Scott Brown 7/e Vol. 3, p 3283*
    - In normal persons during BERA testing, 7 waves are produced in the first 10 milli seconds
    - The 1st, 3rd and 5th wave are the most stable and are used in measurements
    - These waves are studied for:
        - Absolute latency
        - Inter wave latency (between wave I and V)
        - Amplitude

Site of Origin of Waves			
Wave	I	Distal part of (**E**ighth nerve)	**E**
Wave	II	Proximal part of **E**ighth cranial nerve	**E**
Wave	III	**C**ochlear nucleus	**C**
Wave	IV	Superior **o**livary complex	**O**
Wave	V	**L**ateral lemniscus	**L**
Wave and	VI VII	**I**nferior colliculus	**I**

    Mnemonic **EE COLI**

40. **Ans. is d i.e. ABC test** *Ref. Dhingra, 6/e, p 22*
    - As discussed earlier absolute bone conduction test is a tuning fork test in which bone conduction of the patient is compared with BC of the examiner after occluding the external auditory meatus of both patient and examiner
    - Bone conduction is a measure of cochlear function.
    Hence, ABC test is used to detect damage to cochlea.
    Rinne's test ⎫
    Weber's test ⎭ — Measure air conduction
    Caloric test – assesses vestibular function

41. **Ans. is a i.e. Middle ear** *Ref. Dhingra 5/e, p 26*
    Threshold for air conduction is increased *(i.e. low frequency sounds are not heard well)* whereas that of bone conduction in normal, i.e. Bone conduction > air conduction which is seen in conductive deafness. Conductive deafness occurs in lesions of either external ear, tympanic membrane, middle ear or ossicles up to stapediovestibular joint.

42. **Ans. is d i.e. VII and VIII nerves** *Ref. Dhingra 6/e, p 25*

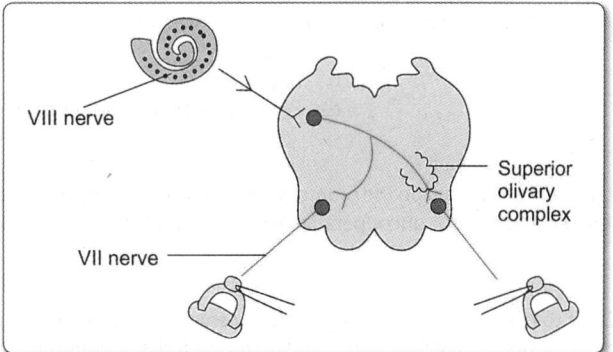

43. **Ans. is c i.e. Inferior vestibular nerve** *Ref. Current Otolaryngology 3/e, p 641*

    Vestibular Evoked Myogenic Potentials
    - The vestibular evoked myogenic potential (VEMP) are short latency electromyograms that are evoked by acoustic stimuli in high intensity and recorded from surface electrodes over the tonically contracted sternocleido mastoid muscle.
    - The origin of VEMP is the saccule.
    - The response pathway consists of:
        - Saccule; Inferior Vestibular Nerve, Lateral Vestibular Nucleus, Lateral Vestibulospinal Tract and Sternocleidomastoid muscle.
    - The test provides diagnostic information about saccular and/or inferior vestibular nerve function.
    - An intact middle ear is required for the response quality.

Waveform of the response

The VEMP waveform is characterized by a
- Wave I – positive peak at 13-15 (p13)
- Wave II – negative peak at 21-24 ms (p23)

Peak to peak amplitude of p13-23 is measured and asymmetries between the right and left side is noted (by calculating asymmetry ratio AR)

Abnormal AR is seen a case of:
- Saccular hydrops (AR > 36%)
- Vestibular schwannoma originating from inferior vestibular nerve.
- Vestibular neuronitis
- Superior canal dehiscence syndrome.

44. **Ans. is b i.e. Outer hair cells are mainly responsible for cochlear microphonix and summation potential.**

Ref. Mohan Bansal, Textbook of Diseases of ENT 1/e, p 24,25 and 145

45. **Ans. is d i.e. Evoked potential generated in cochlea are auditory nerve**

Electrocochleography (EcoG) **measures electrical potentials, which arise in cochlea and CN VIII (Auditory nerve)** in response to auditory stimuli within first 5 milliseconds. It consists of following three types of responses:
1. Cochlear microphonics
2. Summating potentials
3. Action potential of 8th nerve

Endocochlear potential, cochlear microphonics (CM) and summating potential (SP) are from cochlea while the compound action potential (AP) is from the cochlear nerve fibers. Both CM and SP are receptor potentials similar to other sensory end-organs.

- **Endocochlear Potential:** This resting potential of +80 mV direct current (DC) is recorded from scala media. This energy source for cochlear transduction is generated from stria vascularis by Na+/K+ -ATPase pump. Endolymph has high K+ concentration. It acts as a battery and helps in driving the current through the hair cells when they move after exposure to any sound stimulus.
- **Cochlear Microphonics:** Cochlear microphonics (CM) is an alternating current (AC) potential. Basilar membrane moves in response to sound stimulus. Changes occur in electrical resistance at the tips of OHC. Flow of K+ through the outer hair cells produces voltage fluctuations and called CM.

  Cochlear microphonics is absent in the part of cochlea where the outer hair cells are damaged.
- **Summating Potential:** Summating potential (SP) is a DC potential, which may be either negative or positive. It is produced by hair cells. It follows the "envelop" of stimulating sound and is superimposed on cochlear nerve action potential. This is a rectified derivative of sound signal. Probably it arises from IHCs with a small contribution from OHCs.

  Summating potential of cochlea helps in the diagnosis of Ménière's diseases.
- **Compound (Auditory Nerve) Action Potential:** It is the neural discharge of auditory nerve. It follows all or none phenomena so has all or none response to auditory nerve fibers. Each nerve fiber has optimum stimulus frequency for which the threshold is lowest. Amplitude increases while latency decreases with intensity over 40–50 dB range. The following features differentiate it from CM and SP:
    a. No gradation
    b. Latency
    c. Propagation
    d. Post-response refractory period

Method

The recording electrode (a thin needle) is placed on the promontory through the tympanic membrane. The test can be done under local anesthesia, however, children and anxious uncooperative adults need sedation or general anesthesia which has no effect on EcoG responses.

Uses

The main application of ECOG is to help determine if a patient has Meniere's disease. The amplitude of the summating potential (reflecting activity of the hair cells) is compared with that of the compound action potential (reflecting whole nerve activity). If the ratio is larger than normal (0.3-0.5), it is considered indicative of Meniere's disease. The procedure is considered valid only the patient is symptomatic. Now with this background lets analyze each option separately—
- **Option a** – is incorrect as ECOG is a measure of electrical potential of inner ear (and not middle ear latency).
- **Option b** – is correct as explained above – Outer hair cells are mainly responsible for cochlear microphonics and Summation Potential.
- **Option c** – is incorrect as it is not the summating potential but the action potential which is a compound of synchronous auditory nerve potential.
- **Option d** – is incorrect as Action Potential represents neural potential and not the endocochlear receptor potential which is represented by components arising from organ of corti that i.e. SP and cochlear microphonics.

46. **Ans. is a i.e. Stenger test**
    Nonorganic hearing loss: The term implies that there is no organic cause of hearing loss but the person is malingering. The tests to detect malingering

    - Stenger test
    - Lombard test
    - Stapedial reflex
    - Speech audiometry
    - BERA

47. **Ans. is a i.e. Sensorineural hearing loss of 45 dB in left ear and normal right ear** *Ref. Dhingra 6/e, p 22*
    Sensorineural hearing loss of 45 dB in left ear and normal right ear–will show a positive Rinne's test not the negative.

    > **Remember**
    > Rinne test is positive in normal persons and in SNHL. It is negative in case of conductive hearing loss. Negative Rinne may also be seen in case of prefound SNHL.

    Sensorineural hearing loss of 45 dB in left ear and normal right ear—will show a **positive Rinne's test in both the ears**.
    Conductive hearing loss of 40 dB in both ears will show **negative Rinne's test** in **both the ears**.
    Conductive hearing loss of 40 dB in right ear and left ear normal will show a **positive Rinne's test in left ear** and **negative in right ear**.
    Profound hearing loss may show **a false negative Rinne's test** in the **right ear**.

48. **Ans. is a i.e. As** *Ref. Dhingra 4/e, p 25, 88*
    A **35 years old pregnant female complained of hearing loss,** which was **aggravated during pregnancy**. This patient is most probably suffering from **otosclerosis**, which is **more common in females** and **aggravated during pregnancy**.
    Type As tympanogram is seen in otosclerosis

    > "People of African-American descent rarely have otosclerosis — it is usually a condition found in persons of Caucasian or Oriental descent. Women are affected twice as often as men, and pregnancy often has an adverse effect. Otosclerosis is often discovered during or just after pregnancy. The effect of hormone supplements postmenopause is unknown."-http://american-hearing.org/disorders/otosclerosis/

    "A retrospective study has been made of a sample of 479 women with deafness from otosclerosis, classified according to the number of pregnancies they have had and whether there had been a subjective impression of deterioration of hearing during or immediately after at least 1 pregnancy. The study confirms previous reports that pregnancy does involve a risk of aggravating deafness in clinical otosclerosis."-http://www.ncbi.nlm.nih.gov/pubmed/6883784

Types of Tympanogram	
Type A	• **Normal** tympanogram
Type A_s	• Compliance is lower at or near ambient air pressure • Seen in **fixation of ossicles**, e.g. **Otosclerosis**[Q] or **Malleus fixation**[Q]
Type A_D	• High compliance at or near ambient pressure • Seen in **ossicular discontinuity**[Q] or **thin and lax tympanic membrane**[Q]
Type B	• A flat or dome-shaped graph. No change in compliance with pressure changes • Seen in **middle ear fluid**[Q] or **thick tympanic membrane**[Q]
Type C	• Maximum compliance occurs with negative pressure in excess of 100 mm of H_2O. • Seen in **retracted tympanic membrane**[Q] and may show **some fluid in middle ear**[Q]

Chapter 5

Assessment of Vestibular Function

Derangement of vestibular system is indicated by:
- **Vertigo**
- **Nystagmus**

VERTIGO

It is hallucination of movement, i.e. one feels as if a person is moving as compared to his surroundings or vice versa.

Disorders of Vestibular System

Disorders of vestibular system causing vertigo can be divided into:
1. **Peripheral causes** are causes which involve vestibular end organs and their 1st order neurons (i.e. the vestibular nerve). The pathology lies in the internal ear or the VIII nerve. They are responsible for 85% of all cases of vertigo.
2. **Central causes**—which involve CNS after the entrance of vestibular nerve in the brainstem and involve vestibulo ocular and other pathways.

Causes of Vertigo

Peripheral
- Meniere's disease
- Benign Paroxysmal Positional Vertigo
- Vestibular neuronitis
- Labyrinthitis
- Vestibulotoxic drugs
- Head trauma
- Perilymph fistula
- Syphilis
- Acoustic neuroma

Central
- Vertebrobasilar insufficiency
- Posterior inferior cerebellar artery syndrome
- Basilar migraine
- Cerebellar disease
- Multiple sclerosis
- Epilepsy
- Tumors of brainstem and fourth ventricle

Note:
BPPV

It is a condition in which otoconia/debris get dislodged and moves from the utricle into posterior semicircular canal. It is characterized by vertigo when head is placed in a certain critical position, such that posterior semicircular canal comes in a dependent position. The vertigo disappears when the debris settles down in 10–20 seconds.

There is no hearing loss or other associated neurologic symptom. The diagnosis is made by **Dix-Hallpike maneuver**. Treatment of BPPV is by **Epley's maneuver**.

NYSTAGMUS

It is involuntary, rhythmical, oscillatory movements of eyes away from direction of gaze.
- Nystagmus is produced due to stimulation of semicircular canals. The direction of nystagmus depends on the plane of canal being stimulated. The nystagmus is horizontal from horizontal (lateral) canal, rotatory from superior semicircular canal and vertical from posterior semicircular canal.
- Peripheral nystagmus is due to lesions of labyrinth and CN VIII while central vestibular nystagmus is due to lesions in central neural pathways (vestibular nuclear, brainstem and cerebellum).
- In irritative lesions or stimulation of labyrinth (BPPV), the direction of nystagmus is towards the side of lesion.
- In paretic lesions (trauma to labyrinth, damage to CN VIII) nystagmus is in opposite direction.

Nystagmus has 2 components
- Quick (fast) component
- Slow component

Note:
- Nystagmus is named after quick component.
- It is eliminated under the effect of anesthesia.

Tests for Vestibular Functions: For Spontaneous Nystagmus

Clinical tests	Laboratory test
• Fistula test[Q]	• Caloric test
• Romberg test	– Cold caloric tests with ice cold water modified (Kobrak's test)
• Gait	– Fitzgerald-Hallpike test (Bithermal caloric test)
• Past-pointing and falling[Q]	– Temperature of water used is + 7°C from normal body temperature
• Hallpike maneuver (positional test)	– Cold-air caloric test by Dundas-Grant method. Done in case of perforation of tympanic membrane.
	• Electronystagmography
	• Optokinetic test
	• Rotation test
	• Galvanic test[Q]
	• Posturography

Chapter 5: Assessment of Vestibular Function

> **Point to Remember**
> - **Fistula test** is done by pressing the tragus and alternately releasing it or by compression of air by Siegle's speculum. Positive test is indicated by vertigo and nystagmus and signifies presence of fistulous communication between middle ear and labyrinth. Negative test signifies normal ear or dead labyrinth. Positive test is seen in case of (1) Labyrinthine fistula (2) Perilymphatic fistula, i.e opening in oval or round window (3) Fenestration operation.
> - **Galvanic test** is the only vestibular test which helps in differentiating an end organ lesion from that of vestibular nerve leison.
> - **Hennebert's sign:** This is positive fistula test in the absence of fistula. The causes include congenital syphilis (utricular adhesions to stapes) and some cases of Meniere's disease.
> - **Romberg's sign:** It is indicative of not the cerebellum lesions but the dorsal column (somatosensory) lesions.
> - **Frenzel glass:** Nystagmus is best observed in the darkened room by illuminated Frenzel glass, which is nothing but a 20 diopters lens.
> - **Causes of ipsilateral (same direction) nystagmus:** Irrigation of ear with warm water and serous labyrinthitis.
> - **Causes of contralateral (opposite direction) nystagmus:** Purulent labyrinthitis, labyrinthectomy and irrigation of ear with cold water.
> - **Dix-Hallpike maneuver:** DIX-Hallpike maneuver is done is BPPV. The patients head is turned 45° right and then later left, while patient is sitting and then repeated with patient lying supine and his head hanging 30° below the horizontal. **The test is reported positive, if while doing this maneuver, vertical upbeat nystagmus occurs.**
> - **Fitzgerald Hallpike Bithermal caloric test:** The lateral (horizontal) semicircular canal (SCC) is stimulated (tested) by irrigating cold (30°C) and warm (44°C) water in the external auditory canal. Cold water induces opposite side nystagmus while warm water results into the same side nystagmus [COWS (Cold, opposite, Warm, same)]. In a sitting position with head tilted 60° backward, lateral semicircular canal is stimulated during caloric testing. To bring the lateral SCC in vertical position, patient's head is raised 30° forward if she is in supine position but in a sitting position the head is tilted 60° backward..

NEW PATTERN QUESTIONS

Q N1. True about central nystagmus is:
a. Duration not limited
b. Direction fixed
c. Latency present
d. Suppressed by visual fixation

Q N2. True about peripheral nystagmus is:
a. Duration not limited
b. Direction fixed
c. No latency
d. Vertigo not present

Q N3. BPPV of posterior semicircular canal produces:
a. Horizontal nystagmus
b. Pure vertical nystagmus
c. Pendular nystagmus
d. Torsional vertical nystagmus

Q N4. Dunda's grant apparatus is used in:
a. Cold air caloric test
b. Fitzgerald Hallpike's test
c. Bithermal caloric test
d. Rinne test

Q N5. M/C type of nystagmus seen in central vestibular lesions:
a. Pure vertical
b. Pure horizontal
c. Pure torsional
d. Vertical and torsional

Q N6. Which of the following is being done in the figure?

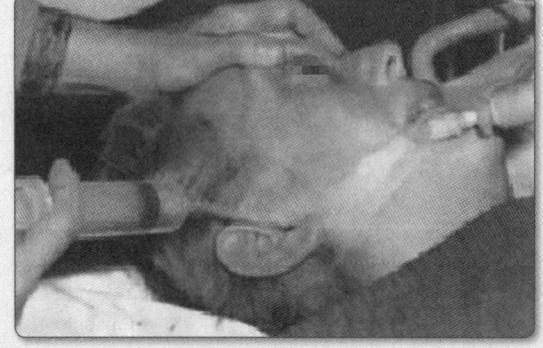

See Color Plate 5

a. Determining Eustachian tube patency
b. Testing vestibulo-ocular reflex by injecting cold water
c. Politzerization
d. Syringe of ear in patient with CSOM and meningitis

Q N7. Fistula test stimulates:
a. Lateral SCC
b. Posterior SCC
c. Anterior SCC
d. Cochlea

Q N8. False positive fistula test is associated with:
a. Perilymph fistula
b. Malignant sclerosis
c. Congenital syphilis
d. Cholesteatoma

Section 1: Ear

Q N9. Identify the procedure being done in the figure:

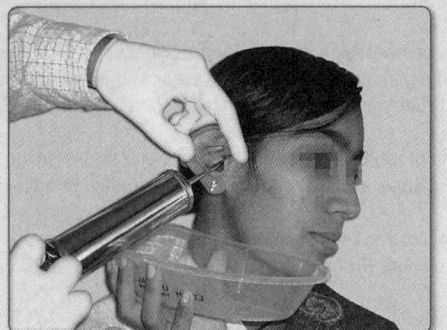

See Color Plate 6

a. Determining Eustachian tube patency
b. Syringing
c. Politzerization
d. Fitzgerald test

Q N10. Identify the instrument shown in the figure:

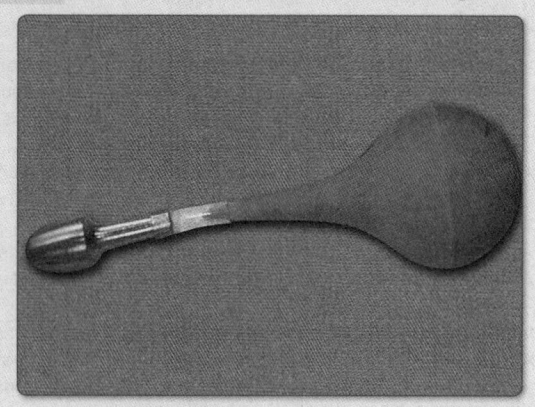

See Color Plate 7

a. Otoendoscope   b. Siegel speculum
c. Politzer bag   d. Otoscope

Explanations and References to New Pattern Questions

N1. Ans. is a i.e. Duration not limited

N2. Ans. is b i.e Direction fixed   *Ref. Essential of Mohan Bansal, p 133*

Distinguishing characteristics of peripheral and central vertigo

Features	Peripheral vertigo	Central vertigo
Nystagmus		
Type	Combined horizontal and torsional	Purely vertical (most common), horizontal, or torsional
Direction	One direction	May change direction
Visual fixation	Inhibits	No change
Fatigable	Yes	No
Latency	Present	Absent
Imbalance	Mild to moderate but able to walk	Severe and unable to stand or walk
Nausea and vomiting	Usually present and severe	Varies
Hearing loss, tinnitus	Common	Rare
Neurologic symptoms (motor and sensory deficiencies, ataxia, Horner's syndrome)	Absent	Common
Recovery	Begins within days	Slow
Head thrust sign	Present	Absent
Common causes	Benign paroxysmal positional vertigo, vestibular neuritis, Meniere's disease, trauma to labyrinth, infection and drugs	Vertebrobasilar insufficiency, cerebrovascular accidents, multiple sclerosis, brain tumors and cerebellar disorders

Friends Note: Peripheral nystagmus has both torsional and either horizontal component or vertical component whereas central nystagmus has single component.

N3. Ans. is d i.e. Torsional vertical nystagmus   *Ref. Essentials of Mohan Bansal, p 132*
Torsional nystagmus with vertical or horizontal component: signifies peripheral cause of nystagmus.

Chapter 5: Assessment of Vestibular Function

> **Remember**
> - BPPV of posterior semicircular canal leads to combined vertical upbeat and torsional nystagmus
> - BPPV of superior semicircular canal lesion leads to torsional vertical downbeat nystagmus
> - Horizontal semicircular canal lesion leads to torsional horizontal nystagmus

Only vertical or horizontal nystagmus without torsion or only torsional without vertical and horizontal nystagmus is seen in central causes of nystagmus.

> **Point to Remember**
> - Pure vertical nystagmus is seen in medullary pons or cerebellar lesions or vertebrobasilar insufficiency.
> - Purely downbeating vertical nystagmus is seen in cerebellar degenerative lesions and Arnold Chiari malformation.
> - Purely upbeating vertical—is seen in lesions of pontomedullary junction, pons and midbrain
> - Purely rotatory seen in syringomyelia and pendular syringomyelia
> - Pure horizontal nystagmus is seen in cerebral lesions.

N4. Ans. is a i.e. Cold air caloric test *Ref. Dhingra 6/e, p 43; Essential of ENT, Mohan Bansal, p 134*

Cold caloric test—employs **Dundas Grant tube**, which is a coiled tube wrapped in cloth. The air in the tube is cooled by pouring ethyl chloride and then blown into the ear.

N5. Ans. is a i.e Pure vertical *Ref. Essentials of ENT, Mohan Bansal, p 132*

Central lesions always lead to pure nystagmus.
The M/C variety being purely vertical (mostly in down beating direction).
Vertical and rotatory nystagmus indicate peripheral cause of nystagmus like BPPV.

N6. Ans. is b i.e Testing vestibulo-oculo reflex by injecting cold water

N7. Ans. is a i.e Lateral semicircular canal *Ref. Tuli 1/e, p 939*

Fistula test stimulates lateral semicircular canal.

N8. Ans. is c i.e Congenital syphilis

False fistula test	Seen in
1. False positive fistula test **(Hennebert sign)**	- Congenital syphilis (here stapes footplate is hypermobile, so even small pressure changes in ear, can lead to excessive movement of stapes footplate and excessive stimulation of utricular macula - 25% cases of Meniere's disease (in these 25% cases, fibrous bands are formed connecting the utricular macule to stapes footplate
2. False negative test	- It is seen when cholesteatoma covers the site of fistula and does not allow pressure changes to be transmitted to the labyrinth

N9. Ans. is b i.e Syringing

The process being done in the figure is syringing. The auricle is pulled upward and backward and direction of ear syringe is postero-superior.

N10. Ans. is c i.e Politzer bag

QUESTIONS

1. Which of the following statement regarding eustachian tube dysfunction is wrong? [AP 2000]
    a. Undistorted light image on the anterior quadrant of tympanic membrane
    b. No movement of the tympanic membrane on Siegel's method
    c. Malleus is easily visible
    d. Lusterless tympanic membrane
2. Common cause of Eustachian diseases is due:
    a. Adenoids   b. Siegle's
    c. Otitis media   d. Pharyngitis
3. All are tests to check Eustachian tube patency *except*: [AIIMS]
    a. Valsalva maneuver   b. Fistula's test
    c. Frenzel's maneuver   d. Tonybee's maneuver
4. Eustachian tube function is best assessed by: [AIIMS May 2015]
    a. Politzer test
    b. VEMP
    c. Rhinomanometry
    d. Tympanometry
5. Positive Romberg test with eyes closed detects defect in: [AIIMS May 09]
    a. Proprioceptive pathway   b. Cerebellum
    c. Spinothalamic tract   d. Peripheral nerve
6. Site of lesion in unilateral past pointing nystagmus is: [AIIMS June 97]
    a. Posterior semicircular canal
    b. Superior semicircular canal
    c. Flocculonodular node
    d. Cerebellar hemisphere
7. Post-traumatic vertigo is due to: [PGI June 06, 03]
    a. Perilymphatic fistula
    b. Vestibular neuritis
    c. Secondary endolymphatic hydrops
    d. Ossicular discontinuity
    e. Benign positional vertigo
8. Positional vertigo is: [UP 2001]
    a. Lateral   b. Superior
    c. Inferior   d. Posterior
9. What is the treatment for Benign Positional vertigo? [APPG 06]
    a. Vestibular exercises   b. Vestibular sedatives
    c. Antihistamines   d. Diuretics
10. Latest treatment in BPPV is: [Kerala 03]
    a. Intralabyrinthine streptomycin
    b. Intralabyrinthine steroids
    c. Valsava maneuver
    d. None of the above
11. Vestibular function is tested by: [PGI Dec 02]
    a. Galvanic stimulation test b. Acoustic reflex
    c. Fistula test   d. Impedance audiometry
    e. Cold caloric test
12. On otological examination all of the following will have positive fistula test *except*: [AI 02]
    a. Dead ear
    b. Labyrinthine fistula
    c. Hypermobile stapes footplate
    d. Following fenestration surgery
13. A positive fistula test during Siegelization indicates: [2000]
    a. Ossicular discontinuity
    b. Paralabyrinthitis due to erosion of lateral semicircular canal
    c. CSF leak through the ear
    d. Fixation of stapes bone
14. False positive fistula test is associated with: (TN 2005)
    a. Perilymph fistula   b. Malignant sclerosis
    c. Congenital syphilis d. Cholesteatoma
15. Hallpike test is done for: [DNB 2002]
    a. Vestibular function   b. Corneal test
    c. Cochlear function   d. Audiometry
16. Fitzgerald's caloric test uses temperature at: [JIPMER 92]
    a. 30°C and 44°C   b. 34°C and 41°C
    c. 33°C and 21°C   d. 37°C and 41°C
17. At what angle is Hallpike thermal caloric test done: [APPGI 06]
    a. 15°   b. 30°
    c. 45°   d. 60°
18. Cold caloric test stimulates: [AP 2008]
    a. Cochlea
    b. Lateral semicircular canal
    c. Posterior semicircular canal
    d. All of the above
19. In 'cold caloric stimulation test1, the cold water, induces movement of the eye ball in the following direction:
    a. Towards the opposite side   [AI 99]
    b. Towards the same side
    c. Upwards
    d. Downwards
20. In Fitzgerald Hallpike differential caloric test, cold-water irrigation at 30 degrees centigrade in the left ear in a normal person will include: [2000]
    a. Nystagmus to the right side
    b. Nystagmus to the left side
    c. Direction changing nystagmus
    d. Positional nystagmus
21. Which of the following is not true of caloric test? [MH 2005]
    a. Induction of nystagmus by thermal stimulation
    b. Normally, cold water induces nystatmus to opposite side and warm water to same side.
    c. In canal paresis the test is inconclusive
    d. None of the above

Chapter 5: Assessment of Vestibular Function

22. **Caloric test has:** *[Delhi 96]*
    a. Slow component only
    b. Fast component only
    c. Slow + Fast component
    d. Fast component occasionally
23. **Spontaneous vertical nystagmus is seen in the lesion of:** *[Kolkata 2005]*
    a. Midbrain
    b. Labyrinth
    c. Vestibule
    d. Cochlea
24. **True about central nystagmus:**
    a. Horizontal
    b. Direction fixed
    c. Direction changes
    d. Not suppressed by visual fixation
    e. Suppressed by visual fixation
25. **Third window effect is seen in:** *[AIIMS Nov 2012]*
    a. Perforated tympanum
    b. Dehiscent superior semicircular canal
    c. Round window
    d. Oval window
26. **Features of superior canal dehiscence are:** *[PGI 2010]*
    a. Positive Romberg's sign
    b. Positive Tullio's phenomenon
    c. Positive Hennebert's sign
    d. Oscillopsia
    e. Positive Dix-Hallpike Maneuver
27. **Vertigo is defined as:** *[FMGE 2013]*
    a. Subjective sense of imbalance
    b. Objective sense of imbalance
    c. Both of the above
    d. Round movement
28. **Calorie test based on thermal stimulation stimulates of which part of the semi circular canals:** *[FMGE 2013]*
    a. Posterior
    b. Anterior
    c. Lateral
    d. All of the above
29. **Nystagmus is associated with all *except*:** *[AP 2003]*
    a. Cerebellar disease
    b. Vestibular disease
    c. Cochlear disease
    d. Arnold Chiari malformation
30. **Spontaneous pure vertical nystagmus is seen in the lesion of:** *[Kolkata 2005]*
    a. Medulla
    b. Labyrinth
    c. Middle ear
    d. Cochlea
31. **Destruction of right labyrinth causes nystagmus to:** *[DPG 2009]*
    a. Right side
    b. Left side
    c. Pendular nystagmus
    d. No nystagmus
32. **Positional vertigo is due to stimulation of:** *[UP 2001]*
    a. Lateral semicircular canal
    b. Superior semicircular canal
    c. Inferior semicircular canal
    d. Posterior semicircular canal
33. **In cold caloric stimulation test, the cold water, induces movement of the eye ball in the following direction:** *[New Pattern]*
    a. Towards the opposite side
    b. Towards the same side
    c. Upwards
    d. Downwards
34. **Epley's maneuver is done in:** *[New Pattern]*
    a. Positional vertigo
    b. Otosclerosis
    c. ASOM
    d. CSOM
35. **A person has vertigo without CNS involvement. Causes is/are:** *(PGI May 2016)*
    a. Perilymph fistula
    b. Otolithiasis
    c. Vestibular neuritis
    d. Meniere's disease
    e. Multiple sclerosis

Explanations and References

1. **Ans. is a i.e. Undistorted light image on the anterior quadrant of tympanic membrane**
   Ref. Dhingra 5/e, p 66,61; 6/e, p 55, 57-59

   Eustachian Tube Dysfunction
   - Normally Eustachian tube (ET) is closed and opens intermittently during yawning, swallowing and sneezing through active contraction of Tensor vili palatini muscle
   - It serves important functions like

   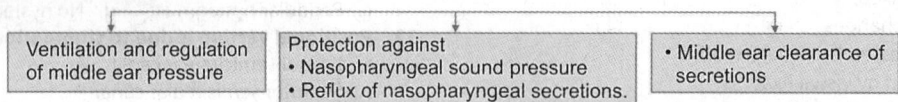

   - When ET is blocked it leads to negative pressure in middle ear and retraction of tympanic membrane.

   Symptoms
   - Otalgia/ear pain[Q]
   - Hearing loss[Q]
   - Popping sensation[Q]
   - Tinnitus
   - Disturbance of equilibrium or vertigo.

   O/E
   - Tympanic membrane is retracted [Q] (i.e. cone of light will be distorted obviously)
   - Congestion along the handle of malleus (i.e. malleus will be easily visible)
   - Transudate will be visible behind the tympanic membrane imparting it an amber color (i.e. it will be lusterless)
   - In severe cases as in barotraumas, there may be visible hemorrhages /hemotympanum or even perforation of the tympanic membrane.

   Friends here it is very important to know **features of Retracted Tympanic membrane:**

1. It appears dull and lusterless
2. Cone of light is absent or interrupted
3. Handle of malleus appears foreshortened
4. Lateral process of malleus becomes more prominent
5. Anterior and posterior malleal folds become sickle shaped.

   So even if we do not know anything about Eustachian tube blockage – then also, by just remembering the features of retracted tympanic membrane, we can solve this one.

2. **Ans. is a i.e Adenoids**
   Ref. Dhingra 5/e, p 67; 6/e, p 60

Eustachian tube dysfunction is commonly caused by:
• Adenoids/allergy
• Barotrauma
• Cleft palate
• Down syndrome
• Nasal condition like: – Polyps
– Sinusitis
– DNS
– Nasopharyngeal tumor/mass

3. **Ans. is b i.e. Fistula's test**
   Ref. Dhingra 5/e, p 65, 66; 6/e, p 59

4. **Ans. is d. i.e. Tympanometry**
   Ref. Essentials of ENT, Mohan Bansal, p47

   This question can be solved even, if we do not know all tests for Eustachian tube patency, because we know fistula test is for assessing vestibular functions and not for Eustachian tube patency. Still it is worthwhile knowing tests for Eustachian tube patency.

Chapter 5: Assessment of Vestibular Function

Tests for Eustachian Tube Patency

Mnemonic	PMT is So Very Furiously Complicated
P	**P**olitzer test[Q]
M	**M**ethylene blue test[Q]
T	**T**oynbee test[Q]
Is	**I**nflation, Deflation test[Q]
So	**So**notubometry[Q]
Very	**V**alsalva test[Q]
Furiously	**F**renzel maneuver[Q]
Complicated	**C**atheterization[Q]
Test	**T**ympanometry

The best test is tympanometry as it can be performed in perforated ear also.

5. **Ans. is a i.e. Proprioceptive pathway** *Ref. Essential of Mohan Bansal, p 134*
   - **The Romberg is a test of proprioceptive function:**
     – "The Romberg test explores for imbalance due to proprioceptive sensory loss. The patient is able to stand with feet together and eyes open but sways or falls with eyes closed; it is one of the earliest sings of posterior column disease."
     – DeJong's the neurologic examination By William Wesley Campbell, Russell N. DeJong, Armin F. Haerer 6/e p 447
   - **Proprioceptive pathway:**
     – Proprioception is the ability to sense the position of one's extremities without the aid of vision.
     – The peripheral sense organs are located in the muscle, tendons, and joints. The first cell body is situated in the dorsal root ganglion, going without a synapse to the ipsilateral fasiculi cuneatus and gracilis (**dorsal column**) to the lower medulla where the synapse occurs. Following a decussation of the internal arcuate fibers, the impulses ascend in the **medial lemniscus** to the thalamus, terminating in the parietal lobe, posterior to those that convey touch.

Note: Romberg's test is not a test of cerebellar function. Patients with cerebellar ataxia will, generally, be unable to balance even with the eyes open.

6. **Ans. is d i.e. Cerebellar hemisphere** *Ref. Ganong 22/e, p 221, 222; Dhingra 6/e, p 46*

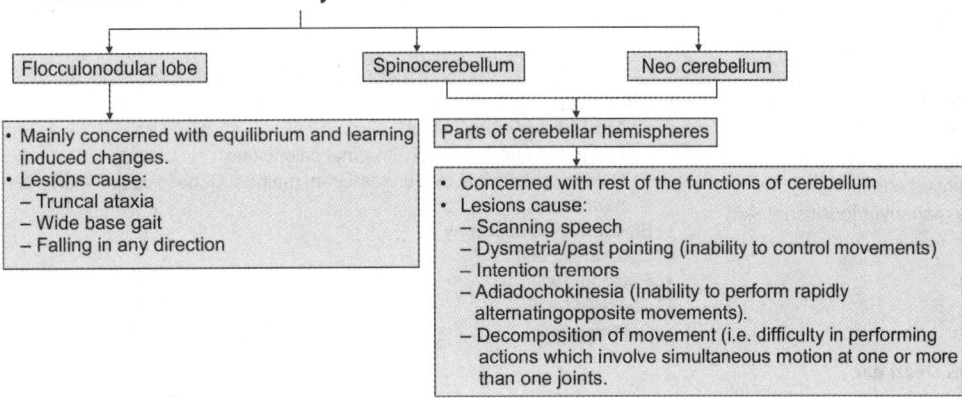

Nystagmus can occur in both midline or hemispheral disease, but past pointing indicates hemispheral lesion.

7. **Ans. is a, c and e i.e. Perilymphatic fistula, Secondary endolymphatic hydrops and Benign positional vertigo**
   Ref. Dhingra 6/e, p 46; Current otolaryngology 2/e, p 714

   Post traumatic vertigo can be seen in:
   - Severe trauma to parietal skull bone
   - Longitudinal temporal bone #   cause concussion of labyrinth or completely
   - Whiplash injury   disrupt bony labyrinth or cause injury of VIII
   - Barotrauma   nerve or cause a perilymphatic fistula
   - Severe acoustic trauma

In case of acoustic trauma vertigo can be due to disturbance in the vestibular end organs, i.e. otolitis.
- **Secondary endolymphatic hydrops** *(secondary Meniere's disease)* is clinical presentation of Meniere's disease viz episodic vertigo, fluctuating hear loss, tinnitus and ear fullness due to conditions like head trauma or ear surgery, viral infection *(measles/mumps)* syphilis and Logan's syndrome.
- **Benign paraxysmal positional vertigo:** It is most common type of peripheral vertigo which arises due to collection of debris in posterior semicircular canal. 20% patients of BPPV have an antecedant h/o head trauma.

8. **Ans. is d i.e. Posterior**
9. **Ans. is a i.e. Vestibular exercises**
10. **Ans. is d i.e. None of the above** *Ref. Dhingra 5/e, p 51; 6/e, p 45; Current Otolaryngology 2/e, p 713, 714*

Benign Paroxysmal Positional Vertigo

- Characterized by vertigo when the head is placed in certain critical position.
- Not associated with hearing loss or any other symptom.
- **Caused by disorder of posterior semicircular canal**^{Q} (generally debris is collected in it)
- Average age of presentation -5th decade
- History of head trauma/ear infections may be present in 20% cases.
- Vertigo is fatiguable
- Vertigo may be associated with nausea
- Characteristic nystagmus (latent, geotropic, fatigable) with Dix Halpike test

Management

Vestibular exercises *(Epley's maneuver)* done to reposition the debris in the utricle is the only current treatment of choice. In some patients labyrinthine sedatives like prochlorperazine, promethazine may be given.

Role of Surgery in BPPV

Surgery is reserved only for those very rare patients who have no benefit from vestibular exercises and have no intracranial pathology on imaging studies.
Surgery of choice: Posterior semicircular canal occlusion.

11. **Ans. is a, c and e i.e. Galvanic stimulation test, Fistula test, and Cold caloric test** *Ref. Dhingra 5/e, p 46-50; 6/e, p 43,44*

Tests for Vestibular Function

Clinical tests	Laboratory test

• Fistula test^Q
 • Romberg test
 • Gait
 • Past-pointing and falling^Q
 • Hallpike maneuver (positional test)
	• Caloric test
	   – Modified (Kobrak's test)
	   – Fitzgerald-Hallpike test (Bithermal caloric test)
	   – Cold-air caloric test by Dundas-Grant method. Done in case of perforation of tympanic membrane.
	 • Electronystagmography
	 • Optokinetic test
	 • Rotation test
	 • Galvanic test^Q
	 • Posturography

12. **Ans. is a i.e. Dead ear**
13. **Ans. is b i.e. Paralabrynthitis due to erosion of lateral semicircular canal** *Ref. Dhingra 5/e, p 46; 6/e, p 41; Tuli 1/e, p 39*

Fistula test is done to Assess the Vestibular Function

- **Basis:** In case of fistulous communication between middle ear and labyrinth
↓
Any pressure change in
External auditory canal (produced by pressing tragus or by Siegel's speculum)
↓
will stimulate lateral semicircular canal *(Ref: Tuli 1/e p. 939)*
↓
Produce nystagmus/vertigo

Chapter 5: Assessment of Vestibular Function

Fistula Test is

Positive	Negative	False positive	False negative
• (Means labyrinth is functioning and a fistulous communication is present between middle ear and labyrinth) • In erosion of **lateral semicircular canal as in cholesteatoma** (Ans 13) • Abnormal opening in oval window - post stapedectomy fistula. • Abnormal opening in round window • Hypermobile stapes footplate • Fenestration operation	• In normal individuals • In dead labyrinth (Ans 12)	(i.e. positive fistula test without the presence of fistula is called as **Hennebert's Sign**) Seen in: **Congenital syphilis and Meniere's disease**	(i.e. fistula is present but still fistula test is negative) • When cholesteatoma covers the site of fistula • Ill fitting speculum.

14. **Ans. is c i.e. Congenital syphilis** *Ref. Dhingra 5/e, p 47*
    Already explained.
15. **Ans. is a i.e. Vestibular function** *Ref. Dhingra 5/e, p 47*
    For details see preceding text.
16. **Ans. is a i.e. 30°C and 44°C**
17. **Ans. is b i.e. 30°**
18. **Ans. is b i.e. Lateral semicircular canal** *Ref. Dhingra 5/e, p 48; 6/e, p 43; Maqbool 11/e, p 43*

Caloric Tests: Important points
- **Principle:** to induce nystagmus by thermal stimulation of vestibular system.
- Lateral semicircular canal^Q is commonly tested by all these tests
- There are 3 methods of performing these tests:

Cold caloric test (modified Kobrak test)	Fitzgerald: (Hallpike test (bithermal caloric test)	Cold air caloric test
Patient position: patient is seated with head tilted 60°C backwards (to place horizontal canal in vertical position) Temperature of water used - ice cold water.	Patient position: patient lies supine with head tilted 30 Temperature of water = **30°C and 44°C**	Done when there is perforation of tympanic membrane (as irrigation with water is contraindicated in these cases) Air cooled by ethylchloride is blown into the ear by Dundas Grant tube

19. **Ans. is a i.e Towards the opposite side** *Ref. Dhingra 5/e, p 48; 6/e, p 43*
20. **Ans. is a i.e. nystagmus to the right side**

In caloric test: Hallpike Fitzegerald test

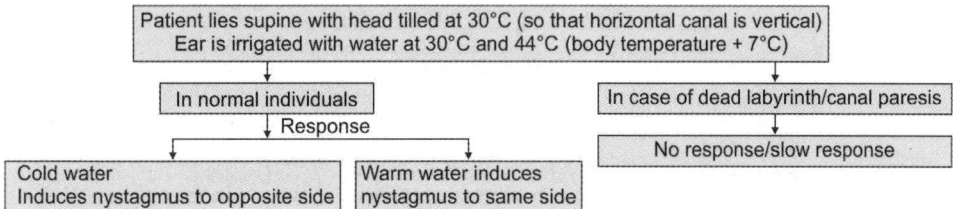

Mnemonic

COWS
Cold water induces nystagmus to Opposite side whereas Warm water to Same side.

In Q 20:
Since cold water is used to irrigate left side: Nystagmus will be towards opposite side, i.e. right side

21. **Ans. is c i.e. In canal paresis the test is inconclusive** *Ref. Scott Brown 7/e vol-3, p 3727*
    As discussed in previous question:
    - *Nystagmus can be induced both by cold as well as thermal stimulation*
    - *Cold stimulation causes nystagmus towards opposite side while thermal stimulation causes nystagmus towards same side (COWS)*
    - *In canal paresis either there is a reduced or absent response (causes of U/L canal paresis are–U/L vestibular Schwannoma or vestibular neuritis)*
    - *B/L absence of caloric nystagmus is seen in case of aminoglycoside ototoxicity or postmeningitis.*

22. **Ans. is c i.e. Slow + Fast component** *Ref. Dhingra 5/e, p 48; 6/e, p 43; Maqbool 11/e, p 43*
    Caloric test is used to test vestibular function/labyrinthine function
    So nystagmus induced by it is vestibular in origin.
    Vestibular nystagmus has both fast (of cerebral origin) and a slow component (of vestibular origin).

23. **Ans. is a i.e. Midbrain** *Ref. Scotts Brown 7/e, Vol 3, p 3922*
    "Vertical nystagmus means vertical displacement of the eye, not side to side nystagmus when attempting upward or downward gaze. As defined vertical nystagmus always indicates brainstem dysfunction". *Ref. Scott Brown 7/e, Vol 3, p 3922*

24. **Ans. is a, c and d i.e. Horizontal , Direction changes and Not suppressed by visual fixation**
    Ref. PL Dhingra 5/46, 6/e, p 42; Harrison 17/e, p 144, 45 www.jeffmann.net/NeuroGuidemaps/nystagmus.html; Maqbool III/e, p 43; Scotts Brown 7/e, vol 3, p 3724

Features	Peripheral	Central
Form	Torsional with horizontal or vertical component	Purely horizontal or vertical (No torsional component)
Direction of nystagmus^Q	Direction fixed	Direction changing^Q
Latency	2-20 seconds	No latency
Duration	Less than 1 minute	More than 1 minute
On visual fixation	Nystagmus disappears	Does not disappear
Accompanying symptoms	Tinnitus, vertigo	None
Fatiguability	Fatiguable	Non fatiguable
Example	BPPV, labyrinthitis, Meniere's disease labyrinthine fistula	Vertebrobasilar insufficiency, tumors

25. **Ans. is b i.e. Dehiscent superior semicircular canal** *Ref. Current Otolaryngology 3/e, p 737, 738*

26. **Ans. is b, c and d i.e. Positive Tullio's phenomenon, Positive Hennebert's sign and Oscillopsia**
    Ref. Current Otolaryngology 3/e, p 737, 738
    In 1998, Lloyd minor and colleagues described sound and/or presssure induced vertigo associated with bony dehiscence of the superior semicircular canal.
    - **Third window effect takes place in case of dehiscent superior semicircular canal whereby the dehiscent part of semicircular canal acts as a third window of inner ear.** As a result, endolymph within the labyrinthine system continues to move in relation to sound or pressure changes which causes activation of the vestibular system.

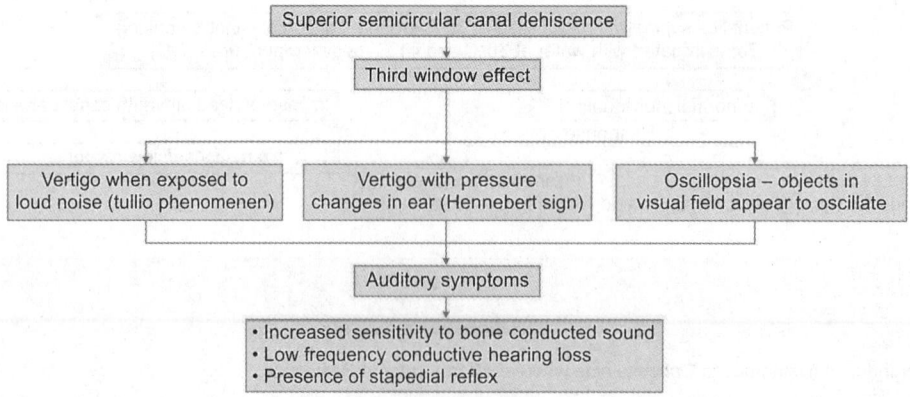

 Note: The presence of stapedius reflex with low-frequency conductive hearing loss should prompt radiological imaging of the inner ear to exclude the possibility to dehiscence of the inner ear.

Chapter 5: Assessment of Vestibular Function

Patient profile
- **Age:** Although dehiscence of the superior canal may be congenial symptoms and signs usually do not present early in life; the youngest patients have been in their teen. Median age at diagnosis is 40 years.
- **Sex:** SCDS appears to affect males and females equally.
- **Symptoms:** Patients may complain of vestibular symptoms only, auditory and vestibular symptoms, or, less commonly, isolated auditory symptoms.
  - Patients report increased sensitivity to bone-conducted sounds.
  - Inner ear conductive hearing loss is common.
  - Stapedial reflex is present.
- **Pathology:** The dehiscent portion of the superior canal acts as a third mobile window allowing acoustic energy to be dissipated there. As a result, endolymph within the labyrinthine system continue to move in relation to sound or pressure, which causes an activation of the vestibular system.
- **Imaging studies of choice** is high-resolution CT of the temporal bone.
- **Audiologic testing** demonstrates low-frequency conductive hearing loss with the presence of stapedius reflex Differential diagnosis for the condition is -Otosclerosis where although low frequency conductive hearing loss is seen but due to fixation of the stapes footplate, the stapedial reflex is absent.

Also know

"**Oscilopsia**" is visual disturbance in which objects in the visual field appear to oscillate. The severity of the effect may range from a mild blurring to rapid and periodic jumping. Oscillopsia may be caused by loss of the vestibulo-ocular reflex, involuntary eye movements such as nystagmus, or impaired coordination in the visual cortex (especially due to toxins) and is *one of the symptoms of superior canal dehiscence syndrome.* Sufferers may experience dizziness and nausea. Oscillopsia can also be used as a quantitative test to document aminoglycoside toxicity"–*en.wikipedia.org/Oscillopsia.*

> **Other causes leading to third window effect:**
> 1. Anatomical third window
> 2. Diffuse third window
>   A. Semicircular window
>   - Superior canal dehiscence
>   - Posterior canal dehiscence
>   - Posterior canal dehiscence
>   - Lateral canal dehiscence
>   B. Vestibule
>   - Large vestibular aqueduct syndrome
>   - Inner ear malformation causing a dehiscence between internal auditory canal and dehiscence
>   C. Cohlea
>   - Dehiscence between carotid canal and scala vastibule
>   - Inner ear malformation causing a dehiscence between internal auditory canal and scala vestibule.

27. **Ans. is a i.e. Subjective sense of imbalance** *Ref. Mohan Bansal 1/e, p 227*
    Vertigo is a subjective sense of imbalance or false sense of motion felt by patient.

    Vertigo can be

    Peripheral (M/C = 85% cases)
    - Involves vestibular end organs and their 1st order neurons (i.e. the vestibular nerve)
    - Cause lies in the internal ear or VIIIth nerve.

    Central (15%)
    - Involves central nervous system after the entrance of vestibular nerve in the brainstem and involves vestibulo-ocular and vestibulospinal pathways

28. **Ans. is c i.e. Lateral** *Ref. Mohan Bansal 1/e, p 236; Point 12*
    Fitzgeraled Hallpike Bethernal caloric test: the lateral semicircular canal (SCC) is stimulated (tested) (horizontal) by irrigating cold (30°C) and warm water (44°C) in the external avditoy canal warm. *Ref. Mohan Bansal 1/e, p 236*

29. **Ans. is c i.e. Cochlear disease** *Ref. Dhingra 6/e, p 45*
    Cochlear problems is associated with hearing loss and not nystagmus.
    Rest all are associated with nystagmus.

30. **Ans. is a i.e. Medulla**
    (Read explanation of N3 for explanation)

31. **Ans. is b i.e. Left side** *Ref. Essentials of ENT Mohan Bansal, p 131*
    Remember the following FUNDA

    > - In destructive lesions or paretic lesions e.g. trauma to labyrinth, the nystagmus is towards the opposite side.
    > - In irritative lesions, e.g. serous labyrinthitis, fistula of labyrinth, the nystagmus is towards ipsilateral side.

32. **Ans. is d i.e. Posterior semicircular canal** *Ref. Dhingra 6/e, p 45*
    BPPV is due to stimulation of posterior semicircular canal.

33. **Ans. is a i.e. Towards the opposite side** *Ref. Dhingra 6/e, p 43*
    As discussed previously:
    The mnemonic 'COWS' (cold-opposite; warm–same side) is very helpful to remember the direction in which water induces nystagmus in caloric test.

34. **Ans. is a i.e. Positional vertigo** *Ref. Dhingra 6/e, p 45*
    Benign paroxysmal positional vertigo (BPPV) is characterized by vertigo when the head is placed in a certain critical position, and can be treated by Epley's maneuver.
    The principle of this maneuver is to reposition the otoconial debris from the posterior semicircular canal back into the utricle.
    After maneuver is complete, patient should maintain an upright posture for 48 hours. Eighty per cent of the patients will be cured by a single maneuver.

35. **Ans. is a, b, c and d i.e. Perilymph fistula, Otolithiasis, Vestibular neuritis and Meniere's disease**
    See the text for explanation

Chapter 6

Diseases of External Ear

Normal Commensal Flora of the External Ear
- Staphylococcus epidermidis
- Corynebacterium species
- Staphylococcus aureus
- Streptococcus viridans

Inflammatory Conditions of the External Ear

■ OTITIS EXTERNA

Any inflammatory condition of the skin of the external auditory canal is otitis externa

Classification

a. **Localized** – furunculosis
b. **Diffuse otitis externa**
 - Idiopathic
 - Traumatic
 - Irritant
 - Bacterial
 - Fungal (most common cause)
 - Environmental
c. **Part of generalized skin conditions–**
 - Seborrheic dermatitis
 - Allergic dermatitis
 - Atopic dermatitis
 - Psoriasis
d. **Malignant necrotizing** – otitis externa
e. **Other** (keratosis obturans)

A. Fungal

- **Otomycosis (fungal otitis externa)**
  - It is seen in hot and humid climate

> **Point to Remember**
> ➢ M/C cause of otitis externa is fungal i.e. otomycosis.

Most Common Organisms
- *Aspergillus niger* appearing as black-headed filamentous growth
- *Candida albicans* appearing white and creamy deposit
- **Others**
  - *A. fumigatus* – Green/Blue growth
  - Dermatophytes – Actinomyces (wet blotting paper appearance)

Symptoms:
- Intense itching
- Pain
- Watery discharge with musty odor

Treatment:
- Ear toileting to remove all discharge and epithelial debris
- Antifungal ear drops
- Antibiotics: As they help to reduce edema and inflammation and thus permit better penetration of anti-fungal agents

B. Bacterial

- **Furunculosis (localized acute otitis externa)**

Most common organism: *Staphylococcus aureus*
Site: Hair bearing area of the cartilaginous part of the external auditory canal

Symptoms:
- Discomfort and pain
- Aggravated by jaw/pinna movement
- May have associated deafness if canal gets occluded due to edema

Signs:
- Tragal sign positive
- In severe cases:
  a. **Retroauricular sulcus is obliterated**
  b. Forward displacement of the pinna

Treatment:
- Local—10% ichthammol glycerin pack
- Oral antibiotics → if local cellulitis is present
- Oral analgesics
- Incision and drainage → if abscess formation
- In recurrent furunculosis – Rule out diabetes mellitus

- **Diffuse otitis externa: (Tropical/Singapore ear/Telephonist ear)**

Most common organisms:
- *Pseudomonas pyocyaneas*
- *Bacillus proteus*
- *Staphylococcus aureus*
- *E. coli*

Diffuse otitis externa can be:
i. **Acute** – Signs and symptoms similar to furunculosis
ii. **Chronic** – Symptoms:
 - Irritation in the ear
 - Constant desire to itch

Signs:
- Scanty discharge in the externa auditory canal
- Dried crusts
- Scaling and fissuring in the canal wall

Treatment:
- Ear toileting most important step
- Medicated wicks (antibiotic + steroids)
- Oral antibiotic are indicated in case of cellulitis and lymphadenitis
- Analgesics for relief of pain

- **Malignant otitis externa/necrotising otitis externa**
Progressive debilitating and sometimes fatal infection of the external auditory canal, characterized by granulation tissue in external auditory canal at the junction of bone and cartilage.

Most common organism: *Pseudomonas aeruginosa*
Others: – S. aureus
  – S. epidermidis
  – Aspergillus
  – Actinomyces

Pathologically: Characterized by necrotizing vasculitis
Features: Occurs commonly in:
- Elderly diabetic
- Immunosuppressed patient/use of immunosuppressive drugs
- Patients who have received radiotherapy to skull base

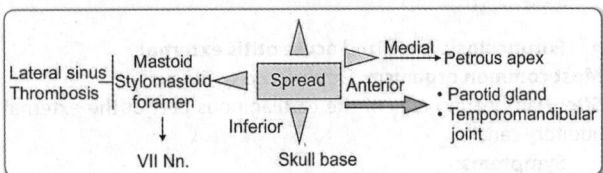

Fig. 6.1: Spread of malignant otitis externa

Spread of the infection: See Fig. 6.1
- **Nerves commonly involved:**

Most common nerve involved	– VII.
Others	– IX, X, XI, XII,

- **Investigation:** CT scan, gallium and technetium-99 scintigraphy
- **For early diagnosis:** Tc 99 scan is used but the test remains positive for a year or so, hence cannot be used to monitor the disease
- **For monitoring the disease:** Gallium citrate (Ga) 67 scan is done. Indium (in III) labelled leucocyte scan is equally sensitive but more specific than Ga 67 scan
- **Other Ix:** Culture and sensitivity
- **CT** and **MRI** are equally sensitive to assess the extent of disease.
- **Biopsy** is done to rule out malignancy
- **ESR** is often raised and can be used to monitor the progress of disease
- **Prognosis:**
  • It has high mortality rate (so termed as malignant)
  • Death due to intracranial complications like sigmoid sinus thrombosis

Treatment: Includes correction of immunosuppression (when possible), local treatment of the auditory canal, long-term systemic antibiotic therapy, and in selected patients, surgery.
- In all cases, the external ear canal is cleansed and a biopsy specimen of the granulation tissue sent for culture.
- IV antibiotics is directed against the offending organism.

- For pseudomonas aeruginosa, the most common pathogen, the regimen involves an antipseudomonal penicillin or cephalosporin *(3rd generation piperacillin or ceftazidime)* with an aminoglycoside. A fluoroquinolone antibiotic can be used in place of the aminoglycoside.
- Ear drops containing antipseudomonal antibiotic e.g. ciprofloxacin plus a glucocorticoid is also used.

- Extensive surgical debridement once an important part of the treatment is now rarely needed.

- **Perichondritis**
  - It mostly occurs due to infection secondary to either blunt trauma or iatrogenic trauma.
  - M/C organism: Pseudomonas
  - Pinna becomes red, hot and stiff
  - **Treatment:** Systemic antibiotics + local application of 4% aluminium acetate. If abscess has formed incision and drainage should be done.

C. **Viral**
- **Herpetic otitis externa:**
Organism: H. simplex
    H. zoster

Features of *H. zoster*/Ramsay Hunt syndrome
- Site of affection:
  • Geniculate ganglion of the facial nerve
  • May also involve the V and VIII nerves

Symptoms:
- Severe otalgia
- Vesicular eruptions on pinna of the affected ear.
- Facial nerve palsy (LMN type)
- May show associated vesicular eruption in the buccal mucosa, hard palate and hypopharynx.

Treatment:
- Oral acyclovir
  (to be started within 72 hours of the onset of rash)

- **Bullous myringitis: Otitis externa hemorrhagica**
Organism: Viral or mycoplasma pneumoniae
Features: Hemorrhagic blebs on the lateral surface of the tympanic membrane and the skin of the external auditory canal.
- It is painful condition^Q

Treatment:
- Analgesics
- Antibiotic: Only in case of secondary ear infection
- Blebs NOT to be incised

NEW PATTERN QUESTIONS

Q N1. Malignant otitis externa is:
  a. Malignancy of external ear
  b. Caused by hemophilus
  c. Blackish mass of Aspergillus
  d. Pseudomonas infection in diabetic patients

Q N2. IOC for early diagnosis of malignant otitis externa:
  a. Tc-99 scan
  b. Ga-67 scan
  c. In 111 labelled leukocyte scan
  d. MRI

Chapter 6: Diseases of External Ear

Q N3. IOC to detect the intracranial complications of malignant otitis externa:
a. CT scan b. MRI
c. Biopsy d. Tc-99 scan

Q N4. IOC for resolution of infection in malignant otitis externa:
a. CT scan b. MRI
c. Ga-67 scan d. Tc-99 scan

Q N5. IOC to detect the extent of bone erosion in malignant otitis externa:
a. CT scan b. MRI
c. Ga-67 scan d. Tc-99 scan

Q N6. Diffuse otitis externa is also known as:
a. Glue ear b. Malignant otitis externa
c. Telephonist's ear d. ASOM

Q N7. Regarding necrotizing otitis externa all are true *except*:
a. Caused by pseudomonas
b. Surgery never done
c. Facial nerve involved
d. Common in diabetics

TUMORS OF THE EXTERNAL AUDITORY CANAL

Benign:
- Papilloma
- Adenoma ─┐
- Fibroma ──┼─ Ceruminoma
- Exostoses ┘
- Osteoma ─── Sebaceous adenoma

Exostoses (most common benign tumor of external auditory canal)	Osteoma
• Multiple	• Rounded, pedunculated
• Sessile hemispherical elevations	• U/L condition
• B/L condition	• Arises at the junction of bony and cartilaginous meatus
• Arises in the bony meatus	

MISCELLANEOUS CONDITIONS OF EXTERNAL EAR

IMPACTED WAX/CERUMEN

- Secreted by ceruminous and sebaceous glands in the cartilaginous part of external canal.
- **Clinical features:** Sense of blockage
  Itching
  ↓ hearing
  Tinnitus
  Vertigo
- **Treatment:** If hard, soften it by wax solvents like soda glycerin and removed by syringing with sterile water at body temperature, or with wax hook.

 Note: For syringing pinna is pulled upward^Q and backward^Q and a stream of water from the ear syringe is directed along the posterior superior wall of the meatus^Q

Complications: Syringing can lead to vertigo, rupture of the tympanic membrane and reactivation of quiescent otitis media.

Contraindications of syringing:
- H/O ear surgery
- Perforation of TM
- Acute inflammation
- Grommet inserted

TRAUMA TO EAR

Hematoma

- It is collection of blood between the auricular cartilage and its perichondrium.
- Mostly it is the result of blunt trauma and is seen in boxers, wrestlers and rugby players.
- Extravasated blood may clot and then organize, resulting in a typical deformity called *Cauliflower ear* (pugilistic or boxer's ear)
- If Hematoma gets infected. Severe perichondritis may set in.
- Treatment is aspiration of the hematoma under strict aseptic precautions and a pressure dressing.
- When aspiration fails, incision and drainage should be done and pressure applied by dental rolls tied with through and through sutures.
- All cases should receive prophylactic antibiotics.

KERATOSIS OBTURANS

It is accumulation of desquamated keratin in the external auditory meatus. Also called as *canal wall cholesteatoma* M/C in young patients.

Clinical Features

- Severe ear pain
- Mild/moderate conductive hearing loss
- Associated sinusitis or bronchitis

Management

- Surgical removal under GA
- In recurrent cases—canal plasty can be done
- Mastoidectomy should be performed in cases with primary cholesteatoma of external canal.
- Recurrence is common.

IMPORTANT POINTS

- Syringing is indicated in patients with ear symptoms where wax obstructs the view of the tympanic membrane.

- Malignant otitis externa is caused by pseudomonas and is seen in diabetic patients.
- Herpes zoster oticus also called Ramsay Hunt syndrome is caused by chickenpox virus, varicella and affects geniculate ganglion.
- **Cholesteatoma of external auditory meatus is also called Keratosis obturans** and is characterized by hyperemia and irritability of canal skin.
- **Singapore ear** also known as **Telephonist ear or Tropical** ear is a type of diffuse otitis externa due to hot and humid climate
- Exostosis is the most common benign tumor of the external auditory meatus.
- Osteomas are usually single and arise at bony and cartilaginous junction of external auditory canal, while exostosis are multiple bony outgrowths from bony meatus.
- The M/C congenital anomaly of ear is Bat ear.
- The rarest congenital anomaly of ear is **Polyotia**.

NEW PATTERN QUESTIONS

Q N8. Chondritis of aural cartilage is most commonly due to:
- a. Staphylococcus
- b. Pseudomonas
- c. Candida
- d. Streptococcus

Q N9. Otitis externa hemorragica is caused by:
- a. Influenza
- b. Proteus
- c. Staph
- d. Streptococcus

Q N10. Congenital displacement of the pinna is:
- a. Coloboma lobuli
- b. Melotia
- c. Scroll ear
- d. Cleft pinna

Q N11. Blue drum is seen in:
- a. Tympanosclerosis
- b. Secretory otitis media
- c. Otosclerosis
- d. Myringitis bullosa

Q N12. Keratosis obturans is:
- a. Foreign body in external auditory canal
- b. Desquamated epithelial cell + cholesterol
- c. Cholesterol crystals surrounded by calcium
- d. Wax in ext. auditory canal

Chapter 6: Diseases of External Ear

Explanations and References to New Pattern Questions

N1. Ans. is d i.e. Pseudomonas infection in diabetic patients
See the text for explanation.

N2. Ans. is a i.e. Tc-99 scan

N3. Ans. is b i.e. MRI

N4. Ans. is c i.e. Ga-67 scan

N5. Ans. is a i.e. CT scan

Investigations done in malignant otitis externa	
• For early diagnosis	Tc-99 scan
• For resolution of disease	Ga-67 scan
• For intracranial extension of disease	MRI
• For detecting extent of bone erosion	CT scan
• To rule out malignancy	Biopsy

N6. Ans. is c i.e. Telephonist's ear

Diffuse otitis externa is known as tel\ephonist ear or singapore ear or tropical ear.

N7. Ans. is b i.e. Surgery never done   *Ref. Dhingra 6/e, p 52*

Its not that surgery is never done, but yes surgery is not the first option since all the other 3 options are correct, we will take it as the answer because it is partially incorrect.

N8. Ans. is b i.e. Pseudomonas   *Ref. Dhingra 6/e, p 50*

Read the text for explanation.

N9. Ans. is a i.e. Influenza   *Ref. Dhingra 6/e, p 52*

Otitis externa hemorrhagica is most commonly caused by influenza virus and is characterized by formation of hemorrhagic bullae on the tympanic membrane.

N10. Ans. is b i.e. Melotia

Congenital malformations	Definition
Anotia	Congenital absence of pinna
Macrotia	Congenitally enlarged pinna
Microtia	Congenitally small pinna
Melotia	Congenital displacement of pinna-ear located on cheek due to lack of aural ascent
Low set ears	Ear which is set below an arbitrary line drawn between the lateral canthus of eye and occipital protuberance
Synotia	Both ears very close to each other
Coloboma lobuli	Congenital fissure of the ear lobe
Lop ear	The external ear stands away from the head at a greater angle (normal angle = in males = 25° and in females = 18°)
Polyotia	Additional pinna on one or both sides
Scroll ear	Helix of pinna round forward and inward

N11. Ans. is b i.e. Secretory otitis media

Normally tympanic membrane is pearly white in color:

Abnormal color	Seen in
Red	• Acute otitis media • Glomus jugulare
Blue	• Secretory otitis media • High jugular bulb

N12. Ans. is b i.e. Desquamated epithelial cell and cholesterol

See the text for explanation.

QUESTIONS

1. **Common causes of otitis externa:** [PGI 08]
   a. Aspergillus   b. Mucor
   c. Candida   d. Pseudomonas
   e. Klebsiella
2. **External otitis is also known as:** [DNB 2003]
   a. Glue ear   b. Malignant otitis externa
   c. Telephonist's ear   d. ASOM
3. **Causes of otomycosis:** [PGI-08]
   a. Candida   b. Aspergillus
   c. Thermophilus   d. Staphylococcus
4. **Fungus causing otomycosis most commonly is:**
   a. Aspergillus fumigatus   b. Candida   [Delhi 96]
   c. Mucor   d. Penicillin
5. **Myringitis bullosa is caused by:** [AI 93]
   a. Virion   b. Fungus
   c. Bacteria   d. Virus
6. **In Ramsay Hunt syndrome, all nerves are involved except**
   a. 5   b. 7   [RJ 2002]
   c. 8   d. 9
7. **Hemorrhagic external otitis media is caused by:**
   [PGI Dec. 98]
   a. Influenza   b. Proteus
   c. Staphylococcus   d. Streptococcus
8. **A patient has come with furuncle of ear. What is the commonest method of treatment?**
   a. Ear pack with 10% ichthammol in glycerin wick
   b. Antibiotic and rest   [Orissa 99]
   c. Antibiotic and drainage
   d. Analgesic
9. **Malignant otitis externa is caused by:** [AP 96; Comed 07]
   a. S. aureus   b. S. albus
   c. P. aeruginosa   d. E. coli
10. **True statement about malignant otitis externa is:**
    a. Not painful   [PGI 96]
    b. Common in diabetics and old age
    c. Caused by streptococcus
    d. All of the above
11. **Malignant otitis externa is:** [PGI Dec. 99]
    a. Malignancy of external ear
    b. Caused by hemophilus influenzae
    c. Blackish mass of aspergillus
    d. Pseudomonas infection in diabetic patient
12. **Malignant otitis externa is characterized:**
    [PGI Dec. 03; June 06]
    a. Caused by pseudomonas aeruginosa
    b. Malignancy of external auditory canal
    c. Granulation tissue is seen in the floor of external auditory canal
    d. Radiotherapy can be given
    e. Gallium scan is helpful for monitoring treatment
13. **All of the following are true about malignant otitis externa except:**
    a. ESR is used for follow-up after treatment
    b. Granulation tissues are seen on superior wall of the external auditory canal
    c. Severe hearing loss is the chief presenting complaint
    d. Pseudomonas is the most common cause
14. **An elderly diabetic present with painful ear discharge and edema of the external auditory canal with facial palsy, not responding to antibiotics. An increased uptake on technetium bone scan is noted. The most probable diagnosis is:** [AI 12]
    a. Malignant otitis external
    b. Malignancy of the middle ear
    c. Infective disease of the middle ear
    d. Malignancy of nasopharynx with Eustachian tube obstruction
15. **A 75-year-old diabetic patient presents with severe ear pain and granulation tissue at external auditory canal with facial nerve involvement. The most likely diagnosis is:**
    a. Malignant otitis externa
    b. Nasopharyngeal carcinoma
    c. Acute suppurative otitis media
    d. Chronic suppurative otitis media
16. **An old diabetic male presented with rapidly spreading infection of the external auditory canal with involvement of the bone and presence of granulation tissue. The drug of choice for this condition is:** [AIIMS May 08]
    a. Ciprofloxacin   [May 2014]
    b. Penicillin
    c. Second generation cephalosporin
    d. Aminoglycosides
17. **Which of the following is not a typical feature of malignant otitis externa?** [AIIMS May 06]
    a. Caused by *Pseudomonas aeruginosa*
    b. Patients are usually old
    c. Mitotic figures are high
    d. Patient is immunocompromised
18. **Facial nerve palsy is seen in:** [Jipmer 03]
    a. Seborrheic otitis externa
    b. Otomycosis
    c. Malignant otitis externa
    d. Eczematous otitis externa
19. **Keratosis obturans is:** [TN 2007]
    a. Foreign body in external auditory canal
    b. Desquamated epithelial cell + cholesterol
    c. Cholesterol crystals surrounded by calcium
    d. Wax in external auditory canal
20. **Chalky white tympanic membrane is seen in:** [RJ 2001]
    a. ASOM   b. Otosclerosis
    c. Tympanosclerosis   d. Cholesteatoma
21. **A 60-year-old man presented with left sided ear discharge for 7 years with dull earache. O/e intact tympanic membrane on both sides, mass is seen in the posterior canal wall on left side. Diagnosis is?** [AIIMS May 2013]
    a. Keratosis obturans
    b. CSOM

Chapter 6: Diseases of External Ear

c. External otitis
d. Carcinoma of external auditory canal

22. **Cauliflower ear is:** [Manipal 06]
   a. Keloid
   b. Perichondritis in Boxers
   c. Squamous cell carcinoma
   d. Anaplastic cell carcinoma

23. **Not true about auricular hematoma:** [PGI May 2011]
   a. All case should receive antibiotic
   b. Commonly seen in rugby player
   c. Resolve spontaneously

24. **Direction of water jet while doing syringing of ear should be:** [Mahara 02]
   a. Anteroinferior
   b. Posterosuperior
   c. Anterosuperior
   d. Posteroinferior

25. **All are true regarding foreign body impaction in ear except:** (PGI Nov 2016)
   a. Syringing is used for removing vegetative foreign body
   b. Syringing uses room temperature water
   c. Blunt hook is used to remove rounded foreign body
   d. Objects located medial to isthmus of canal is difficult to remove
   e. GA is preferred in children to remove foreign bodies

26. **A newborn presents with bilateral microtia and external auditory canal atresia. Corrective surgery is usually performed is:** [AI 07]
   a. < 1 year of age
   b. 5–7 years of age
   c. Puberty
   d. Adulthood

27. **Features of moderately retracted tympanic membrane are all except:** [MH 2005]
   a. Handle of malleus appearance foreshortened
   b. Cone of light is absent or interrupted
   c. Lateral process of mallous becomes more prominent
   d. None

28. **Dysfunction of tympanic membrane is characterized by all except:** [AP 2000]
   a. Normal 'cone of light'
   b. Retracted TM
   c. Non prominent umbo
   d. Prominent malleolar folds

29. **True statement regarding wax in ear:** [PGI Nov 2016]
   a. Syringing and instrumental manipulation are generally done to remove impacted wax
   b. If wax is hard and impacted, ceruminolytic substances is used to soften wax
   c. In syringing fluid is injected along the lower wall of the meatus
   d. Wax has antibacterial property

Explanations and References

1. **Ans. is a, c and d i.e. Aspergillus, Candida and Pseudomonas** *Ref. Current Otolaryngology 2/e, p 629, 630*
   - Otitis externa is an inflammatory and infectious process of the external auditory canal which is seen in all ages and both sexes.
   - M/C organism causing otitis externa are:
     a. Pseudomonas aeruginosa^Q
     b. Staphylococcus aureus
   - Less commonly isolated organisms are:
     a. Proteus species
     b. Staphylococcus epidermidis
     c. Diphtheroids
     d. E. coli

Fungal Otitis Externa/Otomycosis
   - In 80% of cases organism is **aspergillus**^{Q}
   - 2nd M/C organism is **candida**

Other more rare fungal pathogens include
   - Phycomycetes
   - Rhizopus
   - Actinomyces
   - Penicillium

2. **Ans. is c i.e. Telephonist's ear** *Ref. Internet search*
   Humidity and hot climate are one of the predisposing factors for otitis externa. Hence – otitis externa is also k/a Singapore ear (where climate is hot and humid) or Telephonist ear as talking on phone causes humidity around ear) or Swimmers ear.

   > **Also know**
   > Pseudomonas aeruginosa is a normal inhabitant of external ear. Its numbers are kept in balance by the normal acidity of EAC. Prolonged swimming or abusive use of cotton typed ear buds can alter the pH, producing a more basic environment in which pseudomonas grows rapidly.

3. **Ans. is a and b i.e. Candida and Aspergillus**
4. **Ans. is a i.e. Aspergillus fumigatus**   *Ref. Dhingra 5/e, p 58, 6/e, p 52; Current Otolaryngology 2/e, p 630; Scotts Brown 7/e, vol 3 p 3355*
   M/C cause of fungal otitis externa or otomycosis is - Aspergillus niger 2nd M/C cause is candida.
5. **Ans. is d i.e. Virus**   *Ref. Turner 10/e, p 323; Dhingra 5/e, p 62, 6/e, p 55*
   Myringitis bullosa hemorrhagica is a painful condition.
   It is characterized by formation of hemorrhagic blebs on tympanic membrane and deep meatus. It is probably caused by virus or mycoplasma pneumoniae   *(Dhingra 6/e, p 62)* but according to *Turner 10/e p 323*
   "Myringitis bullosa hemorrhagica occurs in presence of viral infection, usually influenzae."

Note: Myringitis granulosa is associated with impacted wax, long standing foreign body or external ear infection.

External ear condition	Most common organism
Furunculosis	Staphylococcus
Otomycosis	Aspergillus niger (M/C); Candida albicans (2nd M/C)
Otitis externa hemorrhagica	Influenza virus
Myringitis bullosa	Influenza virus Less commonly mycoplasma pneumoniae Pseudomonas aeruginosa
Malignant otitis externa	Pseudomonas
Perichondritis	Impacted wax
Myringitis granulosa	Foreign body

6. **Ans. is d i.e. 9**   *Ref. Dhingra 5/e, p 107, 6/e, p 52, 96; Scotts Brown 7/e, vol 3 p 260, 3379-3382*
   Herpes zoster oticus / Ramsay Hunt syndrome –
   – It is herpetic vesicular rash on the cochlea, external auditory canal or pinna with lower motor neuron palsy of the ipsilateral facial nerve.
   – It is k/a Ramsay Hunt syndrome following the first description of 60 cases by John Ramsay hunt in 1907.
   – It may be accompanied by anesthesia of face, giddiness and hearing impairment due to involvement of Vth and VIIIth nerve.
7. **Ans. is a i.e. Influenza**   *Ref. Dhingra 5/e, p 58, 6/e, p 52*
   Hemorrhagic external otitis media: (Otitis externa hemorrhagia) is **caused by influenza virus.**
   • Characterised by formation of haemorrhagic bullae on tympanic membrane.
   • **Clinical features:** severe pain and blood stained discharge.
   • **Treatment:** Analgesics + antibiotics.
8. **Ans. is a i.e. Ear Pack with 10% ichthammol in glycerin wick**   *Ref. Dhingra 5/e, p 57, 51; Turner 10/e, p 272*
   Furuncle (boil) is due to staphylococcal infection of the hair follicle.

   Management
   • Local heat + sedatives
   • Packs of 10% ichthammol (acts as antiseptic) and glycerine (hygroscopic action decreases edema). It is the commonest treatment and most of the furuncles burst spontaneously by this treatment.
   • Antibiotics (Flucloxacillin) is given for 5 days
   • If abscess is formed: Incision and drainage is done
   • In case of recurrent furunculosis - Rule out diabetes and staphylococcal skin infection.
9. **Ans. is c is P. aeruginosa**
10. **Ans. is b i.e. Common in diabetics and old age**
11. **Ans. is d i.e. Pseudomonas infection in diabetic patient**
12. **Ans is a, c and e i.e. Caused by pseudomonas aeruginosa; Granulation tissue is seen in the floor of external auditory canal; and Gallium scan helpful for monitoring treatment**
      Ref. Dhingra 5/e, p 58, 6/e, p 52 Scott's Brown 7/e, vol 3 p 3336-3339; Harrison 17/e, p 208
    For details see preceding text
13. **Ans. c. Severe hearing loss is the chief presenting complaint**   *Ref. Dhingra 5/e, 58*
    Severe hearing loss is not the chief presenting complaint in malignant otitis externa.

Chapter 6: Diseases of External Ear

A patient of malignant otitis externa presents with:
- **Severe, unrelenting, deep-seated otalgia, temporal headaches, purulent otorrhea,** possibly dysphagia, **hoarseness,** and/or **facial nerve dysfunction.**

> - The pain is out of proportion to the physical examination findings.
> - **Marked tenderness** is present in the soft tissue **between the mandible ramus and mastoid tip.**
> - **Granulation tissue** is present at the **floor of the osseocartilaginous junction.** This finding is **virtually pathognomonic of malignant external otitis.**

Rest of the options i.e. pseudomonas is the M/C cause, granulation tissue seen on superior wall of the external auditory canal and ESR used for follow-up are correct.

14. **Ans. a i.e. Malignant otitis externa** *Ref. Dhingra 5/e, p 58, 6/e, p 52 Scott's Brown 7/e, vol 3 p 3336-3339*

An elderly diabetic patient
+
Painful ear discharge
+
Facial N palsy   All are highly suggestive of malignant otitis externa
+
No Response to treatment
+
↓'ed uptake on Technetium bone scan

Note:
- Gold standard for diagnosis of malignant otitis externa is technetium 99 scan
- In refractory cases of otitis externa if it is not responding to antibiotics even after 7–10 days of treatment always suspect malignant otitis externa
- M/C organism causing malignant otitis externa = Pseudomonas

15. **Ans. a. Malignant otitis externa** *Ref. Dhingra 5/e, p 58*
Presence of a **painful lesion** in the **external ear** with the **evidence of granulation tissue** and associated **cranial nerve palsies (VII nerve)** in a **diabetic** (or **immunocompromised**) patient do not leave any doubt about a diagnosis of **malignant otitis externa.**

16. **Ans. is b i.e. Pencillin** *Ref. Harrison 17/e, p 208*
Rapidly spreading infection of external auditory canal, seen in diabetic patient with involvement of bone and presence of granulation tissue point towards malignant otitis externa as the diagnosis.

Treatment
- Includes correction of immunosuppression (when possible), local treatment of the auditory canal, long-term systemic antibiotic therapy, and in selected patients, surgery:
- In all cases, the external ear canal is cleansed and a biopsy specimen of the granulation tissue sent for culture.
- IV antibiotics is directed against the offending organism.
- For Pseudomonas aeruginosa, the most common pathogen, the regimen involves an antipseudomonal penicillin or cephalosporin (3rd generation piperacillin or ceftazidime) with an aminoglycoside. A fluoroquinolone antibiotic can be used in place of the aminoglycoside.
- Ear drops containing antipseudomonal antibiotic e.g. ciprofloxacin plus a glucocorticoid is also used.
- **Extensive surgical debridement once an important part of the treatment is now rarely needed.**

17. **Ans. is c i.e. Mitotic figures are high** *Ref. Dhingra 5/e, p 52, 6/e, p 52; Harrison 17/e, p 208*
"Malignant otitis externa is a misnomer where the term malignant doesnot indicate malignant pathology". **It is an inflammatory condition caused by pseudomonas infection.** *(So high mitotic figures will not be seen).*

18. **Ans. is c i.e. Malignant otitis externa**
Malignant otitis externa—can cause destruction of tissues of canal, pre and postauricular region by various enzymes like leuthinase and hemolysis. Infection can spread to skull base and jugular foramen causing multiple cranial palsies in which most common is facial nerve palsy.

19. **Ans. is b i.e. Desquamated epithelial cell + cholesterol** *Ref. Scott's Brown 7/e, Vol-3 p 3342; Dhingra 5/e, p 61*
20. **Ans. is c i.e. Tympanosclerosis**
See the text for explanation

21. **Answer is a i.e. Keratosis obturans** *Ref. Dhingra 6/e, p 108, 54*
Presence of mass seen in the ear canal, with a long history of symptoms rules out carcinoma of ext. auditory canal.
Option d:—
- **Carcinoma of external ear canal**
  Squamous carcinoma is the most frequent neoplasm in the external auditory canal (EAC), about four times more common than basal carcinomas. This ratio is reversed in the pinna.
  Basal cell carcinoma, adenocarcinoma, ceruminoma, and malignant melanoma are the other types of cancers seen in external auditory canal.
  Most squamous cell carcinomas occur in the fifth and sixth decades of life. Foul smelling blood stained discharge is the primary symptom, and there is severe otalgia, hearing loss, and bleeding.
  These tumors have an aggressive nature and spread along preformed vascular and neural pathways, invading adjacent structures like facial nerve labyrinthine, cranial nerves IX, X, XI and XII. Treatment usually combines surgery with free margins and radiotherapy.
  Duration of the symptoms being 7 years and these features not occurring, rules out this option.
- **Option b:** CSOM
  Normal tympanic membrane and absence of deafness are against CSOM.
- **Option c:** Presence of mass does not support the diagnosis of chronic external otitis.
  Thus by exclusion our answer is keratosis obturans (option a).
- **Keratosis Obturans:** Also known as **canal wall cholesteatoma**.
  It is seen commonly in younger age groups, due to defective epithelial migration from the tympanic membrane to posterior meatal wall, which results in collection of pearly white epithelial debris in deep meatus.
  Usually patients with conductive deafness and earache.

Note:
- Keratosis obturans should be differentiated from primary canal cholesteatoma which is characterized by invasion of squamous tissue from the external ear canal into a localized area of bone erosion.

22. **Ans. is b i.e. Perichondritis in Boxers** *Ref. Dhingra 5/e, p 56, 6/e, p 50; Current Otolaryngology 2/e, p 649*

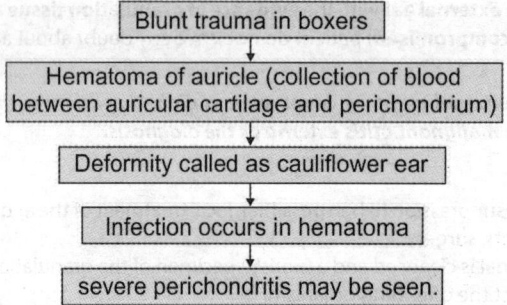

23. **Ans. is c i.e. Resolve spontaneously** *Ref. Current Otolaryngology 2/e, p 649; Dhingra 5/e, p 54, 6/e, p 49*
Hematoma of auricle
- M/C seen in boxers, wrestlers and rug by players
- Accumulation of blood in subperichondrial space, secondary to blunt trauma lifting the perichondrium away from cartilage
- As cartilage lacks its own blood supply and relies on the vascularity of the perichondrium
- It leads to necrosis of cartilage and predisposing to infection
- New cartilage may then form at the pericondrium creating a rather thick deformed, unattractive ear called as cauliflower ear
- Treatment is aspiration of hematoma under aseptic condition and carefully packing the auricle
- All cases should receive prophylactic antibiotics

24. **Ans. is b i.e. Posterosuperior** *Ref. Dhingra 5/e, p 60, 6/e, p 53*
In syringing *(done to remove impacted wax)* pinna is pulled upwards and backwards and a stream of water from the ear syringe is directed along the posterosuperior wall of the meatus.

Chapter 6: Diseases of External Ear

25. **Ans. All are true regarding foreign bodies**

    Method

    Pinna is pulled upwards and backwards and a stream of water from the ear syringe is directed along **posterosuperior wall of meatus**. Pressure of water, built up deeper to the wax, expels the wax out.

    For syring water at room temperature is to be used. Too hot or too cold water can result in vertigo.

26. **Ans. is b i.e. 5-7 years of age** *Ref. Current Diagnosis and Treatment in Otorhinology 2/e, p 627*

    Treatment of Microtia

    Classical treatment involves auricular reconstruction in multiple stages. Patients undergo observation until the age of 5 years to allow for growth of rib cartilage which is harvested for reconstruction. This approach offers the benefit of reconstruction with autogenous material which ultimately requires little or no maintainance. Typically reconstruction occurs in 4 stages.

27. **Ans. is d i.e. None** *Ref. Dhingra 5/e, p 61-62, 6/e, p 55*

28. **Ans. is a i.e. Normal cone of light.**

    Retracted Tympanic Membrane

    It is the result of negative intratympanic pressure when Eustachian tube is blocked

    Characteristics
    - It appears dull and lusterless^Q
    - Cone of light is absent or interrupted^Q
    - Handel of malleus appears foreshortened^Q
    - Lateral process of malleus becomes more prominent^Q
    - Anterior and posterior malleal folds become sickle shaped^Q
    - It is immobile or has limited mobility when tested with pneumatic otoscope or siegle's speculum.

    Features of Normal Tympanic Membrane
    - It is shiny and pearly grey in colour
    - Has concavity on its lateral surface
    - Cone of light seen in antero – inferior quadrant
    - It is transparency varies
    It is mobile when tested with pneumatic otoscope or siegle's speculum.

29. **Ans. is a, b and d i.e. syringing and instrumental manipulation are generally done to remove impacted wax, if wax is hard and impacted cerumenolytic substances is used to soften the wax and wax has antibacterial property.** *Ref. Dhingra 6/e, p 53*

    Impacted wax or cerumen:
    - Wax is composed of secretions of sebaceous gland, ceruminous gland, hair, keratin and dirt.
    - Wax has protective function as it lubricates the ear canal and entraps any foreign material that enters the canal
    - It has acidic pH and is bacteriostatic and fungistatic (i.e. option d is correct)
    - Management = syringing
    If wax is hard then it might have to be softened with wax solvents containing cerumenolytic agents prior to syringing (option b is correct).

Chapter 7

Diseases of Middle Ear

1. *Otitis media refers to an inflammatory process within the middle ear cleft.*
   Otitis media can be either acute or chronic. There is no absolute time limit, but in general, disease that persists for more than 3 months should be considered as chronic.
2. Eustachian tube is central to the pathogenesis of all forms of OM (with the possible exception of cholesteatoma). Any anatomic or functional obstruction of Eustachian tube can cause otitis media.
3. The more acute angle of ET in children as compared to adults is responsible for more prevalence of OM in children
4. In patients of Down syndrome, ET is abnormally patent or short and it loses its normal protective function against reflux of nasopharyngeal contents which results in more cases of OM in this population.

ACUTE SUPPURATIVE OTITIS MEDIA (ASOM)

Acute inflammation of middle ear cleft < 3 weeks, infective in origin.

Organism

- Streptococcus pneumoniae *(Most common)*
- H. influenzae (2nd most common)
- Moraxella catarrhalis
- Viral
  - Synctial virus
  - Influenza virus
  - Rhino and adeno virus
- It is one of the most common infectious diseases seen in children
- Peak incidence – first 2 years of life
- M/C route of infection is through Eustachian tube.

Table 7.1: Stages of ASOM

Stage of tubal Occlusion	Stage of Pre-suppuration	Stage of Suppuration	Stages of Resolution/complication
Symptoms: Deafness, *Earache*	• Deafness • Deafness • Fever	• Excruciating pain • Tympanic membrane bulges and finally ruptures • Fever	• Earache is relieved

Signs

- *Tympanic membrane appears red and bulging with loss of landmarks* (**cartwheel appearance seen**)^Q.
- 85% of the tympanic membrane rupture occurs in the antero-inferior quadrant.
- There is collection of pus behind the tympanic membrane. Thus pus comes out under pressure and synchronizing with each arterial pulse, called as **pulsatile otorrhea or light-house sign**.
- *Closure of the perforation in 90% of cases occurs in one month.*
- *Tuning fork tests show conductive deafness.*
- *Facial paralysis in ASOM is rare.*

Treatment

- **Watchful waiting**
  The current practice guidelines advise on an initial watchful waiting without antibiotic therapy for healthy 2-year-old or older children with non-severe illness (mild otalgia and fever < 39°C) because AOM symptoms improve in 1-3 days. Watchful waiting is not recommended for children < 2 years even in case of uncertain diagnosis.
- **Antibiotics:** Penicillin group – *Amoxicillin (80 mg/kg/d)* given in 3 divided doses × 10 day is the drug of choice
- Analgesics
- Aural toileting
- **Myringotomy:** It is done in the posterior inferior quadrant by a 'circumferential (*see* Fig 7.3A)' incision.

Point to Remember

Indications of Myringotomy
- Tympanic membrane bulging and there is acute pain.
- Incompelete resolution with antibiotics and patient complains of persistent deafness.
- Persistent effusion >12 weeks.
- ASOM with facial nerve palsy.

Prognosis

Most of the cases resolve without any adverse outcome. Rarely, it may lead to the following complications.

Point to Remember

- Recurrent AOM is defined as > 3 episodes of ASOM in a 6 month period or > 4 episodes in a 12 month period, with complete resolution of symptoms and signs in between the episodes.

Chapter 7: Diseases of Middle Ear

NEW PATTERN QUESTIONS	
Q N1.	**Myringotomy is:** a. Surgical opening in Eustachian tube b. Surgical opening in tympanic membrane c. Surgical opening in semicircular canal d. None
Q N2.	**For ASOM Myringotomy is done in which quadrant:** a. Antero-inferior b. Antero-superior c. Postero-superior d. Postero-inferior
Q N3.	**Light house sign is seen in ASOM in which stage:** a. Stage of suppuration b. Stage of hyperemia c. Stage of resolution d. Stage of pre-suppuration
Q N4.	**M/c organism of AOM:** a. Pneumococcus b. Staphylococcus c. Streptococcus d. H. influenzae

ACUTE NECROTIZING OTITIS MEDIA

Variant of ASOM, often seen in children suffering from measles, scarlet fever or influenza.

Organism	: β hemolytic Streptococcus
Age group	: Infants, young children
Predisposing factor	: Children acutely ill with scarlet fever, measles, pneumonia, influenzae
Features	: Necrosis and sloughing of the tympanic membrane, leading to marginal perforation, necrosis of Ossicles and VII N palsy seen
Symptoms	: Profuse foul smelling discharge (due to necrosis of the tympanic mucoperiosteum)
Treatment	: IV penicillin *In fulminant cases:* IM gamma globulin is given *In resistant cases:* If acute mastoiditis supervenes cortical mastoidectomy is done

NONSUPPURATIVE OTITIS MEDIA

A. Serous Otitis Media/Secretory Otitis Media/Otitis Media with Effusion/Mucoid Otitis Media/Glue Ear/ Silent Otitis Media

- Characterized by accumulation of nonpurulent effusion in middle ear cleft.
- It is common in 2–6 years of age.

Causes

- Malfunctioning of Eustachian tube:
  – Adenoid hyperplasia.
  – Benign and malignant tumors of the nasopharynx.
  – Cleft palate and palatal paralyses
  – Otitic barotrauma
  – Chronic rhinitis and sinusitis
  – Chronic tonsillitis
  – Viral infections–Adenoviruses and rhinoviruses
- It can also occur subsequent to inadequate treatment of ASOM.

Point to Remember

- M/c cause of serous otitis media in children is hypertrophlied adenoids.
- M/c cause of U/L serous otitis media in adults is nasopharyngeal carcinoma.

Symptoms

- Painless condition.
- **M/c symptom** is **painless insidious onset fluctuating deafness** of conductive variety. It is mild and often detected only with audiogram. It is B/L (it is the most common cause of hearing loss in children in the developed world).
- Delayed and defective speech.
- Feeling of blocked ears.

Signs

- *Tympanic membrane* appears dull with thin leash of blood vessels at the periphery.
- It is yellow/dull gray in color
- **Light reflex is absent**
- Tympanic membrane retracted with mobility restricted
- Fluid levels and air bubbles are seen through it (see Fig. 7.1).

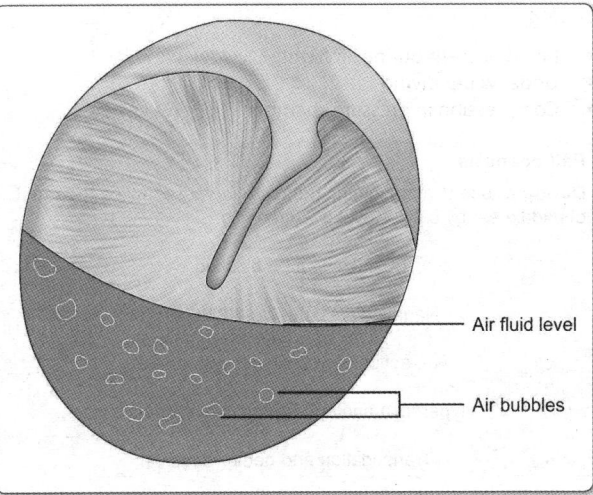

Fig. 7.1: Secretory otitis media with air fluid level and air bubbles

Note:
- In case of glue ear - fluid is sterile.
- There is no perforation

Investigations
- Tuning fork test: Conductive hearing loss (20–40 db)
- Impedance audiometry shows Type B curve, i.e. a flat curve. It is a very useful investigation in children
- In very early stages before effusion, type C tympanogram may be obtained
- X-ray mastoid: Clouding of air cells.

Treatment
- *Medical:*
  - Topical decongestants
  - Antiallergics
  - Antibiotics – effect is short lived
- *Surgical:* Surgery is done if SOM does not resolve within 3–6 months of medical management, myringotomy is done and fluid removed and grommet inserted.
  In SOM the myringotomy incision is a **radial incision given** in **anteroinferior quadrant**. (*see* Fig 7.3B)
  - Surgical management of causative factor is also done, i.e. adenoidectomy/tonsillectomy.

NEW PATTERN QUESTION

Q N5. Gold standard investigation for otitis media with effusion:
a. Pneumatic otoscopy b. Tympanometry
c. Audiometry d. None

B. Aero-otitis Media/Ottic Barotrauma

Etiology
- Rapid descent during air flight
- Under water diving
- Compression in pressure chamber

Pathogenesis
During descent atmospheric pressure increases more than that of middle ear by critical level of 90 mm Hg.
↓
Eustachian tube blocked
↓
Negative pressure in middle ear
↓
Retraction of tympanic membrane
↓
Hyperemia and engorgement of vessels
↓
Transudation and hemorrhage

Symptoms
- Severe earache
- Deafness
- Tinnitus

Signs
Air bubbles or hemorrhagic effusion in middle ear.

Treatment
Medical: • Oral and topical decongestants
• Antihistaminics
Surgical: • Myringotomy

Preventive Measures
- Avoid air travel in presence of upper respiratory infection.
- Do not sleep during descent.
- Chewing gum exercises should be done during descent so that Eustachian tube remains open
- Autoinflation of Eustachian tube by valsalva should be done.
- Use vasoconstrictor nasal spray and systemic decongestant half an hour before descent in case of previous history of similar episode.

Note:
- Barotrauma cannot occur in these who have perforation of tympanic membrane
- During ascent, the atmospheric pressure is lower as compared to middle ear.
- Thus Eustachian tube opens and passively moves air from middle ear to nasopharynx. So otitic barotrauma does not usually occur during ascent.

Point to Remember

Extra Edge
- **Lighthouse sign and pulsating otorrhea** are seen in ASOM and acute mastoiditis following ASOM.
- Silent otitis media or otitis media with effusion (OME) shows fluid level and air bubbles with no perforation in TM with B type (flat) curve on impedance audiometry.
- In **chronic adhesive otitis media,** adhesions form between drum and middle ear, while in atelectatic ear there is complete collapse of thin drum on the promontory.
- Best treatment of **adhesive otitis media** is hearing aid.
- **Fluctuating deafness of conductive** nature is seen in secretory otitis media, **while fluctuating SNHL** is a feature of Meniere's disease.
- *Potbelly tympanic membrane is a feature of secretory otitis media*.

NEW PATTERN QUESTIONS

Q N6. M/c cause of conductive deafness in children is:
a. Secretory otitis media
b. Otosclerosis
c. Congenital stapes fixation
d. Trauma

Q N7. Otitic barotrauma results due to:
a. Ascent in air
b. Descent in air
c. Linear acceleration
d. Sudden acceleration

Q N8. Eustachian tube gets blocked if pressure difference is more than:

   a. 15 mm Hg   b. 30 mm Hg
   c. 50 mm Hg   d. 90 mm Hg

CHRONIC SUPPURATIVE OTITIS MEDIA

CSOM is chronic infection of the middle ear and mastoid. It is characterized by a permanent perforation in Tympanic membrane.

Generally, a perforation of TM heals by 6–12 weeks. Therefore any perforation which persists for ≥ 12 weeks is considered as permanent and leads to CSOM.

It is of two Types: A. Tubotympanic
B. Atticoantral

A. Tubotympanic Type (Safe CSOM)

- It is particularly prevalent in developing countries and is most common in low socioeconomic group
- Most common organisms isolated are – P. aeruginosa, S. aureus and proteus species.
- It is safe or benign type of CSOM and involves anteroinferior part of middle ear cleft, i.e. Eustachian tube and mesotympanum.
- **Here perforation occurs in any part of pars tensa except margins.**
- There is no risk of serious complication.
- M/c in children.

Pathogenesis of Tubotympanic Type

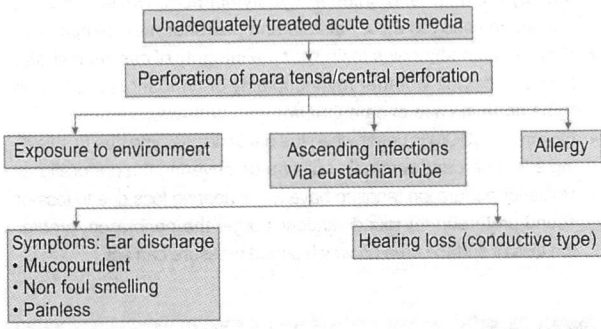

Flowchart 7.1: Pathogenesis of tubotympanic variety

Complications: In long standing cases of Tubotympanic variety of CSOM, necrosis of ossicles can occur due to repeated infection. The M/C ossicle to necrose is Incus (long process).

Treatment

(a) Medical Treatment (Treatment of Choice)

- Aural toilet – It is an important step in treatment and should not be missed
- Topical and systemic antibiotic

(b) Surgical Treatment

Surgical treatment is done at a later stage to correct the hearing loss

Prerequisites
- Ear dry for 6 weeks without antibiotics
- Eustachian tube function normal
- Normal middle ear mucosa

Procedure of choice: Myringoplasty – if ossicle chain is intact; (Details see later)

Tympanoplasty – if ossicular chain is disrupted

B. Atticoantral Type: Unsafe or Dangerous Type

- Involves posterosuperior part of middle ear cleft, i.e. attic, antrum and mastoid
- Associated with an attic or a marginal perforation.
- Associated with cholesteatoma formation
- Risk of complication is high like brain abscess and other intracranial complications

Cholesteatoma is the presence of keratinizing stratified squamous epithelium within the middle ear cleft. (It is not cholesterol nor a tumor).

Cholesteatoma can either be congenital or acquired.

- **Congenital Cholesteatoma:** It arises from the embryonic epidermal cell rests in the middle ear cleft or temporal bone. Congenital cholesteatoma occurs at three important sites: I. Middle ear, II. petrous apex, III. cerebellopontine angle.

  A middle ear congenital cholesteatoma presents as a white mass behind an intact tympanic membrane and causes conductive hearing loss. It may sometimes be discovered on routine examination of children or at the time of myringotomy.

  It may also spontaneously rupture through the tympanic membrane and present with a discharging ear indistinguishable from a case of chronic suppurative otitis media.

Levenson Criteria for Congenital Cholesteatoma
➤ White mass medial to normal TM
➤ Normal pars flaccida and tensa
➤ No history of otorrhea or perforations
➤ No prior otologic procedures
➤ Prior bouts of otitis media (not excluded)

- **Acquired Cholesteatoma:** Acquired cholesteatoma could be primary or secondary.
- **Primary acquired cholesteatoma:** It is called primary as there is no history of previous otitis media or a pre-existing perforation. Theories on its genesis are:
  - **Invagination of pars flaccida:** Persistent negative pressure in the attic causes a retraction pocket which accumulates keratin debris. When infected, the keratin mass expands towards the middle ear. Thus, attic perforation is in fact the proximal end of an expanding invaginated sac.
  - **Basal cell hyperplasia:** There is proliferation of the basal layer of pars flaccida induced by subclinical childhood infections. Expanding cholesteatoma then breaks through pars flaccida forming an attic perforation.
  - **Squamous metaplasia**
- **Secondary acquired cholesteatoma:** In these case, there is already a pre-existing perforation in pars tensa. This is often associated with posterosuperior marginal perforation or sometimes large central perforation. It arises due to migration of squamous epithelium (Habermann's theory)

Pathogenesis: See Flowchart 7.2.

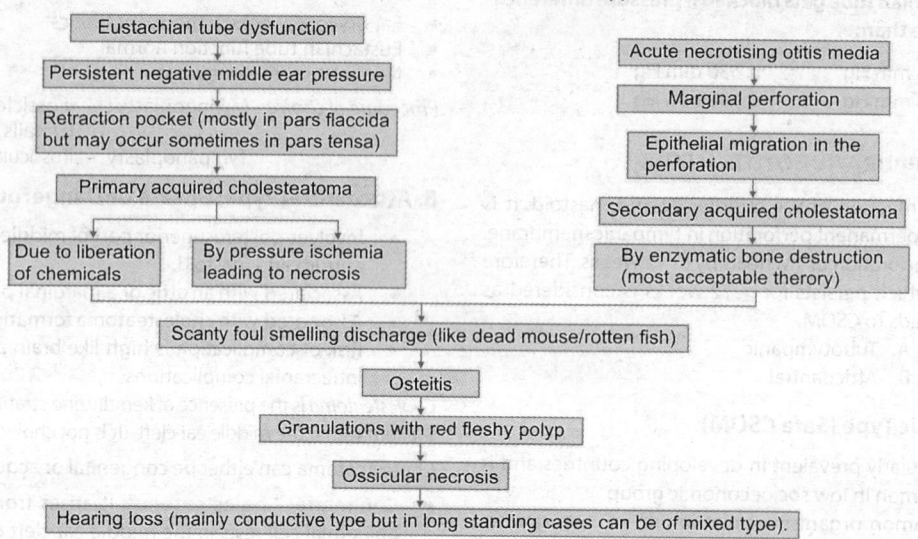

Flowchart 7.2: Pathogenesis of atticoantral type of CSOM.

NEW PATTERN QUESTIONS

Q N9. Witt-Mack's theory of cholesteatoma formation is related to:
a. Squamous metaplasia
b. Basal cell hyperplasia
c. Invagination of pars flaccida
d. None of the above

Q N10. Which is true of cholesteatoma?
a. Physiological
b. Erodes bone
c. Benign neoplasm
d. Contains cholesterol

Clinical Features

- Scanty foul smelling painless discharge.
- Conductive type of hearing loss (If ossicles get eroded then mixed hearing loss occurs)
- Tinnitus may be present
- Bleeding: in case of polyps/granulation tissue
- It can lead to facial nerve twitching, palsy or paralysis.

Signs

- Marginal posterosuperior or attic perforation with granulation tissue or pearly white flakes of cholesteatoma
- **Imaging study:** CT scan is the investigation of choice.

Table 7.2: Features of safe and unsafe CSOM

Feature	Safe CSOM	Unsafe CSOM
Discharge	Copious, odorless	Scanty, foul smelling
Perforation	Central (in pars tensa)	Attic or marginal (in pars flaccida)
Polyp	Pale colored	Fleshy
Cholesteatoma	Absent	Present
Complications	Rare	Common

Treatment

- **Surgical:** It is the mainstay of treatment.^{Q}
- Primary aim is removal of disease by mastoidectomy to make ear safe followed by reconstruction of hearing at a later stage.
- **Surgery of choice:** Modified Radical mastoidectomy^Q.

> **Extra Edge**
>
> - Ciliated columnar epithelium lines the Eustachian tube, anterior mesotympanum and inferior hypotympanum, while cuboidal epithelium lines the attic, mastoid and posterior mesotympanum.
> - Simple patch test helps to find out the integrity of ossicular chain, hence to decide whether myringoplasty or tympanoplasty needs to be done in case of safe CSOM.
> - Hearing in CSOM is better when the ear is discharging due to shielding effect of round window or discharge covering the perforation.
> - Posterior perforation tends to have more hearing loss due to loss of sound protection for round window. Larger the perforation, greater the loss of surface area on which sound pressure can act.

NEW PATTERN QUESTIONS

Q N11. Cholesteatoma is commonly caused by:
a. Atticoantral perforation
b. Tubotympanic disease
c. Central perforation of tympanic membrane
d. Meniere's disease

Q N12. TOC of perforation in pars flaccida of tympanic membrane with cholesteatoma is:
a. Myringoplasty
b. Modified radical mastoidectomy
c. Antibiotics
d. Radical mastoidectomy

Chapter 7: Diseases of Middle Ear

The newer classification of Chronic otitis media

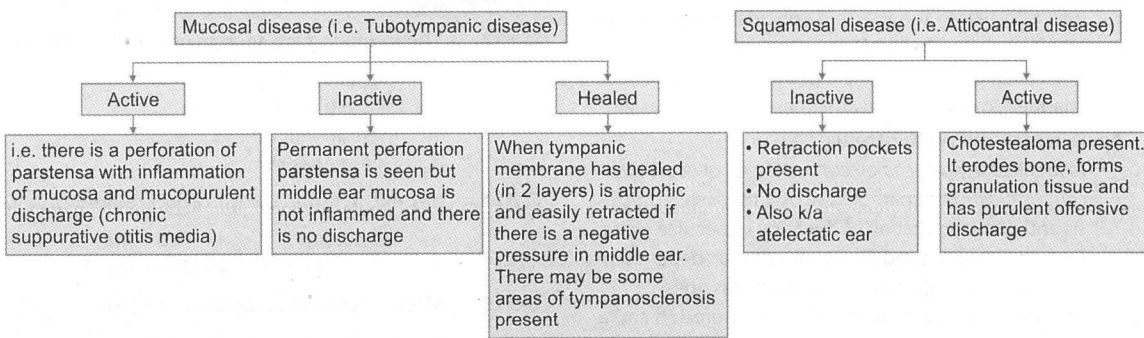

- **Mucosal disease (i.e. Tubotympanic disease)**
  - **Active**: i.e. there is a perforation of parstensa with inflammation of mucosa and mucopurulent discharge (chronic suppurative otitis media)
  - **Inactive**: Permanent perforation parstensa is seen but middle ear mucosa is not inflamed and there is no discharge
  - **Healed**: When tympanic membrane has healed (in 2 layers) is atrophic and easily retracted if there is a negative pressure in middle ear. There may be some areas of tympanosclerosis present
- **Squamosal disease (i.e. Atticoantral disease)**
  - **Inactive**:
    - Retraction pockets present
    - No discharge
    - Also k/a atelectatic ear
  - **Active**: Chotestealoma present. It erodes bone, forms granulation tissue and has purulent offensive discharge

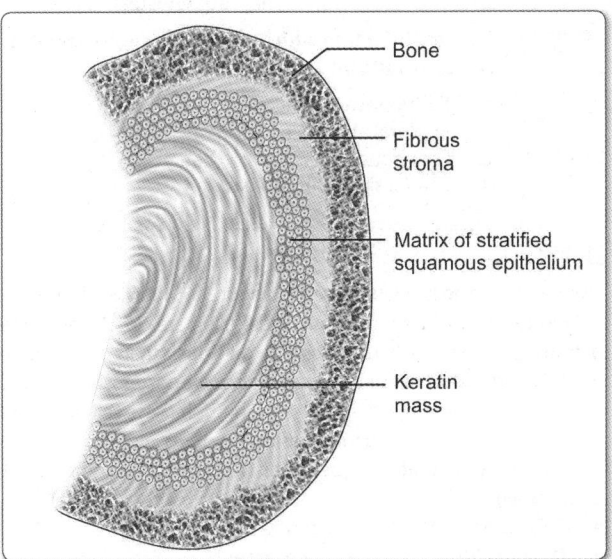

Fig. 7.2: Cholesteatoma structure. Stroma, matrix and keratin mass

(Labels: Bone, Fibrous stroma, Matrix of stratified squamous epithelium, Keratin mass)

COMPLICATIONS OF OTITIS MEDIA

Extracranial (Intratemporal) complications	Intracranial complications
• Mastoiditis • Petrositis/Gradenigo syndrome • Facial paralysis • Labyrinthitis • Osteomyelitis of temporal bone • Septicemia or pyemia • Otogenic tetanus	• Meningitis • Extradural abscess • Subdural abscess • Otogenic brain abscess • Lateral sinus thrombophlebitis • Otitic hydrocephalus

ACUTE MASTOIDITIS

- M/C extracranial (intratemporal) complication of acute otitis media.
- Inflammation of the mucosal lining of the mastoid antrum and its air cell system.
- **Organism (most common):** B hemolytic *Streptococcus pneumoniae*.

Symptoms

- Persistence of pain, fever and discharge even after 3 weeks of ASOM.

Note: Any persistence of discharge beyond 3 weeks, in a case of acute otitis media points to mastoiditis.

Signs

- Tenderness over the mastoid antrum/suprameatal triangle
- **Ironed out appearance of skin over mastoid due to thick periosteum is the first sign of acute mastoiditis**
- *Condutive type of hearing loss present.*
- *Retroauricular swelling:* Over the mastoid which pushes pinna forwards and downwards and the retro auricular sulcus appears deepened.
- Mucopurulent discharge seen in EAC.
- P*ostero-superior canal wall sagging*
- *Tragal sign –ve*
- *Movement of pinna is not painful.*

Point to Remember

➤ **Mastoid Reservoir sign**: Positive, i.e. meatus fills up immediately with pus after cleaning.
➤ **Light house sign**: The purulent discharge is often pulsatile and comes out through the perforation of pars tensa.

X-ray Mastoid

- Clouding of air cells due to collection of exudates in them
- Bony partition between the cells becomes indistinct.
- Best view to know the extent of pneumatization and destruction in mastoid is lateral oblique view called as **Schuller's view/Law's view**.

Type of Acute Mastoiditis

- Acute mastoiditis can be staged as:
  1. **Acute mastoiditis without periostitis/osteitis**
     – It is the extension of the pathological process of acute middle ear infection. No periostitis or osteitis of the mastoid is present.

2. **Acute mastoiditis with periostitis**
   - Infection within the mastoid spreads to periosteum covering the mastoid process. The route of infection from the mastoid cells to the periosteum is by venous channels, mot commonly the mastoid emissary vein.
3. **Acute mastoiditis with osteitis**
   - Also called as *acute coalescent mastoiditis* or *acute surgical mastoiditis*. Basic pathology is osteitis, in which necrosis and demineralization of the bony trabeculae occur. From this stage onward disease progression depends on the direction in which the erosive process goes:
     * Most commonly, mastoid cortex is eroded and a subperiosteal abscess develops.
     * Medial progression causes petrositis and Gradenigo's syndrome.
     * Anterior progression can compromise the fallopian canal or labyrinth causing facial palsy or vertigo.
     * Infection in the cranium causes intracranial complications meningitis, abscess, lateral sinus thrombophlebitis, otitic hydrocephalus.
   - Classically, the term mastoiditis referred to acute coalescent mastoiditis with superiosteal abscess lateral to the mastoid cortex occurring 2 weeks after onset of ASOM.

Abscesses in Relation to Mastoid Infection

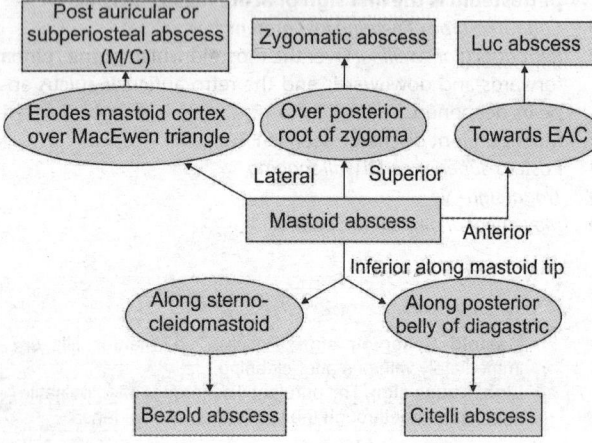

Treatment
- IV antibiotics
- Myringotomy: If pus is under tension
- Cortical mastoidectomy:
  - In case of intracranial/intratemporal complications
  - If patient's condition deteriorates after 24 hours despite adequate treatment

Note: If a subperiosteal abscess or an intracranial extension of disease is suspected, surgery in combination with high dose IV antibiotics should be 1st line of therapy.

NEW PATTERN QUESTIONS

Q N13. The following are seen in mastoiditis *except*:
  a. Light house sign
  b. Mastoid reservoir sign
  c. Mastoid tenderness
  d. Griesinger's sign

Q N14. M/c extracranial complication related to ASOM:
  a. Mastoiditis   b. Petrositis
  c. Labyrinth   d. Facial N palsy

Q N15. M/c abscess following mastoiditis:
  a. Bezold   b. Citelli
  c. LUC   d. Subperiosteal

Q N16. Mastoid infection which erodes through the outer cortex results in:
  a. Subperiosteal abscess
  b. Epidural abscess
  c. Perichondritis
  d. Lateral sinus thrombosis

PETROSITIS/GRADENIGO'S SYNDROME

The petrous bone is pneumatized in about 30% individuals. The CN VI (abducens) and/ CN V (trigeminal) ganglion are closely related to petrous apex. There are two groups of air cells' tracts that communicate mastoid and middle ear to the petrous apex viz posterosuperior and antero inferior tract. Infection may pass through these cell tracts and reach petrous apex leading to petrositis.

Classical presentation of petrositis is Gradenigo's syndrome, i.e. triad of **(3D)**
- Persistent ear **D**ischarge: Otorrhea
- **D**iplopia (due to VI nerve involvement)
- **D**eep seated orbital or retro-orbital pain (due to Vth nerve involvement)

Sudden disappearance of symptoms in Gradenigo syndrome suggests intracranial rupture.

Note:
- Persistent ear discharge in cases of cortical or modified redical mastoidectomy is due to Petrositis
  Ref: Essential of MB Pg. 122
- CT of temporal bone confirms the diagnosis.

FACIAL PARALYSIS

For details see chapter: Facial Nerve and its disorders.

LATERAL SINUS THROMBOPHLEBITIS/SIGMOID SINUS THROMBOSIS

May occur as a complication of:
- Acute coalescent mastoiditis
- CSOM and cholesteatoma

Clinical Features

Patient presents with:
- *Picket fence type of fever* with rigors, i.e. fever rises twice during day reaching 104° or 105°F and comes to normal.
  - Fever coincides with release of septic embolic into blood stream.
  - Patient is alert with sense of well-being in between bouts of fever.
- *Headache*
- *Progressive anemia.*

Symptoms of septic emboli, headache and papilledema may indicate extension to involve the cavernous sinus.

Signs

Progressive anemia and emaciation:
- *Torticollis of neck*
- **Griesinger's sign**: Due to thrombosis of mastoid emissary vein. There is edema over posterior part of mastoid.
- **Tobey-Ayer test (queckenstedt's test)**: Compression of jugular vein on thrombosed side does not produce any change in CSF pressure. Whereas compression of jugular vein on healthy side raises CSF pressure.
- **Crow - Beck test**

> *Compression of jugular vein on healthy side*
> ↓
> *Engorgement of retinal veins and supraorbital veins. If there is a thrombosed sinus, no such change is seen.*

- Tenderness along jugular vein.
- Contrast enhanced CT shows a typical **delta sign**. It is a triangular area with rim enhancement and central low density area is seen in posterior cranial fossa on axial cut.
- MRI is more sensitive than CT.

Management

Parenteral antibiotics and possible surgical exploration via mastoidectomy. It may require ligation of internal jugular vein in recalcitrant disease.

NEW PATTERN QUESTIONS

Q N17. Tobey-Ayer test is positive in:
  a. Lateral sinus thrombosis
  b. Petrositis
  c. Cerebral abscess
  d. Subarachnoid haemorrhage

Q N18. Appearance of fever with rigor in a person with otitis media should make you suspect:
  a. Cerebellar abscess
  b. Extradural abscess
  c. Lateral sinus thrombosis
  d. Apex petrositis

INTRACRANIAL COMPLICATIONS

■ EXTRADURAL ABSCESS

It is collection of pus between bone and dura. It is called:

Epidural abscess	Perisinus abscess
↓	↓
If abscess lies medial to sigmoid sinus	If abscess, encloses the sinus

■ SUBDURAL ABSCESS

Collection of pus between dura and arachnoid.

■ MENINGITIS

> - *It is the most common intracranial complication of suppurative otitis media*   *Essential of ENT, Mohan Bansal, 1/e p 123*

- **In infants and children, meningitis is often a complication of AOM while in adults it occurs due to cholesteatoma.**
- **One-third cases of meningitis are otogenic in origin.**
- **Most common organism responsible for otic meningitis are – S. pneumoniae and – H. influenza Type B**
- **Positive Kernig's sign**, i.e. painful extension of leg on flexed thigh
- **Positive Brudzinski's sign**, i.e. flexion of neck causes flexion of hip and knee.
- **Positive Babinski sign**, i.e. extension of big toe on stimulation of lateral aspect of sole.
- Imaging modality of choice: HRCT temporal bone.

NEW PATTERN QUESTION

Q N19. M/c intracranial complication of CSOM is:
  a. Meningitis
  b. Brain abscess
  c. Lateral sinus thrombosis
  d. Subdural abscess

■ BRAIN ABSCESS

- Infections are the most common cause of brain abscess.
  ...*Turner 10/e, p 311-312*
- 50% brain abscess in adults and 25% brain abscess in children are otogenic in origin. In adults cholesteatoma and in children AOM are the M/C causes.

Brain abscess is of 2 types	
Cerebral abscess (*M/C temporal abscess*)	Cerebellar abscess

- **Cerebral abscess** is seen twice as frequently as cerebellar abscess and M/C site of cerebral abscess is Temporal lobe
- Cerebellar abscess can develop as direct extension through Trautmann's triangle.
- **Microbiology:** G-ve organisms (proteus, E. coli, Pseudomonas and anaerobic bacteria along with staphylococci)

Clinical Features

- **Temporal lobe abscess can present as:**
  - **Nominal aphasia**
  - **Homonymous hemianopia** (earliest focal sign).
  - **Contralateral motor paralysis**
  - Epileptic fits
  - Hallucinations of taste and smell
  - Occulomotor palsy
- **Cerebellar abscess:**
  - Ipsilateral spontaneous nystagmus
  - Ipsilateral ataxia
  - Past pointing
  - Intentional tremors
  - Dysdiadochokinesia

Investigation

- CT scan—It reveals the site and size of abscess. **'Ring sign'** i.e. hypodense area surrounded by an area of edema is seen.

Treatment

- *Medical* = high dose IV antibiotics + for raised ICT→ dexamethasone or mannitol.
- *Surgical*
- Drainage of abscess
- In the associated ear = Modified Radial mastoidectomy in CSOM with cholesteatoma.

OTITIS HYDROCEPHALUS

Rare complication:
- Characterized by raised intracranial pressure with normal CSF findings.
- Caused due to thrombus extending to superior sagittal sinus which impedes the function of arachnoid villi to absorb CSF and therefore cause ICT.

Point to Remember
> MRI is the IOC in extradural, Bezold and cerebral abscess. CT is the IOC in cases of coalescent mastoiditis.

SURGICAL MANAGEMENT OF MIDDLE EAR SUPPURATION

INCISIONS FOR EAR SURGERY

- Postaural (William Wilde's) and endaural (Lempert's) incisions are used in mastoidectomy and tympanoplasty.
- Endomeata (Rosen's) incision is used in stapedectomy and in tympanoplasty.

MYRINGOTOMY

- Incising the tympanic membrane to drain the middle ear.
- Can be coupled with insertion of ventilation tube (grommet).

Indication

1. Acute otitis media: Indications in AOM are:
   - Severe pain (bulging red tympanic membrane)
   - AOM going in for complications
   - Unresolved AOM
   - AOM occurring during antibiotic therapy
   - AOM in immunodeficiency
   - **Recurrent AOM** (along with grommet insertion): More than 3 episodes of ASOM in 6–6 episodes in 12 months. Patient should be free of infection in between the episodes. Predisposing causes include adenoid hypertrophy, nasal allergy, chronic sinusitis, cleft palate, and other causes of velopharyngeal insufficiency, craniofacial anomalies, immunodeficiency, and GERD.
2. Otitic barotrauma for drainage and unblocking Eustachian tube.

Myringotomy is coupled with grommet insertion in:
- Suppurative or serous otitis media
- Recurrent Acute otitis media
- Adhesive otitis media
- Meniere's disease

Preferred Site for Myringotomy (Figs. 7.3A and B)

Condition	Site
Acute Suppurative Otitis Media (ASOM) **A**	**Circumferential** incision is made in the posterior-inferior quadrant of tympanic membrane, midway between handle of malleus and tympanic annulus.
Serous Otitis Media ± grommet insertion **B**	A small radial incision is given in antero-inferior quadrant.

Figs. 7.3A and B: Sites of myringotomy

Note:
- Myringotomy was first performed by Astley Cooper for serous otitis media
- Myringotomy is contraindicated in case of suspected intratympanic glomus tumor- In such a case tympanotomy should be done.

MYRINGOPLASTY

Repair of defect of tympanic membrane (In Pars tensa)
- Commonest graft material used is temporalis fascia.
- Other materials include tragal perichondrium, Fat and vein (autografts), or cadaveric dura and vein (homografts).
- It is done using an operating microscope with focal length 200–250 mm.

Indication

A perforated tympanic membrane with only mild conductive hearing loss, which implies a normal ossicular chain.

Techniques

- **Underlay technique:** In this technique, the graft is placed medial to the tympanic annulus, i.e. under it.
- **Overlay technique:** In overlay technique the graft is placed lateral to the tympanic annulus, i.e. over it.

Contraindications

- Active discharge from middle ear
- Nasal allergy
- Otitis externa
- Ingrowth of squamous epithelium into the middle ear
- When the other ear is dead or not suitable for hearing aid rehabilitation
- Children < 3 years

Complications

- Underlay technique:
  1. Middle ear becomes narrow
  2. Graft may adhere to promontory
  3. Can lead to atelectasis of middle ear cavity.
- Overlay technique:
  1. Blunting of anterior sulcus
  2. Lateralization of graft

NEW PATTERN QUESTION

Q N20. Myringotomy is contraindicated in case of:

a. Aero otitis media
b. Glomus tumor
c. Bulging ear drum
d. Atelectatic ear

TYMPANOPLASTY

Eradication of disease from middle ear along with repair, which includes ossicular reconstruction with myringoplasty. Possibly it is the commonest surgery done in CSOM.

Types of Tympanoplasty

Wullstein and Zollner (1953) classified tympanoplasty into following types:

- **Type I:** It differs from simple closure of perforation (myringoplasty) in that here middle ear is also examined to rule out any pathology.
- **Type II:** It is done where there is disease in atticoantral region with mild erosion of malleus or incus Temporalis fascia graft is placed on the incus or remnant of malleus.
- **Type III:** M/c type of tympanoplasty (Columellar type or effect): It is done when malleus and incus are destroyed but stapes is healthy. Graft is placed on the head of stapes. It is also called **myringostapediopexy/columella effect**. This columellar effect is usually present in birds.
- **Type IV:** All ossicles including stapes head are eroded. Graft is placed in such a way that a small air-containing cavity with Eustachian tube and round window is created (cavum minor). Footplate of the stapes should be mobile and is left exposed to sound waves.
- **Type V:** It is also **called fenestration operation**. Here footplate of stapes is fixed, but round window is functioning. In such cases another window is created on horizontal semicircular canal. Commonest ossiculoplasty material is autograft incus.

Extra Edge

Graft materials used during ossiculoplasty:

- **Autografts:** The most commonly used are autograft ossicles (incus) and tragal cartilage or septal cartilage.
- **Homograft:** Ossicles and membrane.
- **Prosthetic implants:** They are made of ceramic (hydroxy appetite), teflon, gold and titanium.
  - **Total ossicular replacement prosthesis (TORP):** It bridges the gap between TM and stapes footplate. Done when all 3 ossicles necrosed
  - **Partial ossicular replacement prosthesis (PORP):** It provides a direct contact between TM and stapes head done when only malleus and incus are necrosed.

NEW PATTERN QUESTIONS

Q N21. Tympanoplasty is mainly used for:

a. Otosclerosis
b. CSOM
c. ASOM
d. None

Q N22. What is tympanoplasty:

a. Eradication of middle ear disease with reconstruction of tympanic membrane and ossicles
b. Eradication of disease from internal ear
c. Eradication of middle ear disease with repair of tympanic membrane only
d. Eradication of middle ear disease with repair of ossicles only

Q N23. Austin's classification for ossicular chain defects depends on:

a. Malleus head and stapes footplate
b. Malleus handle and stapes suprastructure
c. Malleus head and stapes suprastructure
d. Malleus head and stapes head

Q N24. A 3 years old child presents with fever and ear ache. After a course of antibiotic, his condition is still not relieved. What is the next step in management?

a. Myringotomy with antibiotics
b. Myringotomy with grommet insertion
c. Oral antibiotics and decongestants
d. Anti-allergic and decongestants only

Q N25. Myringostapediopexy is classified as which type of tympanoplasty:

a. Type 1
b. Type 2
c. Type 3
d. Type 4

Q N26. Temporal fascia is used in tympanoplasty operations because:
   a. It is closer to the ear
   b. It is easy to remove
   c. It has low metabolic rate
   d. Has some consistency as that of tympanic membrane

Q N27. Tympanoplasty is most commonly performed for tympanic membrane perforation greater than:
   a. 10–20% of the size of tympanic membrane
   b. 20–30% of the size of tympanic membrane
   c. 30–40% of the size of tympanic membrane
   d. 40–50% of the size of tympanic membrane

CORTICAL MASTOIDECTOMY/SIMPLE MASTOIDECTOMY/SCHWARTZ OPERATION

Simple mastoidectomy/Schwartz operation. Involves exenteration of all accessible mastoid air cells without taking down the posterior meatal wall.

Indications

- Acute coalescent mastoiditis
- Incompletely resolved otitis media with reservoir sign
- Masked mastoiditis
- As an initial step to perform:
  - Endolymphatic sac surgery
  - Decompression of facial nerve
  - Translabyrinthine or Retrolabyrinthine procedure, for acoustic neuroma.

Steps

> **Mastoid surgery:**
> - Mastoid exploration is the initial step in all mastoidectomies.
> - It is done using an operating microscope (Focal length 200–250 mm) and drill.
> - The site for drilling – Mc Ewans triangle.
> - **Techniques which are used to control bleeding from bone during mastoid surgery,** include bone wax, bipolar cautery over the bleeding area and using diamond drill, cutting drill over the bleeding area will not control bleeding

RADICAL MASTOIDECTOMY

Aims at exenteration and exteriorization. No reconstruction is attempted.

The disease from the middle ear and mastoid is exenterated, middle ear, attic, antrum, and mastoid air cells are converted into a single cavity by taking down the posterior canal wall and thus exteriorized. The whole mucosa of the middle ear, remnants of tympanic membrane, and ossicles except stapes are removed. The middle ear is closed off by curetting the Eustachian tube and plugging with muscle. No attempts are made to pressure hearing.

Indications

- Malignancy of the external ear and middle ear.
- Unresectable cholesteatoma, scarring, Eustachian tube orifice, and producing severe sensorineural hearing loss.
- If previous attempts to eradicate cholosteatoma have failed.

Another way of classifying mastoidectomy is based on the approach to mastoid		
Canal wall up procedure (Intact canal wall)	**Canal wall down procedure**	
• Posterior canal wall is left intact • Middle ear is approached through facial recess in mastoid	Posterior canal wall is removed thereby exteriorizing the mastoid into the external ear. It can be done as	
• Includes posterior tympanotomy and simple/cortical *mastoidectomy (Schwartz operation)* Consists of complete exenteration of all accessible mastoid air cells and converting them into a single cavity • Middle ear structures are not disturbed Indications – (MAM) M Acute coalescent mastoiditis A Acute otitis media with reservoir sign M Masked mastoiditis	**Modified radical mastoidectomy** Attempt is made to preserve as much hearing as possible. Steps: • Post meatal wall and lateral attic wall are removed • TOE, i.e. Tympanic membrane remnant, Ossicles and Eustachian, Tube functions are preserved.	**Radical mastoidectomy** No attempts are made to preserve hearing Steps: • Post meatal wall is removed • TOE are all removed • Entire area of middle ear, attic, antrum and mastoid are converted to a single cavity
Drawback: Associated with high incidence of residual/recurrent cholesteatoma	**Indications:** • Cholesteatoma confined to attic and antrum • Localized chronic otitis media	**Indications:** • When cholesteatoma can not be removed safely or if previous attempts have failed

"A canal wall up mastoidectomy with ossicular reconstruction may be considered only in patients with chronic otitis media without any evidence of evidence of cholesteatoma"....
Otology and Neurology, Inc, Vol. 2615, Sept. 05, p 1045-1051
More importantly canal up technique is the surgical approach for cochlear implant

Modified Radical Mastoidectomy

- Here in addition to exenteration and exteriorization, reconstruction of the hearing mechanism is also attempted. So in addition to creating an open cavity as in radical mastoidectomy all healthy mucosa, remnants of tympanic membrane and ossicles are preserved to facilitate tympanoplasty later on.
- This is the treatment of choice for attico antral disease and resectable cholesteatoma of middle ear and mastoid including complications.

Measures to avoid Injury to Facial Nerve during Mastoidectomy

- Change to higher power of microscope near facial nerve.
- Adequate irrigation to avoid thermal injury.
- Avoid using cutting burr near the nerve, use diamond burr instead.
- Use the burr along the direction of the nerve – never across.
- Never pull out granulations on the nerve.

> **Point to Remember**
> - Mastoidectomy is one of the commonest causes of iatrogenic facial palsy
> - Commonest site of injury to the facial nerve during mastoidectomy is the 2nd genu).
> - **Focal length of the objective lens of the operating microscope used for ear surgeries**
>   200–250 mm.
>   **Note:** It is 300 mm for nasal surgeries and 400 mm for microlaryngeal surgeries

IMPORTANT LANDMARKS TO REMEMBER WHILE DOING MASTOIDECTOMY

1. Suprameatal (MacEwen's) Triangle

It is bounded superiorly by the supra mastoid crest, anteriorly by the posterosuperior canal wall and a trangential line from here to the supramastoid crest completes the triangle. Antrum lies approximately 1.5 cm deep to the triangle in adults. It is the Surgical Landmark for Mastoid Antrum during Mastoidectomy.

2. Citelli's Angle

Citelli's angle is **sino dural angle** (angle between the plate of bone separating the sigmoid sinus from the mastoid cavity (sinus platel) and the plate of bone separating middle cranial fossa dura from the mastoid cavity [dural plate]). This is a common site of residual/recurrent disease after surgery.

3. Trautmann's Triangle

- This bony plate of posterior surface of petrous bone lies behind the mastoid antrum. It is bounded by:
  - Sigmoid sinus
  - Bony labyrinth
  - Superior petrosal sinus.

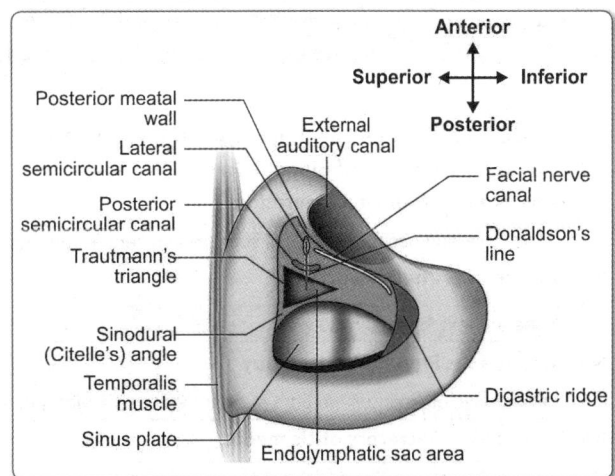

Fig. 7.4: Cortical mastoidectomy cavity—landmarks and structures seen

4. Donaldson's Line

- This line passes through the lateral semicircular canal bisecting the posterior semicircular canal. The endolymphatic sac is situated inferior to Donaldson's line.

Instruments used in Mastoid Surgery

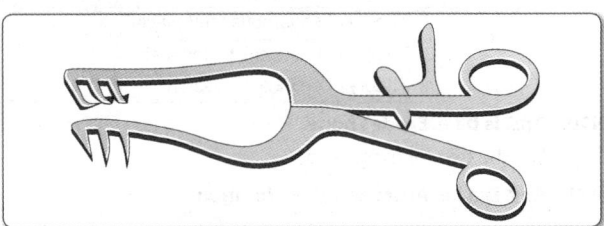

Fig. 7.5: Mollison Mastoid retractor

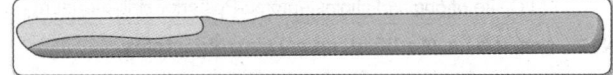

Fig. 7.6: Mastoid gouge

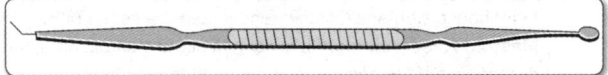

Fig. 7.7: Mastoid seeker with scoop

NEW PATTERN QUESTION

Q N28. TOC of CSOM with vertigo and facial nerve palsy is:
a. Antibiotics and labyrinthine sedative
b. Myringoplasty
c. Immediate mastoid exploration
d. Labyrinthectomy

Explanations and References to New Pattern Questions

N1. Ans. is b i.e. **Surgical opening in tympanic membrane** *Ref. Dhingra ENT 6/e, p 78*

N2. Ans. is d i.e. **Posteroinferior quadrant** *Ref. Dhingra ENT 6/e, p 378*

N3. Ans. is a i.e. **Stage of suppuration**

> Pus formation occurs in stage of suppuration, hence, light house sign is seen in this stage.

N4. Ans. is a i.e. **Pneumococcus**

> See the text for explanation

N5. Ans. is a i.e. **Pneumatic otoscopy** *Ref. Essentials of ENT, Mohan Bansal*

> Pneumatic otoscopy is the gold standard for the diagnosis of otitis media with effusion.

N6. Ans. is a i.e. **Secretory otitis media**

> See the text for explanation

N7. Ans. is b i.e. **Descent in air** *Ref. Dhingra ENT 6/e, p 66*

> Otitic barotrauma or Aero otitis media results due to rapid descent during air flight, underwater divising or compression in pressure chamber.

N8. Ans. is d i.e. **90 mm Hg** *Ref. Dhingra ENT 6/e, p 66*

> Eustachian tube gets blocked when atmospheric pressure is higher than that of middle ear by critical level of 90 mm Hg.

N9. Ans. is c i.e. **Invagination of pars flaccida** *Ref. Tuli, 2/e, p 69; Dhingra 6/e, p 67*

Theory Related to Cholesteatoma formation	Proposed by
1. Invagination of pars flaccida to form retraction pockets (M/C accepted theory)	Wittmack
2. Theory of squamous metaplasia	Sade
3. Theory of basal cell hyperplasia	Ruede
4. Theory of epithelial invasion	Haberman's theory

N10. Ans. is b i.e. **Erodes bone**

See the text for explanation

N11. Ans. is a i.e. **Atticoantral perforation**

Atticoantral disease in which perforation is located in the attic region is associated with development of cholesteatoma and has higher risks of complications like brain abscess and other intracranial infections.

> M/C site of origin of cholesteatoma-Posterior epitympanum (Prussak space).

N12. Ans. is b i.e. **Modified radical mastoidectomy**

Perforation in pars flaccida indicates unsafe CSOM which is managed by modified radical mastoidectomy.

N13. Ans. is d i.e. **Griesinger's sign** *Ref. Disease of ENT Tuli, 2/e, p 62*

> Light house sign and Mastoid tenderness are seen in mastoiditis (as discussed in the text)
> **Mastoid Reservoir sign**: It is seen in acute mastoiditis. There is immediate filling of the deep auditory meatus with pus after cleaning or mopping of the pus.

N14. Ans. is a i.e. **Mastoiditis**

N15. Ans. is d i.e. **Subperiosteal**

> - M/C extracranial complication of CSOM: mastoiditis
> - M/C abscess associated with mastoiditis–post aural subperiosteal abscess
> - M/C Intracranial complication of CSOM- Meningitis
> - M/C nerve involved in CSOM—Facial Nerve

N16. Ans. is a i.e. **Subperiosteal abscess**

> See the text for explanation

Chapter 7: Diseases of Middle Ear

N17. Ans. is a i.e. Lateral sinus thrombosis

Features of lateral sinus thrombosis
1. Picket fence type of fever
2. Griesinger's sign
3. Tobey-Ayer test (Queckenstedt's test)
4. Crowe-Beck test
5. Delta sign: Seen in CT in case of lateral sinus thrombosis

N18. Ans. is c i.e. Lateral sinus thrombosis
See the text for explanation

N19. Ans. is a i.e. Meningitis

See the text for explanation

N20. Ans. is b i.e. Glomus tumor *Ref. Essential of ENT Mohan Bansal, p 432*

- Myringotomy/grommet insertions are contraindicated in suspected cases of intratympanic glomus tumor because they can cause profuse bleeding in such cases.
- **Also know**: In atelectatic ear— Grommet insertion is indicated for long term aeration purpose.

N21. Ans. is b i.e. CSOM *Ref. Dhingra ENT 6/e, p 72*

Tympanoplasty is the M/C surgery done for CSOM.

N22. Ans. is a i.e. Eradication of middle ear disease with reconstruction of tympanic membrane and ossicles *Ref. Dhingra ENT 6/e, p 400*

Tympanoplasty (Tympanum = Middle ear)
It is an operation in which reconstructive procedure is limited to repair of tympanic membrane perforation.
Myringoplasty
It is an operation in which reconstructive procedure is limited to repair of tympanic membrane perforation.
Meatoplasty
Meatoplasty is an operation in which a crescent of conchal cartilage is excised to widen the meatus.

N23. Ans. is b i.e. Malleus handle and stapes suprastructure

Austin classified the ossicular erosions into four types. This classification is based on the presence or absence of malleus handle and stapes suprastructure

Type	Structure absent	Structure present	Management
Type A	Incus	Malleus handle Stapes suprastructures	Incus prosthesis
Type B	• Incus • Stapes • Suprastructures	Malleus handle	TORP
Type C	• Incus • Malleus handle	Stapes suprastructure	PORP
Type D	• Incus • Malleus handle • Stapes suprastructure	—	TORP

Note: In all cases, incus was assumed to be absent, since it is the first ossicle to get eroded.

Stapes suprastructures include:
• Head
• Neck
• Anterior crura
• Posterior crura

N24. Ans. is b i.e. Myringotomy with grommet insertion *Ref. Dhingra ENT 6/e, p 63*
A child presenting with AOM and not responding to medicines, should be managed with myringotomy so that the pus could be drained.

N25. Ans. is c i.e. Type 3
See the text for explanation

N26. Ans. is c i.e. It has low metabolic rate

Temporal fascia is used as it is thin but tough, can be obtained in the same incision, has low O_2 demand, low metabolic rate and after healing looks like tympanic membrane.

N27. Ans. is a i.e. 10-20% of the size of tympanic membrane

Tympanoplasty is most commonly performed for tympanic membrane perforations greater than 10–20% of the size of the entire tympanic membrane. It is done under general anesthesia. M/c approach for tympanoplasty—post auricular approach.

N28. Ans. is c i.e. Immediate mastoid exploration.

Always remember: Following CSOM – if a patient develops vertigo, it is a case of labyrinthitis. Patient is presenting with facial nerve palsy and labyrinthitis i.e. a cholesteatoma or unsafe CSOM is the cause. So, management would be immediate mastoid exploration to remove the cholesteatoma.

Chapter 7: Diseases of Middle Ear

QUESTIONS

ACUTE SUPPURATIVE OTITIS MEDIA

1. **Throat infection causes Ear infection through:** *[PGI 2008]*
   a. Blood spread
   b. Eustachian tube
   c. Nasocranial spread
   d. Simultaneous infection
2. **Commonest cause of acute otitis media in children is:**
   [AIIMS June 00; Delhi- 06; UP-03]
   a. H. influenzae
   b. S. pneumoniae
   c. S. aureus
   d. Pseudomonas
3. **Commonest causative organism for ASOM in 2 years child is:** *[AIIMS Dec. 95; 91]*
   a. Pneumococcus
   b. H. influenzae
   c. Staphylococcus
   d. Streptococcus
4. **True statement about ASOM is:** *[AI 99]*
   a. Most frequently it resolves without sequelae
   b. Commonly follows painful parotitis
   c. Radical mastoidectomy is required for treatment
   d. Most common organism is pseudomonas
5. **Cart Wheel sign is seen in:** *[MP 2008]*
   a. ASOM
   b. AOM
   c. OME
   d. CSOM
6. **Acute suppurative otitis media is treated using all except:** *[AIIMS 91]*
   a. Erythromycin
   b. Penicillin
   c. Streptomycin
   d. Cephalosporin
7. **A child presents with barotrauma pain. There is no inflammation of middle ear, management is:** *[Jharkhand 03]*
   a. Antibiotics
   b. Paracetamol
   c. Suppurative
   d. Grommet tube insertion
8. **Pulsatile otorrhea seen in:** *[AP 97]*
   a. Glomus tumour
   b. CSF otorrhea
   c. ASOM
   d. Fistula
9. **Most common perforation site in tympanic membrane in ASOM:**
   a. Antero-inferior
   b. Postero-inferior
   c. Antero-superior
   d. Postero-superior
10. **Light house sign is seen in:**
    a. ASOM
    b. CSOM
    c. Menieres disease
    d. Cholesteatoma

NONSUPPURATIVE OTITIS MEDIA

11. **A boy with ASOM undergoing treatment with penicillin therapy for 7 days now presents with subsidence of pain and persistence of deafness, diagnosis is:** *[Kolkata 2003]*
    a. Ototoxicity
    b. Secretory otitis media
    c. Adhesive otiti media
    d. Tympanosclerosis
12. **Cause of U/L secretory otitis media in an adult is:** *[PGI Dec. 99 / UP-04]*
    a. CSOM
    b. Nasopharyngeal carcinoma
    c. Mastoiditis
    d. Foreign body of external ear
13. **Acute non suppurative otitis media in adults is due to:** *[UP 2003]*
    a. Allergic rhinitis
    b. URTI
    c. Trauma
    d. Malignancy
14. **Glue ear:** *[DNB 2003]*
    a. Is painful
    b. Is painless
    c. Radical mastoidectomy is required
    d. NaF is useful
15. **Secretory otitis media is diagnosed by:** *[PGI June 98]*
    a. Impedance audiometry
    b. Pure tone audiometry
    c. X-ray
    d. Otoscopy
16. **True about Secretory otitis media:** *[PGI Nov 2016]*
    a. Type C tympanogram may be seen in early stage of otitis media with effusion
    b. Flat tympanogram is present
    c. Leads to conductive deafness
    d. Presence of cleft palate reduces its chance
    e. Most common cause is Eustachian tube dysfunction
17. **Bluish tympanic membrane is seen in:** *[JIPMER 93]*
    a. Early ASOM
    b. Glue ear
    c. Cholesteatoma
    d. Cholesterol granuloma
18. **Treatment of choice for glue ear is:** *[AIIMS May 07]*
    a. Myringotomy with cold knife
    b. Myringotomy with diode laser
    c. Myringotomy with ventilation tube insertion
    d. Conservative treatment with analgesics and antibiotics
19. **A 6-year-old child with recurrent URTI with mouth breathing and failure to grow with high arched palate and impaired hearing is:** *[AIIMS May 07]*
    a. Tonsillectomy
    b. Grommet insertion
    c. Myringotomy with grommet insertion
    d. Adenoidectomy with grommet insertion
20. **A child presenting with recurrent respiratory tract infection, mouth breathing and decreased hearing Treatment is:** *[PGI- 08]*
    a. Tonsillectomy
    b. Adenoidectomy
    c. Grommet insertion
    d. Myringotomy
    e. Myringoplasty
21. **Following statements are true about otitis media with effusion in a child:** *[PGI Dec. 03]*
    a. Immediate myringotomy is done
    b. Type B tympanogram
    c. The effusion of middle ear is sterile
    d. Most common cause of deafness in a child in day care patients

22. **Myringotomy is done after how long of medical management:** [AI Dec 2013]
    a. 1 month
    b. 3 months
    c. 6 months
    d. 1 year
23. **In serous otitis media which one of the following statements is true?** [2000]
    a. Sensorineural deafness occurs as a complication in 80% of the cases
    b. Intracranial spread of the infection complicates the clinical courses
    c. Tympanostomy tubes are usually required for treatment
    d. Gram-positive organisms are grown routinely in culture in the aspirate
24. **Medical treatments is NOT effective in which type of suppurative media:** [UP 07]
    a. Tuberculous OM
    b. Secretory OM
    c. Acute suppurative OM
    d. Chronic suppurative OM
25. **Which of the following is characteristic of T. B otitis media:** [AIIMS May 95]
    a. Marginal perforation
    b. Attic perforation
    c. Large central perforation
    d. Multiple perforation
26. **Tuberculous otitis media is characterized by all except:** [(AIIMS 1994) (AMU 2000)(AP 1996) (Delhi 1985, 1991, 1992, 2003) (Kerala 1998) (PGI 1999 Dec, PGI 1996) (AP 2004)]
    a. Multiple perforations
    b. Pale granulations
    c. Pain
    d. Thin odorless fluid
27. **True about tubercular otitis media:** (PGI May 2016)
    a. Multiple hole in tympanic membrane
    b. Pale granulation mass seen in middle ear
    c. No extra-auricular complication
    d. Corticosteroid is used in treatment
    e. Painless
28. **A child presents with barotrauma pain without middle ear inflammation. Management is:** [Jharkhand 2003]
    a. Antibiotics
    b. Myringotomy
    c. Supportive
    d. Grommet
29. **To do myringotomy in ASOM, the incision is given in posteroinferior region, this is the preferred region for all the following reasons except.** [AI 2007]
    a. It is easily accessible
    b. Damage to ossicular chain does not occur
    c. Damage to chorda tympani is avoided
    d. It is the very vascular region

CHRONIC SUPPURATIVE OTITIS MEDIA

30. **Ossicle M/c involved in CSOM:** [Kolkatta 04]
    a. Stapes
    b. Long process of incus
    c. Head of malleus
    d. Handle of malleus
31. **True about safe CSOM:** [PGI Dec. 00]
    a. Etiology is multiple bacteria
    b. Oral antibiotics are not affective
    c. Ear drops have no role
    d. Ottic hydrocephalus is a known complication
    e. Common in females than males
32. **Treatment of choice in central safe perforation is:** [AI 94]
    a. Modified mastoidectomy
    b. Tympanoplasty
    c. Myringoplasty
    d. Conservative management
33. **What is true in case of perforation of pars flaccida?** [AIIMS May 93]
    a. CSOM is a rare cause
    b. Associated with cholesteatoma
    c. Usually due to trauma
    d. All of the above
34. **Perforation of tympanic membrane with destruction of tympanic annulus is called:** [Bihar 2004]
    a. Attic
    b. Marginal
    c. Subtotal
    d. Total
35. **Cholesteatoma is commonly caused by:** [AI 94]
    a. Attico-antral perforation
    b. Tubotympanic disease
    c. Central perforation of tympanic membrane
    d. Meniere's disease
36. **Cholesteatoma is usually present at:** [Delhi 01]
    a. Anterior quadrant of tympanic membrane
    b. Posteroinferior quadrant of tympanic membrane
    c. Attic region
    d. Central part
37. **Cholesteatoma occurs in:** [AIIMS May 94]
    a. CSOM with central perforation
    b. Masked mastoiditis
    c. Coalescent mastoiditis
    d. Acute necrotizing otitis media
38. **Cholesteatoma is seen in:** [RJ 2006]
    a. ASOM
    b. CSOM
    c. Secretory ottitis media
    d. Osteosclerosis
39. **Most accepted theory for the formation of secondary cholesteatoma:** [DNB 2001]
    a. Congenital
    b. Squamous metaplasia
    c. Ingrowth of squamous epithelium
    d. Retraction pocket
40. **Levinson's criteria for diagnosing congenital cholesteatoma includes:** [PGI Nov. 2010]
    a. Whitish mass behind intact TM
    b. Normal pars tensa and pars flaccida
    c. Recurrent attacks of otorrhea
    d. Prior otitis media is not an exclusion criteria
41. **Prior H/O ear surgery Scanty, foul smelling, painless discharge from the ear is characteristic feature of which of the following lesions:** [AIIMS Nov. 00; 04]
    a. ASOM
    b. Cholesteatoma
    c. Central perforation
    d. Otitis externa
42. **True about cholesteatoma is/are:** [PGI Dec. 02; 06]
    a. It is a benign tumor
    b. Metastasizes to lymph node
    c. Contains cholesterol
    d. Erodes the bone
    e. Malignant potential

Chapter 7: Diseases of Middle Ear

43. Cholesteatoma commonly perforates: [PGI 00]
    a. Lat. Semicircular canal   b. Sup. semicircular canal
    c. Promontory   d. Oval window
44. Cholesteatoma (Atticoantral) true about: [PGI June 06]
    a. Scanty, malodorous discharge
    b. Otalgia
    c. Central perforation
    d. Ossicular involvement
    e. Eustachian tube dysfunction
45. The treatment of choice for atticoantral variety of chronic suppurative otitis media is: [AIIMS Nov. 02]
    a. Mastoidectomy
    b. Medical management
    c. Underlay myringoplasty
    d. Insertion of ventilation tube
46. Treatment of choice for Perforation in pars flaccida of the tympanic membrane with cholesteatoma is: [AI 96]
    a. Myringoplasty
    b. MRM
    c. Antibiotics
    d. Radical mastoidectomy
47. The posterosuperior retraction pocket, if allowed to progress, will lead to: [AI 03]
    a. Sensori-neural hearing loss
    b. Secondary cholesteatoma
    c. Tympanosclerosis
    d. Tertiary cholesteatoma
48. Most difficult site to remove cholesteatoma in sinus tympani is related with: [Kolkatta 2001]
    a. Anterior facial ridge   b. Posterior facial ridge
    c. Epitympanum   d. Hypotympanum
49. A child presents with ear infection with foul smelling discharge. On further exploration a small perforation is found in the pars flaccida of the tympanic membrane. Most appropriate next step in the management would be: [AIIMS Nov. 07]
    a. Topical antibiotics and decongestants for 4 weeks
    b. IV antibiotics and follow-up after a month
    c. Tympanoplasty
    d. Tympano-mastoid exploration
50. A 5-year-old boy has been diagnosed to have posterior superior retraction pocket. All would constitute part of the management except: [AI 03]
    a. Audiometry   b. Mastoid exploration
    c. Tympanoplasty   d. Myringoplasty

COMPLICATION OF OTITIS MEDIA

51. The most common complication of chronic suppurative otitis media is: [UPSC 05]
    a. Meningitis   b. Intracerebral abscess
    c. Cholesteatoma   d. Conductive deafness
52. Commonest intracranial complication of CSOM is: [Comed 08, DNB-07]
    a. Subperiosteal abscess   b. Mastoiditis
    c. Brain absess   d. Meningitis

53. M/c nerve to get damaged in CSOM is: [Karn 96]
    a. III   b. IV
    c. VI   d. VII
54. Most common complication of acute otitis media in children: [SRMC 02]
    a. Deafness   b. Mastoiditis
    c. Cholesteatoma   d. Facial nerve palsy
55. Extracranial complications of CSOM: [PGI Dec. 02]
    a. Epidural abscess
    b. Facial nerve plasy
    c. Hearing loss
    d. Labyrinthitis
    e. Sigmoid sinus thrombosis
56. Extracranial complication(s) of CSOM: [PGI June 01]
    a. Labyrinthitis
    b. Otitic hydrocephalus
    c. Bezold's abscess
    d. Facial nerve plasy
    e. Lateral sinus thrombophlebitis
57. Most common extracranial complication of ASOM is: [UP 2001]
    a. Facial nerve paralysis   b. Lateral sinus thrombosis
    c. Mastoiditis   d. Brain abscess
58. Mastoid reservoir phenomenon is positive in: [PGI June 99]
    a. CSOM   b. Petrositis
    c. Coalescent otitis media d. Mastoiditis
59. Acute mastoiditis is characterized by all except: [AP 97]
    a. Clouding of air cells
    b. Obliteration of retroauricular sulcus
    c. Deafness
    d. Outward and downward deviation of the pinna
60. Essential radiological feature of acute mastoiditis is: [UP-03]
    a. Temporal bone pneumatisation
    b. Clouding of air cells of mastoid
    c. Rarefaction and tuning of petrous bone
    d. Thickening of temporal bone
61. In Mastoiditis tenderness is/are present at:
    a. Tragus   [PGI Nov. 2010]
    b. Concha
    c. Mastoid tip
    d. Root of Zygoma
    e. Mastoid antrum
62. Mastoid tip is involved in: [UP-06]
    a. Bezold abscess
    b. Luc abscess
    c. Subperiosteal abscess
    d. Parapharyngeal abscess
63. Bezolds abscess is located in: [AIIMS 92, DNB-07]
    a. Submandibular region   b. Sternomastoid muscle
    c. Digastric triangle   d. Infratemporal region
64. Bezold abscess is seen in: (APPG 2016)
    a. Deep part of bony meatus
    b. Preauricular area
    c. Postauricular area
    d. Upper part of neck

65. The diagnosis in a patient with 6th nerve palsy, retro-orbital pain and persistent ear discharge is: [PGI June 99]
    a. Gradenigo's syndrome b. Sjogren's syndrome
    c. Frey's syndrome d. Rendu Osler Weber disease
66. All are true for Gradenigo's syndrome except: [AI 05]
    a. It is associated with jugular vein tenderness
    b. It is caused by an abscess in the petrous apex
    c. It leads to involvement of the Cranial nerves V and VI.
    d. It is characterized by retro-orbital pain
67. Gradenigo's syndrome characterized by all except: [PGI Dec. 02]
    a. Retroorbital pain
    b. Profuse discharge from the ear
    c. VII nerve palsy
    d. Diplopia
68. Treatment of cholesteatoma with facial paresis in child is: [AIIMS 93]
    a. Antibiotics to dry ear and then mastoidectomy
    b. Immediate mastoidectomy
    c. Observation
    d. Only antibiotic ear drops
69. Treatment of choice for CSOM with vertigo and facial nerve palsy is: [AI 96]
    a. Antibiotics and labyrinthine sedative
    b. Myringoplasty
    c. Immediate mastoid exploration
    d. Labyrinthectomy
70. Most potential route for transmission of Meningitis from CNS to Inner ear is: [AI-09]
    a. Cochlear Aqueduct
    b. Endolymphatic sac
    c. Vestibular Aqueduct
    d. Hyrtle fissure
71. Commonest cause of brain abscess: [PGI June 00]
    a. CSOM b. Pyogenic meningitis
    c. Trauma d. Chr. sinusitis
72. True about otogenic brain abscess is are:
    a. H. influenzae is most common causative organism
    b. C.S.O.M. with lat. sinus thrombosis in turn can cause brain abscess
    c. Most common complication of CSOM
    d. Temporal lobe abscess is associated with personality changes
73. Patient is having scanty, foul smelling discharge from middle ear, develops fever, headache and neck rigidity. CT of the temporal lobe shows a localized ring enhancing lesion, which of the following is least likely cause of this condition: [AI 2011]
    a. S. aureus b. Pseudomonas
    c. S. Pneumoniae d. H. influenzae
74. Lateral sinus thrombosis is associated with all except: [AP 2008]
    a. Greisinger sign b. Gradenigo sign
    c. Lily-Crowe sign d. Tobey Ayer test
75. Griesinger's sign is seen in: [TN 03]
    a. Lateral sinus thrombosis b. Meningitis
    c. Brain abscess d. Cerebellar abscess
76. Tobey-Ayer's test is/are used for: [PGI May 2014]
    a. CSF rhinorrhea
    b. Lateral sinus thrombosis
    c. Sigmoid sinus thrombosis
    d. To check patency of Eustachian tube
77. A child was treated for H. influenza meningitis for 6 month. Most important investigation to be done before discharging the patient is: [AI 99]
    a. MRI
    b. Brainstem evoked auditory response
    c. Growth screening test
    d. Psychotherapy
78. A patient of CSOM has cholesteatoma and presents vertigo with. Treatment of choice would be: [AI 98]
    a. Antibiotics and labyrinthine sedative
    b. Myringoplasty
    c. Immediate mastoid exploration
    d. Labyrinthectomy
79. Cranial nerves related to the apex of petrous temporal bone: [PGI 2005]
    a. V b. VI
    c. VII d. VIII
    e. IX
80. Most common nerve to be damaged in CSOM is:
    a. III b. VII
    c. IV d. VI

SURGICAL MANAGEMENT OF MIDDLE EAR SUPPURATION

81. A 7-year-old child presenting with acute otitis media, does not respond to ampicillin. Examination reveals full and bulging tympanic membrane, the treatment of choice is: [AI 98]
    a. Systemic steroid b. Ciprofloxacin
    c. Myringotomy d. Cortical mastoidectomy
82. A 3-year-old child presents with fever and earache. On examination there is congested tympanic membrane with slight bulge. The treatment of choice is: [AI 95]
    a. Myringotomy with penicillin
    b. Myringotomy with grommet
    c. Only antibiotics
    d. Wait and watch
83. Procedure for serous otitis media is: [AP 2002]
    a. Tympanoplasty b. Mastoidectomy
    c. Myringotomy d. Medical treatment
84. Grommet tube is used in: [TN 2002]
    a. Secretory otitis media
    b. Mucoid otitis media
    c. Serous otitis media
    d. All of the above

85. **True about grommet insertion:** [PGI May 2015]
    a. Small plastic tube aerating middle ear
    b. Maximum duration of grommet insertion is 5 months
    c. Healing occurs more quickly after extrusion than after removal
    d. It is placed anteriorly on tympanic membrane
    e. Surgery is always needed to remove it
86. **For ASOM, myringotomy is done in which quadrant:** [AI 95]
    a. Antero-inferior
    b. Antero-superior
    c. Postero-superior
    d. Postero-inferior
87. **Ideal site for myringotomy and grommet insertion:** [CUPGEE 02]
    a. Anterior superior quadrant
    b. Anterior inferior quadrant
    c. Posterior superior
    d. Posterior inferior
88. **Myringoplasty is plastic repair of:** [PGI]
    a. Middle ear
    b. Internal ear
    c. Eustachian tube
    d. Tympanic membrane
89. **Myringoplasty is done using:** [PGI 97]
    a. Temporalis fascia
    b. Dura mater
    c. Perichondrium
    d. Mucous membrane
90. **Material used in Tympanoplasty:** [PGI 98]
    a. Temporalis fascia
    b. Dura mater
    c. Periosteum
    d. Mucous membrane
91. **Which of the following is true regarding myringoplasty:** [AI 2013]
    a. In underlay graft is placed medial to the annulus
    b. In underlay graft is placed lateral to the malleus
    c. In overlay graft is placed lateral to the malleus
    d. In overlay graft is placed medial to the annulus
92. **Columella effect is seen in:** [TN 2005]
    a. Tympanoplasty
    b. Septoplasty
    c. Tracheostomy
    d. None of the above
93. **Surgery on ear drum is done using:** [Kerala 91]
    a. Operative microscope
    b. Laser
    c. Direct vision
    d. Blindly
94. **Which focal length in the objective piece of microscope is commonly used for ear surgery:** [AIIMS May 05]
    a. 100 mm
    b. 250 mm
    c. 450 mm
    d. 950 mm
95. **Schwartz operation is also called as:** [PGI 97]
    a. Cortical mastoidectomy
    b. Modified radical mastoidectomy
    c. Radial mastoidectomy
    d. Fenestration operation
96. **Simple mastoidectomy is done in:** [MP 2004]
    a. Acute mastoiditis
    b. Cholesteatoma
    c. Coalescent mastoiditis
    d. Localized chronic otitis media
97. **Cortical mastoidectomy is indicated in:** [AIIMS 93]
    a. Cholesteatoma without complication
    b. Coalescent mastoiditis
    c. CSOM with brain abscess
    d. perforation in Pars flaccida
98. **Radical mastoidectomy is done for:** [DNB 2000]
    a. ASOM
    b. CSOM
    c. Atticoantral cholesteatoma
    d. Acute mastoiditis
99. **All of the following steps are done in radical mastoidectomy except:** [AI 97]
    a. Lowering of facial ridge
    b. Removal of middle ear mucosa and muscles
    c. Removal of all ossicles of Eustachian tube plate
    d. Maintenance of patency of Eustachian tube
100. **Radical mastoidectomy includes all except:** [AIIMS 00]
    a. Closure of the auditory tube
    b. Ossicles removed
    c. Cochlea removed
    d. Exteriorisation of mastoid
101. **Nerve damaged in radical mastoidectomy is:** [MH 2000]
    a. Facial
    b. Cochlear
    c. Vestibular
    d. All of the above
102. **Modified redical mastoidectomy is indicated in all except:**
    a. Safe SCOM [MP 2000]
    b. Unsafe CSOM with atticoantral disease
    c. Coalescent mastoiditis
    d. Limited mastoid pathology
103. **Complication of modified radical mastoidectomy include(s):** [PGI Nov 2014]
    a. Conductive hearing loss
    b. Facial nerve injury
    c. Change in taste sensation
    d. Sensory hearing loss
104. **Not self retaining hand held retractor(s) is/are:** [PGI Nov 2014]
    a. Mollison's mastoid retractor
    b. Jansen's mastoid retractor
    c. Lempert's endaural retractor
    d. Davis retractor
105. **A 30-yead-old male is having Attic cholesteatoma of left ear with lateral sinus thrombophlebitis. Which of the following will be the operation of choice?** [AI 06]
    a. Intact canal will be the operation of choice
    b. Simple mastoidectomy with Tympanoplasty
    c. Canal wall down mastoidectomy
    d. Mastodidectomy with cavity obliteration

106. All of the following techniques are used to control bleeding from bone during mastoid surgery except:
    [AIIMS Nov. 04]
    a. Cutting drill over the bleeding area
    b. Diamond drill over the bleeding area
    c. Bipolar cautery over the bleeding area
    d. Bone wax
107. Communication between middle ear and Eustachian tube is obliterated in which surgery: [Delhi 2005]
    a. Tympanoplasty
    b. Schwartz operation
    c. Modified radical mastoidectomy
    d. Radical mastoidectomy
108. Otitis media with effusion is also known as: [PGI May 2012]
    a. Serous otitis media
    b. Suppurative otitis media
    c. Mucoid otitis media
    d. Glue ear
    e. Secretory otitis media
109. Mr. Ramu presented with persistent ear pain and discharge, retro-orbital pain, modified radical mastoidectomy was done to him. Patient comes back with persistent discharge, what is your diagnosis?
    a. Diffuse serous labyrinthitis
    b. Purulent labyrinthitis
    c. Petrositis
    d. Latent mastoiditis
110. An intraoperative photograph of cortical mastoidectomy. Which of the following is the lateral semicircular canal?
    [AIIMS Nov 2017]

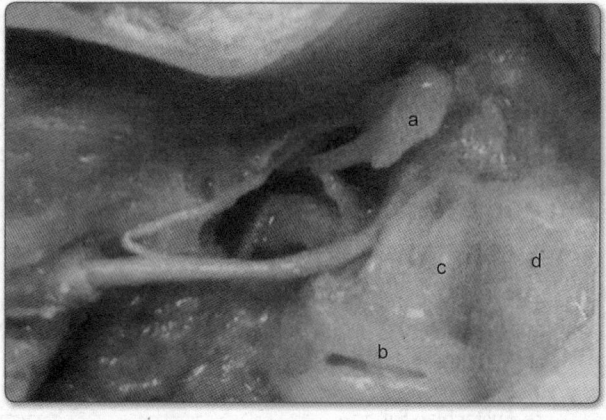

See Color Plate 8

    a. A
    b. B
    c. C
    d. D

Chapter 7: Diseases of Middle Ear

Explanations and References

ACUTE SUPPURATIVE OTITIS MEDIA

1. **Ans. is b i.e. Eustachian tube** *Ref. Dhingra 6/e p 63*
   M/c route of infection in middle ear is Eustachian tube. Infection travels via the lumen of the tube or along subepithelial peritubal lymphatics.
   Eustachian tube in infants and young children is shorter, wider and more horizontal and thus accounts for higher incidence of infections in this age group.

2. **Ans. is b i.e. S. pneumoniae** *Ref. Harrison 17/e, p 208; Current Otolaryngology 2/e, p 656*

3. **Ans. is a i.e. Pneumococcous**
   Most common cause of acute otitis media:
   - Streptococcus pneumonia/pneumococcus (35–40% cases)
   - H. influenza (25–30%)
   - M. catarrhalis (10–20%)

4. **Ans. is a i.e. Most frequently it resolves without sequelae**
   Ref. Turner 10/e, p 424, 428; Dhingra 5/e, p 69, 70, 6/e, p 62, 63; Current Otolaryngology 2/e, p 656-658
   Turner 10/e, p 424, 428 says *"Prognosis of ASOM is good, most cases recover completely. Whether in infants or children."*
   Current otolaryngology 2/e pg-658 says *"The vast majority of uncomplicated episodes of AOM resolves without any adverse outcome"*
   Rest all options are incorrect.

5. **Ans. is a i.e. ASOM** *Ref. Dhingra 5/e, p 70; 6/e, p 62-63*
   Otoscopy Signs for ASOM:
   - There is congestion of pars tensa
   - Leash of blood vessels appear along the handle of malleus and at the periphery giving it a **cartwheel like appearance.**
   - Transluscency is reduced.
   - Later tympanic membrane appears red and bulging with loss of landmarks.
   - Tympanic membrane is immobile n pneumatic ostoscopy

6. **Ans. is c i.e. Streptomycin** *Ref. Turner 10/e, p 281, Dhingra 6/e, p 63*

Medical management is the Treatment of choice in a case of ASOM	
Antibiotics of choice are:	• Ampicillin or amoxicillin (DOC)
Other which can be used	• Cotrimoxazole
	• Cefaclor
	• Erthromycin
	• Penicillin

7. **Ans. is c i.e. Suppurative** *Ref. Turner 10/e, p 349*
   Barotraumatic otitis media
   "Treatment consists of teaching the patient valsalva manoeuvre. If this fails, politzerization or Eustachian tube catheterization is carried out.
   If fluid is present a myringotomy may be necessary and occasionally in resistant cases, grommet insertion may be required until the middle ear mucosa has returned to normal." *Ref. Turner 10/e, p 349*

8. **Ans. is c i.e. ASOM** *Ref. Tuli 1/e, p 53*
   ASOM - In stage of suppuration-**pulsatile otorrhea is present**.
   Light house sign: Seen in ASOM.

9. **Ans. is d i.e. Posterior-superior quadrant** *Ref. Essential of ENT, Mohan Bansal p 110*

10. **Ans. is a i.e. ASOM** *Ref. Tuli 1/e, p 53; Dhingra 5/e, p 86, 6/e, p 62*
    - Light house sign is seen in acute ASOM and in acute mastoiditis following ASOM.
    - There is mucopurulent or purulent discharge, which is often pulsatile
    - On otoscopy examination of ear, this pulsatile discharge reflects light which is called as **light house effect**

NONSUPPURATIVE OTITIS MEDIA

11. Ans. is b i.e. Secretory otitis media *Ref. Dhingra 5/e, p 72, 6/e, p 64*
- Inadequate antibiotic treatment of acute suppurative otitis media may inactivate infection but fail to resolve it completely.
- Low grade infection lingers on which acts as a stimulus for the mucosa to secrete more mucus which leads to development of serous/secretory otitis media.

12. Ans. is b i.e. Nasopharyngeal carcinoma *Ref. Dhingra 5/e, p 72, 6/e, p 251; Current Laryngology 2/e, p 659*
Unilateral serous otitis media in an adult should always raise the suspicion of a benign / malignant tumor of nasopharynx
"In adults presenting with a unilateral middle ear effusion the possibility of a nasopharyngeal carcinoma should be considered".
– *Current Otolaryngology 2/e, p 659*

13. Ans. is d i.e. Malignancy *Ref. Scotts Brown 7/e vol 3 p 3389*
"A high incidence of NPC (Nasopharyngeal Carcinoma) in South East Asia and Southern China correlates with the high incidence of OME (Otitis Media with Effusion) in adults in these regions." –*Scotts Brown 7/e, vol 3 p. 3389*
"Presence of unilateral serous otitis media in an adult should raise suspicion of nasopharyngeal growth". *Ref. Dhingra 6/e p 257*

14. Ans. is b i.e. Is painless *Ref. Dhingra 5/e, p 72, 6/e, p 64; Current Otolaryngology 2/e, p 658*
Glue Ear/serous Otitis Media is a painless condition

15. Ans. is a and d i.e Impedance audiometry and Otoscopy *Ref. Current Otolaryngology 2/e, p 659, 3/e, p 676*
- **Pure tone audiometry:** gives information about the quantity and quality of hearing loss.
- **In secretory otitis media:** conductive deafness of 20–40 dB is seen (which is not a specific finding as conductive deafness can be seen in many other conditions). Therefore, pure tone audiometry is not diagnostic of serous otitis media but provides an assessment of the hearing loss and is therefore important in monitoring the progress of the condition and provides information useful for management decisions
- On otoscopy: Tympanic membrane appears dull, opaque with loss of light reflex
- X-ray mastoid: Shows clouding of air cells. (not diagnostic)
- Impedance audiometry is an accurate way of diagnosing serous otitis media. **It shows type B tympanogram which is diagnostic of fluid in ear**^{Q}.

16. Ans. is a, b, c and e i.e. Type C tympanogram may be seen in early stage of otitis media with effusion, Flat tympanogram is present, Leads to conductive deafness; and Most common cause is Eustachian dysfunction.
Ref. Mohan Bansal Essential of ENT: Pg 105 and 46)
As discussed in the text
- M/C cause of secretory otitis media/otitis media with effusion is Eustachian tube dysfunction (i.e. option **e** is correct)
- Presence of cleft palate increases the chances of ET dysfunction, hence increases chances of otitis media with effusion (i.e. option **d** incorrect)
- Otitis media with effusion leads to conductive deafness in children (i.e. option **c** correct)
- On tympanometry—when there is middle ear effusion, compliance is low and a tympanogram i.e. Type B or flat tympanogram is present. (i.e. option **b** is correct).
However in early stages—when there is eustachian tube dysfunction (just before effusion) at that time. Type C tympanogram may be present.

17. Ans. is b i.e. Glue ear *Ref. Dhingra 5/e, p 72, 6/e, p 64*
In glue ear (serous otitis media) Tympanic membrane is dull opaque with loss of light reflex and appears yellow / grey / blue in color.
- Normal color of tympanic membrane is pearly gray.
- Congested membrane with prominent blood vessels (cartwheel sign) is seen in early stages of acute otitis media.
- Bluish discoloration is seen in hemotympanum.
- Flamingo pink color is seen in otosclerosis.

18. Ans. is c i.e. Myringotomy with ventilation tube insertion
Ref. Logan Turner 10/e, p 437; ENT by Tuli 1/e, p 75-76; Current Otolaryngology 2/e, p 660; Dhingra 6/e, p 64, 5/e, p 73
Treatment of choice for glue ear is **insertion of grommet (i.e., ventilation tube insertion).**
Tympanotomy / cortical mastoidectomy has a very limited role. and is not done nowadays for serious otitis media.
"Myringotomy and aspiration of middle ear effusion without ventilation tube insertion has a short lived benefit and is not recommended"
– *Current otolaryngology 2/e, p 660)*
"From three trials, myringotomy with aspiration has not been shown to be effective in restoring the hearing levels in children with OME" – *Scott Brown 7/e, p 896*

19. Ans. is d i.e. Adenoidectomy with grommet insertion

20. Ans. is a, b, c and d i.e. Tonsilectomy, Adenoidectomy, Grommet insertion; and Myringotomy
Ref. Scott Brown 7/e, vol I p 896-904

Chapter 7: Diseases of Middle Ear

Child is presenting with mouth breathing. Palate is high arched. There is nasal obstruction and recurrent respiratory tract infections along with hearing impairment. All these features are suggestive of adenoid hyperplasia. In case of adenoid hyperplasia impairment of hearing is due to secretory otitis.

Thus the logical step in the management would be myringotomy with grommet insertion (to treat SOM) and adenoidectomy on tonsilectomy (to remove the causative factor). Now since in Q.19 all 4 are given in option, we are going for all four but in Q. 18 choice is between myringotomy with grommet insertion and adenoidectomy and grommet insertion better option is adenoidectomy and grommet insertion (as it is obvious gromet cannot be inserted in tympanic membrane without myringotomy).

21. **Ans. is b, c, and d i.e. Type B tympanogram, The effusion of middle ear is sterile, and Most common cause of deafness in a child in day care patients** *Ref. Dhingra 5/e, p 71-73, 6/e, p 64-65; Current Otolaryngiology 2/e, p 658-659; Ghai 6/e, p 332*

There is no doubt about options b, c and d that they are correct. Option 'a' says – immediate myringotomy should be done. This is incorrect as myringotomy is done only if patient does not respond to medical treatment in 3 months.

According to Ghai

- *If effusion persists beyond 3 months, tympanostomy tube insertion may be considered for significant hearing loss (>25 dB). Other indications of tube placement are ear discomfort or pain, altered behavior, speech delay, recurrent acute otitis media or impending cholesteatoma formation from tympanic membrane retraction".*   ... *Ghai 6/e, p 332*

According to *Current otolaryngology 2nd/ed pg 659*

"A large number of patients with OME (otitis media with effusion) require no treatment, particularly if the hearing impairment is mild. Spontaneous resolution occurs in a significant proportion of patients. A period of watchful waiting for 3 months from the onset (if known) or from the diagnosis if onset unknown), before considering intervention is advisable".

> **Also Know**
>
> *Indications for early insertion of Tympanostomy tube/ grommet tube:*
> - Cases where spontaneous resolution is unlikely as predicted by season of presenting to OPD (i.e. between July to December) and a B/L hearing impairment of >30 dB
> - It is causing significant delay in speech and language development
> - OME is present in an only hearing ear.
> - Recurrent otitis media.

22. **Ans. is b i.e. 3 Months** *Ref. Ghai 6/e, p332; Current otolaryngology 2/e p 659*
 See explanation of Ans 21
23. **Ans. is c i.e. Tympanostomy tubes are usually required for treatment**
 Ref. Scott's Brown 7/e, vol-I p 879-893-896; Current Otolaryngology 2/e, p 658-662; Dhingra 5/e, p 71-72, 6/e, p 64-65
 Lets look at the options one by one:
 Serous otitis media:

Option a

Sensori neural deafness occurs as a complication in 80% of cases
This is **not correct** because serous otitis media leads to conductive type of hearing loss.

Option b

Intracranial spread of the infection complicates the clinical course
This is not true as complications of serous otitis media are:
- Adhesive otitis media
- Atrophy of tympanic membrane
- [Tympanosclerosis (chalky white deposits seen on membrane)
- Atelectasis of middle ear
- Ossicular necrosis
- Cholesteatoma due to retraction pockets
- Cholesterol granuloma due to stasis of secretions

Option c

This is correct because if medical management fails, best treatment is myringotomy with insertion of Tympanostomy tube (Grommet or ventilation tube)

Option d

- Gram positive organism are grown routinely in culture in the aspirate
- Absolutely incorrect because fluid collection in serous otitis media is sterile   —*Dhingra – 5/e, p 71*

Section 1: Ear

24. **Ans. is b i.e. Secretory otitis media** *Ref. Current Otolaryngology 2/e, p 662*
    Treatment summary for otitis media – *Current Otolaryngology 2/e, p 662*

	Acute otitis media	Otitis media with effusion	CSOM
Watchful waiting	Up to 72 hours with analgesia/ antipyretics if non severe and patient > 2 yrs old	For 3 months from onset or diagnosis	N I
Medical therapy	Antibiotic (amoxicillin)	NI	Aural toileting and topical antibiotics (Quinolones)
Surgical intervention	Myringotomy for refractory AOM Cortical mastoidectomy in non-responding cases	VT insertion if unresolved after 3 months Aderoidectomy on second VT insertion	• Tympanoplasty • Tympano mastoid surgery if refractory to medical therapy

NI = not indicated;   VT = ventilation tube

25. **Ans. is d i.e. Multiple perforation**
26. **Ans. is c i.e. Pain** *Ref. Dhingra 5/e, p 83, 6/e, p 74; Scott's Brown 7/e, vol-3 p 3447-3448*
27. **Ans. is a, b and e i.e. Multiple hole in tympanic membrane, Pale granulation mass seen in middle ear, and Painless.**

    Tubercular Otitis Media
    - **Important points:**
        - Seen mainly in children and young adult^Q
        - It is secondary to pulmonary tuberculosis.^{Q}
        - Route of spread - Mainly through Eustachian tube (not blood borne).^{Q}
    - **Symptoms:**
        1. Patients often present with **chronic painless otorrhea** (usually foul smelling) which is resistant to antibiotic treatment^Q
        3. Severe conductive type hearing loss^Q. (sometimes due to involvement of labyrinth may be SNHL)
        4. **Facial nerve palsy may be the presenting symptom in children**^{Q} (Extra auricular symptom)
        5. Cough; fever and night sweats may be present in patients with tuberculous infection in other organ system.
    - **O/E**
        - ***Multiple perforations***^{Q} ***in tympanic membrane*** (This feature was once considered characteristic of TB but now is seldom seen).
        - ***Middle ear and mastoid are filled with pale granulation tissue***^{Q} ***(It is a characteristic of tuberculous otitis media)***^{Q}
    - **Complications:** (Early onset of these symptoms is seen)
        - Mastoiditis
        - Osteomyelitis
        - Postauricular fistula
        - Facial nerve palsy
    - **Management**
        - ATT and mastoidectomy and tympanoplasty.

28. **Ans. is c i.e. Supportive** *Ref. Dhingra 6/e p 66*
    Otitic Barotrauma (Aero otitis media) in mild cases does not require any specific treatment apart from decongestants.
29. **Ans. is d i.e. It is the very vascular region** *Ref. Read below*
    In SOM, myringotomy is done in antero-inferior quadrant because:
    1. It is relatively avascular area ∴ blood loss is less
    2. No important structures are present here ∴ No possibility of them being damaged.
    3. To stimulate Eustachian tube (which also lies in antero inferior quadrant)

CHRONIC SUPPURATIVE OTITIS MEDIA

30. **Ans. is b i.e. Long process of incus** *Ref. Scott's Brown 7/e, vol 3 p 3421*

    > Ossicle M/c involved in CSOM is incus (long process) because of its poor blood supply.

31. **Ans. is a i.e. Etiology is multiple bacteria** *Ref. Dhingra 5/e, p 77, 78, 80, 6/e, p 70*
    - CSOM is caused by multiple bacteria - both aerobic and anaerobic.^{Q} - *Dhingra 5/e p. 78*
    - Their is no sex predilection in CSOM - both sexes are affected equally.^{Q} *Dhingra 5/e, p 77, 6/e, p 70*
    - Treatment of Tubotympanic type of CSOM is aural toileting and antibiotic ear drops. *Dhingra 5/e, p 80, 6/e, p 71*
    As far as oral antibiotics are concerned.
    "They are useful in acute exacerbation of chronically infected ear, otherwise role of systemic antibiotics in the treatment of CSOM is limited." ...*Dhingra 5/e, p 80, 6/e, p 72*
    - Otitic hydrocephalus - is a rare complication of CSOM. ...*Turner 10/e, p 309*

Chapter 7: Diseases of Middle Ear

32. Ans. is d i.e. Conservative management *Ref. Turner 10/e, p 285; Scott's Brown 7/e, vol 3 p 3421 and 3424*

There are 2 schools of thought as far as this question is concerned – Some believe that.
- TOC of central perforation is myringoplasty.
- TOC of central perforation is conservative management.

But according to *Turner 10/e, p 285* - central perforation/ tubo tympanic CSOM are both managed conservatively by antibiotics and by keeping the ear dry.

"If there is recurring discharge or if there is deafness sufficient to cause disability, closure of the perforation by myringoplasty should be considered."

According to Scott's Brown (7/e, vol-3 p 3421)
- Dry perforations that are symptom free do not require usually require closure.
- If the only symptom is a hearing impairment, the chances of improving hearing with surgery should be considered carefully, not just the hearing in the operated ear but the overall hearing ability of the patient.
- In patients with a H/O intermittent activity, surgery to close the perforation is probably indicated to minimize future activity.
- So from all above discussions, it is clear that TOC for central safe perforation is conservative management.

33. Ans. is b i.e. Associated with cholesteatoma *Ref. Dhingra 6/e p59, 5/e p 78*

34. Ans. is b i.e. Marginal

35. Ans. is a i.e. Atticoantral perforation

Tympanic membrane can be divided into 2 parts:

Pars tensa : It forms most of the tympanic membrane. Its periphery is thickened to form fibro cartilaginous ring called as annulus tympanicus.

Pars falccida : It is situated above the lateral process of malleus between the notch of Rivinus and the anterior and posterior malleolar fold.

Perforation in tympanic membrane can be in:

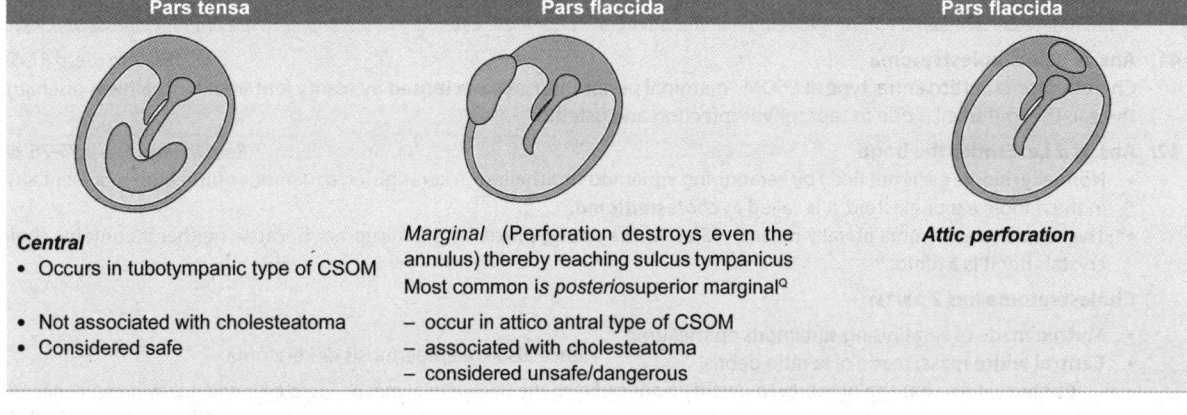

Central
- Occurs in tubotympanic type of CSOM
- Not associated with cholesteatoma
- Considered safe

Marginal (Perforation destroys even the annulus) thereby reaching sulcus tympanicus
Most common is *posterio*superior marginal°
– occur in attico antral type of CSOM
– associated with cholesteatoma
– considered unsafe/dangerous

Attic perforation

 Note: Most common cause of perforation is chronic otitis media.   ... *Dhingra 4/e, p 55*

 Mnemonic

FAMOUS
- **F** – Perforation of Pars **F**laccida.
- **A** – Seen in **A**tticoantral/marginal perforation
- **M** – Associated with CSO**M** (of atticoantral type) or acute necrotizing otitis **m**edia
- **O** – Associated with Ch**o**lesteatoma
- **U** – **U**nsafe type
- **S** – **S**urgery is TOC.

36. **Ans. c i.e. Attic region** *Ref. Dhingra 5/e, p 77, 6/e, p 72*
37. **Ans. is d i.e. Acute necrotizing otitis media**
38. **Ans. is b i.e. CSOM** *Ref. Dhingra 5/e, p 81, 6/e, p 67-68*

Cholesteatoma is presence of keratinising squamous epithelium in middle ear.

Origin

- **Congenital**
- **Primary acquired**
  - No H/O of previous otitis media or pre existing perforation
  - Most common cause is formation of retraction pocket of pass flaccida in which keratin debris accumulates
- **Secondary acquired**
  - Occurs in pre-existing perforation in pars tensa
  - Acute necrotizing otitis media
  - Attico antral/unsafe CSOM
    ↓
  - These perforations result in squamous epithelial migration from tympanic membrane
  - It can also result from implantation of squamous epithelium into the middle ear during surgery.

39. **Ans. is d i.e. Retraction pocket** *Ref. Current Otolaryngology 2/e, p 666*

    Most common accepted theory for formation of **cholesteatoma is formation of a retraction pocket.** According to this theory, chronic negative middle ear pressure (which occurs due to poor Eustachian tube function and chronic inflammation of the middle ear) leads to retractions of the structurally weakest area of the tympanic membrane, the pars flaccida. Once the retractions form, the normal migratory pattern of the squamous epithelium is disrupted, resulting in the accumulation of keratin debris in the cholesteatoma sac.

40. **Ans. is a, b and d i.e. Whitish mass behind intact TM, Normal pars tensa and pars flaccida, Prior otitis media is not an exclusion criteria** *Ref. Internet*

    Levenson Criteria for Congenital Cholesteatoma
    - White mass medial to normal TM
    - No history of otorrhea or perforations
    - Prior bouts of otitis media (not excluded)
    - Normal pars flaccida and tensa
    - No prior otologic procedures

41. **Ans. is b i.e. Cholesteatoma** *Ref. Dhingra 5/e, p 81, 6/e, p 72*

    Cholesteatoma / attico antral type of CSOM / marginal perforation is characterised by scanty foul smelling, painless discharge from the ear. The foul smell is due to saprophytic infection and osteitis

42. **Ans. is d i.e. Erodes the bone** *Ref. Dhingra 5/e, p 75-76, 6/e, p 72*
    - Normally middle ear is not lined by keratinising squamous epithelium. If keratinising squamous epithelium is present anywhere in the middle ear or mastoid, it is called as **cholesteatoma.**
    - The term cholesteatoma literally means - **"Skin in the wrong place."** It is a misnomer because neither it contains cholesterol crystals nor it is a tumor.[Q]

    Cholesteatoma has 2 parts:
    - **Matrix:** made of keratinising squamous epithelium.[Q]
    - **Central white mass:** made of keratin debris. Hence also k/a epidermosis or keratoma
      - Cholesteatoma has the property to destroy bones (due to the various enzymes released by it and not by pressure necrosis).
        – *Dhingra 5/e, p 76, 77, 6/e, p 68*

43. **Ans. is a i.e. Lateral semicircular canal** *Ref. Logan Turner 10/e, p 287*
    - Cholesteatoma has the property to destroy the bone by virtue of the various enzymes released by it.
    - **Structures immediately at the risk of erosion are:**
      - Long process of incus.[Q]
      - Fallopian canal containing facial nerve.[Q]
      - Horizontal/lateral semicircular canal.[Q]

44. **Ans. is a, d and e i.e. Scanty, malodoruos discharge; Ossicular involvement; and Eustachian tube dysfunction**
    Ref. Dhingra 5/e, p 77, 81, 6/e, p 68, 72; Current otolaryngology 2/e, p 666, 3/e, p 683-684; Mohan Bansal p 211
    - Cholestatoma is associated with atticoantral type of CSOM / atticoantral or marginal perforation (and not central perforation).
    - Cholesteatoma leads to destruction of bones therefore there is scanty foul smelling discharge and ossicular necrosis.
    - Hearing loss occurs if ossicles are involved.
    - It is of conductive type but if complications like labyrinthitis intervene, SNHL may also be seen.
    - Bleeding may occur from granulations or polyp.
    - Otalgia is not seen in case of cholesteatoma.

Chapter 7: Diseases of Middle Ear

Note: Cholesteatoma can cause facial nerve palsy and labyrinthitis.

45. Ans. is a i.e. Mastoidectomy *Ref. Dhingra 5/e, p 77, 6/e, p 73*

46. Ans. is b i.e. Modified Radical Mastoidectomy [MRM] *Ref. Dhingra 5/e, p 82, 6/e, p 73; Logan Turner 10/e, p 291*

CSOM is of Two Types

	Tubotympanic or safe type	Atticoantral or unsafe type or dangerous type
Discharge	Profuse, mucoid, odourless	Scanty, purulent, foul- Smelling^Q
Perforation	Central^Q	Attic or posterosuperior marginal^Q
Granulations	Uncommon	Common
Polyp	Pale	Red and Fleshy
Cholesteatoma	Absent	Present^Q
Complications	Rare^Q	Common^Q
Audiogram	Mild to moderate conductive deafness^Q	Conductive or mixed deafness^Q

- TOC for atticoantral variety of CSOM is surgery i.e.
- TOC for tubotympanic type of CSOM is mainly conservative in the form of aural toileting and systemic antibiotics and once the ear is dry myringoplasty can be done.

Note:
- Perforation of pars flaccida leads to attic perforation which is considered dangerous and should be managed with modified radical mastoidectomy

47. Ans. is c i.e. Tympanosclerosis *Ref. Dhingra 4/e, p 60, 5/e, p 76*

In ventilation of the middle ear cleft, air passes from Eustachian tube to mesotympanum, from there to attic, aditus, antrum and mastoid air cell system.
Any obstruction in the pathways of ventilation can cause retraction pockets or atelectasis of tympanic membrane, e.g.:
  i. Obstruction of eustachian tube ® Total atelectasis of tympanic membrane
  ii. Obstruction in middle ear ® Retraction pocket in posterior part of middle ear while anterior part is ventilated
  iii. Obstruction of isthmi ® Attic retraction pocket
Depending on the location of pathologic process, other changes such as thin atrophic tympanic membrane, (due to absorption of middle fibrous layer), cholesteatoma, ***tympanosclerosis.*** and ossicular necrosis
A posterior superior retraction pocket - if allowed to progress leads to primary acquired cholesteatoma and not secondary cholesteatoma.

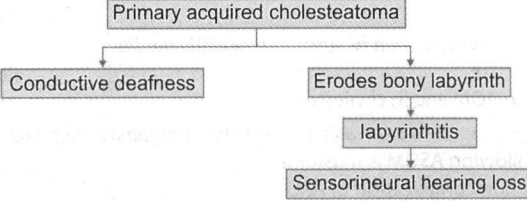

So, tympanosclerosis and sensorineural hearing loss are both correct but tympanosclerosis is a better option than SNHL (which occurs very late when retraction pocket gives rise to cholesteatoma which later causes labyrinthitis)

ALSO KNOW

Tympanosclerosis

- It is hyalinisation and later calcification in the fibrous layer of tympanic membrane.
- Tympanic membrane appears as chalky white plaque.
- Mostly, it remains asymptomatic.
- It is frequently seen in cases of serous otitis media, as a complication of ventilation tube and in CSOM
- Tympanosclerosis mostly affects tympanic membrane but may be seen involving ligaments, joints of ossicles, muscle tendons and submucosal layer of middle ear cleft and interferes in the conduction of sound.

48. Ans. is b i.e. Posterior facial ridge *Ref. Scott's Brown 7/e, vol 3 p 3112-3113*

The sinus tympani (Posterior facial ridge) is the posterior extension of the mesotympanum and lies deep to both the promontory and facial nerve.

The medial wall of sinus tympani becomes continuous with the posterior portion of the medial wall of the tympanic cavity. This is the worst region for access because it is above pyramid, posterior to intact stapes and medial to facial nerve.

A retrofacial approach via mastoid is not possible because the posterior semicircular canal blocks the access.

49. **Ans. is d i.e. Tympano-mastoid exploration** *Ref. Dhingra 5/e, p 82, 6/e, p 73*

Child presenting with foul smelling discharge with perforation in the pars flaccida of the tympanic membrane suggests unsafe CSOM. Conservative management is not of much help in these cases; surgery is the mainstay of treatment.

   Tympanomastoid exploration is the ideal option in such cases.
   - Tympanomastiod exploration can be done through various procedures:
     - ***Canal wall down procedures:*** Atticotomy, and rarely radical mastoidectomy.
     - ***Canal wall up procedures:*** Cortical mastoidectomy
   Preferred treatment would be

   ALSO KNOW
   Reconstruction of hearing mechanism by tympanoplasty is only the second priority.

50. **Ans. is d i.e. Myringoplasty** *Ref. Dhingra 5/e, p 82, 6/e, p 72-73; Logan turner 10/e, p 289*

   Myringoplasty consists of closing a 'central perforation' in the tympanic membrane in the 'tubotympanic type' or 'safe type' of chronic suppurative otitis media. It is not indicated in unsafe or dangerous type of otitis media with posterosuperior atitic perforation.
   - *The patient in question is a case of dangerous or unsafe type of CSOM as signified by the presence of posterosuperior retraction pocket cholesteatoma.*
   - The mainstay in treatment of this type of CSOM is surgery.
     - Primary aim is to remove the disease and render the ear safe.
     Secondary aim is to preserve or reconstruct hearing, but never at the cost of the primary aim.
   - (Mastoid exploration) is the operation of choice.
   - Tympanoplasty: Forms part of secondary aim to reconstruct hearing after a primary mastoid exploration.
     - Dangerous type CSOM is associated with a perforation in attic or posterosuperior region of T.M. along with variable extent of destruction of ossicles and other middle ear contents. Reconstruction of hearing in this type of CSOM thus requires variable extent of ossicular reconstruction besides closure of perforation.
   - *Audiometry* forms an important step in evaluation of disease process preoperatively.
   Although myringoplasty also forms a type of tympanoplasty its use is limited to closure of perforation in the parts tensa of tympanic membrane which is seen in safe type CSOM.

COMPLICATION OF OTITIS MEDIA

51. **Ans. is a i.e. Meningitis**
52. **Ans. is d i.e. Meningitis** *Ref. Essentials of ENT Mohan Bansal, p 123*
    Meningitis: It is the M/c intracranial complication of suppurative otitis media
53. **Ans. is d i.e. VII N** *Ref. Essentials of ENT Mohan Bansal, p 122*
    Facial N paralysis- can occur both in AOM and in cholesteatoma
54. **Ans. is b i.e. Mastoiditis** *Ref: Current Otolaryngology 2/e, p 663, 3/e, p 679; Dhingra 5/e, p 85, 6/e, p 76/77*
    - Most common complication following ASOM is mastoiditis.
    - Facial nerve palsy is an uncommon complication of ASOM.

55. **Ans. is b and d i.e. Facial nerve palsy; and Labyrinthitis** *Ref. Dhingra 5/e, p 85, 6/e, p 75-76; Tuli 1/e, p 66*
56. **Ans. is a, c and d i.e. Labyrinthitis; Bezold's abscess and Facial nerve palsy**

    Extra cranial complications of CSOM are:
    - **P**etrositis (Gradenigo syndrome)
    - **L**abyrinthitis
    - **O**steomyelitis of temporal bone
    - **S**epticemia/pyaemia
    - Otogenic **T**etanus.
    - **F**. Facial nerve palsy
    - Acute **M**astoiditis: – Postaural subperiosteal abscess
        – Zygomatic abscess
        – Luc's abscess
        – Citelli abscess
        – Bezold abscess

    Mnemonic: Pakistan L O S T First Match

Chapter 7: Diseases of Middle Ear

> **Remember**
> M/C Extra cranial complication - mastoiditis (postaural abscess)
> Overall M/C complication - Meningitis

Friends here it is important to note that 'hearing loss' will not be include in the complications of CSOM. As it is a sequalae and not complication of CSOM

Sequelae of CSOM

These are the direct result of middle ear infection and should be differentiated from complications:
- Perforation of tympanic membrane
- Cholesteatoma formation
- Atelectasis and adhesive otitis media
- SNHL
- Learning disabilities
- Tympanosclerosis
- Ossicular erosion
- Conductive hearing loss (d/t ossicular erosion/fixation)
- Speech impairment

Hence – hearing loss, cholesteatoma and conductive deafness are not included in the complications of otitis media.

57. **Ans. is c i.e. Mastoiditis** *Ref: Scott Brown 7/e, vol-3 p 3435*
    Repeat
58. **Ans. is d i.e. Mastoiditis** *Ref. SK De, p 107, 98*
    Mastoid reserve phenomenon is filling up of meatus with pus immediately after cleaning. It is seen in mastoiditis.
59. **Ans. is b i.e. Obliteration of retroauricular sulcus**
60. **Ans. is b i.e. Clouding of air cells of mastoid**
61. **Ans. is c, d and e i.e. Mastoid tip, Root of zygoma and Mastoid antrum**
    Ref. Dhingra 5/e, p 86, 6/e, p 76; Current Otolaryngology 2/e, p 663, 3/e, p 679
    See the text for explanation
62. **Ans. is a i.e. Bezold abscess**
63. **Ans. is b i.e. Sternomastoid muscle** *Ref. Dhingra 5/e, p 87, 6/e, p 78-79; Tuli 1/e, p 56*
64. **Ans. is d i.e. upper part of neck**
    Bezold abscess – Pus passes through the **tip of mastoid** into the sternocleidomastoid muscle in the upper part of neck.
    Some of you may confuse the Bezold abscess with Cielli's abscess – this is because the language given in Dhingra is very confusing.
    For all purposes

> **Remember**
> - In citelli's abscess – pus is seen in digastric triangle after passing through inner table of mastoid process.

> **Note:**
> - M/c site for subperiosteal abscess: Postauricular

65. **Ans. is a i.e. Gradenigo's syndrome**
66. **Ans. is a i.e. It is associated with jugular vein tenderness**
67. **Ans. is c i.e. VII nerve palsy** *Ref. Dhingra 5/e, p 89, 6/e, p 79*
    See the text for explanation
68. **Ans. is b i.e. Immediate mastoidectomy** *Ref. Dhingra 5/e, p 90, 6/e, p 80*
69. **Ans. is c i.e. Immediate mastoid exploration** *Ref. Dhingra 5/e, p 90, 6/e, p 80*

Facial Palsy and CSOM

In CSOM, facial palsy may be due to erosion of fallopian canal by cholesteatoma (which erodes fallopian canal) osteitis, or demineralization. The treatment should be urgent mastoid exploration, with decompression of the facial nerve in the fallopain canal.

> **Note:**
> - However, the scenario is not the same in ASOM. An acute inflammatory process cannot effectively erode the bony fallopian canal within the short period of time. Hence, the only possibility in a patient with ASOM to develop facial palsy is the presence of a congenitally dehiscent fallopian canal (facial nerve without a bony canal), which is the commonest congenital malformation of temporal bone.
> - Thus in this case, the treatment is myringotomy to relieve pressure on the exposed nerve or sometimes cotical mastoidectomy.

70. **Ans. is a i.e. Cochlear Aqueduct** *Ref: Dhingra 5/e, p 11, 12, 6/e, p 9, 10 Current, Diagnosis and Treatment in Otorhinology 2/143*
Cochlear aqueduct is a bony canal that connects the cochlea to the intracranial subarachnoid space. Perilymph within the cochlear aqueduct is in direct continuation with the CSF and hence Cochlear Aqueduct is the most important route for meningitis to spread to the inner ear.

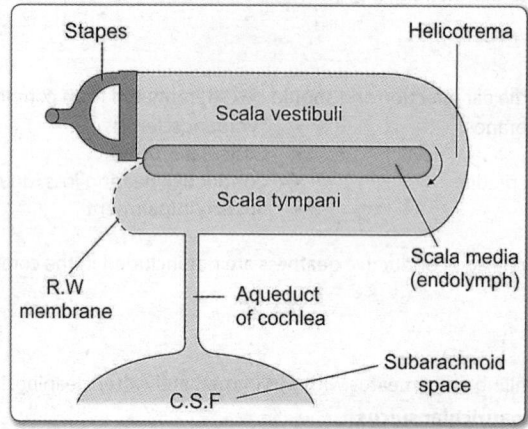

Vestibular Aqueduct

- Vestibular Aqueduct is also a bony connection between the cerebral subarachnoid space and the inner ear.
- Vestibular Aqueduct contains the endolymphatic duct which contains the endolymph. The endolymph within the endolymphatic duct does not however communicate freely with the CSF as it forms a closed space and ends in a cul-de-sac.
- Because the endolymph does not directly communicate with the CSF. Vestibular aqueduct is less important in allowing spread of meningitis from CSF to inner ear than Cochlear Aqueduct.

Hyrtle's Fissure

- Hyrtle's fissure is an embryonic remnant that normally obliterates by 24 weeks.
- When persistent, Hyrtle's fissure provides a connection from the middle ear to the subarachoid space
- Hyrtle's fissure does not directly communicate the internal ear with CSF and usually obliterates early in life and hence is not an important route of spread of infection from CSF to internal ear.

Endolymphatic Sac

Endolymphatic sac is a cul-de-sac containing endolymph that does not directly communicate with CSF.

71. **Ans. is a i.e. CSOM**

72. **Ans. is b and c i.e. CSOM with lateral sinus thrombosis in turn can cause brain abscess and Most common complication of CSOM** *Ref. Turner 10/e, p 311-312; Dhingra 5/e, p 92-93, 6/e, p 82*
    - Commonest organisms in otogenic brain abscess include gram-negative (Proteus, E.coli, Pseudomonas) and anaerobic *bacteria along with Staphylococcus and Pneumococci.*
    - M/C complication of CSOM = Brain abscess.
    - Lateral sinus thrombosis is usually preceded by a perisinus abscess, which may lead later on to cerebeller abscess.
    - Temporal lobe abscess is usually associated with hallucinations, visual field defects, and nominal aphasia, while personality change is not a feature feature of temporal lobe abscess. (It is a feature of frontal lobe abscess.)

73. **Ans. d i.e. H. influenzae** *Ref. Dhingra 5/e, p 92-93, 6/e, p 82; Turner 19/e, p 311-312*
    - Commonest organisms in otogenic brain abscess include gram negative (Proteus, E coli, Pseudomonas) and anaerobic bacteria along with Staphylococcus and Pneumocci.
    - *H. Influenza infection is a rare cause of otogenic abscess.*

74. **Ans. is b i.e. Gradenigo sign**

75. **Ans. is a i.e. Lateral sinus thrombosis** *Ref. Dhingra 5/e, p 95, 6/e, p 84*

76. **Ans. is b i.e. Lateral sinus thrombosis** *Ref. Dhingra 6/e,pgs84; 164*
    See the text for explanation

Chapter 7: Diseases of Middle Ear

77. Ans. is b i.e. Brainstem evoked auditory response *Ref. Ghai 6th/ed p 518; Dhingra 5th/ed p 132*

H. influenza Type Meningitis

"It is frequent in children between the ages of 3 and 12 months. Residual auditory deficit is a common complication."

... *Ghai 6th/ed p 518*

- Since, residual auditory deficit is a common complication of H. influenza meningitis so audiological test to detect the deficit should be performed before discharging any patient suffering from H. influenza meningitis.
- In children best test to detect hearing loss is brainstem evoked auditory response.

"Auditory brainstem response is used both as screening test and as a definitive hearing assessment test in children".

... *Dhingra 4th/ed p 117*

78. Ans. is c i.e. Immediate mastoid exploration *Ref. Turner 10th/ed p 301; Scott's Brown 7th/ed Vol 3 p 3437*
Repeat

79. Ans. is a and b i.e. V and VI nerve. *Ref. Dhingra 6/e p79*
The classical presentation of petrositis is Gradenigo syndrome which is characterised by:
1. External rectus palsy (VI nerve palsy) leading to diplopia
2. Deep seated ear or retro orbital pair (due to V nerve involvement)
3. Persistent ear discharge

80. Ans. is b i.e. VII nerve *Dhingra 6/e p80*
Facial nerve is the M/C nerve to be damaged in CSOM.

SURGICAL MANAGEMENT OF MIDDLE EAR SUPPURATION

81. Ans. is c i.e. Myringotomy *Ref. Dhingra 5th/ed pg 71, 6th/ed p 63*
Child presenting with acute otitis media which is not relieved by antibiotics and bulging tympanic membrane is an indication for myringotomy.

Indications of myringotomy in acute otitis media:
- Drum is bulging + acute pain.
- Incomplete resolution despite antibiotics when drum remains full with persistent conductive deafness.
- Persistent effusion beyond 12 weeks.

82. Ans. is a i.e. Myringotomy with Penicillin *Ref. Dhingra 5th/ed pg 71, 6th/ed p 63*
Fever + earache + congested and bulging tympanic membrane in a four years old child points towards Acute suppurative otitis media as the diagnosis.

- Antibiotics (Penicillin) form the mainstay of treatment of acute otitis media and should be administered in a child with Acute otitis media and once tympanic membrane is bulging, my ringotomy should be done.
- Grommet insertion is not indicated in Acute suppurative otitis media. It may be used in cases of myringotomy for serous or secretory otitis media.

83. Ans. is c i.e. Myringotomy *Ref. Dhingra 5th/ed p 407, 6th/ed p 65; Scotts Brown 7th/ed vol 1 pg. 896 and vol 3 pg 3392*

In Children

TOC of serous otitis media → myringotomy + insertion of grommet (ventilation tube) along with adenoidectomy (if features of adenoid hyperplasia are present) or tonsillectomy

In Adults (*Scotts Brown 7th ed vol 3 pg. 3392*)

In case of serous otitis media without nasopharyngeal carcinoma.
Myringotomy with ventilation tube insertion is done (In adults ventilation tube improves hearing for a very short term < 1 yr)

If there is nasopharyngeal cancer along with serous otitis media
Then there are two treatment options: (i) Hearing aid (ii) Myringotomy without ventilation tube insertion
Recently, CO_2 laser assisted tympanic membrane ventilation has been advocated for the treatment of adult OME.

84. Ans. is d i.e. All of the above *Ref. Dhingra 5th/ed p 71, 73, 6th/ed p 65, 66; Scotts Brown 7th/ed vol/pg 896-897*
As discussed in the text

Myringotomy is coupled with grommet tube insertion in:
1. Serous otitis media (also k/a mucoid otitis media/glue ear)
2. Adhesive otitis media

3. Recurrent acute otitis media
4. Meniere's disease

85. Ans. is a, c and d i.e. Small plastic tube aerating middle ear, Healing occurs more quickly after extrusion than after removal and It is placed anteriorly on tympanic membrane *Ref. Turner 10/e/pgs/438-39*
- Grommet is a small plastic tube aerating ear. (option a)
- The question of whether or not to insert a grommet tube to ventilate the middle-ear cavity after routine myringotomy & aspiration is debated in literature. Shah examined a series in whom a grommet had been inserted anteriorly in one year. He found in period **between 6 weeks & 6 months** postoperatively 80% of the ears with the grommet had normal hearing compared with 20% of cases with no grommet.
- If a grommet is inserted it may be placed posteriorly or anteriorly depending upon the preference of the surgeon
- **Those who place it anteriorly take this as being more physiological** because air normally enters the tympanum through an anterior orifice & it is in the anterior part of the tympanum that the secretory cells are found and have to be dried off
- The grommet **is either rejected spontaneously or may be removed**, preferably under an anesthetic agent because this is momentarily painful. Healing occurs more quickly after extrusion than after removal
- Thin scars on the tympanic are more frequent in the ears that have grommets which suggests that grommets may inhibit healing
- Recurrence (after initial myringotomy, aspiration and grommet insertion) are once again treated by myringotomy and at the second or certainly at the third myringotomy, most surgeon require a second grommet and 11% need a third.

86. Ans. is d i.e. Posteroinferior

87. Ans. is b i.e. Anterior inferior quadrant *Ref. Dhingra 5th/ed p 71, 73, 6th/ed p 65, 398; S1B 7/ed Vol, pg 896-897*
- As discussed- Ideal site for incision in ASOM is postero inferior quadrant
- For serious otitis media/Grommet insertion, ideal site is anterio inferior quadrant (though Dhingra says it can be posterior inferior also) as is proven by the following lines from scotts brown:
  Site of insertion of grommet
  "Insertion of the ventilation tube posterosuperiorly is not recommended because of the potential for damaging the ossicular chain. It makes no difference to the extrusion rate as to whether the tube is inserted through a radial or circumferential incision and whether sited anterosuperiorly rather than antero-inferiorly."
- *Placement antero-inferiorly compared with placement postero-inferiorly lengthens the time a ventilation tube is in situ. To maximize the duration of potential tube function, the preferred insertion site is anteroinferior through a circumferential or radial incision.* *Ref. Scott Brown 7/e, vol/p 896-897*

88. Ans. is d i.e. Tympanic membrane

89. Ans. is a and c i.e. Temporalis fascia and Perichondrium *Ref. Dhingra 5/e, p 409, 416, 6/e, p 406-407*

90. Ans. is a and b i.e. Temporalis fascia and Dura mater
- Myrirgoplasty is repair of a perforation of the tympanic membrane (the pars tensa).
- Tympanoplasty is ossicular reconstruction with myringoplasty.

> - Myringoplasty is done using the graft made of either of the following materials.
>   - Temporalis Fascia (most common)
>   - Tragal cartilage
>   - Perichondrium from tragus
>   - Vein

91. Ans. is a i.e. In underlay graft is placed medial to annulus *Ref. Essentials of ENT Mohan Bansal, p 439*

> **Remember**
> In underlay technique, the graft is placed medial to the annulus whereas in overlay technique, the graft is placed lateral to the annulus

92. Ans. is a i.e. Tympanoplasty *Ref. Dhingra 5/e, p 35, 6/e, p 30; Tuli 1/e, p 491*
As discussed- columella effect is seen in Type III tympanoplasty
Type III tympanoplasty is also the M/C type of tympanoplasty performed

93. Ans. is a i.e. Operative microscope *Ref. Maqbool 11/e, p 62*
Myringotomy i:e surgery on Ear Drum is performed under the operating microscope under general anesthesia.

94. Ans. is b i.e. 250 mm *Ref. Temporal Bone Surgery by MS Taneja 1/e, p 16*

> **Focal length of objective lens:**
> - For ear surgery - 200 mm/250 mm
> - For Laryngeal surgery-400 mm
> - For Nose / Paranasal sinus surgery - 300 mm

95. Ans. is a i.e. Cortical mastoidectomy

96. **Ans. is c i.e Coalescent mastoiditis**
97. **Ans. is b i.e Coalescent mastoiditis** *Ref. Dhingra 5/e, p 411, 6/e, p 401*
    Schwartz operation in another name for cortical/sample mastoidectomy
    See preceding text for indications of cortical mastoidectomy
98. **Ans. is c i.e. Atticoantral cholesteatoma**
99. **Ans. is d i.e Maintenance of patency of Eustachian tube**
100. **Ans. is c i.e Cochlea removed** *Ref. Dhingra 5/e, p 413-414, 6/e, p 405*
     - Radical mastoidectomy is a procedure to eradicate disease from middle ear and mastoid without any attempt to reconstruct hearing.
     - It is rarely done these days – Its only indications are:
       – Malignancy of middle ear
       – When cholesteatoma cannot be removed safely e.g. if it invades eustachian tube, round window or perilabrynthine cells
       – If previous attempts to eradicate cholesteatoma have failed

     Following steps are done in radical mastoidectomy:
     1. **Posterior meatal wall is removed** and the entire area of middle ear, attic, antrum and mastoid is converted into a single cavity, by removing the bridge and lowering the facial ridge.
     2. All remnants of tympanic membrane, ossicles (except the stapes foot plate) and mucoperiosteal lining are removed (Not cochlea)
     3. Eustachian tube is obliterated by a piece of muscle or cartilage
     4. The diseased middle ear and mastoid are permanently exteriorised for inspection and cleaning.

     > **Remember**
     > Bridge is the most posterosuperior part of bony meatal wall lateral to aditus and anturm, which overlies the Notch of Rivinus while facial ridge lies lateral to fallopian canal. Bridge is removed and ridge is lowered in radical or modified radical operation.

101. **Ans. is a i.e. Facial nerve** *Ref. Scotts Brown 7/e vol 3 p 3434*
     Complications of mastoid surgery- are actually very uncommon
     1. Facial palsy (rare)
     2. Total hearing loss/dead ear

      Note: The incidence of facial palsy is widely accepted to be rare in the hands of expert surgeons, however, total loss of hearing also occurs in the hands of expert.

102. **Ans. is c i.e. Coalescent mastoiditis** *Ref. Dhingra 5/e, p 411, 6/e, p 400*
     Now, this is one of those questions where we can get the answer by exclusion.
     Here we know- management of coalescent mastoiditis is cortical mastoidectomy so obviously modified radical mastoidectomy is not done in this case.

103. **Ans. (All)**
     Complication of Radical Mastoidectomy/Modified Radical Mastoidectomy *Dhingra 5/e,pgs414*
     - **Facial paralysis**
     - Perichondritis of pinna
     - Injury to duramater or sigmoid sinus
     - Labyrinthitis, if stapes gets disclosed
     - Meningitis
     - **Severe** conductive **deafness** of 50 dB or more. This is due to removal of all ossicles & tympanic membrane
     - Chocolate or mucous cyst in the radial cavity
     - Cavity problems: Twenty five percent of the cavities do not heal & continue to discharge requiring regular after-care
     - Sensorineural hearing loss occur in up to six percent of patients (Internet Search)
     - Vertigo (dizziness; it may persist for several days) (Internet Search)
     - Tinnitus
     - Temporary loss of taste on the side of the tongue (Internet Search)

104. **Ans. d. i.e. Davis retractor** *Ref. Essential of ENT, MB page 465 Dhingra 5/e,pgs463; http://en.wikipedia.org/wiki/List_of_instruments_used_in_otorhinolaryngology*

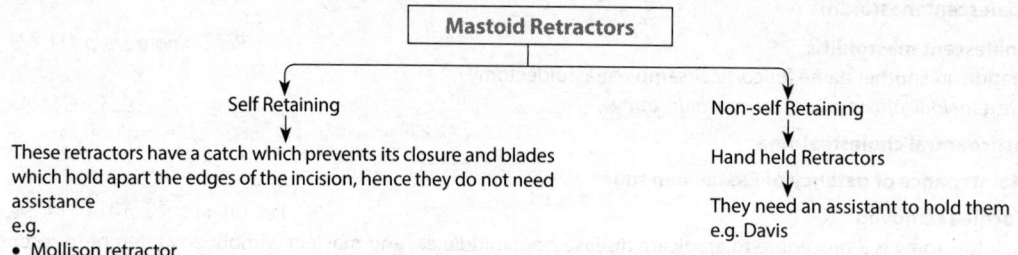

These retractors have a catch which prevents its closure and blades which hold apart the edges of the incision, hence they do not need assistance
e.g.
- Mollison retractor
- Jarson retractor
- Lemperts endaural retractor
- Wullstein retractor
- Plester

They need an assistant to hold them
e.g. Davis

Mollison's mastoid retractor. Used in mastoidectomy to retract soft tissues after incision and elevation of flaps. It is self-retaining and haemostatic.

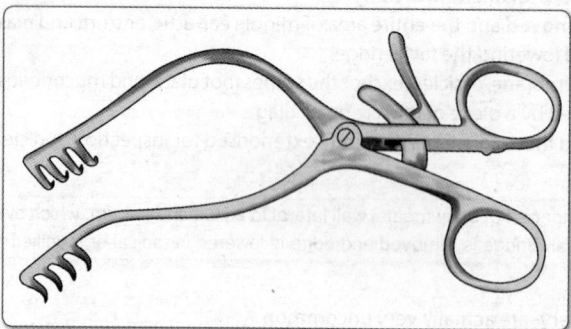

Jansen's self-retaining mastoid retractor. Used in mastoidectomy similar to Mollison's retractor.

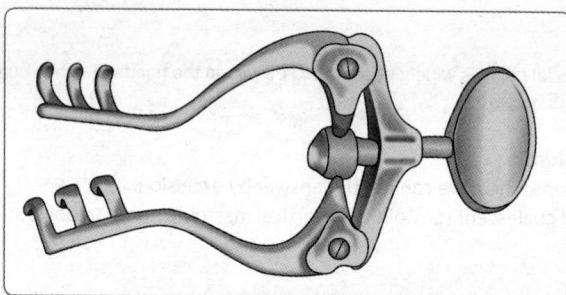

Lempert's endaural retractor. Used for endaural approach to ear surgery. It has two lateral blades which retract the flaps and a third central blade with holes. The central blade retracts the temporalis muscle. The central blade can be fixed to the body of the retractor by its hole.

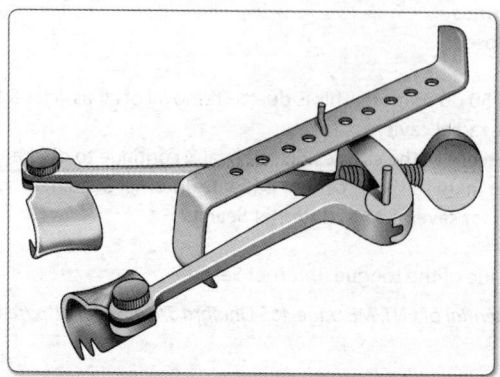

Chapter 7: Diseases of Middle Ear

105. **Ans. is c i.e. Canal wall down mastoidectomy**
    Ref. Dhingra 5/e, p 82, 6/e, p 73; Turner 10/e, p 304; Current Otolaryngology 2/e, p 670 5/e; 7/e Vol 3, p 3432-3433
    As discussed in aitic cholesteatoma we do and if cholesteatoma invades Eustachian tube or perilabyrinthine tissue then management is Radial Mastoidectomy. Now whether we perform radical mastoidectomy or modified radical mostoidectomy both are canal wall down procedures.

106. **Ans. is a i.e. Cutting drill over the bleeding area** *Ref. Essential of ENT Mohan Bansal, p 437*
    Here the answer is obvious as Cutting drill over the bleeding area will increase the bleeding instead of stopping it.
    - Diamond drill over the bleeding area will produce heat and stop the bleeding.
    - Bipolar cautery can be used to control bleeding during mastoid surgery (Not monopolar cautery).
    - Bone wax is also commonly used to control bleeding during mastoid surgery(It seals the bleeding site).

107. **Ans. is d i.e. Radical mastoidectomy** *Ref. Dhingra 6/e, p 403*
    In radical mastoidectomy, the opening of Eustachian tube is closed by curetting its mucosa and plugging the opening with tensor tympani muscle or cartilage.

108. **Ans. is a, c, d and e i.e. Serous otitis media, Mucoid otitis media, Glue ear and Secretary otitis media** *Dhingra 6/e, p 64*
    Otitis media with effusion is also called as serous otitis media, secretory otitis media, mucoid otitis media and glue ear.

109. **Ans. is c, i.e. Petrositis** *Ref. Dhingra 6/e, p 79*
    In the question patient is a case of CSOM, with local spread of infection.
    Dhingra clearly mentions in a patient with CSOM, persistent ear discharge with or without deep seated pain in spite of an adequate cortical or modified mastoidectomy points towards petrositis.
    Persistent ear discharge with or without deep seated pain in spite of an adequate cortical or modified radical mastoidectomy also points to petrositis.

Petrositis: Important Points
- Spread of infection from middle ear and mastoid to the petrous part of temporal bone is petrositis
- It can also involve adjacent 5th cranial nerve and 6th cranial nerve when it produces classical triad of symptoms – 6th nerve palsy, retro orbital pain (5th nerve) and persistent discharge from the ear, known as **Gradenigo's syndrome**

Note: All the three classical components of Gradenigo's syndrome are not needed for diagnosing petrositis.
- Treatment
  Adequate drainage is the mainstay of treatment along with specific antibiotic therapy. Modified radical or radical mastoidectomy is often required if not done already. The fistulous tract should be identified, curetted and enlarged to provide free drainage.

110. **Ans. is c i.e. C**
    Now in the figure we can identify facial nerve very easily. The canal for facial nerve lies above oval window in the medial wall of ear. In the figure we can identify incus and stapes. The foot plate of stapes lies over the oval window.
    Always above the facial canal is a bulge which is due to lateral semicircular canal. Hence in figure C is lateral semicircular canal, also remember the ossicle which lies close to lateral/horizontal semicircular canal is always incus.
    I am showing you another view—here also observe the above said structures.

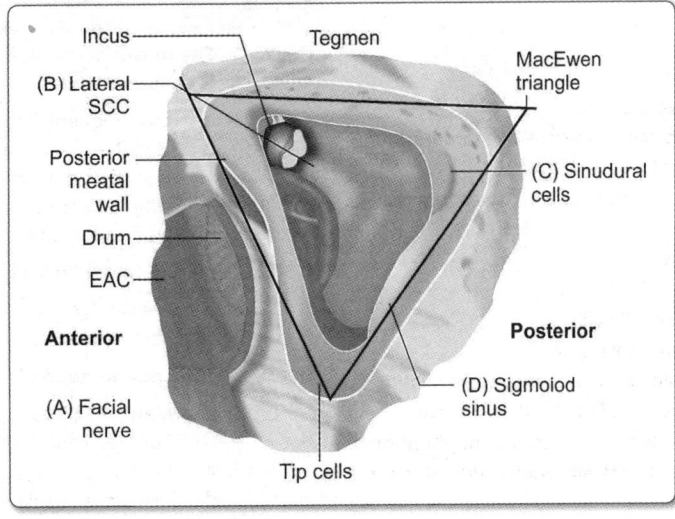

Chapter 8

Meniere's Disease

MENIERE'S DISEASE (ENDOLYMPHATIC HYDROPS)

It is a disease of the membranous inner ear characterized by triad of episodic vertigo followed by fluctuating deafness and fluctuating tinnitus. The additional symptom of aural fullness has been added to the current definition.

Meniere's disease is known after the name of Dr Prosper Meniere who described it in 1861.

Incidence

- **Males affected more than females.**
- **Age of onset:** 35–60 years (*Peak:* 5–6th decade)
- **Generally unilateral** (no predilection for left or right side)
- It may have genetic predisposition which might be caused by mutations on **short arm of chromosome 6**.

Pathology

Membranous labyrinth contains endolymph and in Meniere's disease the membranes containing this endolymph, i.e. membranous labyrinth are dilated like a balloon due to increase in pressure. This is called **hydrops**. So, the main pathology in Meniere's disease is distension of endolymphatic system mainly affecting the cochlear duct (scala media) and the saccule, and to a lesser extent the utricle and semicircular canals. Therefore, Meniere's disease is also called **endolymphatic hydrops**.

Pathophysiology

See Flowchart 8.1:

Clinical Features

- **1st Symptom Vertigo:** Onset sudden
  - Episodic in nature. It typically increases over a period of minutes and usually lasts for several hours.
  - Associated with nausea, vomiting, pallor, sweating, diarrhea and bradycardia
  - **No loss of consciousness.**
- **Fluctuating Hearing loss:**
  - **Fluctuant and progressive SNHL**
    Initially – low frequency losses
    Later – both high and low frequency are involved
- **Diplacusis:** Patient perceives sound louder than normal
  - Intolerance to loud sounds due to recruitment phenomenon (therefore these patients are poor candidates for hearing aids).

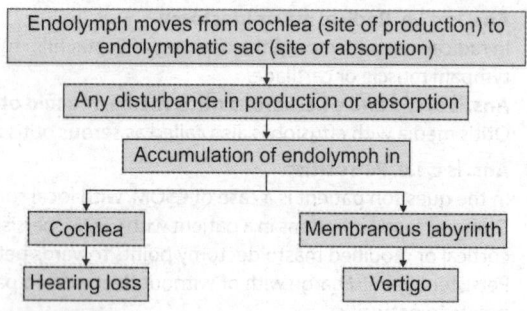

Flowchart 8.1: Pathophysiology Meniere's disease

- **Tinnitus:** roaring type and fluctuating in nature.
- **Aural fullness.**

Other Features

- **Tullio's phenomenon** is seen in some cases of **Meniere's disease:** Subjective imbalance and nystagmus is observed in response to loud, low frequency noise exposure. It is due to distended saccule lying against the stapes footplate.
- **Hennebert's sign:** False positive fistula test seen in Meniere's disease.
- **Drop crisis (otolithic crisis of Tumarkin):** There is sudden drop attack without loss of consciousness. There is no vertigo or fluctuation in hearing loss. Possible mechanism is deformation of the otolithic membrane of the utricle or saccule due to their dilatation.

NEW PATTERN QUESTIONS	
Q N1.	The sensor neural hearing loss in Meniere's disease is characterized by:
	a. Low frequency hearing loss initially
	b. High frequency hearing loss initially
	c. Both high and low frequencies affected simultaneously
	d. No hearing loss at all
Q N2.	Fluctuating hearing loss is a feature of:
	a. Meniere's disease b. Labyrinthine fistula
	c. Lermoyez syndrome d. All of the above
Q N3.	Tulio phenomenon is seen in all *except*:
	a. Meniere's disease
	b. Superior canal dehiscence
	c. Otosclerosis
	d. Perilymph fistula

- Nystagmus:

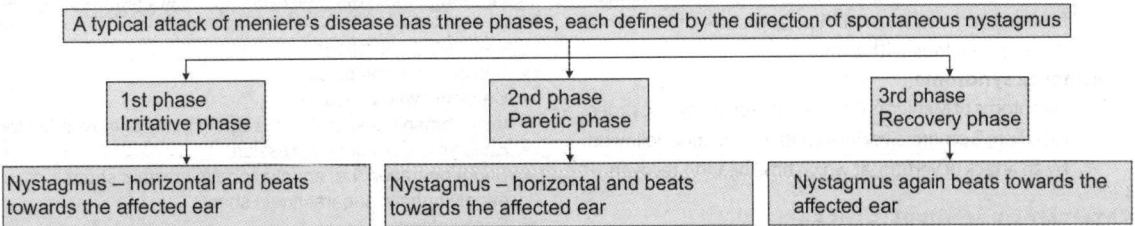

Investigations

- **Tuning fork tests:** Show sensorineural hearing loss, i.e. Rinne test Positive, weber test – towards normal ear, schwabach–shortened.
- **Pure tone audiometry:** SNHL with affection of lower frequencies in early stages and the curve is of rising type or upsloping type. When higher frequencies are involved, curve becomes flat or falling type.
  - 42% Flat audiogram
  - 32% Peaked pattern
  - 19% Downward sloping
  - 7%   Rising pattern
  - Speech audiometry – Discrimination score 55-85%
- **Recruitment:** Present
- **BERA:** Shows reduced latency of wave V
- **Electrocochleography (ECoG):** *Most sensitive and diagnostic.* Records the action potential and the summating potential of the cochlea through a recording electrode placed over the round window area.
  - Normal width of summating potential/action potential = 1.2-1.8 msec.
    Widening greater than 2 msec is usually significant
  - Summating potential (SP)/Action potential (AI) = 1:3 = 0.33
    (Normal)   < 30%
    In Meniere's > 30-40%

The sensitivity of the test can be increased by giving the patient 4 g of oral sodium chloride for 3 days prior to electrocochleography.

- **Caloric tests:** shows canal paresis (reduced response on affected side).
- **Glycerol test:**
  - Glycerol is given parenterally.
  - It produces a decrease in the intralabyrinthine pressure and also improves the cochlear blood flow resulting in improvement of hearing loss or increase in discrimination score by 10.
- **Reverse glycerol test:**
  - Performed using acetazolamide
  - Shows deterioration in the pure tone thresholds and speech discrimination scores.

NEW PATTERN QUESTIONS

Q N4. Chromosome responsible for hereditary Meniere's disease is:
  a. 6   b. 9
  c. 11   d. 14

Q N5. Diagnostic test for Meniere's disease:
  a. BERA
  b. PTA
  c. Electrocochleography
  d. CT

 Note:
- The diagnostic evaluation in Meniere's disease primarily includes (1) Audiometry (2) Fluorescent treponemal antibody absorption (FTA – ABS) to rule out syphilis as syphilis can imitate Meniere's disease.

- Committee on Hearing and Equilibrium of the American Academy of Otolaryngology—Head and neck surgery (AA OHNS) classified the diagnosis of Meniere's disease as follows:

1. **Certain:** Definite Meniere's disease confirmed by histopathology.
2. **Definite:** Two or more definitive spontaneous episodes of vertigo lasting 20 mm or longer.
   a. Audiometrically documented hearing loss on at least one occasion.
   b. Tinnitus or aural fullness in the affected ear.
   c. All other causes excluded.
3. **Probable:**
   a. One definitive episode of vertigo.
   b. Audiometrically documented hearing loss on at least one occasion.
   c. Tinnitus or aural fullness in the treated ear.
   d. Other causes excluded.
4. **Possible:**
   a. Episodic vertigo of Meniere's type without documented hearing loss (vestibular variant) or
   b. Sensorineural hearing loss, fluctuating or fixed, with disequilibrium but without definitive episodes (cochlear variant).
   c. Other causes excluded.

Variants of Meniere's Disease

- There are some variants of Meniere's disease in which clinical presentation is not that classical of Meniere's disease. These variants are:
  1. **Cochlear hydrops**
     - Only the cochlear symptoms and signs of Meniere's disease are present. Vertigo is absent and it appears only after several years. There is block at Ductus reuniens, therefore increased endolymphatic pressure is confined to cochlea only.

2. **Vestibular hydrops**
   - Patient gets typical episodes of vertigo while cochlear function remains normal. Typical picture of Meniere's disease develops with time.
3. **Lermoyez syndrome**
   - Symptoms of Meniere's disease are seen in reverse order. First there is progressive deterioration of hearing, followed by an attack of vertigo, at which time hearing recovers.

TREATMENT OF MENIERE'S DISEASE

I. Medical Management
II. Labyrinthine Exercises
III. Surgical Management

I. Medical Management

- *Initial treatment of Meniere's disease* is with medical management.
- Medical treatment controls the condition in over two third of patients.
- Medical management includes:
  1. *Antihistamine labyrinthine sedatives (vestibular sedatives)*
     - Many cases can be controlled by vestibular sedatives like prochlorperazine, promethazine, and cinnarizine.
  2. *Anxiolytic and tranquilizers*
     - Many patients are anxious, therefore they may be helped by anxiolytic and tranquilizers like diazepam.
  3. *Vasodilators*
     - **Betahistine hydrochloride** the most useful recent addition to the medical management and is routinely prescribed for most patients. It increases labyrinthine blood flow by releasing **histamine**.
     - **Other vasodilators employed include nicotinic acid, thymoxamine, inhaled carbogen** (5% CO_2 with 95% O_2), and **histamine drip**.
     - *Vasodilators increase vascularity of endolymphatic sac and its duct and thereby increases reabsorption of endolymphatic fluid.*
  4. *Diuretics (furosemide)*
     - Diuretics with fluid and salt restriction can help to control recurrent attacks if not controlled by vestibular sedatives or vasodilators.
  5. *Other drugs*
     - Propantheline bromide, phenobarbitone and hyoscine are effective alternatives.
  6. Avoid alcohol, smoking, excessive tea intake and coffee intake during treatment. Avoid excessive salt.

> **Meniett device**: It is seen that intermittent pressure delivered to inner ear, improves symptoms of Meniere's disease as well as improves hearing. This is the principle applied in device called Meniett device whereby intermittent positive pressure is appeared through this instrument.

II. Labyrinthine Exercises

Cawthorne-Cooksey exercise for adaptation of labyrinth:

III. Surgical Management

Surgery in Meniere's disease can be conservative or destructive (Table 8.1).

Table 8.1: Surgical management of Meniere's disease

Surgical
Conservative operations
• Stellate ganglion block
• Cervical sympathectomy
• Intratympanic gentamicin therapy (chemical labyrinthectomy)
• Endolymph sac decompression
• Shunt operation, i.e. endolymphatic mastoid shunt endolymphatic subarachnoid shunt
• Sacculotomy
Destructive operations
• Labyrinthectomy (hearing loss is permanent)
• Vestibular nerve section
• LASER/ultrasonography cause partial destruction of labyrinth without hearing loss.

Procedures of some therapies

1. *Intratympanic Gentamicin Therapy (Chemical Labyrinthectomy)*: Gentamicin is mainly vestibulotoxic. It has been used in daily or biweekly injections into the middle ear. Drug is absorbed through the round window and causes destruction of the vestibular labyrinth. Total control of vertigo spells has been reported in 60–80% of patients.

   Micro Wick: It is a small wick made of polyvinyl acetate and measures 1 mm × 9 mm. It is meant to deliver drugs from external canal to the inner ear and thus avoid repeated intratympanic injections. It requires a tympanostomy tube (grommet) to be inserted into the tympanic membrane and the wick is passed through it. When soaked with drug, wick delivers it to the round window to be absorbed into the inner ear. It has been used to deliver steroids in sudden deafness and gentamicin to destroy vestibular labyrinth in Meniere's disease.

2. *Endolymphatic sac decompression:*
   - By this operation pressure in the sac is relieved and patient becomes free of symptoms.
   - Briefly the procedure is done under local or general anesthesia.
   - A simple mastoidectomy is done and three SCC are delineated.
   - Endolymphatic sac lies close to posterior SCC keeping in mind the Donaldson's line.
   - Bone in this area is drilled with a diamond burr to expose the sac, which gets decompressed thus relieving the symptoms without affecting the hearing.

3. *Endolymphatic shunt operation*: A tube is put between subarachnoid space and endolymphatic sac for drainage of excessive fluid.

4. *Sacculotomy (Fick procedure)*: Saccule is punctured with a needle through stapes footplate. Cody's tack procedure, places a stainless steel tack to periodically decompress the sac.

SECONDARY ENDOLYMPHATIC HYDROPS OR D/D OF MENIERE'S DISEASE

Endolymphatic hydrops is not unique to Meniere's disease. Meniere's disease also called as Primary Endolymphatic hydrops as the cause of Meniere's disease is not known. Other conditions producing endolymphatic hydrops (*secondary endolymphatic hydrops*) are viral infection, syphilis, endocrine (hypothyroidism), autoimmune, trauma, allergy, Paget's disease, acoustic neuroma, vertebrobasilar insufficiency and migraine (CNS disease).

Explanations and References to New Pattern Questions

N1. Ans. is a i.e. Low frequency hearing loss initially *Ref. Dhingra 6/e, page 101*

Initially hearing loss is Meniere's disease affects lower frequencies later involves higher frequencies also. This is because in Meniere's, there is accumulation of endolymph which starts from the apex of cochlea (scale media), thus affecting the lower frequencies initially.

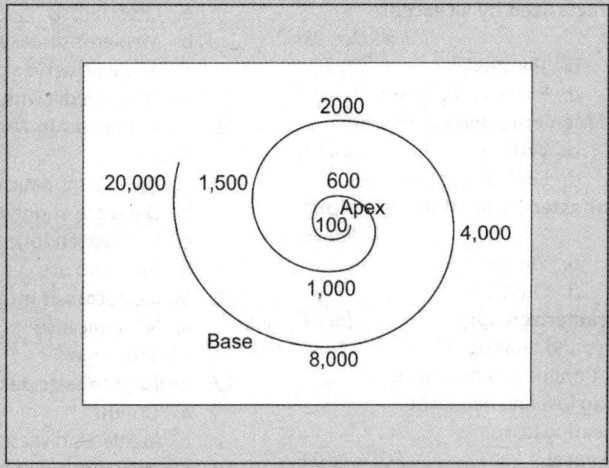

Frequency localization of Cochlea

Higher frequencies are localized in the basal turn and lower ones in the apex.

N2. Ans. is d i.e. All of the above *Ref. TB of ENT, Tuli 2/e, p 115*

Fluctuating hearing loss can be seen in

 Mnemonic: Google SPAM

- **G**oogle = **G**lue ear
- **S** = **S**yphilitic labyrinthitis
- **P** = **P**erilymph fistula (labyrinthine fistula)
- **A** = **A**utoimmune diseases of inner ear
- **M** = **M**eniere's disease and its variant–Lermoyez syndrome

N3. Ans. is c i.e. Otosclerosis

Tullio phenomenon refers to a condition, where exposure to loud sound can result in vertigo, nystagmus, postural imbalance and oscillopsia.

It is seen in:

- **Meniere's disease**
- Superior canal dehiscence
- Perilymph fistula

N4. Ans. is a i.e. 6

Genetically inherited Meniere's disease may be due to mutation on short arm of chromosome 6.

N5. Ans. is c i.e. Electrocochleography *Ref. Dhingra 6/e, p 101*

Electrocochleography is the diagnostic test for Menieres disease. Normally, ratio of summating action potential to action potential (AP) is 30%.
In Meniere disease SP/AP is greater than 30%.

QUESTIONS

1. **Which of the following is not a typical feature of Meniere's disease?** [AIIMS May 06]
   a. Sensorineural deafness b. Pulsatile tinnitus
   c. Vertigo d. Fluctuating deafness

2. **Meniere's disease is characterized by all except:** [AIIMS Dec. 98]
   a. Diplopia b. Tinnitus
   c. Vertigo d. Fullness of pressure in ear

3. **All are manifestations of Meniere's disease except:** [AI 97]
   a. Tinnitus b. Vertigo
   c. Sensorineural deafness d. Loss of consciousness

4. **Meniere's disease is manifested by all of the symptoms except:** [Delhi 96]
   a. Tinnitus b. Vertigo
   c. Deafness d. Otorrhea

5. **Meniere's disease is characterized by:** [AI 04]
   a. Conductive hearing loss and tinnitus
   b. Vertigo, ear discharge, tinnitus and headache
   c. Vertigo, tinnitus, hearing loss and headache
   d. Vertigo, tinnitus and hearing loss

6. **True about Meniere's disease:** [PGI June 03]
   a. Tinnitus b. Episodic vertigo
   c. Deafness d. Diarrhea
   e. Vomiting

7. **Meniere's disease is characterized by:** [PGI Dec. 03]
   a. Fluctuating hearing loss
   b. Also called endolymphatic hydrops
   c. Tinnitus and vertigo are most common symptoms
   d. It is a disease of inner ear
   e. Endolymphatic decompression is done

8. **All are true about Meniere's disease except:**
   a. Triad of recurrent vertigo, fluctuating sensorineural hearing loss, and tinnitus are found
   b. Treatment consists of use of thiazide
   c. Drop attack occurs
   d. Onset only after > 50 years

9. **The dilatation of Endolymphatic sac is seen in:** [AI 2011]
   a. Meniere's disease b. Otosclerosis
   c. Acoustic neuroma d. CSOM

10. **Meniere's disease is:** [PGI June 99]
    a. Perilymphatic hydrops b. Endolymphatic hydrops
    c. Otospongiosis d. Coalescent mastoiditis

11. **True about Endolymphatic hydrops:** [PGI June 06]
    a. B/L Condition b. Females more common
    c. 3rd to 4th decades d. Conductive deafness

12. **Glycerol test is done in:** [AP 1995, TN 2000]
    a. Otosclerosis b. Lateral sinus thrombosis
    c. Meniere's disease d. None of the above

13. **In a classical case of Meniere's disease which one of the following statements is true?** [Karn 01]
    a. Carhart's Notch is a characteristic feature in puretone audiogram
    b. Schwartz's sign is usually present in the tympanic membrane
    c. Low frequency sensorineural deafness is often seen in pure tone audiogram
    d. Decompression fallopian canal is the treatment of choice

14. **Recruitment phenomenon is seen in:**
    a. Otosclerosis [DNB 2007/Kolkata 2002]
    b. Meniere's disease
    c. Acoustic nerve schwannoma
    d. Otitis media with effusion

15. **Vasodilators in Meniere's disease are useful because they:** [Kerala 94]
    a. Dilate lymphatic vessels
    b. Decrease endolymph secretion
    c. Increase endolymph reabsorption
    d. Are of no use

16. **Vasodilators of internal ear is:**
    a. Nicotinic acid b. Histamine
    c. Serotonin d. Kinin

17. **Endolymphatic decompression is done in:** [Delhi 2006]
    a. Tinnitus b. Acoustic neuroma
    c. Meniere's disease d. Endolymphatic fistula

18. **Destructive procedure for Meniere's disease is:**
    a. Fick's procedure
    b. Cody tack procedure
    c. Vestibular neurectomy
    d. Trans-labyrinthine neurectomy
    e. Labyrinthectomy

19. **Differential diagnosis of Meniere's disease are all except:** [UP 07]
    a. Acoustic neuroma b. CNS disease
    c. Labyrinthitis d. Suppurative otitis media

20. **A 55-year-old female presents with tinnitus, dizziness and n/o progressive deafness. Which of the following is not a D/D?** [AIIMS 2001]
    a. Acoustic neuroma b. Endolymphatic hydrops
    c. Meningitis d. Histiocytosis 'X'

21. **Initial mechanism of action of intra-tympanic gentamicin microwick catheter inserted into inner ear in treatment of Meniere's disease:** [AIIMS Nov. 2012]
    a. Damage outer hair cell
    b. Binds to hair cell Na^+-K^+ ATPase channel
    c. Acts on mechanoreceptors of outer hair cell
    d. Bind to Mg^{2+} channel

22. **Which of the following is true about Meniere's disease?**
    a. Surgery is the mainstay of treatment [AIIMS Nov. 2014]
    b. Electrocochleography is the gold standard investigation for diagnosis
    c. Semont's maneuver is used for treatment
    d. In initial stages, inverted 'V' shaped audiogram is seen

23. **Auditory neurotherapy is an effective modality of treatment for which of the following abnormalities of hearing?**
    a. Meniere's disease b. Malignant Otitis Externa
    c. CSOM d. Otosclerosis

Explanations and References

1. **Ans. is b i.e. Pulsatile tinnitus**
2. **Ans. is a i.e. Diplopia**
3. **Ans. is d i.e. Loss of consciousness**
4. **Ans. is d i.e. Otorrhea**
5. **Ans is c i.e. Vertigo, tinnitus, hearing loss and headache**
6. **Ans. is a, b, c, d, e i.e. Tinnitus; Episodic vertigo; Deafness; Diarrhea; and Vomiting**

Ref. Dhingra 5/e, p 112, 6/e, p 100, 101; Tuli 1/e, p 127; Harrison 17/e, p 202, Turner 10/e, p 335

Meniere's Disease is characterized by
- **Episodic vertigo** (accompanied by *nausea*, *vomiting* and vagal disturbances like abdominal cramps, diarrhea and bradycardia)
- **Fluctuating deafness of sensorineural type**
- **Fluctuating tinnitus**
- **Aural fullness**
- **Emotional disturbances, headache and anxiety.**

Note:
- Pulsatile tinnitus is seen in Glomus jugulare, AV shunts, aneurysms, stenotic arterial lesions. It may also occur in secretory otitis media
- In the early stages of disease most patients are well in between the attack. As the disease progresses patients may have persistent hearing loss, tinnitus and postural imbalance between the attacks of vertigo
- Some patients in the later stages develop drop attacks k/a **Tumarkin or otolithic crisis due to otolith dysfunction**
- During this attack patient simply drops without a warning. **There is no associated vertigo or loss of consciousness.**

7. **Ans. is a, b, c, d and e i.e. Fluctuating hearing loss; Also called endolymphatic hydrops, Tinnitus and vertigo are most common symptoms; It is a disease of inner ear; and Endolymphatic decompression is done** *Ref. Dhingra 6/e, p 100-101*

   Read the preceding text for explanation.
8. **Ans. is d i.e. Onset only after >50 years** *Ref. Dhingra 6/e, p 100-105*
   See text for explanation
9. **Ans. is a > c i.e. Meniere's disease > Acoustic neuroma** *Ref. Dhingra 5/e, p 111, 6/e, p 103*
10. **Ans. is b i.e. Endolymphatic hydrops** *Ref. Dhingra 5/e, p 111, 6/e, p 103*

    Meniere's disease, which is an idiopathic lesion, is a clinical diagnosis. The following conditions, which are included in Meniere's syndrome or secondary Meniere's disease, can mimic the clinical features of Meniere's disease and should be kept in mind.
    - Migraine and basilar migraine
    - Autoimmune disease of inner ear and otosclerosis
    - Syphilis and Cogan's syndrome
    - Cardiogenic
    - Vertebral basilar insufficiency
    - Trauma: Head injury or ear surgery
    - Acoustic neuroma

    ### Also Know
    - **Lermoyez syndrome** is a variant of Meniere's disease, where initially there is deafness and tinnitus, vertigo appears later when deafness improves.

11. **Ans. is c i.e. 3rd to 4th decades** *Ref. Dhingra 5/e, p 112, 6/e, p 100-101*
    - **Meniere's disease** lead to sensorineural hearing loss and not conductive type.
    - Generally unilateral
    - Age = *Most common* 35-60 years.
    - It is more common in males

Also remember:		
	Otosclerosis	– Bilateral condition, more common in females
	Bell's palsy	– Unilateral condition with equal sex distribution
	Acoustic neuroma	– Unilateral with condition equal sex distribution
	Glomus tumor	– More common in females

12. **Ans. is c i.e. Meniere's disease** *Ref. Dhingra 5/e, p 113, 6/e, p 102*

    Glycerol is a dehydrating agent. When given orally, it reduces endolymph pressure and causes improvement in hearing as evidenced by an improvement of 10 dB or 10% gain in discrimination score in Meniere's disease patients.

13. **Ans. is c i.e. Low frequency sensorineural deafness is often seen in pure tone audiogram**

    Ref. Dhingra 5/e, p 113, 6/e, p 101
    - Carhart's notch and Schwartz's sign are seen in otosclerosis *Ref. Dhingra 5/e p 98-99, 6/e, p 87*
    - Decompression of endolymphatic sac (and not fallopian canal) is done in Meniere's disease. *Ref. Dhingra 5/e p 116, 6/e, p104*
    - Decompression of Fallopian canal is done in traumatic facial nerve palsy.

    > - Meniere's disease is associated with – SNHL which affects low frequencies first, followed by higher frequencies later. This is visible on pure tone audiogram.

14. **Ans. is b i.e. Meniere's disease** *Ref. Dhingra 5/e, p 31,113, 6/e, p 101*

    ### Recruitment Phenomenon
    - It is a phenomenon of abnormal growth of loudness^Q
    - The ear which does not hear low intensity sound begins to hear greater intensity sounds as loud or even louder than normal hearing ear
    - Thus a loud sound which is tolerable in normal ear may grow to abnormal levels of loudness in the recruiting ear and thus become intolerable^Q
    - Recruitment is typically seen in lesions of cochlea^Q, i.e. Meniere's disease^Q, presbycusis.^{Q}
    - Patients with recruitment are poor candidates for hearing aids. ^{Q}

15. **Ans. is c i.e. Increase endolymph reabsorption** *Ref. Dhingra 5/e, p 115, 6/e, p 104*

16. **Ans. is a and b i.e. Nicotinic acid and Histamine**

    Ischemia of endolymphatic sac
    ↓
    ↓ absorption of endolymph
    ↓
    Endolymphatic hydrops/Meniere's disease

    Vasodilators improve labyrinthine circulation, so, increase endolymph reabsorption.

    > **Vasodilators Used**
    > **During acute attack:**
    > - Carbogen (95% O_2 + 5% CO_2)
    > - Histamine (contraindicated in asthmatics)
    >
    > **During chronic attack:**
    > - Nicotinic acid
    > - Betahistine

17. **Ans. is c i.e. Meniere's disease** *Ref. Dhingra 5/e, p 116, 6/e, p 104*

    As explained in Text:
    - Decompression of endolymphatic sac is done in Meniere's disease.

18. **Ans. is e i.e. Labyrinthectomy** *Ref. Dhingra 5/e, p 116, 6/e, p 104*

    See text for explanation

19. **Ans. is d i.e. Suppurative otitis media**

    ### Differential Diagnosis of Vertigo + Tinnitus + SNHL Deafness – Includes:
    - Meniere's disease (Endolymphatic hydrops)
    - Syphilis
    - Labyrinthitis
    - Labyrinthine trauma due to fracture of temporal bone, postoperatively after stapedectomy
    - Cogan syndrome
    - Labyrinthine hemorrhage due to blood dyscrasia
    - Acoustic neuroma/meningioma (CP angle lesion)
    - Multiple sclerosis
    - Hypothyroidism/Hyperlipidemia.

Note: In serous otitis media these symptoms may be seen but then hearing loss will be of conductive variety and not SNHL.

Chapter 8: Meniere's Disease

20. **Ans. is d i.e. Histiocytosis 'X'** *Ref. Current Otolaryngology 2/e, p 616*

    Delayed Endolymphatic Hydrops
    - Hydrops sometimes develop in patients who have lost their hearing in one or both ears previously. The causes of hearing loss vary, from head injury, meningitis or any other etiology. Patient subsequently develops attacks of vertigo similar to that seen in Meniere's disease in a delayed fashion.
    - Histiocytosis X belongs to the group of disorders collectively termed inflammatory reticuloendotheliosis characterized by multiple osteolytic lesions involving skull, temporal bone, long bones, ribs, and vertebrae. There is generalized lymphadenopathy, hepatosplenomegaly, and in severe cases involvement of the bone marrow. Involvement of temporal bone leads to features mimicking complicated like otorrhea, mastoiditis, facial palsy, and labyrinthitis.

21. **Ans. is a i.e. Direct damage to outer hair cell** *Ref. Dhingra 5/e, p 116, 6/e, p 104*

    Intratympanic Gentamicin Therapy
    - Gentamicin is mainly vestibulotoxic
    - It has been used in daily or biweekly injection into the middle ear
    - Drug is absorbed through round window and causes destruction of vestibular labyrinth
    - Total control of vertigo spells has been reported in 60–80% of patients with some relief from symptoms in others
    - Hearing loss, sometimes severe and profound, has been reported in 4 to 30% of patients treated with mode of therapy.

22. **Ans. is b i.e. Electrocochleography is the gold standard investigation for diagnosis** *Ref. Dhingra 6/e, p 100-104, 5/e, p 112-113; Logan-Turner 10/e, p 335*

    "Electrocochleography" is the gold standard investigation for diagnosis in Meniere's disease.

    > "Electrocochleography" is diagnostic in Meniere's disease, Ratio of Summating Potential (SP) to Action Potential (AP) is greater than 30%

    - Initial management of Meniere's disease is medical management and not surgery
    - In initial stages: An upsloping audiogram in seen, as lower frequencies are affected earlier
    - Later when higher frequencies are also affected, then a flat audiogram is seen.

23. **Ans. is a i.e. Meniere's disease** *Ref. Scott-Brown's Otorhinolaryngology and Head and Neck Surgery 7/e, p3570*

    Among the given options, only Meniere's disease involves the vestibular system of inner ear. Hence a neurotherapy, i.e. direct nerve stimulation is going to be useful only in Meniere's disease.

Chapter 9

Otoclerosis

ANATOMY OF LABYRINTH

- **Otic labyrinth:** Also called **membranous labyrinth or endolymphatic labyrinth**. It consists of utricle, saccule, cochlea, semicircular ducts, endolymphatic duct and sac. It is filled with endolymph.
- **Periotic labyrinth or perilymphatic labyrinth (or space):** It surrounds the otic labyrinth and is filled with perilymph. It includes vestibule, scale tympani, scale vestibuli, peri-lymphatic space of semicircular canals and the priotic duct, which surrounds the endolymphatic duct of otic labyrinth.
- **Otic capsule:** It is the bony labyrinth. It has three layers—
  a. **Endosteal:** The innermost layer. It lines the bony labyrinth.
  b. **Enchondral:** Develops from the cartilage and later ossifies into bone. It is in this layer that some islands of cartilage are left unossified that later give rise to **otosclerosis**.
  c. **Periosteal:** Covers the bony labyrinth.

OTOSCLEROSIS

It is a hereditary localised disease of the bony labyrinth (bony otic capsule) characterised by alternating phases of bone resorption and formation. Here the normal dense enchondral layer of the bony otic capsule gets replaced by irregularly laid spongy bone.

Etiology
- Autosomal dominant[Q] (50% cases are hereditary)
- Male: Female ratio is 1:2
- Age group affected
  - 20–45 years (maximum between 20 and 30 years)
- Puberty, pregnancy and menopause accelerate the condition.
Triggering factor: Viral infection
- Races:
  - White > Negroes
  - More in the Caucasians
- In 70–85% cases it is bilateral.

> **Point to Remember**
> ➤ Site—*Most common* is fissula ante fenestram (anterior to the oval window).[Q]

Other sites:
- Round window area
- Internal auditory canal
- Stapedial footplate
- Semicircular canal

Types of Otosclerosis

Stapedial (Fenestral)	Cochlear (Fenestral)	Histological type
Most common type Most common site is: Fissula ante fenestram[Q]	Involves round window	Lesion detected only on postmortem

- On histopathology *"Blue mantles"* are characteristic.

Clinical Features
Symptoms:

- **Deafness:** Slowly progressive B/L conductive deafness, in a female aggravated by pregnancy generally suggests otosclerosis. U/L hearing loss may occur in 15% cases.

- **Paracusis willisii[Q]:** Patient hears better in noisy surrounding.
- **Tinnitus:** Indicates sensorineural hearing loss *(cochlear otosclerosis).*
- **Voice of the patient:** Quiet voice, low volume speech because they hear their own voices by bone conduction and consequently talk quietly.
- **Vertigo:** Generally not seen.
- In cochlear otosclerosis—there may be vertigo, tinnitus and SNHL (Sensorineural Hearing Loss).

Signs
- **On otoscopic examination:** Tympanic membrane is normal[Q] (pearly white) and mobile in most of the cases.

> **Point to Remember**
> ➤ In 10% cases flamingo-pink blush is seen through the **tympanic membrane called as Schwartz sign.**
> ➤ **Importance of Schwartz sign:** It is indicative of active focus with increased vascularity[Q].
> ➤ Surgery is contraindicated[Q] in patients with Schwartz sign and is an indication for sodium fluoride therapy[Q] such as during pregnancy.[Q]

NEW PATTERN QUESTION

Q N1. Schwartz sign seen in:
  a. Glomus jugulare   b. Otosclerosis
  c. Meniere's diseases d. Acoustic neuroma

Tests
- Tuning fork tests show **conductive type of hearing loss.** Complete fixation of stapes footplate leads to a loss of 80 dB.
  - **Rinne's:** Negative (first for 256 Hz and then 512 Hz).
  - **Weber's:** Lateralised to the ear with greater conductive loss.
  - **Absolute bone conduction:** Normal (can be decrease in cochlear otosclerosis).
  - **Gelles test:** No change in the bone conduction threshold when air pressure is increased by Siegel's speculum. This is because ossicular chain is already fixed.
  - Audiogram shows A-B gap > 15 dB.

Tympanometry/Audiometry

It is one of the important tools in evaluating a patient suspected of otosclerosis:

- **Impedance audiometry:** Patients with early disease may show **Type A tympanogram** (because middle ear aeration is not affected).
  Progressive stapes fixation results in **AS type curve**.
- **Acoustic reflex:** It is one of the **earliest signs of otosclerosis** and precedes the development of an air bone gap.
- **In the normal hearing ear:** The configuration of the acoustic reflex pattern is one of a sustained decrease in compliance owing to the contraction of the stapedial muscle that lasts the duration of stimulus.
- **In otosclerosis:** In early stages.
  A characteristic diphasic on-off pattern is seen in which there is a brief increase in compliance at the onset and at the termination of stimulus occurs. **This is pathognomic for otosclerosis.**^{Q}
- **In later stages:** The Reflex is absent—Stapedial reflex is absent.

Point to Remember

Pure tone audiometry: Normally in otosclerosis—bone conduction is normal but in some cases there is a dip in bone conduction which is maximum at 2000 Hz and is called the **Carhart's notch (Fig. 9.1)**.
Remember: Carhart's notch disappears after successful stapedectomy.

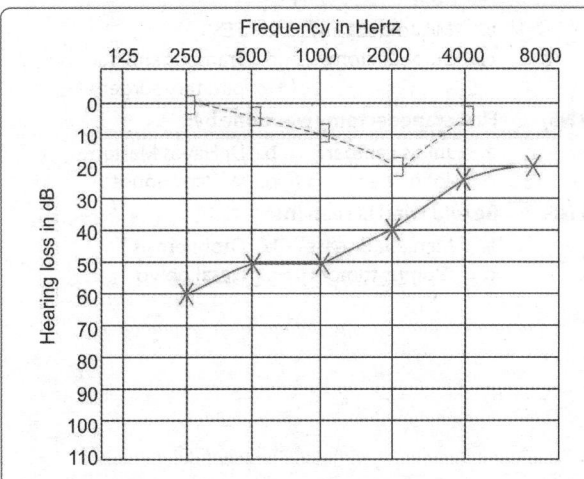

Fig. 9.1: Carhart's notch

In cochlear otosclerosis, cookie bite audiogram seen as bone conduction graph appears like a cookie having better.

NEW PATTERN QUESTIONS

Q N2. A pure tone audiogram with a dip at 2000 Hz is characteristic of:
a. Ototoxicity
b. Noise induced hearing loss
c. Otosclerosis
d. Presbyacusis

Q N3. In otosclerosis the tympanogram is:
a. Low compliance
b. High compliance
c. Normal compliance
d. Any of the above

Extra Edge

- **Histological otosclerosis:** The gold standard for the reporting of the incidence of histological otosclerosis is the study of **bilateral temporal bone**.^{Q}
- **Imaging studies:** Imaging modality of choice is **high resolution CT scan.**^{Q}

Treatment

a. **Observation:**
   - It is the least risky and least expensive option.
   - Preferred for patients with—(i) Unilateral disease (ii) Mild conductive hearing loss.
   - If the patient is not concerned about the hearing loss, then no intervention is required.
   - Audiograms are obtained on yearly basis.
   - Hearing loss typically progresses slowly, ultimately requiring intervention.

b. **Medial therapy:**
   (i) *Sodium fluoride therapy*

Sodium Fluoride Therapy

➢ It is given in doses of 50 to 70 mg/day for 1 to 2 years.

Role

➢ It reduces osteoclastic bone resorption and increases osteoblastic bone formation (It hastens the maturity of active focus).
➢ It inhibits proteolytic enzymes that are cytotoxic to cochlea (may lead to SNHL).

Dangers of Fluoride Therapy

➢ Fracture long bone and spine (due to fluorosis).
➢ So X-ray spine and X-ray of long bones are done as a routine for observing the thickening of trabeculae.

Indications

➢ Cochlear otosclerosis, i.e. Malignant otosclerosis (rapidly progressive cochlear otosclerosis).
➢ Radiologically active focus^Q (new onset disease).
➢ Patients with a positive Schwartz sign^Q.
➢ **Adverse effect**—most common GI disturbances.

Contraindications

➢ Chronic nephritis
➢ Chronic rheumatoid arthritis
➢ Pregnant women/lactating women
➢ Children

(ii) *Bisphosphonates* (e.g. Alendronate, Etidronate)
   – They are anti-resorptive agents that are helpful for the prevention and treatment of osteoporosis and other conditions characterized by increased bone remodeling. They are being tried for use in osteosclerosis. They inhibit osteoclastic activity without affecting bone deposition.
   Main side effect – GI symptoms like nausea and diarrhea

(iii) *Hearing aids:* Most patients with otosclerosis have a normal cochlear function with excellent speech discrimination and are therefore good hearing aid candidates.

Point to Remember
Patients who refuse surgery or are unfit for surgery can use hearing aid.

c. **Surgical treatment:**
- **Selection of patients for stapes surgery**
  - **Air bone gap of at least 25–30 dB** (the larger the air bone gap, the more there is the gain by surgical intervention
  - Hearing threshold should be 30 dB or more.
  - Rinnie negative (both for 256 and 512 Hz.)
  - Speech discrimination score $\geq 60\%$.
  - It is also indicated in patients with profound hearing loss but with good speech discrimination score, so as to enable them to use a hearing aid.)
- **Stapedectomy with prosthesis replacement was earlier the TOC**
  Here the fixed otosclerotic stapes is removed and a prosthesis inserted between the incus and oval window. Prosthesis can be of teflon^Q, stainless steel, platinum or titatinium. Disadvantage—associated with high incidence of perilymph leak and SNHL.
- **New treatment of choice is stapedotomy^Q:** Here a hole is made in centre of footplate of stapes and a **teflon prosthesis** inserted between incus and foot plate.
- **Other surgeries which can be done:**
  - Laser stapedotomy (CO_2 Argon and KTP)
  - Stapes mobilisation
  - **Lempert's fenestration operation:** (outdated procedure).

Point to Remember
Contraindications for surgery
➤ Only hearing ear (**Absolute CI**)
➤ Occupation

  Athletes,   ⎫ Working
  Divers   ⎬ in noisy
  Frequent   ⎪ surroundings
  Air travelers ⎭

➤ Associated Meniere's disease
➤ Pregnancy, young children   ⎫
➤ Otitis externa/Otitis media   ⎬ **Relative**
➤ Tympanic membrane perforation ⎪ **contraindications**
➤ Inner ear malformation/exostosis ⎭
➤ Medically unfit
➤ Active/malignant otosclerosis (It is an indication for fluoride therapy).

Note:
- *Most important complication of stapes surgery* is hearing loss so second operation is considered 6 months to 1 year after first surgery.
- Always the worst ear is operated first.

NEW PATTERN QUESTIONS

Q N4. Wide habenula perforata can lead to problem during which surgery?
  a. Mastoidectomy   b. FESS
  c. Stapedectomy   d. Transsphenoidal pituitary surgery

Q N5. First stapedectomy was done by:
  a. Julius Lempert   b. Dr Hayes Marten
  c. John Shea   d. William House

Q N6. Bezold triad is seen in:
  a. Meniere disease b. Otosclerosis
  c. Glomus tumor   d. Nasal polyp

Chapter 9: Otosclerosis

Explanations and References to New Pattern Questions

N1. Ans. is b i.e. Otoslerosis   *Ref. Dhingra 6/e, p 87*
Schwartz sign is seen in otosclerosis (already discussed).

N2. Ans. is c i.e. Otosclerosis   *Ref. Dhingra 6/e, p 87*
Dip at 2000 Hz in PTA called as Carhart's notch is characteristic of otosclerosis.

N3. Ans. is a i.e. Low compliance
In otosclerosis AS type curve is seen which is a low compliance curve.

> **Remember**
> Type A curve is a normal pressure curve.
> Type Ad curve (seen in ossicular discontinuity) is a high compliance curve.

N4. Ans. is c i.e. Stapedectomy   *Ref. Essentials of ENT Mohan Bansal 1/e, p 56*
Habenula Perforata

> **Habenula perforata** is an opening through which branches of cochlear nerves enter the cochlea. It is associated with congenitally enlarged internal acoustic meatus and stapes fixation.
> If wide, it can lead to perilymph gush in stapes surgery.

N5. Ans. is c i.e. John Shea   *Ref. Wikipedia Internet Search*

> Founder of stapes surgery — Kessel
> Fenestration procedure developed by — Holmgren
> Fenestration procedure popularized by — Lempert
> First stapedectomy done by — John Shea in 1956

N6. Ans. is b i.e. Otosclerosis   *Ref. Tuli ENT 2/e, p 91*

> Bezold triad is seen in otosclerosis and consists of:
> - Negative Rinne
> - Prolonged bone conduction and
> - Raised lower tone limit.

Section 1: Ear

QUESTIONS

1. **Otospongiosis is inherited as:** [AI 95]
   a. Autosomal dominant b. Autosomal recessive
   c. X-linked dominant d. X-linked recessive

2. **True about otosclerosis:** [PGI June 03]
   a. 50% have family history
   b. Males are affected twice than female
   c. More common in Negro's and African's
   d. Deafness occurs in 20–30 years but less in before 10 years and after 40 years
   e. Pregnancy has bearing on it

3. **Common age for otosclerosis is:** [UP-06]
   a. 5–10 years b. 10–20 years
   c. 20–30 years d. 30–45 years

4. **Most common site of otosclerosis is:** [Comed 07]
   a. Round window b. Oval window
   c. Utricle d. Ossicles

5. **The part most commonly involved in otosclerosis is:**
   [PGI June 99/Rohtak 98/UP-08]
   a. Oval window b. Round window
   c. Tympanic membranes d. Malleus
   e. Ossicles

6. **Most common site for the initiation of otosclerosis is:** [Karn 06]
   a. Footplate of stapes b. Margins of stapes
   c. Fissula ante fenestram d. Fissula postfenestram

7. **Otospongiosis causes:** [AI 96]
   a. U/L conductive deafness
   b. B/L conductive deafness
   c. U/L sensorineural deafness
   d. B/L sensorineural deafness

8. **Paracusis willisii is feature of:**
   (MHPGMCET 2002, JIPMER 2000 March, MH 2005)
   a. Tympanosclerosis b. Otosclerosis
   c. Meniere's disease d. Presbycusis

9. **A patient hears better in noise. The diagnosis is:** [Karn. 95]
   a. Hyperacusis b. Hypoacusis
   c. Presbycusis d. Paracusis

10. **Otosclerosis tinnitus is due to:** [Bihar 2005]
    a. Cochlear otosclerosis
    b. Increased vascularity in lesion
    c. Conductive deafness
    d. All of the above

11. **In majority of the cases with otosclerosis the tympanic membrane is:** [Kerala 94]
    a. Normal b. Flamingo-pink
    c. Blue d. Yellow

12. **Schwartz sign seen in:** [MAHE 05, PGI-98]
    a. Glomus Jugulare b. Otosclerosis
    c. Meniere's diseases d. Acoustic neuroma

13. **Which of the following is/are true about Schwartz sign:**
    a. Sign of inactive disease [PGI May 17]
    b. Indication for surgery
    c. More common during pregnancy
    d. Reddish hue over the promontory
    e. Seen in the early stages of the otosclerosis

14. **Gelle's test is for:** [Bihar 2006]
    a. Otosclerosis b. NIHL
    c. Sensorineural deafness d. None of these

15. **Feature in otosclerosis includes:** [AP 2003]
    a. Sounds not heard in noisy environment
    b. Normal tympanum
    c. More common in males
    d. Malleus is most commonly effected

16. **Carhart's notch in audiogram is deepest frequency of:**
    a. 0.5 kHz b. 2 kHz [AI 03; TN 03]
    c. 4 kHz d. 8 kHz

17. **Carhart's notch in audiometry is seen in:** [MAHE 05]
    a. Ocular discontinuity b. Haemotympanum
    c. Otomycosis d. Otosclerosis

18. **In the pure tone audiogram shown below, identify the likely cause:** [AIIMS ....]

    See Color Plate 9

    a. Meniere's disease b. Noise induced hearing loss
    c. Otosclerosis d. Ototoxicity

19. **Acoustic dip occurs at:** [TN 95]
    a. 2000 Hz b. 4000 Hz
    c. 500 Hz d. 1500 Hz

20. **Lady has B/L hearing loss since 4 years which worsened during pregnancy. Type of impedance audiometry graph will be:** [AIIMS May 07]
    a. Ad b. As
    c. B d. C

Chapter 9: Otosclerosis

21. **All are true about otosclerosis except:**
    a. Increased incidence in female [PGI June 06, June 05]
    b. Sensorineural deafness
    c. Irreversible loss of hearing
    d. Carhart's notch at 2000 Hz
    e. Family history positive

22. **Characteristic feature of otosclerosis are all except:**
    [AIIMS June 97]
    a. Conductive deafness   b. Positive Rinne's test
    c. Paracusis willisii   d. Mobile ear drum

23. A 30-year old woman with family history of hearing loss from her mother's side developed hearing problem during pregnancy. Hearing loss is bilateral, slowly progressive, Pure tone audiometry bone conduction hearing loss with an apparent bone conduction hearing loss at 2000 Hz. What is the most likely diagnosis? [AIIMS May 06]
    a. Otosclerosis
    b. Acoustic neuroma
    c. Otitis media with effusion
    d. Sigmoid sinus thrombosis

24. **Medication which may prevent rapid progress of cochlear otosclerosis is:** [Karn. 94]
    a. Steroids   b. Antibiotics
    c. Fluorides   d. Vitamins

25. **All are true statements regarding use of sodium fluoride in the treatment of otosclerosis except:** [AI 2011]
    a. It inhibits osteoblastic activity
    b. Used in active phase of otosclerosis when Schwartz sign is positive
    c. Has proteolytic activity (bone enzymes)
    d. Contraindicated in chronic nephritis

26. A 31-year-old female patient complains of bilateral impairment of hearing for the 5 year. On examination, tympanic membrane is normal and audiogram shows a bilateral conductive deafness. Impedance audiometry shows As type of curve and acoustic reflexes are absent. All constitute part of treatment, except:
    a. Hearing aid   b. Stapedectomy
    c. Sodium fluoride   d. Gentamicin

27. **Following operations are done in case of otosclerosis:**
    a. Stapedectomy   b. Fenestration [PGI Dec. 03]
    c. Stapedotomy   d. Sacculotomy
    e. Mastoidectomy

28. **In otosclerosis during stapes surgery prosthesis used is:** [UP 06]
    a. Teflon piston
    b. Grommet
    c. Total ossicular replacement
    d. All of the above

29. **Which of the following is not resected in stapedotomy?**
    [AIIMS May 2014]
    a. Anterior crus of stapes   b. Posterior crus of stapes
    c. Stapedial ligament   d. Lenticular process of incus

Explanations and References

1. **Ans. is a i.e. Autosomal dominant**   *Ref. Dhingra 5/e, p 97; 6/e, p 86*
   The exact etiology of otosclerosis is not known. In otosclerosis family history/heredity plays an important role. About 50% of patients of otosclerosis have a positive family history.
   - It is an automosal dominant condition^q
   - Shows incomplete penetrance^q and variable expression^q

Also Remember:	It may be associated with **Vander Hoeve syndrome**
	osteogenesis imperfecia
	Blue sclera △ Otosclerosis

2. **Ans. is a, d and e i.e. 50% have family history; Deafness occurs in 20–30 years but less in before 10 years and after 40 years; and Pregnancy has bearing on it**

3. **Ans. is c i.e. 20–30 years**   *Ref. Dhingra 5/e, p 97; 6/e, p 86*
   - 50% of patients of otosclerosis have positive family history.
   - Females are more commonly affected than males (**Note:** unless and until the question says in India always mark female> male as the correct option).
   - Whites are affected more than negroes.
   - Age = most common between 20–30 years (Ans. 3) and is rare before 10 and after 40 years.
   - Deafness is increased by pregnancy, menopause, trauma and major operations.
   - Viruses like measles virus have also been associated with it.

4. **Ans. is b i.e. Oval window**
5. **Ans. is a i.e. Oval window**
6. **Ans. is c i.e. Fissula ante fenestram**   *Ref. Dhingra 5/e, p 97,98; 6/e, p 86, 87*

Most common type of otosclerosis	– Stapedial otosclerosis
Most common site of otosclerosis	– Fissula ante fenestram (i.e. just in front of oval window)
Most common site for stapedial otosclerosis	– Fissula ante fenestram (i.e. just in front of oval window)
Most common site for cochlear otosclerosis	– Round window

7. **Ans. is b i.e. Bilateral conductive deafness**
8. **Ans. is b i.e. Otosclerosis**
9. **Ans. is d i.e. Paracusis**
10. **Ans. is a i.e. Cochlear otosclerosis** *Ref. Dhingra 5/e, p 98; 6/e, p 87; Current Otolaryngology 3/e, p 690*

Symptoms of Otosclerosis

• Hearing loss	– It is the presenting symptom. Hearing loss is painless and has insidious onset. It is bilateral conductive type and usually starts in twenties.
• Paracusis willisii	– Patient hears better in noisy than quiet surroundings
• Tinnitus	– More in cochlear otosclerosis, i.e. it indicates sensorineural degeneration
• Vertigo	– Uncommon
• Speech	– Monotonous, well-modulated soft speech.

Point to Remember

Paracusis	Patient hears better in noise. Seen in otosclerosis.
Presbycusis	SNHL associated with aging. Manifests at 65 years of age (It is physiological).
Hyperacusis	Sensation of discomfort/pain on exposure to loud noises. Seen in injury to nerve to stapedius.
Diplacusis	Patient hears same tone as of different pitches in either ear (distortion of sound). Seen in Meniere's disease.

Extra Edge

- **Paracusis:** Scotts Brown 7th/ed vol-3 pg-3596
- Paracusis refers to auditory dysfunction, in which the perception of volume, pitch, timbre or other quality of sound may be altered.
- In majority of cases, paracusis are attributed to abnormalities at the auditory periphery (as in otosclerosis) However, they have also been reported in CNS lesions including temporal lobe (This is because 'Timbre' of a sound is perceived by well defined regions of posterior Heschl's gyrus and superior temporal sulcus extending into the circular insular sulcus, of both left and right hemisphere).

11. **Ans. is a i.e. Normal**
12. **Ans. is b i.e. Otosclerosis** *Ref. Dhingra 5/e, p 98; 6/e, p 87; Current Otolaryngology 2/e p 674; 3/e, p 690*

In Otosclerosis on Otoscopy

- Tympanic membrane is normal in appearance mostly, middle ear space is well-pneumatized and malleus moves with pneumatic otoscopy (i.e. mobility is normal)
- Sometimes a reddish hue/Flammingo-pink may be seen on the promontory and oval window niche owing to the prominent vascularity associated with an otospongiotic focus. This is known as Schwartz sign.

13. **Ans. is c, d and e i.e. more common during pregnancy, reddish hue over promontory and seen in early stages of the otosclerosis.**

Schwartz sign in otosclerosis

- Refers to reddish/flamingo pink hue of promontory seen through tympanic membrane (i.e. option d correct)
- It indicates active focus with increased vascularity (i.e. option a incorrect)
- Positive Schwartz sign is a relative contraindication for surgery, only once it fades then surgery should be done. i.e. option b incorrect.
- It is an indication for sodium fluoride therapy.
- Schwartz sign is M/C during pregnancy as disease is active (i.e. option c correct).
- Seen in 10% cases.

14. **Ans. is a i.e. Otosclerosis** *Ref. Dhingra 5/e, p 27; 6/e, p 22*

Gelle's Test

This test was earlier done to confirm the presence of otospongiosis. In this test, BC (bone conduction) is tested and at the same time Siegle's speculum compresses the air in the meatus. In normal individuals hearing is reduced after this, i.e. Gelles test is positive but in stapes fixation, sound is not affected, i.e Gelles test is negative.

Chapter 9: Otosclerosis

Basis of the Test

In normal individuals	In case of otosclerosis
↑ in air pressure in ear canal by Siegel's speculum ⇓ Push the tympanic membrane and ossicles inward ⇓ ↑ Intralabyrinthine pressure ⇓ Immobility of basilar membrane ⇓ ↓ hearing (i.e. test is positive)	↑ air pressure in ear canal by Seigel's speculum ⇓ Push the tympanic membrane ⇓ But ossicles are fixed Hence this increased pressure is not transmitted further ⇓ Hence no ↓ in hearing (i.e. test is negative)

 Note: Gelles test will also be negative in case of ossicular discontinuity.

15. Ans. is b i.e. Normal tympanum   *Ref. Dhingra 5/e, p 97, 98; 6/e, p 87; Current Otolaryngology 2/e, p 673,674; 3/e, p 689, 90*
Already explained

16. Ans. is b i.e. 2 kHz

17. Ans. is d i.e. Otosclerosis   *Ref. Dhingra 5/e, p 98; 6/e, p 87; Scott's Brown 7/e, vol-3 p 3461, 3462*

Carhart's notch
- Bone conduction is normal in otosclerosis.
- In some cases there is a dip in bone conduction curve which is maximum at 2000 Hz/2 KHz called as Carharts notch.
- Carhart's notch is seen only in bone conduction curve.
- It disappears after successful stapedectomy/stapedotomy.

Extra Edge
- The reason why it disappears after successful surgery is that when the skull is vibrated by bone—conduction sound, the sound is detected by the cochlea via 3 routes:
  – Route (a)—is by direct vibration within the skull.
  – Route (b)—is by vibration of the ossicular chain which is suspended within the skull.
  – Route (c)—is by vibrations emanating into the external auditory canal as sound and being heard by the normal air-conduction route.
- In a conduction type of hearing loss (as in otosclerosis) the latter two routes are deficient but regained by successful reconstruction surgery. Hence, bone conduction thresholds improve following surgery.

ALSO KNOW
- Dip in noise induced hearing loss is seen at 4 KHz.
- In noise induced hearing loss—Dip is seen in both air and bone conduction curves.
- Trough shaped audiogram is seen in congenital SNHL.
- Flat audiogram with moderate to severes SNHL is characteristic of presbycusis.

18. Ans. is b i.e. Noise induced hearing loss.
In the audiogram—a dip is seen at 4000 Hz which is characteristic of noised induced hearing loss.

19. Ans. is b i.e. 4000 Hz   *Ref. Dhingra 5/e, p 40; 6/e, p 35; Tuli 1/e, p 115*
Acoustic dip is dip seen in pure tone audiometry due to noise trauma, which is seen typically at 4 kHz i.e. 4000 Hz.

20. Ans. is b i.e. As curve   *Ref. Dhingra 5/e, p 97-99; 6/e, p 87, 88; Current Otolaryngology 2/e, p 677; 3/e, p 691*

Lady presenting with hearing loss
+
Bilateral in nature
+
Which worsens during pregnancy

Leaves no confusion—for otosclerosis being the diagnosis.
In otosclerosis—impedance audiometry shows as type of curve.

Note: In the early disease since middle ear aeration is not affected patient shows Type A curve.

21. **Ans. is b and c i.e. Sensorineural deafness; and Irreversible loss of hearing**
    Ref. Dhingra 5/e, p 97-99; 6/e, p 88, 89; Current Otolaryngology 2/e, p 673, 674; 3/e, p 689-691
    - In otosclerosis—50% cases have positive family history.
    - Females are affected more than males.
    - Bilateral conductive deafness seen in otosclerosis is not irreversible as it can be successfully treated by stapedectomy/Stapedotomy.
    - Sensorineural hearing loss occurs when later in the course of time osteosclerotic focus reaches the cochlear endosteum but actually most common hearing loss seen is conductive type.^{Q}
    - Carharts notch is seen in bone conduction curve at 2000 Hz.

22. **Ans. is b i.e. Positive Rinne's test**   *Ref. Dhingra 5/e, p 98, 99; 6/e, p 87, 88; Current Otolaryngology 2/e, p 675-677*
    You are aware of all options given in Question.
    Just remember: The following otoscopic findings in otosclerosis.

    > **Remember**
    > - Tympanic membrane is normal and mobile in 90% cases. (i.e. option d is correct).
    > - Schwartz sign—Flammingo cases pink colour of tympanic membrane is seen in 10% cases. It indicates active focus with increased vascularity.
    > - Stapes footplate—Shows a rice grain/biscuit type appearance
    > - Blue mantles are seen histopathologically.

23. **Ans. is a i.e. Otosclerosis**   *Ref. Dhingra 4/e, p 86, 87; 6/e, p 86, 87; 5/e, p 97-99*

    30 years female
    +
    Bilateral slowly progressive hearing loss
    +
    Positive family history
    +
    Loss apparent during pregnancy
    +
    Cahart's notch at 2000 Hz

    All these leave no doubt about otosclerosis being the diagnosis.

    > **Remember**
    > Otosclerosis is the most common cause of B/L progressive conductive hearing loss in adults.

24. **Ans. is c i.e. Fluorides**
25. **Ans. is a i.e. It inhibits osteoblastic activity**   *Ref. Current Otolaryngology 2/e, p 677; 3/e, p 693; Tuli 1/e, p 81, 82, Otosclerosis and Stapectomy, Diagnosis, Management and Treatment by Gasscocck 1/e, p 61, 62*

    The most useful medication which prevents rapid progression of cochlear otosclerosis is **sodium fluoride**.

    Mechanism of Action
    - It reduces osteoclastic bone resorption and increases osteoblastic bone formation, which promote recalcification and reduce bone remodelling in actively expanding osteolytic lesion.
    - It also inhibits proteolytic enzymes that are cytotoxic to cochlea and lead to SNHL (Hence specially useful in cochlear otosclerosis).
    "Fluoride therapy has been found to significantly arrest the progression of SNHL in the low and high frequencies"
    Ref. Current Otolaryngology 2/e, p 678
    "Sodium fluoride therapy has a role in helping maturity of active focus to arrest cochlear loss"   *Ref. Tuli 1/e, p 82*

26. **Ans. is d i.e. Gentamcin**   *Ref. Dhingra 5/e, p 99; Current Otolaryngology 2/e, p 678, 679*

    Bilateral conductive hearing loss
    +
    Normal tympanic membrane   — Suggest otosclerosis as the diagnosis
    +
    As type of impedance auditometry curve

    Gentamicin is used to treat Meniere's disease. Rest all options are managements for otosclerosis.

Chapter 9: Otosclerosis

27. **Ans. is a, b and c i.e. Stapedectomy, Fenestration and Stapedotomy**

    Ref: Scotts Brown 7/e, vol-3, p 3468 onwards; Current Olotaryngology 2/e, p 678-680

    See text for explanation.

28. **Ans. is a i.e. Teflon piston**   *Ref: Current Otolaryngology 2/e, p 679; Tuli 1/e, p 82; Scotts Brown 7/e, vol-3, p 3479*

    The currently used prosthesis in otosclerosis surgery are:

    - Teflon (M/C used) ⎫
    - Stainless steel   ⎪
    - Platinum   ⎬ All are MRI compatible
    - Gold   ⎪
    - Titanium   ⎭

    The prosthesis is placed between the long process of incus and foot plate of stapes

29. **Ans. d. Lenticular process of incus**   *Ref. Dhingra 5/e, p 100; http://www.audiology.org/news/stapedotomy-versus-stapedectomy#sthash. vipYHiG3.dpuf*

    Lenticular process of incus is not resected in stapedotomy.

    > "A limited opening/hole within the central footplate of the stapes (accomplished via laser or manually with a drill) is referred to as "stapedotomy." Manual footplate perforation is preferred over laser, based on consistent availability of equipment. Fisch advocates leaving the lenticular process (the articulation point between the stapes and the incus) intact during surgery as the prosthesis can be perfectly molded around the incus."-http://www.audiology.org/news/stapedotomy-versus-stapedectomy#sthas. vipYHiG3.dpuf

Chapter 10

Facial Nerve and its Lesions

FACIAL NERVE

- It is the nerve of second brachial arch.
- It is a mixed nerve and has both Motor and sensory components.

Motor component	Sensory component
Supplies the muscles of facial expression (except levator palpebral superioris) and muscles of the 2nd pharyngeal arch	Secretomotor to submandibular, sublingual, salivary and lacrimal glands carries taste fibers from the anterior 2/3rd of the tongue and palate and general somatic sensations from the retroauricular skin

Functional Components and Nuclei of Facial Nerve

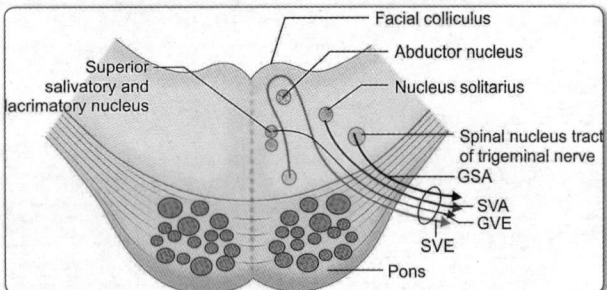

SVE: Special visceral efferent
GVE: General visceral efferent
SVA: Special visceral afferent
GSA: Genral somatic afferent

Component	Origin	Exit from skull	Function
General somatic afferent	Geniculate ganglion	Internal acoustic meatus	Sensation from tympanic membrane and acoustic meatus
Special visceral afferent	Geniculate ganglion	Internal acoustic meatus	Taste from anterior 2/3 of tongue
General visceral efferent	Superior salivatory nucleus	Internal acoustic meatus	Parasympathetic to lacrimal gland and submandibular and salivary gland
Brachial (special nucleus)	Facial nucleus	Internal acoustic meatus	Motor to muscles of facial expression

ALSO KNOW

- At birth facial nerve is located just beneath the skin near the mastoid tip as it emerges from the temporal bone and is vulnerable to the postauricular incision in a young child. As the mastoid tip forms and elongates during childhood, the facial nerve assumes a more medial and protected position.

Course

- **Intracranial part:** From pons to internal autidory meatus (15–20 mm) is intracranial part. The VII nerve after arising from motor nucleus of facial nerve in pons, loops around the abducen nucleus (internal genu), raising facial colliculus (at the floor of fourth ventricle) and exits the brainstem at Ponto-medullary junction to enter the internal auditory meatus.
- **Intratemporal part (longest part):** From internal auditory meatus to stylomastoid foramen. It has 3 subparts as discussed below.
- **Extracranial part:** From stylomastoid foramen to its peripheral branches. At the stylomastoid foramen, the facial nerve passes into parotid gland as a single trunk and then divides into peripheral branches.

Intratemporal part of facial nerve: In the intratemporal part the facial nerve runs through a bony canal (fallopian canal). **The canal is congenitally dehiscent in 50% cases.** The intratemporal has following segments:

- **Meatal segment (8–10 mm):** Within internal acoustic meatus.
- **Labyrinthine segment (4.0 mm):** From meatus to the geniculate ganglion where nerve takes a turn posteriorly forming a "genu" is labyrinthine segment. The labyrinthine segment lies in the inner ear. The nerve in the labyrinthine segment has the narrowest diameter (0.61–0.68 mm) and the bony canal in this segment is also the narrowest. Thus edema or inflammation can easily compress the nerve and cause paralysis. This is also the shortest segment of the nerve.
- **Tympanic or horizontal segment (11.0 mm):** From geniculate ganglion to just above the pyramidal eminence. The tympanic part lies in the middle ear. It lies above the oval window and below the lateral semicircular canal.
- **Mastoid or vertical segment (13.0 mm):** From the pyramid to stylomastoid foramen. Between the tympanic and mastoid segments is the second genu of the nerve.

Chapter 10: Facial Nerve and its Lesions

Table 10.1: Branches of facial nerve

In the Fallopian canal/Intratemporal branches	At its exit from stylomastoid foramen	Communicating branches

Note: From the lateral end of the internal auditory canal to its exit out the stylomastoid foramen, the nerve travels ~3 cm within the fallopian tube.
 	
I. **Greater superficial petrosal nerve** (It arises from geniculate ganglion)
• It joins with deep petrosal nerve to form vidian nerve^q (nerve of pterygoid canal) which supplies:
  – Lacrimal gland
  – Nasal gland
  – Palate gland
  – Pharynx gland
II. **Nerves to stapedius** - arises at the level of 2nd genu (at the level of pyramid) supplies the stapedius muscle. Its injury leads to hyperacusis.
III. **Chorda Tympani** (It arises from the vertical/descending segment of the facial nerve, 4–6 mm above the sylomastoid foramen. As it arises from the facial nerve it makes a 30° angle and delineates a triangular space k/a facial recess.)
• It is the terminal branch of nerves intermedius.
• Enters the tympanic cavity through the posterior canaliculus and exits through the petrotympanic fissure (Canal of Huguier).
• Carries taste fibers from the Anterior 2/3 of the tongue and also supplies secretomotor fibers to submandibular and sublingual glands.
	I. **Posterior auricular nerve:** Supplies posterior auricular muscle, occipital belly of occipitofrontalis along with muscular branches to stylohyoid and posterior belly of digastric	Terminal branches:
		I. **Temporal** (innervate eyebrows and allows for voluntary raising of eye-brows.
		II. **Zygomatic** (innervates orbicularis occuli muscles and is critical for proper eye closure)
		III. **Buccal** (Innervate buccinator and orbicularis oris allowing for proper mouth closure)
		IV. **Mandibular** (innervates platysma)
		V. **Cervical** All terminal branches supply the muscle of face and neck.

NEW PATTERN QUESTIONS

Q N1. Nerve of Wrisberg is:
  a. Sensory part of facial nerve
  b. Motor part of facial nerve
  c. Branch of trigeminal nerve
  d. Branch of vestibular nerve

Q N2. The longest part of facial nerve is:
  a. Intracranial   b. Intratemporal
  c. Extracranial   d. Labyrinthine

Q N3. Facial nerve lies in .... part of Internal Acoustic meatus:
  a. Anterosuperior part
  b. Posterosuperior part
  c. Anteroinferior part
  d. Posteroinferior part

Q N4. Most common segment of facial nerve involved in Bell's Palsy:
  a. Meatal segment
  b. Labyrinthine segment
  c. Horizontal segment
  d. Vertical segment

Q N5. Most common site for congenital dehiscence of fallopian canal:
  a. Meatal segment
  b. Labyrinthine segment
  c. Horizontal segment
  d. Vertical segment

Q N6. Greater superficial petrosal nerve arises from:
  a. Meatal segment
  b. Labyrinthine segment
  c. Horizontal segment
  d. Vertical segment

Q N7. Processus cochleariformis is related to which segment of facial nerve:
  a. Meatal segment   b. Labyrinthine segment
  c. Horizontal segment   d. Vertical segment

Branches of Facial Nerve (see Table 10.1)
Electrodiagnostic Tests to Predict Prognosis in Facial Palsy

- **Electrophysiogical testing:** Includes *electroneuronography, maximal stimulation test,* and *electromyography.*
- These assess the percentage of nerve fibers that have undergone degeneration along with signs of recovery. This is diagnostic as well as prognostic, e.g. in Bell's palsy there is maximum degeneration within the 1st 10 days after which there is recovery. Hence, if degeneration persists beyond 10 days, Bell's palsy is unlikely and it carries a poor prognosis. Hence, electrophysiological testing should be done in those cases of suspected Bell's palsy not responding to steroids.
- This also predicts the feasibility of surgical decompression of facial nerve.

Point to Remember

Site of Injury of Facial Nerve

➤ We have read about the branches of facial nerve and their site of origin. So we can easily make out the site of injury from the symptoms of the patient. First see the major symptoms of facial nerve palsy.
  i. **Loss of lacrimation:** Due to involvement of greater superficial petrosal nerve.
  ii. **Loss of stapedial reflex:** Due to involvement of nerve to stapedius.
  iii. **Lack of salivation:** Due to chordatymapani
  iv. **Loss of taste sensation from Anterior 2/3 of tongue:** Due to chorda tympani.
  v. **Paralysis of muscle of facial expression:** Due to terminal (peripheral) branches.

➤ Now we can make out the site of injury:
  1. **All the 5 symptoms (i to v) are present:** Injury is at or proximal to geniculate ganglion (as all the branches of facial nerve are involved).
  2. **There is no loss of lacrimation (greater superficial petrosal nerve is spared) but symptoms (ii to v are seen)** i.e. stapedial reflex is present: Injury is distal to geniculate ganglion (as there is no loss of lacrimation) but proximal to 2nd genu or pyramid.
  3. If stapedial reflex is present but there is loss of taste sensation from anterior 2/3 of tongue. It means Nerve to stapedius is spared i.e. lesion is distal to 2nd genu (or pyramed) but proximal to orign of chorda tympani.
  4. **Only (vth) symptom is present:** Injury is distal to the origin of chorda tympani, which may be at the level of stylomastoid foramen.

NEW PATTERN QUESTION

Q N8. A patient following injury presents with normal Schirmer test but stapedial reflex is absent on right side. The approximate site of injury of facial nerve is:

a. Intrameatal part   b. Horizontal part
c. Vertical part   d. At stylomastoid foramen

Presentation of Facial Nerve Paralysis

Facial nerve paralysis produces following manifestations:
- Weakness of the muscle of the facial expression and eye closure, which results in:
  i. *Absence of nasolabial fold*
  ii. Epiphora
  iii. Wide palpable fissure
  iv. Voluntary eye closure may not be possible and can produce damage to the conjunctiva and cornea
  v. *Loss of wrinkles of forehead*
  vi. *The face sags and is drawn across to the opposite side on smiling*
  vii. Drooping of angle of mouth.

Concept of Nuclear, Supranuclear, and Infranuclear Facial Nerve Paralysis

The motor nucleus of the facial nerve is located in pons. Facial nerve paralysis occurring due to injury or disease of the facial nucleus is termed as **nuclear paralysis (lower motor neuron type paralysis)**.

The motor nucleus is innervated by corticonuclear fibers **(supranuclear fibers or upper motor neuron fibers)** arising from the contralateral cerebral cortex. A lesion anywhere in the course of upper motor neuron fibers is **supranuclear facial paralysis (upper motor neuron type paralysis)**.

Note: Although the motor nucleus of the facial nerve receives supranuclear fibers arising from the contralateral cerebral cortex; however, a part of the motor nerve nucleus of the facial nerve is innervated by the cortical fibers from the ipsilateral side also. This means a part of the nucleus is bilaterally innervated.

The efferent fibers arising from the facial nerve nucleus are referred to as 'infranuclear' fibers or lower motor neuron fibers. These fibers innervate all facial muscles supplied by the facial nerve. Facial nerve paralysis occurring due to injury or disease of the infranuclear fibers is termed as **infranuclear facial nerve paralysis (lower motor neuron type paralysis)**.

Clinical Correlation

The part of motor nucleus of facial nerve supplying the muscles of the lower part of the face receives the corticonuclear fibers from the opposite cerebral hemisphere, while the part of motor nucleus of facial nerve, which supplies the muscles of the upper part of the face receives corticonuclear fibers from both cerebral hemispheres. As a result in supranuclear lesions (i.e. lesions involving the upper motor neurons) of the facial nerve, the upper half of the face on both sides is spared and the lower half of the face is affected on the opposite side. On the other hand, in nuclear and infranuclear lesions, i.e. lower motor neuron lesions, whole of the face is affected on the side of lesion (Fig. 10.1).

Infranuclear Lesion (Lower Motor Neuron Lesion)

Point to Remember

In Lower Motor Neuron (LMN) Facial Paralysis

➤ *All muscles of the face* are involved on the side of lesion (*Ipsilateral side*)

In the infranuclear paralysis, the nerve is affected near the stylomastoid foramen. Facial muscles can also be paralyzed by interruption of corticonuclear fibers running from the motor cortex to the facial nucleus. This is referred to as supranuclear paralysis.

The effects of paralysis are due to the failure of the muscles concerned to perform their normal actions. Some effects are as follows:
- The normal face is more or less symmetrical. When the facial nerve is paralyzed on one side, the most noticeable feature is the **loss of symmetry**

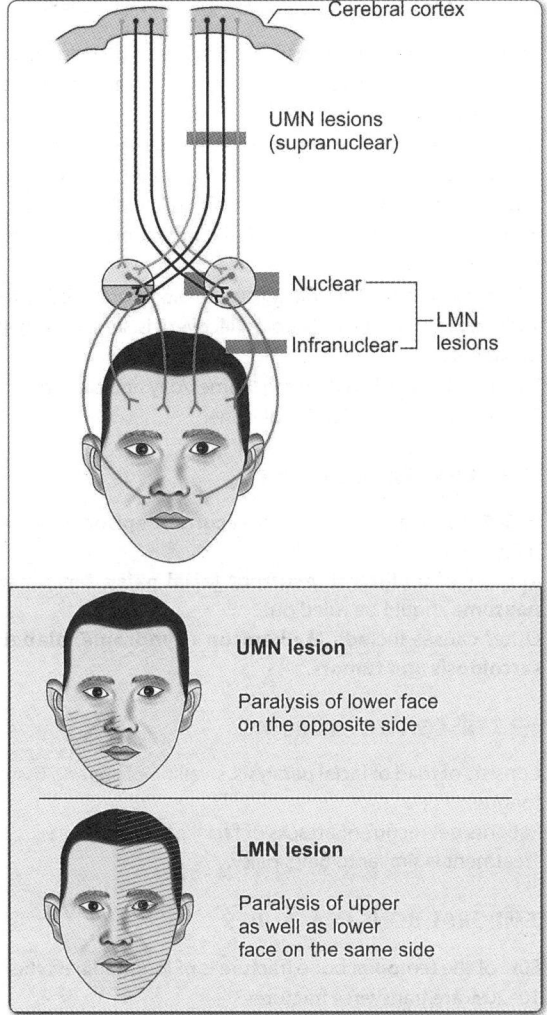

Fig. 10.1: Facial nerve palsy

- **Normal furrows on the forehead are lost** because of paralysis of the occipitofrontalis
- **There is drooping of the eyelid**, and **the palpebral fissure is wider on the paralyzed side**, because of paralysis of the orbicularis oculi. The conjunctival reflex is lost for the same reason
- There is **marked asymmetry of the mouth**, because of paralysis of the orbicularis oris and of muscles inserted into the angle of the mouth. This is most obvious when a smile is attempted. As a result of asymmetry, the protruded tongue appears to deviate to one side but is, in fact, in the midline
- During mastication, **food tends to accumulate between the cheek and the teeth**. This is normally prevented by the buccinator.

Additional effects are observed in injuries to the facial nerve at levels higher than the stylomastoid foramen, as follows:

- If the injury is proximal to the origin of the chorda tympani, there is loss of sensation of taste on the anterior two-thirds of the tongue

- The transmission of loud sounds to the internal ear is normally dampened by the stapedius muscle. When the lesion is proximal to the origin of the branch to the stapedius, this muscle is paralyzed. As a result, even normal sounds appear too loud (**hyperacusis**)
- In fractures of the temporal bone or in lesions near the exit of the nerve from the brain, the vestibulocochlear nerve may also be affected (**leading to deafness**).
- Site of lesion in lower motor paralysis may be:
  i. **Supratemporal:** Lesion is proximal to the bony canal, which may be:
     a. **At the level of nucleus:** There is associated VI nerve involvement
     b. **At the cerebellopontine angle:** There is associated vestibular and auditory defects and other cranial nerve involvement Vth, IXth, Xth, XIth.
  ii. **Intratemporal:** Lesion is in the bony canal, from internal acoustic meatus to stylomastoid foramen.
- The side can be localized by **topodiagnostic tests:**

Topodiagnostic Tests for Intratemporal Lesion

- **Schirmer's test (for lacrimation):** Decreased lacrimation when lesion is at or proximal to geniculate ganglion.
- **Stapedial reflex:** Lost if lesion is proximal to the nerve to stapedius.
- **Taste test:** Impaired taste when lesion is proximal to chorda tympani.
- **Submandibular salivary flow test:** Impaired when lesion is proximal to chorda tympani.

  iii. **Infratemporal:** Lesion is outside the temporal bone in the parotid area. *Only the motor functions of nerve are affected.*
- Test for identifying whether the patient has *upper motor neuron (UMN) or lower motor neuron (LMN)*
  – In an LMN lesion, the patient cannot wrinkle their forehead, i.e. the final common pathway to the muscle is destroyed. Lesion must either in the pons, or outside brainstem (posterior fossa, bony canal, middle ear or outside skull).
  – In a UMN lesion, the upper facial muscles are spared because of alterntive pathways in the brainstem, i.e. the patient can wrinkle their forehead (unless there is bilateral lesion) and the sagging of the face seen with LMN palsies is not as prominent.

Electrophysiological Tests

  – These tests are useful in knowing the severity and prognosis of facial nerve injury
- These include:

Electroneurography (ENoG)

In this evoked electroneurography, the facial nerve is stimulated and the compound action potentials (amplitudes of the summation potentials) from the facial muscles are recorded and measured objectively. Supramaximal level of current is applied over the main trunk of facial nerve. The readings are compared with the normal side.

The peak-to-peak amplitude is directly proportional to the number of intact motor axons. So the test assesses extent of neuronal degeneration. The response of paralyzed side is reported

as a percentage of response on normal side, thus telling the proportion of fibers that have degenerated.
- **Interpretation:** Fall of summating potential to 10% of the normal value is an indication (90% degeneration) for the surgical decompression.
- **Limitation:** It must be done within 2 week of the onset of palsy.

Electromyography (EMG)
It records spontaneous activity of facial muscles at rest and on voluntary contraction. Electrode is directly inserted in to the muscle.

Interpretations
- **Normal:** At rest, normal muscle does not show any electrical activity. On voluntary contraction, normal volitional motor unit potentials are observed.
- **Denervated muscle:** Fibrillation potentials appear within 14–21 days after denervation.
- **Earliest signs of recovery:** Reinnervation potentials can be seen much before (up to 12 weeks) any visible facial movement.

BELL'S PALSY
- Commonest cause of acute onset LMN facial palsy.
- M/c type of infranuclear paralysis
- Sudden in onset
- It is unilateral
- Was thought to be idiopathic, but there are recent evidences indicating Herpes simplex virus as the causative agent.
- H/O viral prodromal symptoms
- Rapidly progresses within 1st 10 days put complete recovery is a rule.
- Facial muscles on one side are paralyzed.
  a. Inability to close eye.
  b. On attempting to close eye, eyeball turns up and out–*Bell's phenomenon*.
- Ipsilateral loss of salivation and lacrimation.
- Hyperacusis is present.
- Taste may be affected.
- Ear and other CNS functions are normal.
- Recurrences both ipsilateral and contralateral occur in up to 12% patients.

Treatment
Conservative:
- **Steroids:** Prednisolone (1 mg/kg/days × 10 days and then taper for next 5 days)
- **Acyclovir:** Adults: 200–400 mg five times/ day
- **Care of the eye**
- Physiotherapy
- Vitamin B1, B6 and B12 combinations.

Surgery (Nerve decompression): It relieves pressure on the nerve fibers and improves microcirculation. *Done if medical therapy fails and there is no recovery in 8–12 weeks.*

> **Point to Remember**
> **Prerequisites for Surgery**
> **BAD syndrome:**
> ➢ Lack of **B**ell's phenomenon
> ➢ Corneal **a**nesthesia
> ➢ **D**ry eyes

HERPES ZOSTER OTICUS/RAMSAY HUNT SYNDROME
- Reactivation of dormant herpes zoster virus in the geniculate ganglion of facial nerve and spiral and vestibular ganglion VIIIth nerve leads to Ramsay Hunt syndrome.
- It is characterized by vesicles around the external ear canal, pinna, and soft palate sensorineural hearing loss and vertigo due to involvement of VIIIth nerve along with ipsilateral facial palsy.
- Besides VIIth nerve it can involve other cranial nerves viz. V, VIII, IX and Xth nerve.
- In comparison to Bell's palsy, progression begins by 11th to 14th day but prognosis is poor. Recovery is seen only in 40% of patients.
- Treatment is acyclovir 800 mg 5 times/day and steroids.
- Surgical decompression is not done.

RECURRENT FACIAL PALSY
- **In 3–10% cases** of Bell's palsy, **recurrent episodes of facial palsy** occur.
- In cases of **unilateral recurrent facial palsy, facial nerve neuroma** should be ruled out.
- Other causes include **Melkersson's syndrome, diabetes, sarcoidosis and tumors.**

MELKERSSON'S SYNDROME
- Consists of triad of facial paralysis, swelling of lips and fissured tongue.
- Patients get recurrent attacks of facial palsy.
- Treatment is similar to Bell's palsy.

TEMPORAL BONE FRACTURES
- 80% of the temporal bone fracture is of longitudinal type^Q.
- 10–20% are transverse fractures^Q.
- 40–50% of the transverse fractures cause facial nerve injury^Q.
- Facial nerve involvement is rare with longitudinal fracture^Q.
  Temporal bone fracture: Clinical features include hearing loss, dizziness, facial weakness, ear bleeding, hemotympanum, raccoon eyes, and/or **bruising over the mastoid cortex (Battle's sign).**
- Radiological investigation: The best radiologic examination is a temporal bone CT scan (HRCT).

Indications for surgical exploration of the facial nerve:
- Immediate onset of complete facial paralysis.
- Delayed onset of complete facial paralysis associated with:
  – Radiologic evidence of a fracture through the Fallopian canal of facial nerve.
  – Poor prognostic testing with electroneuronography or electromyography.

NEW PATTERN QUESTION
Q N9. IOC to detect temporal bone fracture is:
  a. MRI   b. HRCT
  c. X-ray   d. PET scan

IATROGENIC OR SURGICAL TRAUMA

Parotid surgery during tympanoplasty or mastoid surgery. The paralysis may be immediate (needs earliest surgical decompression and repair) or delayed (treated conservatively). The exposed nerve may be pressed by the pressure on ear packing. This just needs removal or ear pack.

SURGICAL TREATMENT OF FACIAL NERVE PALSY

- **Decompression:** The facial nerve is compressed by intraneural edema, hematoma and a fractured bone in the Fallopian canal. The compressed nerve is exposed in surgical decompression. The facial nerve sheath is slit to relieve pressure.

  When electrical tests indicate progressive nerve weakness (> 90%) facial nerve decompression should be done at the earliest in cases of Bell's palsy, Ramsay Hunt syndrome and longitudinal temporal bone fracture.
- **End-to-end anastomosis:** It is a suitable procedure for extratemporal part of facial nerve. The gap between the severed ends of nerves are few millimeters. The two ends should be approximated without any tension. A 9/0 or 10/0 monofilament suture is used to tie the nerve ends.
- **Nerve graft (cable graft):** It is indicated when the gap between severed ends is more and cannot be closed without tension by end-to-end anastomosis. **Nerve graft is usually taken from greater auricular nerve, lateral cutaneous nerve of thigh or the sural nerve.** In the Fallopian canal, graft may not need any suturing.
- **Hypoglossal-facial anastomosis:** It is indicated when proximal facial nerve stump cannot be identified. Anastomosis of hypoglossal nerve to the severed peripheral end of the facial nerve improves the muscle tone and permits some movements of facial muscles.
- **Plastic procedures:** The procedures such as facial slings, face lift operation, slings of masseter and temporalis muscle, improve cosmetic appearance in cases where nerve grafting is not possible or has failed.

NEW PATTERN QUESTION

Q N10. All of the following nerve grafts can be used in facial nerve injury except:
a. Greater auricular N
b. Sural N
c. Lateral cutaneous N of thigh
d. Occipital N

IMPORTANT CLINICAL CONCEPTS FOR NEET

1. Total length of facial nerve is 60–70 mm.
   - Intracranial segment : 15–20 mm
   - Meatal segment : 8–10 mm
   - Labyrinthine segment : 3–5 mm
   - Tympanic segment : 8–10 mm
   - Mastoid segment : 15–20 mm
   - Extratemporal segment : 15–20 mm
2. Vidian nerve[Q] is formed by greater superficial petrosal nerve joining deep petrosal nerve (sympathetic) for supplying the lacrimal glands, mucous glands of nose, palate and pharynx[Q].
3. M/c tumor of facial nerve is Schwannoma.
4. Schirmer's test, taste sensation or salivation test give information about the probable site of lesion in facial nerve injury.
5. Crocodile tears[Q] while eating are due to misdirection of secretomotor impulses meant for salivary gland and are treated by tympanic neurectomy.
6. Melkersson's syndrome[Q] is characterized by recurrent facial nerve palsy, swelling of lips and furrowing of tongue.
7. Heerfordt's syndrome[Q]: There is bilateral parotid enlargement with uveitis and transient facial palsy due to sarcoidosis.
8. Bannwarth's syndrome/Lyme's disease: There is rash, fever, myalgias, arthralgia, pharyngitis and lymphadenopathy with facial nerve palsy. It is due to spirochaetes infection.
9. Genu of facial nerve: The sharp turns made by facial nerve is called as genu. 1st genu is thickened to form the geniculate ganglion, surface landmark being processus cochleariformis. Surface landmark for 2nd genu is horizontal semicircular canal. Tympanomastoid suture line is the landmark for descending portion. These landmarks are used in mastoid surgery. 1st genu is the commonest site of injury to facial nerve in trauma, while 2nd genu is the commonest site of injury to facial neve in mastoid surgery.
10. Facial nerve palsy at stylomastoid foramen causes deviation of angle of mouth to opposite side (due to paralyses of muscles of facial expression) and absence of corneal reflex.
11. Causes of B/L facial palsy: Guillian-Barre Syndrome, infectious mononucleosis, amyloidosis, Sarcoidosis, Skull trauma, acute porphyria, Lyme's disease and botulism.

Explanations and References to New Pattern Questions

N1. Ans. is a i.e. Sensory part of facial nerve *Ref. Dhingra 6/e, p 90*

Nervus intermedius (nerve of Wrisberg) is the part of facial nerve located between motor component of facial nerve and vestibulo-cochlear (VIII) nerve. On reaching facial canal it joins the motor root of facial nerve at geniculate ganglion. It caries fibers for taste, salivation lacrimation and general sensation from external ear, i.e. it is sensory in nature.

N2. Ans. is b i.e. Intratemporal *Ref. Dhingra 6/e, p 60*

See the text for explanation.

N3. Ans. is a i.e. Anterosuperior part *Ref. Essentials of ENT Mohan Bansal, p 165)*

Internal Auditory Canal (See 1.17 of chapter 1)
- Anterosuperior quadrant – Facial Nerve
- Posterosuperior quadrant – superior vestibular
- The two being separated by bills bar nerve.
- Anteroinferior quadrant – cochlear nerve
- Posteroinferior quadrant – Inferior vestibular nerve

N4. Ans. is b i.e. Labyrinthine segment *Ref. Essential of ENT Mohan Bansal, p 149*

The bony fallopian canal in the labyrinthine segment is narrowest and more prone to compression in Bells palsy.

N5. Ans. is c i.e. Horizontal segment *Ref. Essential of ENT Mohan Bansal pg 149: Dhingra 6/e, p 91*

The tympanic part or horizontal part of the facial nerve above the oval window is the M/c site for congenital dehiscence (15–30%). Other sites: being geniculate ganglion and retrofacial mastoid air cells region.

N6. Ans. is c i.e. Horizontal segment *Ref. Essentials of ENT Mohan Bansal, p 149*

Segment of Facial Nerve	Branches
1. Meatal segment	No branch
2. Labyrinthine segment	No branch
3. Horizontal/tympanic segment	Greater superficial petrosal nerve (1st Branch of facial nerve arising from geniculate ganglion)
4. Vertical/mastoid segment	Nerve to stapedius (from the second genu or at the level of praymid) Nerve to chorda tympani

N7. Ans. is c i.e. Horizontal segment *Ref. Essentials of ENT Mohan Bansal, p 150*

Surgical landmarks of facial nerve	
Landmark	Indicates
1. Processes cochleaformis	Beginning of horizontal segment (Trympanic segment) of facial nerve.
2. Oval window and horizontal semicircular canal	Horizontal segment of facial nerve is situated above the oval window and below the horizontal semicircular canal.
3. Short process of incus, pyramid and tympano mastoid suture	Related to vertical segment of facial nerve

N8. Ans. is b i.e. Horizontal part

Schirmer Test: Compares lacrimation of the two sides. Lacrimation is brought about by greater superficial petrosal nerve since it supplies the lacrimal gland.

Hence Schirmer test, tests the function of greater superficial petrosal nerve. If in the patient Schirmer test is normal i.e. greater superficial petrosal nerve is not injured.

Greater superficial petrosal nerve arises from geniculate ganglion. Hence it means the site of lesion is distal to geniculate ganglion. The question further says stapedial reflex is absent.

For stapedial reflex–nerve to stapedius is responsible. If stapedial reflex is absent it means nerve to spadiceus is injured. Nerve to stapedius arises at the level of 2nd genu from pyramid. Hence the lesion should be proximal to it

Thus lesion is occurring in the part beyond geniculate ganglion but before the pyramid, i.e. horizontal part (tympanic part).

Chapter 10: Facial Nerve and its Lesions

N9. Ans. is b i.e. HRCT *Ref. Essential of ENT Mohan Bansal, p 156*

Read the text for explanation.

N10. Ans. is d i.e. Occipital N *Ref. Essential of Mohan Bansal, p 158*

Nerve grafts for facial nerves
1. Greater auricular N (M/c used)
2. Lateral cutaneous N of thigh
3. Sural nerve.

QUESTIONS

BRANCHES AND SITE OF LESION

1. **First branch of the facial nerve is:** [UP. 2004]
   a. Greater petrosal nerve b. Lesser petrosal nerve
   c. Chorda-tympani nerve   d. Nerve to the stapedius

2. **All the following muscles are innervated by the facial nerve except:** [AIIMS May 03]
   a. Occipito-frontalis   b. Anterior belly of digastric
   c. Risorius   d. Procerus

3. **Lacrimation is affected when facial nerve injury is at:** [AI 98]
   a. Geniculate ganglion
   b. In semicirculalr canal
   c. At sphenopalatine gangila
   d. At foramen spinosum

4. **A patient presents with hyperacusis, loss of lacrimation and loss of taste sensation in the anterior 2/3rd of the tongue. Edema extends up to which level of facial nerve:** [2001]
   a. Vertical part
   b. Vertical part beyond nerve to stapedius
   c. Vertical part and beyond nerve to stapedius
   d. Proximal to geniculate ganglion

5. **Dryness of eye is caused by injury to facial nerve at:** [AI 96]
   a. Chorda tympani
   b. Cerebellopontine angle
   c. Tympanic canal
   d. Geniculate ganglion

6. **Hyperacusis in Bell's palsy is due to the paralysis of the follwing muscle:** [AIIMS May 06]
   a. Tensor tympani   b. Levator palatii
   c. Tensor veli palatii d. Stapedius

7. **Intratemporal lesion of chorda tympani nerve results in:** [AIIMS Dec. 94]
   a. Loss of taste sensations from papilla of tongue
   b. Loss of taste sensations from anterior 2/3rd of tongue
   c. Loss of taste sensations from posterior 1/3rd of tongue
   d. Loss of secretomotor fibers to the submandibular salivary gland

8. **Dryness of mouth with facial nerve injury – site of lesion is at:** [UP 2008]
   a. Chorda tympani nerve
   b. Cerebellopontine angle
   c. Geniculate ganglion
   d. Concussion of Tympanic membrane

9. **Facial nerve palsy at sternomastoid canal can cause:** [AIIMS June 99]
   a. Loss of corneal reflex at site of lesion
   b. Loss of corneal taste sensation anterior 2/3 of ipsilateral tongue
   c. Loss of lacrimation at site of lesion
   d. Hyperacusis

CLINICAL FEATURES

10. **Right upper motor neuron lesion of facial nerve causes:** [AIIMS 95]
    a. Loss of taste sensation in right anterior part tongue
    b. Loss of corneal reflex right side
    c. Loss of wrinkling of forehead left side
    d. Paralysis of lower facial muscles left side

11. **Which one of the following statements is correct in facial paralysis?** [MP 2009]
    a. The nasolabial fold is obliterated on the same side
    b. The nasolabial fold is obliterated on the opposite side
    c. The face deviates to the same side
    d. The face deviates to the opposite side

12. **Which test can detect facial nerve palsy occurring due to lesion at the outlet of stylomastoid:** [AIIMS Nov. 93]
    a. Deviation of angle of mouth towards opposite side
    b. Loss of taste sensation in anterior 2/3 of tongue
    c. Loss of sensation over right cheek
    d. Deviation of tongue towards opposite side

13. **Crocodile tears is due to:** (Delhi 2005)
    a. Cross innervation of facial nerve fibers
    b. Cross innervation of trigeminal nerve fibers
    c. Improper regeneration of trigeminal nerve
    d. Improper regeneration of facial nerve

CAUSES OF FACIAL PALSY

14. **Iatrogenic traumatic facial nerve palsy is most commonly caused during:**
    a. Myringoplasty   b. Stapedectomy
    c. Mastoidectomy   d. Ossiculoplasty

15. **Which fracture of the petrous bone will cause facial nerve palsy:** [AI 07]
    a. Longitudinal fractures
    b. Transverse fractures
    c. Mastoid
    d. Facial nerve injury is always complete

16. **Facial nerve palsy is seen in this condition:** [JIPMER 03]
    a. Seborrheic otitis externa b. Otomycosis
    c. Malignant otitis externa   d. Cerebellar abscess

17. **Which part of the facial nerve is commonly exposed through natural dehiscence in the fallopian canal?** [2005]
    a. Horizontal part
    b. Upper half of the vertical part
    c. Lower half of the vertical part
    d. Labyrimthine part

18. **Most common cause of facial palsy:**
    a. Post operative   b. Trauma
    c. Ramsay Hunt syndrome d. Bell's palsy

Chapter 10: Facial Nerve and its Lesions

19. Most common cause of lower motor neuron facial palsy is: [MP 2004]
    a. Cholesteatoma
    b. Cerebello-pontine angle tumours
    c. Bell's palsy
    d. Postoperative (ear surgery)

BELL'S PALSY

20. Bell's palsy is paralysis of: [Comed 07]
    a. UMN V nerve
    b. UMN VII nerve
    c. LMN V nerve
    d. LMN VII nerve
21. True regarding Bell's palsy is all except [AIIMS May 2013]
    a. Steroids are used
    b. U/L facial weakness
    c. Role of herpes simplex in etiology
    d. Immediate surgical decompression is required
22. Which of the following is not true about Bell's palsy? [Delhi 2008]
    a. Acute onset
    b. Always recurrent
    c. Spontaneous remission
    d. Increased predisposition in Diabetes Mellitus
23. Which one of the following statements truly represent Bell's paralysis: [AIIMS May 05; AI 04]
    a. Hemiparesis and contralateral facial nerve paralysis
    b. Combined paralysis of the facial, trigeminal, and abducens nerves
    c. Idiopathic ipsilateral paralysis of the facial nerve
    d. Facial nerve paralysis with a dry eye
24. All of the following are seen in Bell's palsy except: [SGPGI 05]
    a. Ipsilateral-facial palsy
    b. Ipsilateral-loss of taste sensation
    c. Hyperacusis
    d. Ipsilateral ptosis
25. True about lower motor neuron palsy of VIIth nerve: [PGI Nov. 05]
    a. Other motor cranial nerves also involves
    b. Melkersson's syndrome cause recurrent paralysis
    c. Eye protection done
    d. Prognosis can be predicted by serial electrical studies
    e. Bell's palsy is commonest cause
26. Bell's palsy patient comes on day 3. Treatment given would be: [AIIMs Nov 09, May 2010]
    a. Intratympanic steroids
    b. Oral steroids + vitamin B
    c. Oral steroids + Acyclovir
    d. Vitamin B Vasodilator
27. A case of Bell's palsy on steroids, shows no improvement after two weeks. Next step in manangement is: [MP2000]
    a. Vasodilators and ACTH
    b. Physiotherapy
    c. ↓ Steroids dose
    d. Electrophysiological nerve testing
28. Evidence based therapy of Bell's palsy include(s): [PGI May 2016]
    a. Facial nerve massage
    b. Facial nerve stimulation
    c. Steroid
    d. Acyclovir
29. Treatment of choice for mastoid fracture with facial nerve palsy is: [AIIMs June 99, Sept 96]
    a. Nerve decompression
    b. High dose of steroid
    c. Sling operation
    d. Repair the fracture and wait and watch
30. A patient presents with facial nerve palsy following head trauma with fracture of the mastoid: best intervention here is: [AI 01]
    a. Immediate decompression
    b. Wait and watch
    c. Facial sling
    d. Steroids

RAMSAY HUNT SYNDROME

31. A man presents with vesicles over external acoustic meatus with ipsilateral facial palsy of LMN type. The cause is: [AP 2005]
    a. Herpes zoster
    b. Herpes simpex virus-I
    c. Varicella
    d. None of the above
32. Ramsay Hunt syndrome is caused by: [PGI Dec. 98]
    a. H. simplex
    b. H. zoster
    c. Influenza
    d. Adenovirus
33. Ramsay Hunt syndrome all are true except: [SGPGI 05]
    a. VII Nerve is involved
    b. Facial muscle are involved
    c. Facial vesicle is seen
    d. Herpes zoster is etiologic agent
34. All of the following are true for Ramsay Hunt syndrome, except: [AI 02]
    a. It has viral etiology
    b. Involves VIIth nerve
    c. May involve VIIIth nerve
    d. Results of spontaneous recovery are excellent
35. True about Ramsay Hunt syndrome except: [UP 2000]
    a. Involves VII nerve
    b. May involves VIII nerve
    c. Surgical removal gives excellent prognosis
    d. Causative agent is virus

OTHERS

36. True about Mobius syndrome: [PGI Nov. 2014]
    a. 10th N involvement
    b. 7th N involvement
    c. Abduction defect
    d. Esotropia
    e. 6th CN involvement

Explanations and References

1. **Ans. is a i.e. Greater petrosal nerve**   *Ref. Dhingara 5/e, pg102, 6/e, p 90; Current Olotaryngology 2/e, p 836*
   - *Greater superficial petrosal nerve:* It is the *first branch and arises from geniculate ganglion (i.e. first genu).* It joins the deep petrosal nerve to form *vidian nerve* (nerve to pterygoid canal) and carries secretomotor fibers to the *lacrimal gland, nasal gland, Palate gland and pharyngeal gland.*

2. **Ans. is b i.e. Anterior belly of digastric**   *Ref. BDC Vol. III 4/e, p 139-140*

   ### Facial Nerve Supplies

Forget	=	**F**acial muscles except levator palpebrae Superioris (Which is supplied by 3rd nerve).
Pediatric (Pd)	=	**P**osterior belly of **D**igastric
Surgery	=	**S**tapedius
Always	=	**A**uricular muscles
Opt For	–	**O**ccipto **F**rontalis
Plastic	–	**P**latysma
Surgery	–	**S**tylohyoid
Mnemonic:		**Forget Pediatric Surgery Always Opt for Plastic Surgery.**

   Note:
   - Anterior belly of digastric is supplied by nerve to mylohyoid.
   - Procerus and Risorius are muscles of face.

3. **Ans. is a i.e. Geniculate ganglion**   *Ref. Dhingra 5/e, p102, 6/e, p 90-91*
   For lacrimation greater superficial petrosal nerve which is a branch of facial nerve is responsible
   It arises from the geniculate ganglion/any lesion occurring at the level of geniculate ganglion will injure this branch and will lead to dryness of eyes.

   ### ALSO KNOW
   For locating the site of injury of facial nerve:
   - First see the major symptoms of facial nerve palsy:
     i. **Loss of lacrimation:** Due to involvement of greater superficial petrosal nerve.
     ii. **Loss of stapedial reflex:** Due to involvement of nerve to stapedius.
     iii. **Lack of salivation:** Due to Chorda tympani.
     iv. **Loss of taste sensation from Anterior 2/3 of tongue:** Due to chorda tympani.
     v. **Paralysis of muscle of facial expression:** Due to terminal (peripheral) branches.
   - Now you can make out the site of injury:
     – **All the 5 symptoms (i to v) are present:** Injury is at or proximal to geniculate ganglion (as all the branches) of facial nerve are involved)
     – **There is no loss of lacrimation (greater petrosal and nerve to stapedius are spread) but symptoms (ii) to (v) occur:** Injury is distal to geniculate ganglion but proximal to or at the level of second genu from where the nerve to stapedius arises.
     – **Only symptoms (iii) to (v) are present (greater petrosal and nerve to stapedius are spread):** Injury distal to second genu but proximal to origin of chorda tympani, i.e., Injury is between Second genu and mid portion of vertical segment.
     – **Only (vth) symptoms is present:** Injury is distal to the origin of chorda tympani, which may be at the level of stylomastoid foramen.

4. **Ans. is d i.e. Proximal to geniculate ganglion**   *Ref. Current Otolaryngology 2/e, p 836-838, 3/e, p 865-67*
   In the question patient is presenting with
   i. Hyperacusis which means nerve to stapedius is involved which arises from the vertical / descending part of facial nerve.
   ii. Loss of lacrimation – i.e. greater superficial petrosal Nerve which arises from geniculate ganglion is involved.
   iii. Loss of taste sensation in anterior 2/3 of tongue – i.e. chorda tympani nerve which arises from vertical/descending part of facial nerve is involved.

   > **Remember**
   > - Any lesion will lead to paralysis of all Nerves distal to it and will spare proximal nerves
   > - Hence – we will have to look for the most proximal lesion which in this case is geniculate ganglion
   > - So lesion is either at or proximal to geniculate ganglion

Chapter 10: Facial Nerve and its Lesions

5. **Ans. is d i.e. Geniculate ganglion**
6. **Ans. is d i.e. Stapedius** *Ref. Tuli 1/e, p87*

   Hyperacusis (Phonophobia) occurs due to undue sensitivity to loud sounds.
   - Stapedius muscle dampens excessive vibrations of the stapes caused by high pitched sounds in order to protect the internal ear.
   - If this protective reflex is not elicited it indicates stapedius paralysis and results in hyperacusis.

Test	Level of lesion of facial nerve palsy
Schimers test of lacrimation (↓ed on paralyzed side)	Geniculate ganglion
Hyperacusis/Phonophobia (undue sensitivity to loud sounds)	Nerve to Stapedius involved
↓ ed taste sensation	Chorda tympani nerve involved
Salivation test (↓ ed salivation on paralyzed side)	Terminal branches-Nerve to submandibular gland involved

7. **Ans. is d i.e. Loss of secretomotor fibers to the submandibular salivary gland**
8. **Ans is a i.e. Chorda tympani nerve.** *Ref. BDC Vol. III 3/e, p113, 127*

   Chorda Tympani Nerve Carries
   - Preganglionic secretomotor fibers to submandibular ganglion
   - Taste fibers from anterior 2/3rd of tongue
   - Responsible for salivary secretion from submandibular & sublingual gland

   So, Ideally a lesion of chorda tympani should impair both these functions but – sensations from ant 2/3rd of tongue are not impaired as an alternate pathway passing through the nerve of pterygoid canal to the otic ganglion exists *(which does not pass through middle ear)* which is preserved in lesions of chorda tympani.
   Any lesion of chorda tympani thus leads to dryness of mouth

9. **Ans. is a i.e. Loss of corneal reflex at the site of lesion** *Ref. Dhingra 5/e, p 102, 6/e, p 90-91*

   Course of Facial Nerve
   - Below stylomastoid formen, facial nerve gives following branches: Posterior auricular branch, muscular branches (stylohyoid and posterior belly of diagastric) and terminal (peripheral) branches.
   - **Lesion at sternomastoid foramen**
     i. **Will spare:**
        - Greater superficial petrosal nerve → Lacrimation present.
        - Nerve to stapedius → Normal stapedial reflex and no hyperacusis.
        - Chorda tympani → Normal salivation and taste sensation in anterior 2/3 of tongue.
     ii. **Will involve:**
        Terminal (peripheral) branches → Paralysis of muscles of facial expression. **Corneal reflex will also be lost** because efferent fibers of corneal reflex are derived from peripheral branches of facial nerve (it is an LMN type lesion).

Remember	
Corneal Reflex:	• **Afferent:** Trigeminal nerve
	• **Efferent:** Peripheral branches of facial nerve

10. **Ans. is d i.e. Paralysis of lower facial muscles left side**
    Ref. Macleods clinical examination 12/e, p 282, Dhingra 5/e, p 105-106

    It is a General Rule that:
    - UMN lesion cause • Contralateral paresis
    - LMN lesion cause • Ipsilateral paresis

    So, right upper motor neuron lesion of facial nerve will lead to paresis / deformity of left side. (Ruling out **options "a"** and **"b"**)

    In Right UMN Palsy
    - Facial muscles of opposite side (left side) will be affected
    - Upper facial (forehead) muscles will be spared
    - So patient will have paralysis of lower facial muscles on contralateral (left) side.

11. **Ans. is a i.e. Nasolabial fold is obliterated on the same side** *Ref. Dhingra 5/e, p 106*
    Always remember: Lower motor neuron type of facial paralysis is much more common than upper motor neuron type. If any question is asked on facial paralysis unless and until it mentions 'UMN type, all paralysis should be taken as LMN type.
    LMN type facial paralysis causes ipsilateral facial paralysis.

Following features are seen in Facial nerve paralysis:
- Loss of wrinkles (on ipsilateral side in LMN type paralysis)
- Wide palpebral fissure (on ipsilateral side)
- Epiphora (on ipsilateral side)
- Absence of nasolabial fold (on ipsilateral side)
- Drooping of angle of mouth (on ipsilateral side)

Note: In facial nerve paralysis – the peripheral branches supplying the facial muscles will be paralyzed which will lead to, paralysis of facial muscles on the ipsilateral side and angle of mouth will be deviated to opposite side (Not the whole face so option d is incorrect)

12. Ans. is a i.e. Deviation of angle of mouth towards opposite side *Ref. Dhingra 5/e, p 102, 6/e, p95*
- Lesion occurring at the outlet of stylomastoid foramen means **LMN palsy so** face sags and is drawn across to opposite side. Chorda tympani nerve is spared at this level hence taste sensation over anterior 2/3 of tongue preserved

13. Ans. is d i.e. Improper regeneration of facial nerve
Ref. Dhingra 5/e, p110, Current Ololaryngology 2/e, p 839, 3/e, p 870

Crocodile tears (gustatory lacrimation) There is unilateral lacrimation with mastication
- It is due to faulty regeneration of parasympathetic fibers which normally travel through chorda tympani but are misdirected towards greater superficial petrosal nerve and instead of going to salivary glands reach the lacrimal glands.
This results in unilateral lacrimation with mastication
- Treatment – Sectioning the greater superficial petrosal nerve or tympanic neurectomy

ALSO KNOW
- Frey's syndrome (gustatory sweating) – There is sweating and flushing of skin over the parotid area during mastication.

Remember
Irreversible axonal injury and aberrant patterns of regeneration are more common from grade III degree of sunderland classification of facial nerve degeneration[Q]

14. Ans. is c i.e. Mastoidectomy *Ref. Logan Turner 10/e, p 359*
"All ear operations run the risk of facial nerve damage, particularly if the nerve is exposed. In particular a mastoidectomy has a high risk because a sharp cutting rotating burr is used in close proximity to the nerve."

Other Operations where Facial Nerve may be damaged
- Stapedectomy
- Removal of acoustic neuroma

15. Ans. is b i.e. Transverse fractures *Ref. Dhingra 5/e, p 108, 6/e, p97*
Fracture of petrous temporal bone can be longitudnal or transverse. Facial palsy is seen more often with transverse fracture[Q].

	Longitudnal	Transverse
Frequency	Most common (80%)	Less common (20%)
Bleeding from ear	Present	Absent (as tympanic membrane is intact)
CSF otorrhea	Present	Absent
Structures injured	Tegmen, ossicles and Tympanic Membrane	Labyrinth or CN VIII
Hearing loss	Conductive	SNHL
Facial paralysis	Less common, (10% cases)	More common *(40–50%)*
Onset of paralysis	Delayed onset paralysis	Immediate onset of paralysis
Part of facial nerve injured	Distal to geniculate ganglion	Proximal to geniculate ganglion
Vertigo	Less often	More often

In these cases it is important to know whether paralysis was of immediate or delayed onset –
Immediate onset paralysis is treated conservatively.
Delayed onset paralysis – requires surgery in the form of decompression, reanastomosis of cut ends or cable nerve grafts.

16. Ans. is c i.e. Malignant otitis externa *Ref. Dhingra 5/e, p 58, 6/e, p 52*
Facial paralysis is seen in malignant otitis externa as discussed in previous chapters.

17. **Ans. is a i.e. Horizontal part** Ref. Scotts Brown 7/e, vol-3 p 3888; Current Otolaryngology 2/e, p 837
    Explanation: The Horizontal/tympanic part of facial nerve
    - Is most susceptible to injury during surgery.
    - Maximum bone dehiscence occur in this part adjacent to oval window.
18. **Ans. is d i.e. Bell's palsy**
19. **Ans. is c i.e. Bell's palsy** Ref. Scotts Brown 7/e, vol 3 p 3891; Harrison 17/e, p 2585
    "The commonest cause of facial palsy in adults is Bell's palsy" –Scotts Brown 7/e, vol-3 p 3891
    It is unilateral and infranuclear type of palsy. It is also the M/c cause of LMN facial palsy – (Harrison 17/e, p 3891)
20. **Ans. is d i.e. LMN VII nerve**
21. **Ans. is d i.e. Immediate surgical decompression is required.**
22. **Ans. is b i.e. Always recurrent**
    Read text for explanation: Ref. Dhingra 5/e, p 105, 106 , 6/e, p 95; Current Otolaryngology 2/e, p 847, 854, 855;
    Scotts Brown 7/e vol-3 p 3885; Harrison 17/e, p 2584
23. **Ans. is c i.e. Idiopathic ipsilateral paralysis of the facial nerve**
    Ref. Dhingra 5/e, p 105, 6/e, p 95; Harrison 17/e, p 2585; Scott's Brown 7/e, vol-3 p 3883, 3885
    - Bells paralysis is an LMN type of facial nerve palsy of unknown etiology i.e. idiopathic nature.
    - Lower motor neuron type of palsy causes ipsilateral paralysis therefore bells palsy causes ipsilateral facial paralysis.
    - Other neurological examinations are normal in Bells palsy
24. **Ans. is d i.e. Ipsilateral ptosis** Ref. Harrison 17/e, p 2585; Dhingra 5/e, p105-106, 6/e, p 95
    Bell's palsy is an acute onset lower motor neuron type of palsy – their will be Ipsilateral loss of:
    - Taste sensation, lacrimation and salivation
    - Facial paralysis
    - Noise intolerance (hyperacusis)
    - Eye balls will turn up and out (Bells phenomenon) on attempting to close eyes but ptosis will not be seen.

     Note: In Bell's palsy – Facial paralysis is usually preceded by pain behind the ear.

25. **Ans. is a, b, c, d and e i.e. Other motor cranial nerves also involves, Melkersson's syndrome cause recurrent paralysis, Eye protection done, Prognosis can be predicted by serial electrical studies, Bell's palsy is commonest cause**
    Ref. Dhingra 5/e, p 105-06, 6/e, p 95, 96; BDC 4/e, vol III/p 54; Current Otolaryngology 2/e, p847, 3/e, p 876
    - Most common cause of lower motor neuron (LMN) type of facial palsy is Bell's palsy.
    - Melkersson's syndrome consists of a triad of: (i) Facial paralysis, (ii) Swelling of lips, (iii) Fissured tongue, Paralysis may be recurrent.
    - As patient is unable to close the eye, eye protection is required to protect cornea and conjunctiva.
    - The prognosis in acute facial palsy can be accurately determined by serial electrical testing. The response to electrical tests have been found to be most useful in the first 5 days *after the onset.*
    - As far as option 'a' is concerned–other cranial nerves also involved–current otolaryngology 3rd/ed p876 says –
    - "There may also be subtle but frequent associated dysfunction of cranial nerves V, VIII, IX and X in association with Bell's palsy."
      i.e option a is correct.

    ALSO KNOW

    Surgical decompression of facial nerve
    Approaches: Transmastoid, transcanal, via middle fossa

    All indications of facial nerve decompression
    - Complete paralysis (>90% by ENG in case of Bell's palsy)
    - Tumors of facial nerve
    - Cholesteatoma causing facial palsy
    - Traumatic facial palsy.

26. **Ans. is c i.e. Oral steroids + Acyclovir**
    Ref. Current Olotaryngology 2/e, p 856; Scott's Brown 7/e, vol-3 p 3886, 3/e, p884-887

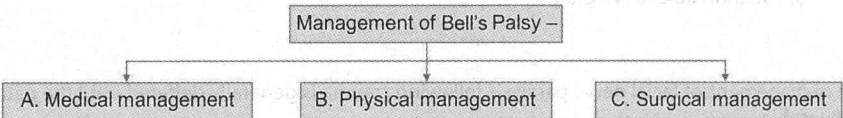

Medical Management

Consists of either steroid on antineural therapy.

The usual recommended regime is prednisolone 1 mg/kg/day for five days followed by a ten day taper and oral acyclovir (200-400 mg 5 times daily) for ten days.

Physical Management

Includes :
- **Electrical stimulation:** It is done to maintain membrane conductivity and reduce muscle atrophy
- It is generally used in patients left with partial defects
- **Eye care:** The cornea is vulnerable to drying and foreign body irritation in acute facial palsy due to orbicularis oculi dysfunction. So measures conferring corneal protection are recommended. Like:
  - Artificial tears drops at daytime
  - Ocular ointment at night
  - Use of sunglasses, etc.

In long standing cases: Reducing the area of exposed cornea by implanting a gold weight in the upper lid (tarsorapphy) is done.

Surgical Management Nerve decompression

27. Ans. is d i.e. Electrophysiological nerve testing   *Ref. Current Otolaryngology 2/e, p 858, 842, 3/e, p. 887, 870, 872*

In a patient who has had no improvement in steroids after 2 weeks of use will not benefit from an increase in dose of steroid
Also vasodilators and ACTH have no role in management of Bell's palsy
Hence they are also ruled out.
So now we are left with 2 options viz-
  i. Electrophysiological nerve testing
  ii. Surgical decompression

Nerve decompression – Surgical management of acute facial nerve palsy is based on the principle that axonal ischemia can be reduced by decompression of nerve segments presumed to be inflamed and entrapped. Nerve decompression is not done in all cases of acute facial palsy.

Prerequisite for Nerve decompression (Read very carefully)
To identify those patients who may benefit from nerve decompression, electrophysiological testing should be done prior to it   *Ref. Current Otolaryngology 3/e, p887*

The test done is – Evoked electro myograpy (EEMG). Surgical treatment is offered when evoked response amplitudes are 10% (or less) of the normal side.
So now after understanding all this lets see the question once again –
It says – a case of bells palsy on steroids, shows no improvement after 2 weeks, **next step in management** would be -
Next step would obviously be electrophysiolgical testing for two reasons:
1. Bell's palsy as a rule recovers after 10 days and responds after steriod, the diagnosis has to reviewed to rule out other causes like herpes zoster oticus (which can be indicated by the pattern of degeneration on electrophysiological nerve testing)
2. If electrophysiological testing predicts poor prognosis for recovery. It is an indication for nerve decomppression.

28. Ans. is c i.e. Steroid   *Ref. NCBI, Internet*

As discussed in the text and previous questions, all the options given are, used for managing Bells palsy. But when question asks specifically about evidence based management then the only proven beneficial result is seen with steroids—Prednisolone.

29. Ans. is a i.e. Nerve decompression   *Ref. Dhingra 5/e, p 107*

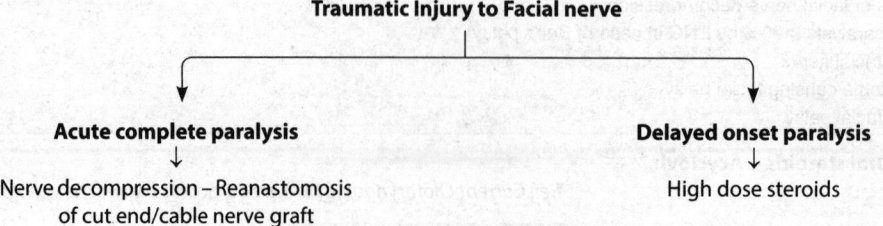

ALSO KNOW

As a general rule management of facial nerve paralysis following trauma is generally deffered until the patient is both medically and neurologically stable.

30. **Ans. is a i.e. Immediate decompression** *Ref. Scotts Brown 7/e, vol- 3 p 3888*
    In case of Temporal bone trauma
    "In case of acute complete paralysis, surgical exploration is warranted if ENOG shows > 90% denervation within 6 days of the onset of paralysis and the patient is neurologically stable"

31. **Ans. is a i.e. Herpes zoster**

32. **Ans is b i.e. H. zoster**   *Ref. Dhingra 5/e, p 107, 6/e, p 96; Scotts Brown 7/e, vol-3 p 3886; Current Otolaryngology 2/e, p 847,849*
    Ramsay Hunt syndrome/Herpes zoster oticus is a lower motor neuron type of facial palsy due to varicella zoster (herpes zoster). It is characterized by vesicles around the external canal, pinna and soft palate, SNHL and vertigo due to involvements of VIIIth nerve along with facial nerve palsy.

33. **Ans. is c i.e. Facial vesicle is seen**   *Ref. Dhingra 5/e, p107, 6/e, p96; Current Otolaryngology 2/e, p 849, 3/e, p 878*
    - Vessicles in Ramsay Hunt syndrome are seen in the preauricular skin, the skin of ear canal the soft palate and not on facial skin
    - All other options are correct and explained in the perceding text.

34. **Ans. is d i.e. Results of spontaneous recovery are excellent**

35. **Ans. is c i.e. Surgical removal gives excellent prognosis**   *Ref. Scotts Brown 7/e, vol-3 p 241*
    See the text for explanation.

36. **Ans. b, c, d and e i.e. 7th CN involvement, Abduction defect, Esotropia and 6th CN involvement.**
    Ref. Nelson 18/e,pgs2450-51,677,2567,2582;emedicinemedscape.com
    Mobius syndrome   *Nelson 18/e,pgs2450-51,677,2567,2582*

    - *"It is characterized by **bilateral facial** weakness **(i.e VII CN)**, which is often associated with **abducens nerve** paralysis **(i.e VI CN)**"* Nelson 18th/2450

    - The facial palsy is commonly bilateral, frequently asymmetric, and often incomplete, tending to spare the lower face and platysma.
    - **Ectropion**, epiphora, and **exposure keratopathy** may develop.
    - The abduction defect may be unilateral or bilateral. Esotropia is common.
    - Whether the primary defect is maldevelopment of cranial nerve nuclei, hypoplasia of the muscles, or a combination of central and peripheral factors is unclear.
    - **Surgical correction of the esotropia** is indicated and amblyopia should also be treated.

CHAPTER 11

Lesion of Cerebellopontine Angle and Acoustic Neuroma

ANATOMY OF INTERNAL AUDITORY CANAL (IAC)

Contents of Internal Auditory Canal

In addition to internal auditory vessels, following nerves enter the IAC (Fig. 11.1):
- **Facial nerve** in anterosuperior quadrant.
- **Superior vestibular nerve** in posterosuperior quadrant.
- **Cochlear nerve** in anteroinferior quadrant.
- **Inferior vestibular nerve** in posteroinferior quadrant.

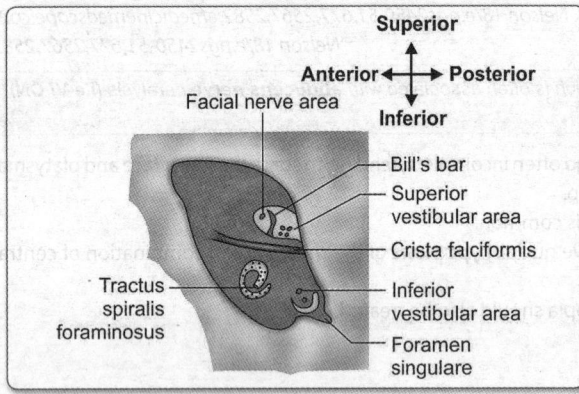

Fig. 11.1: Fundus of right internal auditory canal (IAC) as seen through the IAC
Courtesy: Essentials of Mohan Bansal, Jaypee Brothers Medical Publishers Pvt. Ltd., p 165

ANATOMY OF CEREBELLOPONTINE ANGLE (CPA)

- It is a triangular area bounded anterolaterally by petrous temporal bone, medially by pons and brainstem, posteriorly by cerebellum and flocculus.
- Contents of the angle are: Anterior Inferior cerebellar artery^Q and VII, VIII cranial nerve.^Q
- Immediately superior to is the V cranial nerve and III, IV, VI are further up.
- Inferiorly lies IX, X, XI cranial nerve: Thus in lesions of CPA all these nerves can be involved.

Point to Remember

Lesions of CP angle
- M/C Acoustic neuroma = 80%
- Meningoma = 10%
- Congenital cholesteatoma = 5%
- Others = 5%

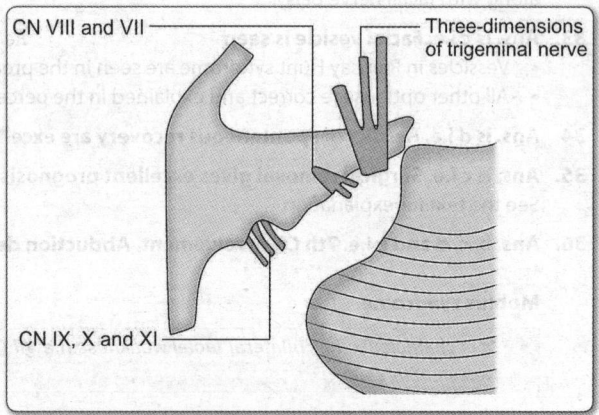

Fig. 11.2: Cerebellopontine angle

VESTIBULAR SCHWANNOMA/ACOUSTIC NEUROMA

- It is the *most common* **intracranial schwannoma.**
- Constitutes **80% of all cerebellopontine angle** tumors^Q (M/C benign tumor of CP angle) and 10% of all brain tumors
- It is **benign**, encapsulated and extremely slow growing tumor. It is locally invasive.
- *Most common* site of acoustic neuroma:
  - Inferior vestibular nerve^Q > superior vestibular nerve^Q > Cochlear nuclei.^Q (rare)
  - Bilateral vestibular schwamoma is *diagnostic* of **Neurofibromatosis 2.**
- It originates in the Schwann cells of the inferior or superior vestibular nerves at the transition zone (**Obersteiner Redlich Zone**) of the central and peripheral myelin, which lies in internal auditory canal.

Growth of Tumor

- The tumor arises from vestibular nerves' parts which are in Internal acoustic meatus (IAM) or Internal auditory canal (IAC).
- It reaches the CPA (Figs. 11.3A to D) after eroding and widening IAM.
- Anterosuperiorly, it involves the CNV (i.e CNV is the earliest nerve to be involved by AN) and inferiorly involves the CN IX, X and XI, which lie in jugular foramen.
- A big AN can displace brainstem and put pressure on cerebellum and raise intracranial tension. Seventy percent of ANs grow slowly over years and 30% remain stable.

- **Fundus examination:** Papilloedema (blurring of disk margins).

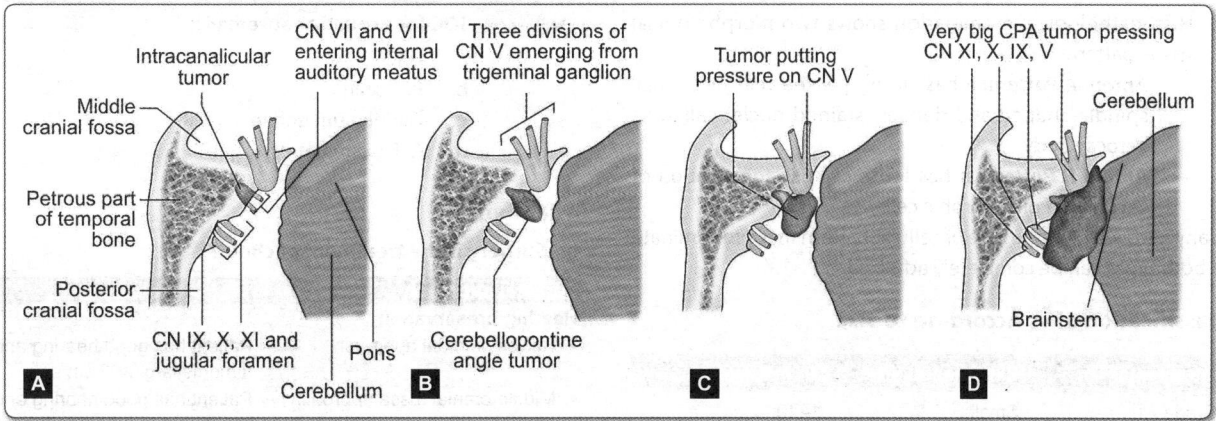

Figs. 11.3A to D: Acoustic neuroma. (A) Intracanalicular tumor; (B) Cerebellopontine angle tumor; (C) Tumor pressing trigeminal nerve; (D) Tumor pressing glossopharyngeal, vagus, and accessory nerves, brainstem and cerebellum
Courtesy: Essential of ENT, Mohan Bansal, Jaypee Brothers Medical Publishers Pvt. Ltd., p 165

Clinical Features

- **Age** most common in 40-60 years^Q (occurs in 20-30 years of age when the tumour is found in association with Neurofibromatosis type 2).
- Both sexes are affected equally^Q.
- Tumour is *radioresistant*^{Q}.
- *In 90% cases it is unilateral*, it may be bilateral in **Von Recklinghausen disease/Neurofibromatosis.**^{Q}

NEW PATTERN QUESTIONS	
Q N1.	**Neurofibromatosis type 2 is associated with:**
	a. B/L acoustic neuroma
	b. Cafe-au-lait spots
	c. Chromosome 22
	d. Lisch nodule
	e. Posterior subcapsular lenticular cataract
Q N2.	**Acoustic schwannoma most common site is:**
	a. CP angle
	b. Fossa of Rosenmuller
	c. Retropharyngeal space
	d. None of the above

Clinical Symptoms

- **Earliest symptom:** Cochleovestibular symptoms (deafness, tinnitus) as tumor arises from IAC.
- **Most common symptom:** Progressive unilateral sensorineural (retrocochlear) hearing loss (present in 95% patients) often^Q accompanied by tinnitus (Present in 65% patients).

Point to Remember
> There is marked difficulty in understanding speech out of proportion to the pure tone hearing loss. This is characteristic of acoustic neuroma^Q.

- May also present with sudden hearing loss (in 20% cases).
- True vertigo is seldom seen^Q.
- In 2% cases, it is asymptomatic.

Features due to involvement of specific structures:

- **Facial nerve:** Sensory fibers are more sensitive and affected early. Motor fibers are more resistant so are affected late.
  - **Histeliberger's sign:** Numbness of posterior aspect of concha, which is supplied by the sensory fibers of the facial nerve.
  - **Electrogustometry:** Loss of taste from anterior 2/3 tongue.
  - **Schirmer's test:** Reduced lacrimation.
  - **Blink reflex:** It is delayed.
- **CN V:** The first extracanalicular nerve to be involved is trigeminal. The tumor is in CPA and of about 2.5 cm size.
  - Reduced corneal sensitivity (earliest sign most common sign of acoustic removal).
  - Numbness or paresthesia of face.
- **CN IX and X**
  - Dysphagia, hoarseness of voice and nasal regurgitation of fluid.
  - Palatal, pharyngeal and laryngeal paralysis.
- **CN XI, XII, III, IV and VI:** They are involved when tumor is very large.
- **Brainstem:** Long motor and sensory tracts are involved.
  - Weakness and numbness of the arms and legs with exaggerated tendon reflexes.
- **Cerebellum:** Finger-nose test, knee-heel test, dysdiadochokinesia, ataxic gait, inability to walk along a straight line with tendency to fall to the affected side.
- **Raised intracranial tension**
  - Blurring of vision, headache, nausea, vomiting, and diplopia (CN VI involvement).
- **Fundus examination:** Papilloedema (blurring of disk margins).
- In terminal stages, there is:
  - Herniation of cerebellar tonsils
  - Failure of the vital centers in the brainstem

Histopathology

- Histopathological examination shows two morphological tissue patterns.
  - **Antoni A Pattern:** It has closely packed cells with small spindle-shaped and densely stained nuclei called as Verocay Body
  - **Antoni B Pattern:** It has loose cellular aggregation of vacuolated pleomorphic cells.

In any particular VS, one type of cellular pattern may predominate or both types can be completely admixed.

Classification of vs According to Size

Intrameatal Tm	Extrameatal size	2n millimetres
Grade I	Small	1–10
Grade II	Medium	11–20
Grade III	Moderately large	21–30
Grade IV	Large	31–40
Grade V	Giant	> 40

Investigations

- **Audiological test: Show features of retrocochlear hearing loss.**
  - Rinne +ve
  - Webers → towards normal side
  - Schwabach → shortened
  - PTA → shows sensorineural hearing loss
  - Tone decay > 30 dB
  - Recruitment negative^Q
  - Speech discrimination score poor^Q (**speech discrimination score becomes worse at higher speech intensity and this phenomenon is called as roll over phenomenon**)
  - BERA - Delay of > 0.2 msec in Wave V between the 2 sides. The best test for acoustic neuroma is BERA.
- **Acoustic reflex:** Shows stapedial reflex decay.
- **Vestibular test:** Caloric test usually show diminished or absent response^Q but may be normal, if tumour is very small.
- This is because caloric test is mainly a test for lateral semicircular canal which is innervated by superior vestibular nerve. Thus, a small tumor arising from inferior vestibular nerve may not lead to any charge in caloric response. Later when superior vestibular nerve is compressed the caloric response is reduced.
- **Investigation of choice = Gadolinium enhanced MRI = 100% diagnostic yield**

NEW PATTERN QUESTION

Q N3. IOC for acoustic neuroma is:
a. HRCT
b. PET scan
c. Gadolinium enhanced MRI
d. CSF examination

Treatment:

- **Surgery is the treatment of choice^Q.**

Surgical approach	Indication
Hearing preservation	
• Retrosigmoidal approach	– Patient has good hearing and tumor is large > 3 cm size
• Middle cranial fossa approach	– Patient has good hearing and tumor size is < 1.5 cm (i.e. small tumors)
• Retro labyrinthine	– Small CPA tumor not extending into lateral part of internal auditory canal
Hearing ablation	
Translabyrinthine approach	– Suitable for tumors < 3 cm but disadvantage is SNHL – M/C approach

Hearing rehabilitation following tumour excision:

- Cochlear implant^Q
- Auditory brainstem implant—In cases of bilateral acoustic neuroma^Q.

Stereotactic radiosurgery/Gamma knife (Radiation is derived with Co-60):

- **Stereottic radiotherapy:** Concentrates high dose radiation on the tumor so that its growth is arrested without affecting surrounding tissue
- Used in patients who refuse surgery^Q
- Source of radiation = Cobalt 60.

Advantages:

- No morbidity of surgery.
- VII nerve functions preserved
- Hearing preserved.

Now due to its low morbidity gamma knife surgery or stereotactic RT is taken as an alternative to surgery in tumors less than 3 cm in size

- Modification of Gamma knife is X-knife where source of radiation is linear accelerator.

Cyber knife:

- It is a type of—Robotic Surgery where the surgery is done by computer controlled robotics

Chapter 11: Lesion of Cerebellopontine Angle and Acoustic Neuroma

---- **Explanations and References to New Pattern Questions** ----

N1. Ans. a, b, c, and e i.e. B/L acoustic neuroma, Cafe-au-lait spots, Chromosome 22 and posterior subcapsular lanticular cataract
Ref: Current Otolaryngology 3/e, p 801, 802

B/L acoustic neuromas are a hallmark of Neurofibromatosis 2
- Neurofibromatosis Type 2 is an autosomal dominant highly penetrant condition
- Gene for NF-2 is located on chromosome 22q.
- Patients with NF2 present in second and third decade of life, rarely after the age of 60.
- M/C symptom/presenting symptom = Hearing loss
- Skin tumors are present in nearly two thirds of patients of NF-2

"Cafe au lait spots, which are a hallmark of NF-1, are also frequently found in patients with NF2. In contrast to patients with NF1, patients with NF 2 invariably have fewer than six of these hyperpigmented lesions. Juvenile posterior sub capsular lenticular opacies are common and have been reported in up to 51% of patients with NF 2."
Ref. Current Otolaryngology 3/e, p 801, 802

So as is clear from above lines–cafe an lait spots and posterior subcapsular lenticular opacity are seen in NF-2 also.

> **Remember**
> **Diagnostic criteria for NF-2**
>   I. **Bilateral acoustic neuroma**
>   or
>   II. **Family hisory of NF-2 and**
>   U/L Vestibular schwannoma/acoustic neuroma
>   or
>   III. **Any two of the following:**
>   Meningioma
>   Glioma
>   Neurofibroma
>   Schwannoma
>   Posterior subcapsular leticular opacity

 Note: In patients of Neurofibromatous-2 operated for B/L acoustic neuroma, best method of hearing rehabilitation is auditory brainstem implant.

N2. Ans. is a i.e. CP angle *Ref. Dhingra 6/e, p 112*
Read preceeding text.

N3. Ans. is c i.e. Gadolinium enhanced MRI *Ref. Dhingra 6/e, p 103*
Gadolinium enhanced MRI is the gold standard for diagnosis of acoustic neuroma. Intracanalicular tumor of even a few millimeters can be detected by this method.

QUESTIONS

1. **Most common cerebellopontine angle tumour is:** [Kerala 91]
   a. Acoustic neuroma
   b. Cholesteastoma
   c. Meningioma
   d. All of the above

2. **Cerebellopontine angle tumor produces:** [PGI 2005]
   a. Tinnitus
   b. Deafness
   c. Absent corneal reflex
   d. Trigeminal neuralgia

3. **Schwannoma involves the:** [AI 99]
   a. Vestibular part of VIIIth nerve
   b. Cochlear part of VIIIth nerve
   c. Vagus nerve
   d. Hypoglossal nerve

4. **Acoustic neuroma commonly arise from:**
   [AI 11, AI 10, AIIMS Nov. 09] [AIIMS Dec. 98, J and K-05]
   a. Superior vestibular nerve
   b. Inferior vestibular nerve
   c. Cochlear nerve
   d. Facial nerve

5. **In acoustic neuroma cranial nerve to be involved earliest is:** [AI 07, UP-08]
   a. 5
   b. 7
   c. 10
   d. 9

6. **The earliest symptom of acoustic nerve tumor is:**
   [AI 95, Delhi-05, Karnatak-09]
   a. Sensorineuran hearing loss
   b. Tinnitus
   c. Vertigo
   d. Otorrhea

7. **Earliest sign seen in Acoustic neuroma is:** [UPSC 05]
   a. Facial weakness
   b. Unilateral deafness
   c. Reduced corneal reflex
   d. Cerebellar signs

8. **Acoustic neuroma causes:** [PGI June 99]
   a. Cochlear deafness
   b. Retrocochlear deafness
   c. Conductive deafness
   d. Any of the above

9. **Hitzelberger's sign is seen in:** [AI 08]
   a. Vestibular schwannoma
   b. Mastoiditis
   c. Bells palsy
   d. Cholesteatoma

10. **In acoustic neuroma all are seen *except*:** [MP 2000]
    a. Loss of corneal reflex
    b. Tinnitus
    c. Facial palsy
    d. Diplopia

11. **In a patient with acoustic neuroma all are seen *except*:** [SGPGI 07]
    a. Facial nerve may be involved unilateral deafness
    b. Reduced corneal reflex
    c. Cerebellar signs
    d. Acute episode of vertigo

12. **Earliest ocular finding in acoustic neuroma:** [PGI 00]
    a. Diplopia
    b. Ptosis
    c. Loss of corneal sensation
    d. Papilloedema

13. **Vestibular neuroma not correct:** [AP 2005]
    a. Nystagmus
    b. High frequency sensorineural deafness
    c. Absence of caloric response
    d. Normal corneal reflex

14. **True about Acoustic neuroma:** [PGI June 04]
    a. Malignant tumor
    b. Arises form vestibular nerve
    c. Upper pole displaces IX, X, XI nerves
    d. Lower pole displaces trigeminal cranial nerve

15. **True about vestibular schwanomma:** [PGI May 2015]
    a. Unilateral hearing loss is common presentation
    b. Mostly malignant
    c. Most common tumour of CP angle
    d. Sensorineural deafness
    e. Uncapsulated

16. **Progressive loss of hearing, tinnitus and ataxia are commonly seen in a case of:** [SGPGI 05]
    a. Otitis media
    b. Cerebral glioma
    c. Acoustic neuroma
    d. Ependymoma

17. **Acoustic neuroma of 1 cm diameter, the investigation of choice:** [Kerala 97]
    a. CT scan
    b. MRI scan
    c. Plain X-ray skull
    d. Air encephalography

18. **A patient is suspected to have vestibular schwannoma the investigation of choice for its diagnosis is:** [AIIMS 04]
    a. Contrast enhanced CT scan
    b. Gadolinium enhanced MRI
    c. SPECT
    d. PET scan

19. **A 70-year-old male presents with loss of sensation in external auditory meatus (Hitselberger sign positive). The likely diagnosis is:** [AI 2008]
    a. Vestibular Schwannoma
    b. Mastoiditis
    c. Bell's palsy
    d. Cholesteatoma

Chapter 11: Lesion of Cerebellopontine Angle and Acoustic Neuroma

Explanations and References

1. **Ans. is a i.e. Acoustic neuroma**
   Ref. Current Otolaryngology 2/e, p 765; 3/e, p 791-92; Turner 10/e, p 39; Dhingra 5/e, p 124; Dhingra 6/e, p 112

   Point to Remember
   - M/C CP angle tumour is Acoustic neuroma = 80%
   - 2nd M/C CP angle tumor is meningoma ≥ 10%

2. **Ans. is a, b, c, d, i.e. Tinnitus, Deafness, Absent corneal reflex and Trigeminal neuralgia**   *Ref. Current Otolaryngology 3/e, p 792*
   The two most common CP angle tumors are:

Acoustic neuromas	Meningomas
• M/C symptom = U/L deafness • 2nd M/C symptom tinnitus • M/C nerve involved = Facial nerve therefore absent corneal reflex is seen	• M/C symptom = U/L deafness (80%) followed by vertigo (75%) and tinnitus = 60% • In meningiomas Unlike Acoustic neuroma – Trigeminal neuralgias, facial paresis, lower cranial nerve deficits and visual disturbances are more common.

   Hence all the above features are seen in CP angle tumors.

3. **Ans. is a i.e. Vestibular part of VIIIth nerve**   *Ref. Logan Turner 10/e, p 339*

4. **Ans. is b i.e. Inferior vestibular nerve**   *Ref. Glasscock-Shambaugh, Surgery of the Ear, 6/e, p 644*
   Historically, the superior vestibular nerve sheath was thought to be the site of origin, giving rise to nearly two-thirds of tumors. More recent reviews show the inferior vestibular nerve to be the predominant site of origin for these tumors.

5. **Ans. is a i.e. 5 Nerve**   *Ref. Dhingra 5th/e, p 124; 6th/e, p 112*

6. **Ans. is a i.e. Sensory neural hearing loss**

7. **Ans. is c i.e. Reduced corneal reflex.**   *Ref. Dhingra 5/e, p 124; Turner 10/e, p 341*

   Remember
• Most common nerve from which vestibular schwannoma arises	• Inferior vestibular nerve
• Earliest symptom	• Progressive unilateral sensorineural hearing loss often accompanied by tinnitus
• Earliest cranial nerve to be involved by acoustic neuroma	• VIII nerve followed by V nerve followed by VII nerve
• Earliest presentation of Vth nerve involvement/ Earliest sign of Acoustic neuroma	• Decreased corneal sensitivity
• Significance of Vth nerve involvement	• Implies that tumor is atleast 2.5 cm in size and occupies cerebellopontine angle
• Earliest presentation of VII nerve involvement	• Involvement of Sensory fibers leading to hypothesia of posterior meatal wall (Hitzelberger sign)

   Note: Although facial nerve is involved facial nerve palsy is rarely seen.

8. **Ans. is b i.e. Retrocochlear deafness**   *Ref. Tuli 1/e, p 114*
   - **SNHL can be:**
     a. **Cochlear SNHL** – Hair cells are mainly damaged.
     b. **Retrocochlear SNHL** – There is lesion of VIIIth nerve or its central connections.
   - Acoustic neuroma cause retrocochlear type of SNHL as it damages VIIIth nerve.
   - Meniere's disease causes cochlear deafness.

Note:
- **Important features of Retrocochlear hearing loss/Acoustic Neuroma:**
  - Sensorineural hearing loss more marked in high frequencies.
  - Poor discrimination score (0-30%).
  - Recruitment phenomenon absent and roll over phenomenon present, i.e. discrimination score further decreases when loudness is increased beyond a particular point.
  - Short increment sensitivity index (SISI) test will show a score of 0-20% in 70-90% cases.
  - Tone decay significant.

9. **Ans. is a i.e. Vestibular Schwannoma** *Ref. Dhingra 5/e, p 124; 6/e, p 112*

    Hitzelberger's sign is hypoaesthesia of posterior meatal wall seen in vestibular Schwanoma /acoustic neuroma due to involvement of sensory fibres of VIIth nerve.

10. **Ans. is c i.e. Facial palsy** *Ref. Scott's Brown 7/e, vol-3, p 3959; Dhingra 5/e, p 124, 125; 6/e, p 112, 113*

    In Acoustic Neuroma
    - Loss of corneal reflex is seen – due to the involvement of tringeminal nerve
    - Tinnitus – due to pressure on cochlear nerve
    - Large tumors can cause diplopia *Ref. Turner 10/e, p 341*

    As far as facial nerve palsy is concerned *Ref. Scott Brown 7th/e, vol-3, p 3931*

    "Vestibular schwannomas, although inevitably grossly distort the VIIth nerve, very rarely present as a VIIth nerve palsy. If there is a clinical evidence of a cerebellopontine angle lesion and if the VIIth nerve is involved, alternative pathology is more likely".

    Hence although Acoustic neuroma may involve the 7 nerve but complete palsy is never seen

11. **Ans. is d i.e. Acute episode of vertigo** *Ref. Dhingra 5/e, p 124*

    Lets see Each Option Separately
    - **Option a** – Facial nerve may be involved –
      This is correct as we have discussed in previous Questions. Facial nerve may be involved but complete palsy doesnot occur
    - **Option b** – Reduced corneal reflex –
      This is correct reduced corneal reflex is the **first sign of trigeminal nerve involvement**
    - **Option c** – Cerebellar signs – This is correct
    - **Option d** – Acute episodes of vertigo
      "Vestibular symptoms seen in acoustic neuroma are imbalance or unsteadiness. True vertigo is seldom seen"
      Ref. Dhingra 5/e, p 124; 6/e, p 112
      Acute episode of vertigo is a rare presenting feature in acoustic neuroma since it is a slow growing tumor so there is adequate time for compensation.

12. **Ans. is c i.e. Loss of corneal sensation** *Ref. Dhingra 5/e, p 124; Turner 10/e, p 341*
    - **Earliest nerve involved by acoustic neuroma** – Vth nerve/trigeminal nerve.
    - Earliest manifestation of Vth nerve involvement is decreased corneal sensitivity leading to loss of corneal reflex.

13. **Ans. is d i.e. Normal corneal reflex** *Ref. Dhingra 5/e, p 125*

    As far as the answer is concerned – I am sure no one has any doubts about it because corneal reflex is absent in acoustic neuroma But lets focus on option c, i.e. Absence of caloric response –

    In acoustic neuroma –

    Caloric test will show diminished or absent response in 96% patients due to vestibular involvement.

    Hence option c, i.e. correct

    Also Know
    Criteria of suspicion for Acoustic neuroma (Turner 10th/ed pg 341)
    - Unilateral deafness of less than 10 years.
    - Sudden deafness with retrocochlear involvement which does not respond to steroids
    - Poor speech discrimination score in relation to pure tone threshold
    - Spontaneous nystagmus with eyes closed on electronystagmography without a history of disequilibrium
    - Absence of caloric response in case of normal hearing
    - Hearing loss with reduced corneal reflex
    - Local pain

Chapter 11: Lesion of Cerebellopontine Angle and Acoustic Neuroma

 Note: If hearing loss is the only symptom and it is of more than 10 years duration, an acoustic neuroma is most **unlikely** as a tumor which has been growing for longer than this period because it will give features of other cranial nerve or brainstem involvement also.

14. **Ans. is b i.e. Arises from vestibular nerve**   *Ref. Dhingra 5/e, p 114; 5/e, p 134*

    Explanation

    Here **Option a**, i.e. malignant tumor is incorrect as acoustic neuroma is a benign tumor.
    Option b: It arises from vestibular nerve is correct
    Option c: Upper pole displaces IX, X and XI nerve–incorrect, as is evident from the diagram given in the text: Upper pole displaces III, IV and V nerve whereas lower pole displaces IX, X and XI nerve.

15. **Ans. is a, c and d i.e. Unilateral hearing loss is common presentation. Most common tumor of CP angle and Sensorineural deafness**   *Ref. Dhingra 6/e, p 112-14; Logan Turner 10/e p. 339-44*
    Already explained.

16. **Ans. is c i.e. Acoustic neuroma**   *Ref. Dhingra 5/e, p 124*
    Already explained.

17. **Ans. is b i.e. MRI scan**

18. **Ans. is b i.e. Gadolinium enhanced MRI scan**   *Ref. Current Otolaryngology 2/e, p 767: Dhingra 5/e, p 126*
    MRI with gadolinium contrast is the gold standard for the diagnosis or exclusion of vestibular Schwannoma.

19. **Ans. is a i.e. Vestibular schwanoma**   *Ref. Dhingra 6/e, p 112*
    This is a case of vestibular schwanoma where involvement of sensory fibres of VIIth nerve leads to anesthesia over the postero superior part of external meatus and canal. This is known as **Hitselberger sign**.

Chapter 12

Glomus Tumor and Other Tumors of the Ear

GLOMUS TUMOUR (PARAGANGLIOMAS)

- Glomus tumor are the **most common benign tumors** of middle ear
- Resemble carotid body therefore also called as **chemodectoma**
- Consists of paraganglionic cells derived from *neural crest* (Paragangliomas)
- It usually *arises* from dome of jugular bulb as **glomus jugulare** or from **promontory** along the course of tympanic branch of IX cranial nerve *(Jacobson's nerve)* and along the course of branch Xth cranial nerve *(Arnold's nerve)* as **glomus tympanicum**
- *Sometimes it may be multicentric (10% cases), i.e originates from more than 1 site*
- Most common site in middle ear: *hypotympanum.*

NEW PATTERN QUESTIONS

Q N1. M/C benign tumor of the external auditory canal is:
  a. Glomus tumor
  b. Exostosis
  c. Osteoma
  d. Hemangioma

Q N2. M/C benign tumor of middle ear is:
  a. Glomus tumor
  b. Hemangioma
  c. Exostosis
  d. Osteoma

Features

- *Slow growing **locally** invasive*, noncapsulated tumor which causes destruction of the bone and facial nerve
- Highly vascular-Main *Blood supply: ascending pharyngeal artery*
- Commonly affect **middle-aged females** (typically in 4th or 5th decade of life)
- *Malignant transformation and metastasis are rare*
- *Less than 10% tumors are associated with catecholamine secretion.*

Pathologically

They originate from the **'chief cell'** which contains acetylcholine, catecholamine and serotonin

- Classic findings are clusters of chief cells k/a **Zellballen**, with a rich vascular plexus throughout the entire Tumor. Therefore, they are highly vascular and may bleed substantially during surgical excision
  - Bilateral tumors occur in 1–2% cases
  - Can be hereditary also
- Also associated with pharamatoses (neurologic disease with cutaneous manifestations like von Recklinghausen neurofibromatosis, Sturge-Weber syndrome, tuberous sclerosis and von Hippel-Lindau disease)
- Also associated with MEN Type I syndrome.

Rule of Ten: For Glomus tumors—10% tumors are familial, 10% secrete catecholamines and 10% are multicentric.

Spread of Tumor

Site of Spread	Presentation
Tympanic membrane	– Vascular polyp
Labyrinth, petrous, pyramid and mastoid	– Hearing loss
Jugular foramen and base of skull	– Cranial nerve palsies VII, VIII, IX to XII
Eustachian tube	– Mass on nasopharynx
Intracranially spreads	
Lung, liver lymph nodes	

Point to Remember

M/C cranial nerve involved = Facial nerve followed by the last four cranial nerves.

Clinical Features

When tumor is intratympanic:

1. Earliest symptoms are deafness (conductive) and tinnitus (pulsatile and of swishing character, synchronous with pulse and can be temporarily stopped by carotid pressure). This is because jugular bulb is related to floor of middle ear.
2. Otoscopy shows **red reflex; rising sun appearance**, tympanic membrane appears **bluish and bulging.**
3. **Pulsation sign/Brown sign/Blanching sing** is positive (when ear canal pressure is raised with Siegel's speculum, tumor pulsates vigorously and then blanches; reverse happens with release of pressure).
4. **Aquino sign** – It is blanching of the mass with manual compression of ipsilateral carotid artery.

When tumor present as polyp:

1. History of *profuse bleeding* from the ear either spontaneously or on attempts to clear it.
2. Dizziness, vertigo, facial paralysis, earache otorrhea.

Chapter 12: Glomus Tumor and Other Tumors of the Ear

- **Audible bruit:** Heard by stethoscope over mastoid at all stages.
- Some glomus tumor secrete catecholamines and produce headache, sweating flushing, etc.
- Patient may show features of cranial nerve IX and X, involvement viz. dysphagia or hoarseness.

Extra Edge

Pulsatile tinnitus: Pulsatile tinnitus is characteristic of glomus tumor but can also be seen in other conditions.
➢ **Other Conditions Causing Pulsatile Tinnitus**
Arterial – Glomus tumor, AV malformation of temporal bone, aberrant internal carotid artery, cartoid/subclavian atherosclerosis
Venous – High jugular bulb, benign ICT.

Investigations

- **Examination under microscope:** Pulsatile mass seen.
- **Catecholamines levels:** Check the levels of serum catecholamines and their breakdown product VMA in urine before surgery for glomus tumor.
- **CT scan:** investigation of choice. Helps to distinguish glomus jugulare from glomus tympanicum with the help of.

Phelp's sign: absence of normal crest between the carotid canal and jugular fossa on lateral tomography, in case of glomus jugulare.

- **HRCT** and *gadolinium enhanced MRI* is used to delineate the intracranial extent of tumor.

A combination of CT scan and contrast MRI is the imaging regimen of choice for glomus jugular tumor.

- **Audiogram** will show conductive deafness if the middle ear space is invaded with tumor. If inner ear is invaded SNHL is seen
- **Angiography:** It is necessary when CT scan shows involvement of jugular bulb, carotid artery or intracranial extension. Following procedures are done:
  - For carotid artery: Carotid arteriography
  - For jugular bulb: Jugular venography
  - For intracranial extension: Vertebral arteriography

Point to Remember

➢ Biopsy is contraindicated in glomus tumors since they are very vascular.

NEW PATTERN QUESTIONS	
Q N3.	IOC for Glomus tumor: a. CT scan b. Catecholamine levels c. MRI d. Biopsy
Q N4.	A 42-year-female presents with U/L progressive conductive hearing loss with pulsatile tinnitus and blood stained discharge. She also complains of headache, sweating and palpitations. All of the following investigations are warranted in this case *except*: a. Otoscopy b. Serum catecholamines c. Urine VMA d. Biopsy
Q N5.	FISCH classification is used for: a. Juvenile nasopharyngeal angiofibroma b. Nasopharyngeal ca c. Vestibular schwannoma d. Glomus tumor

Treatment

Surgery – *Microsurgical total tumor removal is the treatment of choice for most patients.* Patients with functionally secreting tumors need to be alphablocked with phentolamine before and during surgery to prevent life-threatening hypertension as the alpha adrenergic hormones are released with tumor manipulation.

- **Embolization:** *Is the sole treatment in inoperable patients who have received radiation.*
- Preoperative embolization is done to decrease vascularity of tumor before surgery.
- **Radiation:** is reserved for inoperable lesions, old age and unfit patients.

Complications: see Flowchart 12.1

Flowchart 12.1: Complications of Glomus tumor

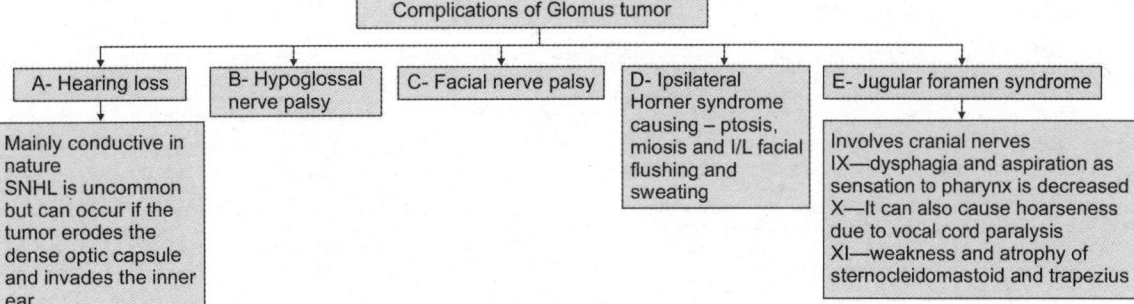

Explanations and References to New Pattern Questions

N1. Ans. is b i.e Exostosis
Ref. Essentials of ENT Mehan Bansal p 160

N2. Ans. is a i.e. Glomus tumor

> Exostoses are the M/C benign tumor of external auditory canal.
> **Important points on Ear Tumors:**
> - Of all the cases of ear carcinomas—85% occur on Pinna, 10% in external canal and 5% in middle ear.
> - M/C benign tumor of external canal—Exostosis.
> - M/C benign tumor of middle ear—Glomus tumor.
> - Exostosis are M/C in divers, swimmers and hence also called as surfers ear.

N3. Ans. is a i.e. CT scan

See the text for explanation

N4. Ans. is d i.e. Biopsy
Ref Dhingra 6/e, p 110

> **Remember**
> A 42-year-old female complaining of U/L conductive hearing loss and pulsatile tinnitus points towards Glomus tumor.
> Otoscopy should be done as it shows characteristic red reflex.
> Patient is complaining of headache, palpitations, etc i.e the tumor is secreting catecholamine, so serum catecholamine and urine VMA levels should be measured.
> Biopsy is contraindicated in Glomus tumors since they are very vascular and can bleed profusely.

N5. Ans. is d i.e. Glomus tumor
FISCH classification of glomus tumor

Type	Extent	Management
Type A	Confined to middle ear	Excised through external auditory meatus i.e. transmeatal route
Type B	Extending to mastoid	Excised through combined approach from meatus and mastoid
Type C	Extending to labyrinth and involving petrous apex	Excised through infratemporal fossa approach
Type D	Intracranial extension	Posterior fossa craniotomy

QUESTIONS

1. **The usual location of Glomus jugular tumor is:**
   [Delhi 90, UP-03]
   a. Epitympanum b. Hypotympanum
   c. Mastoidal cell d. Promontory

2. **Earliest symptom of glomus tumor is:** [UP 06]
   a. Pulsatile tinnitus b. Deafness
   c. Headache d. Vertigo

3. **Pulsatile tinnitus in ear is due to:** [TN 01]
   a. Malignant otitis media b. Osteoma
   c. Mastoid reservoirs d. Glomus jugulare tumor

4. **True about Glomus jugulare tumor:** [PGI June 04]
   a. Most common in male
   b. Arises from non-chromaffin cells
   c. Lymph node metastasis seen
   d. Multicentric
   e. Pulsatile tinnitus and conductive type of hearing loss seen

5. **All are true about glomus jugulare tumors except:** [UP 03]
   a. Common in female
   b. Causes sensory neural deafness
   c. It is a disease of infancy
   d. It invades labyrinth, petrous pyramid and mastoid

6. **Brown sign is seen in:** [AI 07]
   a. Glomus tumor b. Meniere's desease
   c. Acoustic neuroma d. Otoscleorsis

7. **Phelp's sign is seen in:** [AIIMS May 02]
   a. Glomus jugulare b. Vestibular Schawannoma
   c. Maniere's disease d. Neurofibromatosis

8. **The glomus tumor invasion of jugular bulb is diagnosed by?** [UP 05]
   a. Carotid angiography b. Vertebralvenousvenography
   c. X-ray d. Jugular venography

9. **A patient presents with bleeding from the ear pain tinnitus and progressive deafness. On examination, there is a red swelling behind the intact tympanic membrane which blanches on pressure with pneumatic speculum. Management includes all except:**
   [AIIMS Nov. 01]
   a. Radiotherapy b. Surgery
   c. Interferons d. Preoperative embolization

10. **Which is the most pulsatile tumor found in external auditary meatus which bleeds on touch?** [AIIMS 95]
    a. Squamous cell ca of pinna
    b. Basal cell ca
    c. Adenoma
    d. Glomus tumor

11. **Mass in ear, on touch bleeding heavily, causes:** [DNB 01]
    a. Glomus Jugulare b. Ca mastoid
    c. Acoustic neuroma d. Angiofibroma

12. **Most common bony tumour of middle ear is:** [UP 07]
    a. Adenocarcinoma b. Squamous cell carcinoma
    c. Glomus tumor d. Acoustic neuroma

13. **Treatment of middle ear malignancy includes:** [Mahe 07]
    a. Excision of petrous part of temporal bone
    b. Subcortical excision
    c. Modified radical mastoidectomy
    d. None of the above

Explanations and References

1. Ans. is b i.e. Hypotympanum
Ref. Dhingra 5/e, p 120, 6/e, p 109

Glomus tumor is of 2 types:

Glomus jugulare	Glomus tympanicum
Arises from: • Dome of jugular bulb • Hypotympanum *Invades:* • Jugular foramen therefore involves cranial nerves IX to XII and compresses jugular vein *Clinical features:* • Signs of compression of cranial nerves IX to XII	*Arises from:* Promontory of middle ear *Clinical features:* • Aural symptoms sometimes with facial paralysis

2. Ans. is a i.e. Pulsatile tinnitus
Ref. Dhingra 5/e, p 120, 6/e, p 109; Current Otolaryngology 2/e, p 799, 3/e, p 815

"The two most common presenting symptoms of paraganglioma of temporal bone **(Glomus tumor)**[Q] are **conductive hearing loss**[Q] **and pulsatile tinnitus**[Q]"
– Current Otolaryngology 3/e, p 815

Hearing loss is conductive and slowly progressive Tinnitus is **pulsatile**[Q] and of **swishing character**[Q], **synchronous with pulse**[Q], and can be **temporarily stopped by carotid pressure**[Q].

Thus, both pulsatile tinnitus and deafness are seen in glomus tumor.

According to Turner 10/e, p 214

"The earliest symptom of a glomus tumor is pulsatile tinnitus."

3. Ans. is d i.e. Glomus jugulare tumor
Ref. Dhingra 5/e, p 120, 6/e, p 109

Pulsatile tinnitus – Seen in Glomus tumor
Pulsatile otorrhea – Seen in ASOM

4. Ans. is b, d and e i.e Arises from non-chromaffin cells; Multicentric; and Pulsatile tinnitus and conductive type of hearing loss seen
Ref. Dhingra 5/e, p 120, 6/e, p 109-110; Current Otolaryngology 2/e, p 794-800, 3/e, p 814, 815, 816

Explanation

- Glomus tumor is more common in females.
- Glomus tumor is also referred to as chemodectomy or *nonchromaffin paraganglion*.
- Glomus tumor is a benign tumor, therefore lymph node metastats is not present.
- Multicentric tumors are found in 3-10% of sporadic cases and in 25-50% of familial cases.
- Fluctuating (Pulsatile) tinnitus and conductive hearing loss are the earliest symptoms of glomus tumor.

5. Ans. is c i.e. It is a disease of infancy
Ref. Dhingra 5/e, p 120-121, 6/e, p 109-110

Let us see each option separately

Option a – *Common in females*
It is correct as females are affected five times more than males.

Option b – *Causes sensorineural deafness*
This is partially correct as glomus tumor leads to mainly conductive type hearing loss. Sensorineural hearing loss is uncommon but can occur if the tumor erodes the dense otic capsule bone and invades the inner ear.

Option c – *It is a disease of infancy*
This is incorrect as Glomus tumor is seen in middle age (40-50 years)

Option d – *It invades labyrinth, petrous pyramid and mastoid.*
This is correct

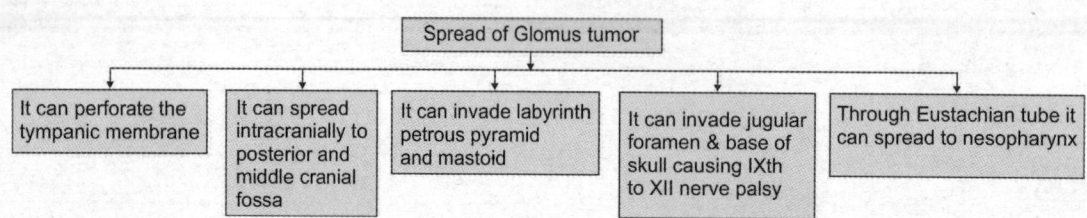

6. **Ans. is a i.e. Glomus tumor** *Ref. Dhingra 5/e, p 120, 6/e, p 109*
7. **Ans. is a i.e. Glomus jugulare** *Ref. internet search*
   Phelp's sign
   Rising sun sign are all seen in Glomus tumor
   Pulsation sign/brown sign
   Aquino sign
   Phelp sign This sign is seen on CT scan
   In CT – in case of glomus jugulare tumor the normal crest between the carotid canal and jugulare tumor is absent whereas it is not so in case of glomus tympanicum
   For details of other sign see the preceding text
8. **Ans. is d i.e. Jugular venography** *Ref. Dhingra 5/e, p 121, 6/e, p 110*
   MRI – gives soft tissue extent of tumor; Magnetic Resonance Angiography (MRA) shows compression of the carotid artery whereas magnetic resonance venography shows invasion of jugular bulb by the tumor (For more details on imaging techniques used in case of Glomus tumor – see the preceding text)

   > **Remember**
   > Preoperative biopsy is never done in case of glomus tumor as it can lead to bleeding.

9. **Ans. is c i.e. Interferons** *Ref. Dhingra 5/e, p 121, 6/e, p 110; Current Otolaryngology 2/e, p 801, 802*

   Patient presenting with progressive deafness, tinnitus and bleeding from ear
   +
   Red swelling behind the intact tympanic membrane (i.e. rising sun sign)
   +
   Swelling blanches on pressure with pneumatic speculum (i.e. Brown's sign)
   ↓
   Indicate Glomus tumor as the diagnosis

   Management options for Glomus tumor

Surgery	Radiotherapy	Embolization

Microsurgical total tumor removal is the TOC	• Does not cure the tumor
	• Reduces the vascularity of tumor and arrests its growth
	• Used for
	  – Inoperable tumor
	  – Residual tumor
	  – Recurrences after surgery
	  – Elderly patients
		• Pre-operative embolization after digital substraction angiography, reduces the vascularity of the tumor prior to surgery
		• Used as sole treatment in inoperable cases who have received prior radiotherapy

10. **Ans. is None or d i.e. Glomus tumor** *Ref. Turner 10/e, p 215; Dhingra 5/e, p 120, 6/e, p 109*
    It is worth noting here that though the glomus tumor is the neoplasm of middle ear, it may perforate the tympanic membrane and appears as a polypus in the *external auditory* meatus which bleeds profusely if touched.
11. **Ans. is a i.e. Glomus Jugulare** *Ref. Dhingra 5/e, p 120, 6/e, p 109*
    The answer to this question is quite obvious as Glomus tumors are highly vascular tumors and bleed on Touch.
12. **Ans. is b i.e. Squamous cell carcinoma**
13. **Ans. is a and c i.e. Excision of petrous part of temporal bone; and Modified radical mastoidectomy**
    Ref. Dhingra 5/e, p 122-123, 6/e, p 110-111
    Most common malignant tumor of middle ear and mastoid is **squamous cell carcinoma**.

    ### Clinical Features
    - It affects age group 40–60 years
    - Slightly more common in females
    - Most important predisposing cause is long standing CSOM
    - Patient may present with chronic foul smelling blood stained discharge
    - Pain is severe and comes at night.
    - Facial palsy may be seen
    - **O/E** – Friable, hemorrhagic granulation or polyp are present.
    - **Diagnosis** – made only on biopsy

    CT and angiography are done to see the extent of disease.
    Metastasis occurs to cervical lymph nodes later.
    Treatment of carcinoma of middle ear is combination of surgery followed by radiotherapy.
    Surgery consists of radical mastoidectomy/subtotal or total petrosectomy depending on the extent of tumor.

Chapter 13

Rehabilitative Methods

HEARING AIDS

Hearing aids are devices to amplify sounds reaching the ear. Suitable for patients with conductive hearing loss. In SNHL, there may be distortion of sound due to recruitment.

Hearing Aid Components

Microphone	Amplifier	Receiver
Collects the sound & transforms into electric energy	Intensifies electrical impulses	Electrical impulses translated to louder sounds

Types of Hearing Aid

- **Conventional type:** Increases the volume of all incoming sounds with minor adjustments.
- **Programmable analogue:** Programmed by computer, has some flexibility for adjustment based on preferences and listening environment.
- **Digital type:** The software is programmed by an audiologist to allow dramatic flexibility in adjustments. Soft sounds are distinguished from loud sounds. Clarity is enhanced.

Hearing Aid Styles

Hearing Aid Styles

Completely in the canal (CIC)
- Smallest type
- Used for mild to moderate hearing loss
- Most difficult to
- Place and adjust.

In the canal type (ITC)
- Larger than CIC
- Used for mild to moderate hearing loss
- Easier to use.

In the ear type (ITE)
- Larger than ITC
- Fills the bowl of the ear
- Used for wide variety of hearing impairment
- Easier to use than CIC and ITC.

Contd...

Contd...

Behind the ear (BTE)
- Circuit and the microphone fit behind the ear
- Used for wide range of hearing loss
- Good for children.

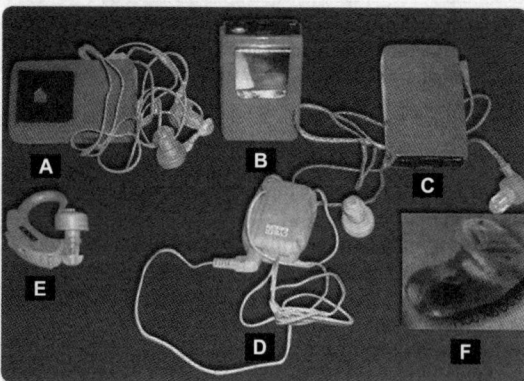

Fig. 13.1: Various types of hearing aids. A, B, C, D—Pocket model type; E–Postaural type; F–In the canal type of the hearing
Courtesy: TB of ENT, BS Tuli 2/e, p 128, Jaypee Brothers Medical Publishers Pvt. Ltd.

Indications

- **Absolute Indication:** Congenital deafness, for proper development of speech and language:
  - Patient who has hearing problem which is not treatable by medical or surgical methods.
  - Conductive deafness patients who do not want surgery/unfit for surgery.

 Point to Remember

In SNHL: Results are not very good particularly in those with recruitment positive.

Disadvantages of conventional hearing aids

- Cosmetically unacceptable due to visibility.
- Acoustic feedback.
- Spectral distortion.
- Occlusion of external auditory canal.
- Collection of wax in the canal and blockage of insert.
- Sensitivity of canal skin to earmoulds.
- Problem to use in discharging ears.

Chapter 13: Rehabilitative Methods

BONE ANCHORED HEARING AID (BAHA)

Newer Advanced Hearing Aid

It acts by directly stimulating cochlea, bypassing external and middle ear since it is anchored to bone. Thus it is useful in patients with conductive hearing loss with good cochlear function.

BAHA device is anchored to the bone of deaf side ear. It collects sound waves and by means of bone conduction transmits it to the cochlea of other side.

Indications for BAHA

1. When air-conduction (AC) hearing aid cannot be used:
   - *Canal atresia, congenital malformation of ear not amenable to treatment.*
   - *Chronic ear discharge, not amenable to treatment.*
   - *Excessive feedback and discomfort from air-conduction hearing aid.*
2. Conductive or mixed hearing loss, e.g. otosclerosis and tympanosclerosis where surgery is contraindicated.
3. Single-sided hearing loss.

NEW PATTERN QUESTIONS

Q N1. A 1-year-child with anotia (absence of Pinna) on right side is brought by the parents to ENT clinic with concern of hearing loss on right side. What is the best device in such a case, if hearing loss is confirmed?
   a. Cochlear implant immediately
   b. Cochlear implant at 6 years
   c. BAHA immediately
   d. BAHA at 6 years of age

Q N2. Ideal time for treatment of hearing loss for language development is:
   a. 6 months
   b. 1 year
   c. 2 years
   d. 3 years

Q N3. Bone anchored hearing aid is composed of all of the following *except*:
   a. Titanium implant
   b. Receiver
   c. External abutment
   d. Sound processor

VIBRANT SOUND BRIDGE/IMPLANTABLE HEARING AID

It is an implantable hearing aid which directly stimulates the ossicles, bypassing external ear and tympanic membrane. The implanted part consists of transducer attached to incus.

Candidate Profile

Appropriate candidates for direct drive middle ear hearing devices include adult aged 18 years and older with moderate-to-severe sensorineural hearing loss. Candidates should have experience of using traditional hearing aids and should have a desire for an alternative hering system.

Advantage

Better sound quality and less wax related problems and less feedback.

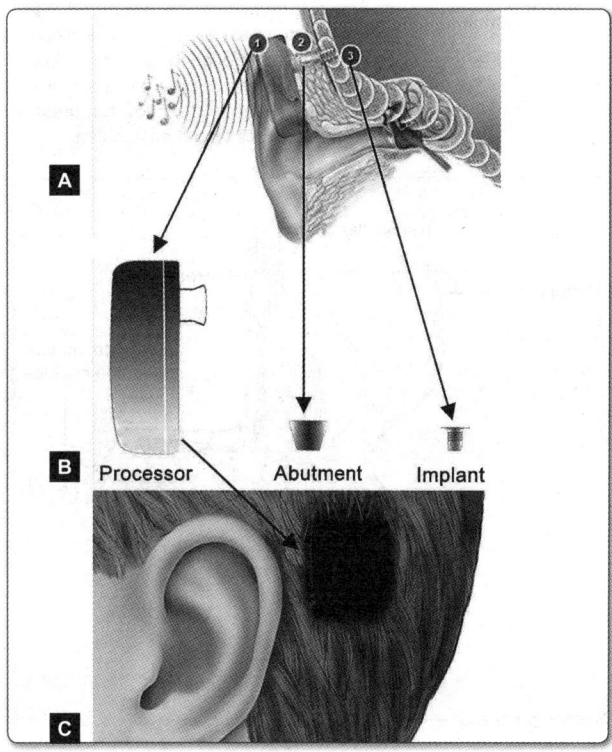

Figs. 13.2A to C: BAHA (A) BAHA system; (B) BAHA parts; (C) BAHA processor in position

Courtesy: Essentials of Mohan Bansal, p 80, Jaypee Brothers Medical Publishers Pvt. Ltd.

COCHLEAR IMPLANTS

Cochlear Implant

It is an electronic device that converts the mechanical sound energies into electrical signals that can be directly delivered into the auditory nerve in severe or profoundly hearing impaired individuals, who cannot benefit from hearing aids (i.e. it bypasses the cochlea). In other words cochlear implant replaces the organ of corti.

Indications

- B/L severe hearing loss (> 70 dB)
- Patients not benefitted by hearing aids given for severe sensorineural hearing loss
- Auditory neuropathy
- Mondini aplasia.

Components of Implants

External component	Internal component
• Microphone • Speech processor • Transmitter • **It remains outside the body**	• Receiver/stimulator (implanted under the skin) • Electrode is implanted in ↓ Scale tympani of the cochlea^Q via cochleostomy and if is not possible it can be assessed through the round window It may be placed at other locations like promontory or round window but these are inferior locations than cochlea.

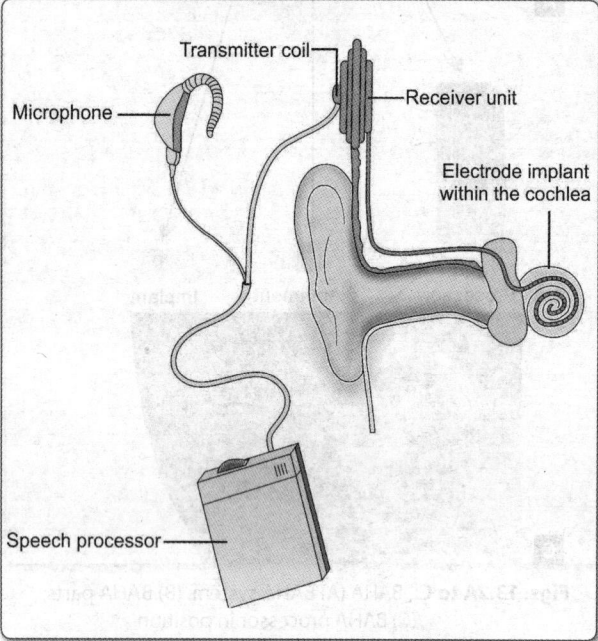

Fig. 13.3: Parts of cochlear implant
Courtesy: Textbook of ENT, BS Tuli 2/e, p 129

Current cochlear devices are FDA approved for implantation in children 12 months and older, with no upper age restrictions. Furthermore, it has been shown that outcomes in adults > 65 years are no better or no worse than those in young adults. The earlier the implantation is done in children, the more favorable the results.

Prerequisites
- Intact VIII nerve and higher auditory pathways
- **At least 1 year of age**
- Postlingual deaf patients tend to do better than prelingual deafs
- The patient should have a speech discrimination score of less than 50%.

 Point to Remember

Surgical approach to place the electrode:
➢ M/C used is facial recess approach (posterior tympanotomy).
➢ Recently Vera technique is gaining popularity.

Contraindications: Deafness due to—
- Absence of cochlea or lesions of cochlea
- Absent cochlear nerve.

Remember: Cochlear implant was invented by Dr William F. House.

NEW PATTERN QUESTIONS

Q N4. Following implantation of cochlear implant, activation of the device is done after:
  a. 1 week   b. 1 day
  c. 2 weeks   d. 3-4 weeks

Q N5. All of the following investigations are done before implanting cochlear implant *except*:
  a. CT
  b. MRI
  c. Pure tone audiometry
  d. X-ray

Q N6. Cochlear implant, which is true:
  a. Not contraindicated in cochlear malformation
  b. Contraindicated in children < 5 years of age
  c. Indicated in mild-moderate hearing loss
  d. Port is inserted through oval window

AUDITORY BRAINSTEM IMPLANTS

- It is designed to **stimulate the cochlear nuclear complex in the brainstem directly by** placing the implant in the lateral recess of fourth ventricle. Such an implant is needed when both CN VIII has been severed in surgery of vestibular schwannoma. In these cases, cochlear implants are of no use.

 Point to Remember

In unilateral acoustic neuroma, ABI is not necessary as hearing is possible from the contralateral side but in bilateral acoustic neuromas as neurofibromatosis type 2 rehabilitation is required by ABI.

- **Site of implant = Lateral recess of fourth ventricle.**

 Note:

In some patients, where auditory brainstem implant is not possible due to tumor induced damage to cochlear nucleus after acoustic neuroma surgery; Inferior colliculus of midbrain can be stimulated—This is called as **Auditory midbrain implant**.

NEW PATTERN QUESTION

Q N7. Site for placing an auditory brainstem implant:
  a. Lateral ventricle   b. Fourth ventricle
  c. Round window   d. Scala tympani

Chapter 13: Rehabilitative Methods

Explanations and References to New Pattern Questions

N1. Ans. is c i.e. BAHA immediately *Ref. Dhingra 6/e, p 122*

> BAHA is primarily suited for people who have unilateral conductive hearing loss as the device is based on bone conduction.
> In the question, child is having ANOTIA on right side (i.e. absent outer ear) with hearing loss on right side (obviously).
> In this case cochlear implants cannot be used as they are suitable for B/L hearing loss.
> BAHA is the best hearing aid in this case. Now comes at what time should it be implanted.
> At 6 years—surgical reconstruction of pinna is done, but if we wait till that time—childs speech will get affected. Hence it is better to put BAHA device as early as possible

N2. Ans. is a i.e. 6 months (Internet)

Babies with hearing loss should begin to get intervention services as soon as possible, but no later than 6 months of age.

N3. Ans. is b i.e. Receiver

BAHA use a surgically implanted abutment to transmit sound by direct conduction through bone to inner ear, by bypassing the external auditory canal and middle ear.

The device is composed of 3 main parts:

> a. A titanium implant
> b. An external abutment
> c. Sound processor

The titanium prosthesis is surgically implanted on to the mastoid bone.

N4. Ans. is d i.e 3-4 weeks *Ref. Dhingra 6/e, p 126*

> Activation of the cochlear implant is done 3-4 weeks after implantation.
> Following this, the implant is programmed (called as mapping). Mapping is done on regular basis during postoperative rehabilitation.

N5. Ans. is d i.e. X-ray *Ref. Dhingra 6/e, p 126*

> **Preoperative Investigations done before Cochlear Implant Surgery:**
> 1. For imaging of temporal bone, cochlear, auditory N and brain:
>   - CT
>   - MRI
> 2. For audiological evaluation:
>   - PTA
>   - Tympanometry
>   - Otoaccoustic emission
>   - Auditory brainstem response
>   - Auditory steady state response.
> 3. Hearing aid trial—speech perception and discrimination score
> 4. Speech aid language evaluation
> 5. Psychological evaluation
>
> **Note:** After cochlear implantation has been done, in postoperative period and later also MRI is contraindicated. CT can be done.

N6. Ans. is a i.e. Not contraindicated in cochlear malformation

- Cochlear implants are not contraindicated in cochlear malformations.
- They are contraindicated in children <12 months of age (not 5 years)
- Indicated in severe SNHL
- Port is inserted via cochleostomy and if not possible through round window.

N7. Ans. is a i.e. Lateral ventricle *Ref. Dhingra 6/e, p 127*

> See the text for explanation.

QUESTIONS

1. Which of the following would be the most appropriate treatment for rehabilitation of a patient, who has bilateral profound deafness following surgery for bilateral acoustic schwannoma: [AIIMS Nov 03]
   a. Bilateral high powered digital hearing aid
   b. Bilateral cochlear implant
   c. Unilateral cochlear implant
   d. Brainstem implant

2. A child aged 3 years, presented with severe sensorineural deafness was prescribed hearing aids, but showed no improvement. What is the next line of management:
   a. Fenestration surgery   b. Stapes mobilisation
   c. Cochlear implant   d. Conservative

3. A 10-year-old boy Rajan is having sensorineural deafness, not benefited by hearing aids. Next best management is: [AIIMS 01]
   a. Cochlear implant   b. Stapes fixation
   c. Stapedectomy   d. Fenestration

4. In cochlear implants electrodes are most commonly placed at:
   a. Oval window
   b. Round window
   c. Horizontal semicircular canal
   d. Cochlea

5. Cochlear implant is done in: [Bihar 05]
   a. Scala vestibuli
   b. Scala tympani
   c. Cochlear duct
   d. Endolymphatic duct

6. Which of the following statement regarding cochlear implant is true: [AIIMS Nov 10]
   a. Cochlear malformation is not a CI to its use
   b. Contraindicated in children < 5 yrs of age
   c. Indicated in mild-moderate hearing loss
   d. Approached through oval window

7. Cochlear implant is done if the following is intact: [AIIMS Nov 12]
   a. Outer hair cell   b. Inner hair cell
   c. Spiral ganglion cell   d. Auditory nerve

8. Contraindication of cochlear implantation is/are:
   a. Mondini deformity   [PGI May 2017]
   b. Intracochlear ossification
   c. Chronic suppurative otitis media
   d. Agenesis of cochlear nerve

9. Which intervention is best in patients operated for bilateral acoustic neuroma for hearing rehabilitation:
   a. Brainstem hearing implant   [PGI Nov 2012]
   b. Bilateral cochlear implant
   c. Unilateral cochlear implant
   d. High power hearing aid
   e. Myringoplasty

10. True about BAHA: [AIIMS May 13]
    a. Useful in canal atresia and microtia
    b. Useful in bilateral severe SNHL
    c. Useful after surgery in neurofibromatosis 2 for acoustic neuroma
    d. It can bypass cochlea

11. Father of neuro-otology is: [AIIMS May 2013]
    a. William F House
    b. Julius Lempert
    c. John Shea
    d. Hayes Martin

12. All are true about cochlear implant except: [AIIMS 2009]
    a. Minimum age is 1 year
    b. PTA of 70 dB or more
    c. Switch on is done after 3 weeks
    d. MRI has no role in preop assessment

13. A two year old child was planned for brainstem implant. All are indications of brainstem implant except: [AIIMS 2004]
    a. B/L neurofibromatosis
    b. Absent auditory nerves
    c. Absent cochlea
    d. Mondini deformity

14. Which of the following part of cochlear implant is implanted during surgery: [AIIMS May 2014]
    a. Receiver stimulator   b. Transmitting coil
    c. Microphone   d. Speech processor

15. What is placed during surgery for cochlear implant: [AIIMS Nov 2013]
    a. Microphone   b. Speech processor
    c. Transmitting coil   d. Receiver stimulator

Explanations and References

1. **Ans. is d i.e. Brainstem implant** *Ref. Harrison 17/e, p 204*

Hearing loss	Rehabilitative measure
• Conductive hearing loss	• Corrective surgery/Hearing aids
• Mild/moderate SNHL	• Hearing aids
• Bilateral severe to profound SNHL with word recognition score < 30%	• Cochlear implants
• Bilateral damage to eight nerve by trauma /bilateral vestibular schwannoma	• Brainstem auditory implants (placed near cochlear nucleus)

2. **Ans. is c i.e. Cochlear implant** *Ref. Dhingra 5/e, p 139, 6/e, p 125; Current Otolaryngology 2/e, p 882*

3. **Ans. is a i.e. Cochlear implant**

   B/L severe or profound hearing loss not benefited by hearing aid it is an indication for use of cochlear implants.

4. **Ans. is b i.e. Round window** *Ref. Dhingra 5/e, p 140, 6/e, p 126*

5. **Ans. is b i.e. Scala tympani**

   M/C Surgical approach for placing cochlea implant = Facial Recess approach (Posterior tympanotomy) which involves doing a cortical mastoidectomy. From the middle ear the electrodes are then introduced into the **scala tympani** through the **round window**. Recently Veria technique (Non-mastoidectomy technique) is gaining popularity for cochlear implantation. It uses transcanal approach.

   ### Advantage of Vera technique
   - Simple
   - Less chances of injuring facial nerve
   - Suitable in young children where mastoid has not developed fully
   - Minimal bone trauma ∴ fast healing and less complication rate

6. **Ans. is a i.e. Cochlear malformation is not a CI to its use** *Ref. Current Otolaryngology 3/e, p 856; Dhingra 5/e, p 139, 140*

   ### Explanation
   - As discussed earlier Cochlear implants are useful in B/L severe to profound hearing loss and not in mild-moderate hearing loss
     ∴ **Option C is incorrect** *Ref. Dhingra 6/e, p 125*
   - Cochlear implants can be implanted in children at 12 months of age, rather early implantation gives better results.
     Ref. Dhingra 5th/ed, p 139, 6th/ed, p 125

     "*The timing of implantation is very important*. Earlier implantation in children generally yields more favorable results and many centers roultinely implant children under 12 months of age." *Ref. Current Otolaryngology 3/e,, p 856.*
     So friends—Option b—C/I in children < 5 years of age is incorrect.
   - Approach for cochlear implants is via facial recess, where a simple cortical mastoidectomy is done first and short process of incus and lateral semicircular canal is identified.
     The facial recess is operated by performing a posterior tympanotomy. A cochleostomy is then done inferior to round window (Not oval window) with the goal of affording access to scale tympani (where the electrode has to be placed).
     Thus option d i.e. it is approached through oval window is incorrect.
     So by exclusion are answer is a i.e. cochlear malformation is not a contradiction to its use.

7. **Ans. is d i.e. Auditory nerve** *Ref. TB of Mohan Bansal, Textbook of Diseases of Ear, Nose and Throat 1/e, p 178*

   ### Cochlear Implants
   "*They are indicated for patients of profound binaural SNHL (with nonfunctional cochlear hair cells) who have intact auditory nerve functions and show little or no benefit from hearing aids.*" *Ref. Mohan Bansal 1/e, p 178*

8. **Ans. is b, c and d i.e. Intracochlear ossification, CSOM and agenesis of cochlear nerve**
   Cochlear Implantation

Contraindications

Absolute	Relative
• Cochlear nerve aplasia (option d) • Complete agenesis of cochlea (i.e. Michael aplasia) (option a ruled out) • Severe mental disease/mental retardation such that patient is unable to cooperate with speech training	• Significant intracochlear ossification (option b) • Active chronic otitis media (option c) • Medical contraindications like pulmonary, cardiac conditions, uncontrolled epilepsy etc • Post lingually deaf adult

Note: **In mondini dysplasia**
The cochlea has 1.5 turns or only basal coil is present. The condition can be unilateral or bilateral
In Mondini dysplasia, cochlear implant has given excellent results.

> **Remember**
> Michael Aplasia = cochlear implant contraindicated
> Mondini dysplasia = cochlear implant not contraindicated
> CSOM – cochlear implant contraindicated
> Serous/secretory otitis media – cochlear implant not contraindicated.

9. Ans. a i.e. Brainstem hearing implant   *Ref. Dhingra 6/e, p 127*

Auditory brainstem implant (ABI)

"This implant is designed to stimulate the cochlear nuclear complex in the brainstem directly by placing the implant in the lateral recess of the fourth ventricle. Such an implant is needed when CN VIII has been severed in surgery of vestibular schwannoma. In these cases, cochlear implants are obviously of no use".

"In unilateral acoustic neuroma, auditory brainstem implant (ABI) is not necessary as hearing is possible from the contralateral side but in bilateral acoustic neuroma as in neurofibromatosis-2, rehabilitation is required by ABI"   *Ref. Dhingra 6/e, p127*

Note: Brainstem implant is currently used only in patients with NF-2 and is always implanted simultaneously with tumor removal (usually during excision of the patient's second tumor). *It is useful in patients who have had both cochleovestibular nerves sacrificed, since this implant stimulates the cochlear nuclear complex in the brainstem directly.*

10. Ans. is a i.e. Useful in canal atresia and microtia   *Ref. Dhingra 6/e, p 122, 123*

BAHA: Bone anchored hearing aid is a type of hearing aid which is based on the principle of bone conduction. BAHA uses a surgically implanted abutment to transmit sound by direct conduction through bone to cochlea, bypassing the external auditory canal and middle ear.

> **Indications for BAHA**
> • When air-conduction (AC) hearing aid cannot be used:
>   – Canal atresia, congenital or acquired, not amenable to treatment.
>   – Chronic ear discharge, not amenable to treatment.
>   – Excessive feedback and discomfort from air-conduction hearing aid.
> • Conductive or mixed hearing loss, e.g. otosclerosis and tympanosclerosis where surgery is contraindicated.
> • Single-sided hearing loss.

Note: For severe bilateral SNHL—Cochlear implant is used.
For bilateral acoustic neuromas in Neurofibromatosis – auditory brainstem implant is used.

11. Ans. is a i.e. William F House   *Ref: Internet search*

12. Ans. is d i.e. MRI has no role in preop assessment
Lets see each option separately
Option a: Minimum age 1 year– correct
Option b: PTA of 70% dB or more – correct as cochlear implant is useful in B/L severe hearing loss > 70 dB.
Option c: Switch on is done after 3 weeks – correct. Remember after placing an implant, a gap of 2–3 weeks is given for the wound to heal before the implant is to activated. Activation does not produce instant hearing.
Option d: MRI has no role is preop assessment – incorrect

Chapter 13: Rehabilitative Methods

> Preop investigation done before an implant is placed:
> - Complete audiological evaluation
> - HRCT
> - MRI.

13. Ans. is d i.e. Mondini deformity *Ref: Dhingra 6/e, p 115*

In Mondini deformity the defect is at the level of cochlea, which can be corrected by cochlear implant.

14. Ans. is a i.e. Receiver stimulator *Ref: Dhingra 6/e, p 124*

15. Ans. d i.e. Receiver stimulator *Ref. Dhingra 4/e, p 121-123*

A cochlear implant has an external and internal component *Dhingra 6/e, p124*

> **Receiver/Stimulator** *(Implanted* **under the skin)** *and* **Electrode array** *(implanted in the* **scala tympani of the cochlea)** *are the part of* **internal component of cochlear implant,** *which are fitted* **inside the body.**

Microphone, Speech-processor and Transmitter are the part of **external component of cochlear implant,** which remain **outside the body.**

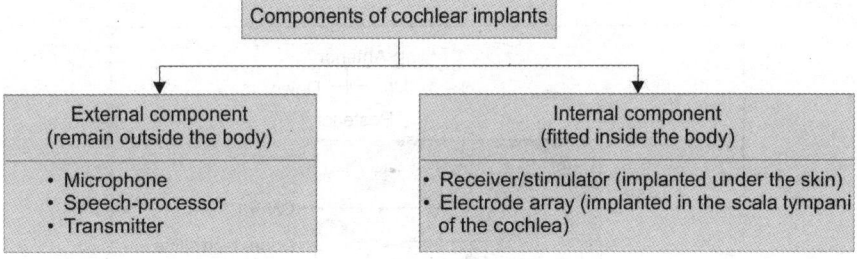

Chapter 14

Miscellaneous

1. **Citelli's angle is:**
   a. Sold angle
   b. CP angle
   c. Sinodural angle
   d. Part of MC Evans triangle

   Ans. is c i.e. Sinodural angle
   Ref. Dhingra 6/e, p 402; Fig. 79.5
   As seen from the figure Citelli's angle is Sinodural angle

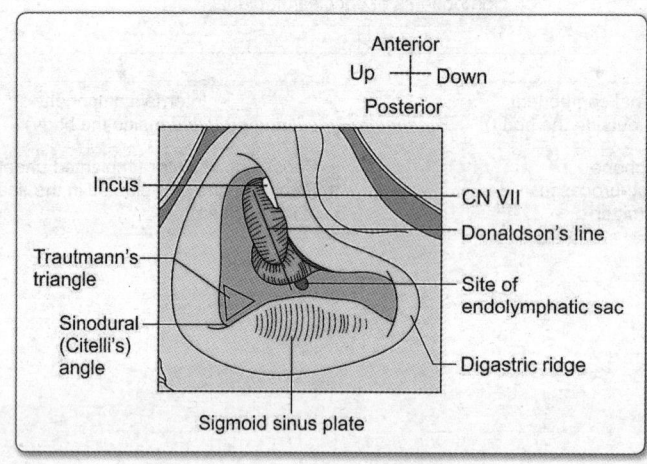

2. **Which of the following is a feature of tympanic membrane perforation (printed esophageal rupture in paper)?** [UP 00]
   a. Tinnitus
   b. Vertigo
   c. Conductive deafness
   d. Fullness in ear

   Ans. is c i.e. Conductive deafness
   Ref. Dhingra 5/e, p 34; Turner 10/e, p 284
   Tympanic membrane perforation is associated with a conductive hearing loss of 10–40 dB.

3. **Use of Siegel's speculum during examination of the ear provides all except:**
   a. Magnification
   b. Assessment of movement of the tympanic membrane
   c. Removal of foreign body from the ear
   d. As applicator for the powdered antibiotic of ear

   Ans. is c i.e. Removal of foreign body
   Ref. Dhingra 5/e, p 383; SR Mowson Disease of Ear 4/e, p 93-94; Maqbool 11/e, p 34

   Uses of Siegel's Pneumatic Speculum

   Mnemonic: 3T - 3 M

   3T's are:
   - Fistula **t**est
   - Gelle's **t**est
   - Powder **t**est

   3M's are:
   - For **m**agnification
   - For instillation of **m**edicines into middle ear
   - To assess the **m**obility of tympanic membrane

    Note: Periphery of tympanic membrane has maximum mobility[Q].

Chapter 14: Miscellaneous

4. **The focal length of the mirror used in head lamp:** [APPGI 06]
   a. 85 mm
   b. 150 mm
   c. 250 mm
   d. 400 mm

   Ans. is c i.e. 250 mm Ref. Dhingra 5/e, p 379
   - Head mirror is a concave mirror used to reflect light from the bull's eye lamp onto the part being examined
   - It has focal length of ~ 25 cm (= 10 inch) The examiner sees through the hole in the center of the mirror
   - Diameter of central hole = 19 mm (3/4 inch)

5. **Focal length of head mirror used in ENT-OPD:** [Bihar 2005]
   a. 9 inch
   b. 10 inch (25 cm)
   c. 11 inch
   d. 12 inch

   Ans. is b i.e. 10 inch (25 cm) Ref. Dhingra 4/e, p 336, 5/e, p 379

6. **Diameter of head mirror in ENT is:** [Bihar 2005]
   a. 20 cm
   b. 22 cm
   c. 10 cm
   d. 26 cm

   Ans. is c i.e. 10 cm Ref. Dhingra 4/e, p 336, 5/e, p 379
   Diameter of the head mirror used in ENT is 89 mm (3 and half inch).

7. **Impedance denotes:** [PGI 99]
   a. Site of perforation
   b. Disease of cochlea
   c. Disease of ossicles
   d. Higher function disorder

   Ans. is c i.e. Disease of ossicles Ref. Tuli 1/e, p 35
   "Impedance audiometry, measures the resistance of tympanic membrane and middle ear and also compliance of tympanic membrane and ossicular chain to sound pressure transmission. Tympanogram is the graphic representation of compliance and impedance of tympanic ossicular system with air pressure changes."
   From above text it is quite obvious that impedance is for disease of ossicles.

8. **During normal conversation sound heard at 1 meter distance is:** [Bihar 2004, 05]
   a. 80 dB
   b. 60 dB
   c. 90 dB
   d. 120 dB

   Ans. is b i.e. 60 dB Ref. Dhingra 4/e, p 20, 5/e, p23

Whisper	30 dB
Normal conversation	60 dB
Shout	90 dB
Discomfort of the ear	120 dB
Pain in the ear	130 dB

9. **Prolonged exposure to noise levels greater than the following can impair hearing permanently:** [Karnat 96]
   a. 40 decibels
   b. 85 decibels
   c. 100 decibels
   d. 140 decibels

   Ans. is c i.e. 100 decibels Ref. Park 19/e, p 599

   "Repeated or continuous exposure to noise around 100 decibels may result in a permanent hearing loss." Ref. Park 19th/e, p 599
   "A noise of 90 dB SPL, 8 hours a day for 5 days per week is the maximum safe limit as recommended by Ministry of Labour, Govt of India-rules under Factories Act." Ref. Dhingra 4/e, p 35; 5/e, p 40

    Note: Impulse noise (single time exposure) of more than 140 dB is not permitted.

10. **A man Rajan, age 70 years, presents with tinnitus. Most probable diagnosis is:** [AIIMS Nov 00]
    a. Acoustic neuroma
    b. ASOM
    c. Labyrinthitis
    d. Acoustic trauma

    Ans. is a i.e. Acoustic neuroma Ref. Dhingra – read below

Condition	Points in favor	Points against
Acoustic neuroma	Presenting symptom • Tinnitus • Age of patient	Associated with SNHL hearing loss (which is not given in the question) • No history of ear ache, fever and hearing loss • Tinnitus is not the presenting symptom

Condition	Points in favor	Points against
ASOM *(Dhingra 4th/ed p 61)*	Tinnitus may be seen in stage of presuppuration	• It is common in infants and children
Labyrinthitis	Tinnitus may be seen	• Tinnitus is not seen
Acoustic trauma		• No history of trauma • It is associated with varying degree of hearing loss which is not given

Amongst the options given, acoustic neuroma is the best option here. If presbycuses would have been given in the options, we would have chosen it

11. Gustatory sweating and flushing (Frey's syndrome) follows damage to the: [JIPMER 80; DNB 91]
   a. Trigeminal nerve
   b. Facial nerve
   c. Glossopharyngeal nerve
   d. Vagus nerve
   e. Auriculotemporal nerve

   Ans. is e i.e. Auriculotemporal nerve *Ref. Maqbool 11/e, p 276; S. Das Short Cases of Clinical Surgery 3/e, p 82*

   Auriculotemporal syndrome (Syn. Frey's Syndrome)
   Partial injury to the auriculotemporal nerve gives rise to such syndrome. This type of injury:
   - May be congenital, possibly due to birth trauma.
   - May be accidental injury.
   - May be caused by inadvertent incision for drainage of parotid abscess.
   - May occasionally follow superficial parotidectomy.

   Clinical features: There is flushing and sweating of the skin innervated by the auriculotemporal nerve particularly during meal and presence of cutaneous hyperesthesia in front and above (the ear the area supplied by the auriculotemporal nerve.)

   The Explanation of this syndrome is:
   – The postganglionic parasympathetic fibers become united to the sympathetic nerves from the superior cervical ganglion which are concerned to supply vessels and sweat glands of that region. This causes flushing and sweating of the skin.
   – Following injury to the auriculotemporal nerve, postganglionic parasympathetic fibers from the otic ganglion grow down the sheaths of the cutaneous filaments, so hyperesthesia follows stimulation of the secretomotor nerves.

   Treatment: If the symptoms persist, the treatment is avulsion of the auriculotemporal nerve in front of the auricle where it lies just posterior to the superficial temporal vessels.

12. A patient has bilateral conductive deafness, tinnitus with positive family history. The diagnosis: [AIIMS 93]
   a. Otospongiosis
   b. Tympanosclerosis
   c. Menitere's disease
   d. Bilateral otitis media

   Ans. is a i.e. Otospongiosis *Ref. Dhingra 5/e, p 97-98*

13. Presbycusis is: [TN 2007, 205]
   a. Loss of accommodation power
   b. Hearing loss due to aging
   c. Noise induced hearing loss
   d. Congenital deafness

   Ans. is b i.e. Hearing loss due to aging *Ref. Dhingra 5/e, p 41; Scott-Brown's Otolaryngology 7/e, vol 3,Chap 238 p 3539*
   It is mid to late adult onset, bilateral, progressive sensorineural hearing loss, where underlying causes have been excluded.

14. Second primary tumor of head and neck is most commonly seen in malignancy of: [AIIMS May 2012]
   a. Oral cavity
   b. Larynx
   c. Hypopharynx
   d. Paranasal sinuses

   Ans. is a i.e. Oral cavity *Ref. Internet search*
   - Patients with **head and neck squamous cell carcinoma (HNSCC)** are at increased risk for the development of second primary malignancies compared with the general population.
   - These second primary malignancies typically develop in the **aerodigestive tract** (lung, head and neck, esophagus).
   - The most frequent second primary malignancy is lung cancer.
   - The highest relative increase in risk is for a second head and neck cancer.
   - The site of the index cancer influences the most likely site of a second primary malignancy.
     – In patients with an index malignancy of the larynx, the second primary tumor was commonly seen in lung, while
     – In patients with an index malignancy of the oral cavity, the second primary tumor was commonly seen in head and neck or esophagus.

   The criteria for classifying a tumor as a second primary malignancy are:
   - Histologic confirmation of malignancy in both the index and secondary tumors.
   - There should be at least 2 cm of normal mucosa between the tumors. If the tumors are in the same location, then they should be separated in time by at least five years.
   - Metastatic tumor should be excluded.

SECTION 2

Nose and Paranasal Sinuses

Section Outline

15. Anatomy and Physiology of Nose
16. Diseases of External Nose and Nasal Septum
17. Granulomatous Disorders of Nose, Nasal Polyps and Foreign Body in Nose
18. Inflammatory Disorders of Nasal Cavity
19. Epistaxis
20A. Diseases of Paranasal Sinus—Sinusitis
20B. Diseases of Paranasal Sinus—Sinonasal Tumor

CHAPTER 15

Anatomy and Physiology of Nose

ANATOMY OF NOSE

Nose consists of:
- External nose
- Internal nose consisting of
  - Nasal vestibule
  - Nasal cavity

■ EXTERNAL NOSE

External nose is a pyramidal structure and its skeletal framework is made of bone and cartilage. The upper angle of the nose where it is continuous with forehead is called as **root of the nose**. The base of the nose which is directed downwards has 2 openings called **anterior nares or nostrils**. The two nares are separated by the **columella**. These nares lead to skin lined part of the nasal cavities called as **vestibule of the nose**.

Skeletal framework of external nose: It consists of upper 1/3rd bony part and lower 2/3rd cartilaginous part.
A. Bony part consists of:
   1. Paired nasal bone
   2. Paired frontal process of the maxilla
   3. Nasal process of the frontal bone.

The nasal bone articulates with the nasal process of the frontal bone superiorly, frontal process of the maxilla laterally, inferiorly with the upper lateral cartilage and medially with nasal bone of the other side. The junction between the two nasal bones forms the **nasal bridge**.

B. Cartilaginous part is made of following cartilages:
   1. Paired upper lateral cartilage
   2. Paired lower lateral cartilage (alar cartilage)
   3. Paired sesamoid cartilage
   4. Unpaired anterior part of septal cartilage.

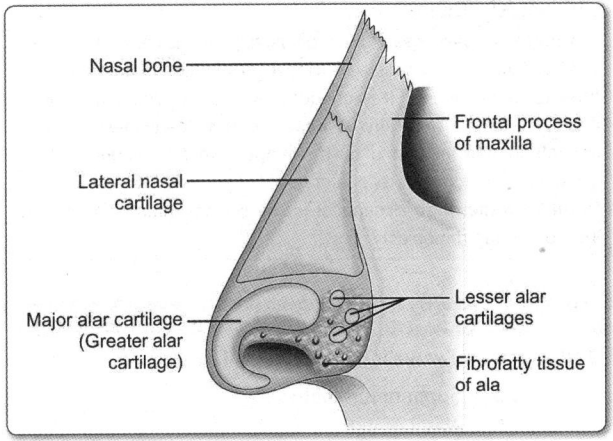

Fig. 15.1: Skeletal framework of external nose

Muscles of external nose are procerus and nasalis consisting of compressor and dilator naris. These muscles are *supplied by facial nerve*.
- **Nerve supply of the external nose:** Nose receives its sensory supply from the ophthalmic nerve (which supplies tip of nose) and the maxillary division of trigeminal nerve (which supplies side and ala of nose).
- **Lymphatics:** drain into submandibular and preauricular group of lymph nodes.

> **Points to Remember**
> - Nose is made of 4 cartilages (mainly hyaline)—3 paired (upper lateral, lower lateral or alar cartilage, sesamoid cartilage) and one unpaired (i.e. septal) cartilage.
> - Sesamoid cartilages or lesser alar cartilages may be 2 or more in number and are present just lateral to lower lateral cartilages.
> - The alar cartilage is a U shaped and comprises of medial and lateral crus. The medial crura of two sides meets in midline to from the **columella**. The lateral crura are the lower lateral catilages.
> - **Rhinion**—the point where the lower end of internasal suture meets with the lower cartilaginous part of the nose.
> - The groove between upper and lower lateral cartilages is called **Limen nasi** which is the site for inter cartilaginous incision.
> - The septal cartilage supports the dorsum of nose. In case of septal abscess or during submucous resection of septum when excessive septal cartilage is removed—there is **supratip depression of nose**.

NEW PATTERN QUESTIONS		
Q N1.	The shape of septal cartilage is:	
	a. Triangular	b. Quadrilateral
	c. Rectangle	d. Pyramidal
Q N2.	The part between the 2 nasal vestibules is called as:	
	a. Rhinon	b. Nasion
	c. Columella	d. Root of nose
Q N3.	Osseocartilaginous junction on the dorsum of nose is:	
	a. Nasion	b. Rhinion
	c. Columella	d. Glabella
Q N4.	Sensory epithelium of nose is derived from:	
	a. Neural crest	b. Neural tube
	c. Endoderm	d. Mesoderm

INTERNAL NOSE

The septum divides the internal nose into right and left nasal cavity.

Nasal cavity has 2 parts—anteriormost part vestibule and rest-nasal cavity proper.

Nasal Vestibule

- It is a skin lined entrance to the nasal cavity i.e. it is lined by stratified squamous epithelium.
- It contains hair follicles, hair *(called Vibrissae)*, sebaceous glands and sweat glands.

Clinical Correlation

Furuncle of nose arises from the vestibule and is called as **nasal vestibulitis**. M/c cause is staphylococcal infection of hair follicle.
Internal nasal valve: It is bounded laterally by limen nasi and inferior turbinate, **medially by nasal septum** (cartilaginous part) and inferiorly by the floor of **pyriform aperture**. It is the area of the greatest constriction of respiratory tract.
Point to remember—limennasi is the site for intercartilaginous incision during rhinoplasty.

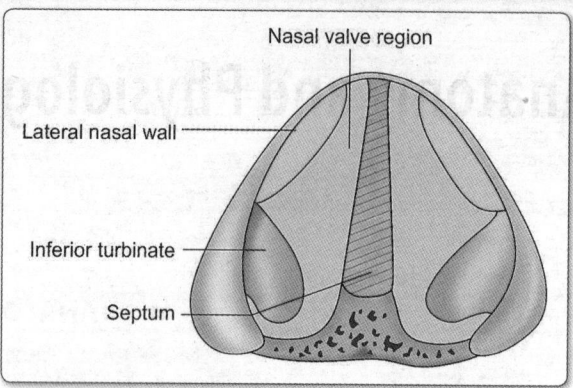

Fig. 15.2: Internal nasal valve region

- The inferior turbinate is a separate bone, while rest of the turbinates are a part of ethmoidal labyrinth.^{Q}
- Below and lateral to each turbinate is the corresponding meatus.
- Sometimes a *fourth turbinate* is also present just above superior turbinate. This fourth turbinate is known as **supreme turbinate**. Supreme (fourth) turbine is found in 30% of population.

 Point to Remember
➤ The largest turbinate is inferior turbinate.

NEW PATTERN QUESTIONS

Q N5. Nasal valve is bounded by all *except*:
a. Superior turbinate
b. Nasal septum
c. Upper lateral cartilage
d. Pyriform aperture

Q N6. Internal nasal valve is bounded by:
a. Septal cartilage
b. Lower lateral cartilage
c. Upper lateral cartilage
d. Alae

Q N7. Patency of nasal valve is checked by:
a. Caloric test   b. Rhinoscopy
c. Cottle test   d. Probing

NEW PATTERN QUESTIONS

Q N8. Which of the following is an independent bone?
a. Superior turbinate
b. Middle turbinate
c. Inferior turbinate
d. All of the above

Q N9. Supreme turbinate is another name for:
a. Superior turbinate
b. Middle turbinate
c. Inferior turbinate
d. None of the above

Q N10. Sphenopalatine foramen is related to .... turbinate:
a. Superior turbinate
b. Middle turbinate
c. Inferior turbinate
d. None of the above

Nasal Cavity

Each nasal cavity has a lateral wall, medial wall, a roof and floor.

Lining

The upper one-third of nasal cavity is lined by olfactory epithelium.

Rest of the lining is pseudostratified ciliated columnar epithelium containing mucous glands (called as **Schneiderian membrane**).

Lateral Nasal Wall

- It has 3 bony projections called as turbinates or conchae.
- The turbinates increase the surface area of nose.
- From below upward they are inferior, middle and superior turbinates.

Inferior meatus

- It is the largest meatus.
- Its highest point is the junction of anterior and middle one third.
- Nasolacrimal duct opens in the inferior meatus just anterior to its highest point *(it is closed by a mucosal flap called* **Hasner's valve**). The direction of Nasolacrimal duct is downward, backward and laterally from lacrimal sac to nose and has a length of 1.8 cm.

Chapter 15: Anatomy and Physiology of Nose

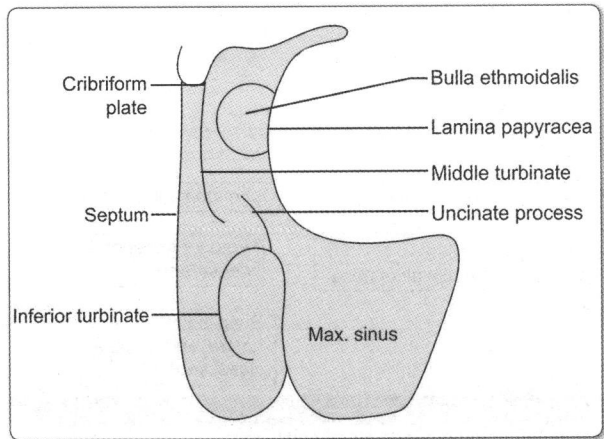

Fig. 15.3: Coronal section showing relationships of uncinate process, bulla ethmoidalis, middle turbinate, maxillary sinus, orbit and cribriform plate

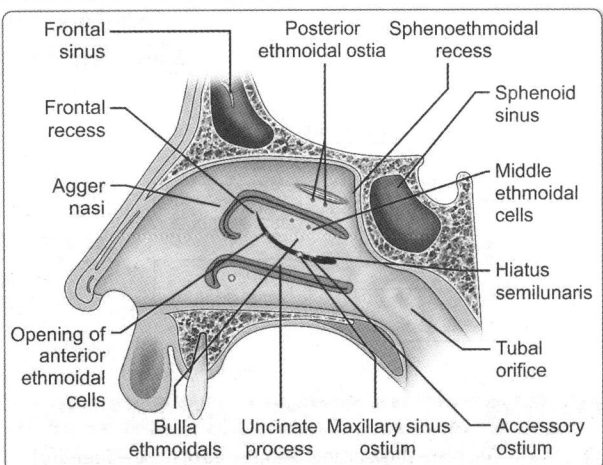

Fig. 15.4: Coronal section showing relationships of uncinate process, bulla ethmoidalis, middle turbinate, maxillary sinus, orbit and cribriform plate

Middle meatus

- Lies lateral to the middle turbinate.
- **In the middle meatus is the opening of anterior group of sinuses viz maxillary sinus, frontal sinus and anterior ethmoids.**
- The forward continuation of the middle meatus is called **atrium** of the nasal cavity.
- A curved ridge above the atrium is called the agger nasi and it may get pneumatized from the ethmoid and is known as **agger nasi air cell**.
- Just beneath the attachment of the middle turbinate, is a small thin plate of bone covered by mucoperiosteium. This sickle shaped thin bone is called the **uncinate process**.
- Posterosuperior to the uncinate process, a rounded prominence is seen called the **bulla ethmoidalis**. It represents the middle ethmoidal air cells. Below the bulla ethmoidalis, a slit-like semilunar shaped opening is present and is called as hiatus **semilunaris**. This leads to a narrow three-dimensional space between the uncinate process and the bulla ethmoidalis laterally and middle turbinate medially and is called **the ethmoidal infundibulum**.
- The frontal sinus drains into the infundibulum through the frontal recess or through the anterior ethmoidal air cells.
- The natural ostium of the maxillary sinus opens into the hiatus and is located between the anteroinferior part of the bulla and the uncinate process.
- These important structures within the middle meatus as described above constitute the **osteomeatal complex**.

Superior meatus

- It lies lateral to superior turbinate.
- Posterior ethmoidal sinus open into it.

Sphenoethmoidal recess

Lies above the superior turbinate and receives the opening of the sphenoid sinus.

 Points to Remember

- The middle turbinate is not usually pneumatised.
- Pneumatisation of middle turbinate is called **concha bullosa**.

Osteomeatal Complex Area (Picadli's Circle)

- It is that area of middle meatus where sinus ostia of anterior group of sinuses (frontal/anterior ethmoidal/maxillary) are surrounded by uncinate process, ethmoidal infundibulum and bulla ethmoidalis.
- **Structures contributing to its formation are:**
  - Uncinate – Process
  - Bulla – Ethmoidalis
  - Ethmoidal – Infundibulum
  - Hiatus – Semilunaris
  - Frontal – recess

Even a minor pathology in this area can lead to secondary sinusitis in major sinuses by obstruction to sinus ostia. ∴ This is the site of pathogenesis of sinusitis.

Ethmoidal air cells: They give a Honeycomb appearance.

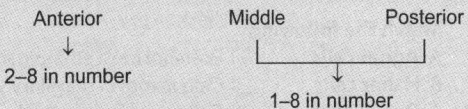

- In **anterior ethmoid** cells named are:
  - Bulla ethmoidalis
  - Agger nasi – cells anterior to attachment of middle turbinate.
  - **Haller cells:** These are ethmoidal cells in floor of orbit and root of maxillary sinus.
- In **posterior ethmoid** cells are:
  - **Onodi cells:** They, are the most posterior ethmoidal air cells. They are surgically important as they are related to optic nerve and internal carotid artery.
- The arterior ethmoidal cells open into the ethmoidal infendibulum (middle meatus).
- The middle ethmoidal cells opens into the ethmoidal bulla.
- The posterior ethmoidal cells open into the superior meatus.

Section 2: Nose and Paranasal Sinuses

Flowchart 15.1: Blood supply of nose

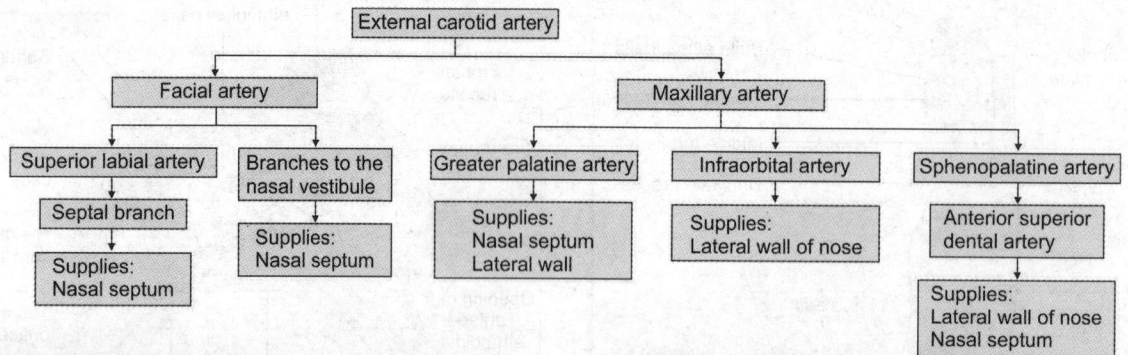

NEW PATTERN QUESTIONS

Q N11. The plate show an important area of nose—identify it:

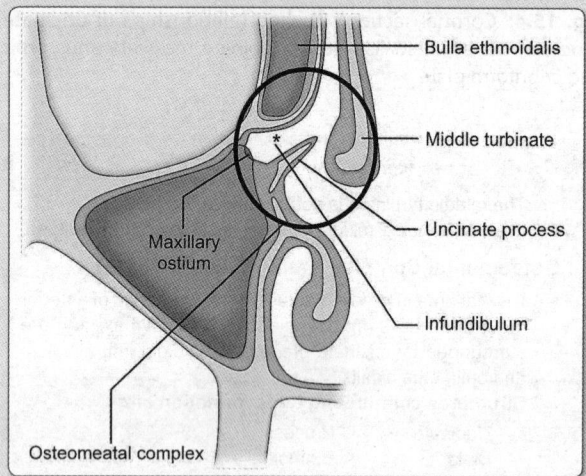

See Color Plate 10

a. Nasal valve b. Columella
c. Osteomeatal complex d. Vestibule

Q N12. All of the following drain in middle meatus *except*:
a. Maxillary sinus b. Frontal sinus
c. Ethmoidal sinus d. Nasolacrimal duct

Q N13. Match the following:
A Agger cells   I Posterior most ethmoidal cells
B Haller cells   II Cells in roof of maxillary sinus
C Onodi cells   III Cells anterior to attachment of middle turbinate
D Concha bullosa   IV Pneumatisation of middle-turbinate

a. A III B I C II D IV   b. A I B II C III D II
c. A III B II C I D IV   d. A II B III C I D IV

Medial Wall of Nose/Nasal Septum
Parts

Columellar septum
Formed by medial crura of the alar cartilage.
Membranous septum
Double layer of skin with no bony/cartilaginous support.

Septum proper
- Septal cartilage/quadrilateral cartilage
- Perpendicular plate of ethmoid
- Vomer

Other bony minor contributors are:
- Nasal spine of frontal bone
- Crest of palatine bone
- Crest of maxilla
- Rostrum of sphenoid bone

> **Point to Remember**
> ➤ Amongst all—the nasal septum is mainly formed by vomer, perpendicular plate of ethmoid and septal cartilage.

Blood Supply of Nose

The nose is supplied by both internal and external carotid artery. Main supply is by external carotid artery. A good guidline for the students to remember is that the middle turbinate is the dividing line—the area of nose above the middle turbinate is supplied by internal carotid artery (mainly) and below it by external carotid artery (mainly).

- The external carotid artery gives 2 main branches facial artery and maxillary artery (*see* Flowchart 15.1 for details).

Blood Supply of the Nasal Septum (Flowchart 15.2)

Flowchart 15.2: Blood supply of the nasal septum

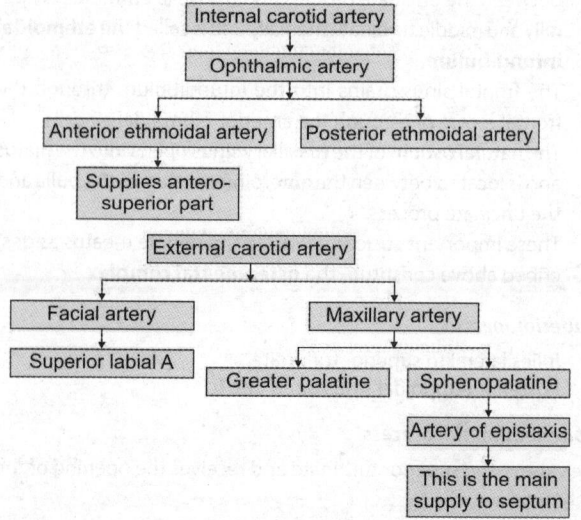

Chapter 15: Anatomy and Physiology of Nose

> **Point to Remember**
>
> ➤ **Little's area** is the most vascular area on the anteroinferior part of nasal septum. Branches of *anterior ethmoidal, sphenopalatine (artery of epitaxis), superior labial* and *greater palatine* and their corresponding veins anastomose here to form a vascular plexus called "*Kiesselbach plexus*". Blood vessels at this site lack cushioning effect and are liable to trauma causing epistaxis.

NEW PATTERN QUESTION

Q N14. Anterior ethmoidal artery arises from:
a. Maxillary artery
b. Mandibular artery
c. Superficial temporal artery
d. Ophthalmic artery

Nerve Supply of Nasal Cavity

- Nasopalatine/Branches of sphenopalatine ganglia supply *majority of the septal area.*
- Anterior ethmoidal nerve supplies the *anterosuperior part.*
- Anterior superior alveolar nerve supplies *anteroinferior portion.*
- General sensory nerves derived from the branches of trigeminal nerve are distributed to the whole of the lateral wall.

> **Point to Remember**
>
> **Secretomotor supply** of nose is through the vidian nerve (also k/a nerve of pterygoid).
> ➤ Vidian nerve is the nerve of pterygoid canal formed by the union of Superficial Petrosal nerve and Deep Pterosal nerve. This is the main parasympathetic supply of nose.

Clinical Correlation

In vasomotor rhinitis where there is an imbalance between sympathetic and parasympathetic system, one of the surgical options is Vidian Neurectomy.

Lymphatic Drainage of Nasal Cavity

- Lymphatics from external nose and *anterior part* of nasal cavity drain into **submandibular lymph nodes** while those from the *rest of nasal* cavity drain into **upper jugular nodes** either directly or through the retropharyngeal node.

IMPORTANT CLINICAL VIGNETTE

■ DANGEROUS AREA OF FACE (FIG. 15.5)

Dangerous area of face includes upper lip and anteroinferior part of nose including the vestibule. This area freely communicates with the cavernous sinus through a set of valveless veins, anterior facial vein and superior ophthalmic vein. Any infection of this area can thus travel intracranially leading to meningitis and cavernous sinus thrombosis.

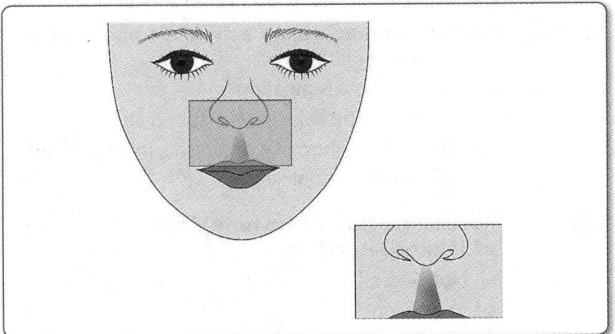

Fig. 15.5: Dangerous area of face

■ ETHMOID BONE AND NOSE

The ethmoid bone is an important bone of nose.

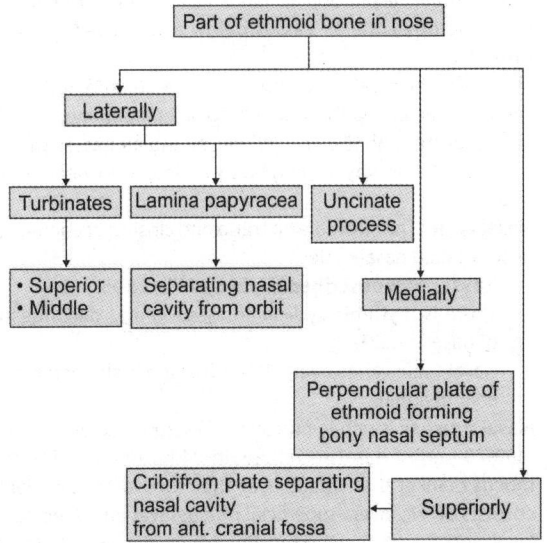

■ IMPORTANT MEASUREMENTS

- Length of nasal cavity – 8 cm
- Area of olfactory epithelium
  - 2 cm² - 5 cm²
  - Capacity of maxillary sinus - 15 cc

Gateways: There are a number of routes by which nerves and vessels enter and leave the nasal cavity—

Gateway	Structures passing through it
• Cribriform plate	• Olfactory nerve
• Sphenopalatine foramen	• Sphenopalatine branch of maxillary artery
	• Nasopalatine branch of maxillary nerve
	• Superior nasal branch of maxillary nerve
• Incisive canal	• Nasopalatine nerve (from nasal cavity to oral cavity)
	• Greater palatine artery (from oral cavity to nasal cavity)

PHYSIOLOGY OF NOSE

FUNCTIONS OF NOSE

The functions of nose are:
1. Olfaction
2. Respiration
3. Airconditioning of respired air
4. Protection of lower airway
5. Vocal resonance
6. Nasal reflex

Important points:
1. Newborns are obligatory nose breathers and therefore B/L choanal atresia may asphyxiate them to death if immediate airway management is not done
2. During quite respiration air passes between turbinates and nasal septum. Little air passes below and above the level of turbinates
3. The roof of the nasal cavity and area above superior turbinate is lined by olfactory epithelium. During quiet breathing, very little air passes through this area. While sniffing air passes through this area, that is why sniffing helps in detecting weak odours also.
4. **Nasal cycle:** The alternate opening and closing of each side of nose is called nasal cycle:
   - **Kayser first described nasal cycle in 1895**
   - There is rhythmic cyclical congestion and decongestion of nasal mucosa
   - Nasal cycle varies **every 2½–4 hrs** and is characteristic of an individual.
5. **Nasal mucosa** is rich in mucous and serous secretory glands (600-700 ml of nasal secretions in 24 hours), which form a mucus blanket that spread over the mucosa. Mucus blanket consists of two layers superficial mucus layer and deep serous layer and floats **(5–10 mm/minute)** on the cilia. Cilia beat constantly (10–20 times per second at room temperature) like a "conveyer belt" towards the nasopharynx. The complete sheet of mucus blanket reaches into the pharynx in 10–20 minutes. This viscous mucus blanket entraps bacteria, viruses and dust particles from the inspired air and carries them into pharynx and gets swallowed into stomach and digested.

6. **Kartagener's syndrome:** In this *immotile cilia syndrome* cilia are defective and cannot beat effectively and lead to stagnation of mucus. There is absence of dynein arm on the peripheral ciliary microtubules. Patient presents with triad of—
   - Chronic rhinosinusitis (mucus accumulation in nose)
   - Bronchiectasis and
   - Situs inversus
7. **Olfactory system** is an important constituent of limbic system.
   - **Olfactory receptor cells:** Olfactory epithelium in the olfactory region of nose contains millions of olfactory receptor cells, mucosal surface and expand into a ventricle that have several cilia and receive odorous substances.
   - **Olfactory nerves:** Central processes of the olfactory cells make olfactory nerves.
   - **Olfactory bulb:** Olfactory nerves pass through the cribriform plate of ethmoid and end in the mitral cells of the olfactory bulb.
   - **Olfactory tract:** Axons of mitral cells traverse in olfactory tract.
   - *Cerebrum:* Olfactory tract carries smell to the prepiriform cortex and the amygdaloid nucleus.

NEW PATTERN QUESTIONS

Q N15. Which of the following is not a function of nose?
   a. Olfaction
   b. Air pressure control
   c. Humidification of air
   d. Temperature control of inspired air

Q N16. Ciliary movement rate of nasal mucosa is:
   a. 1–2 mm/min   b. 2–5 mm/min
   c. 5–10 mm/min   d. 10–12 mm/min

Q N17. Parosmia is:
   a. Perversion of smell sensation
   b. Absolute loss of smell sensation
   c. Decreased smell sensation
   d. Perception of bad smell

Q N18. Nasal cycle is the cyclical alternate nasal blockage occurring:
   a. Every 6-12 hours   b. Every 2-4 hours
   c. Every 4-8 hours   d. Every 12-24 hours

Q N19. Function of mucociliary action of upper respiratory tract is:
   a. Temperature regulation
   b. Increased the velocity of inspired air
   c. Traps the pathogenic organisms in inspired air
   d. Has no physiological role

Q N20. Movement of mucous in nose is by:
   a. Mucociliary action
   b. Inspiration
   c. Expiration
   d. Both inspiration and expiration

Q N21. Odour receptors are present in:
   a. Olfactory epithelium   b. Olfactory tract
   c. Amygdala   d. Olfactory bulbs

Chapter 15: Anatomy and Physiology of Nose

EXAMINATION OF NOSE

ANTERIOR RHINOSCOPY

- It is done using thudichum nasal speculum (Fig. 15.6) or Vienna type speculum.
- Used to visualize nasal cavity
- Nasal cavity, septum, floor of nose, inferior and middle turbinate, inferior and middle meatuses can be visualized by it.

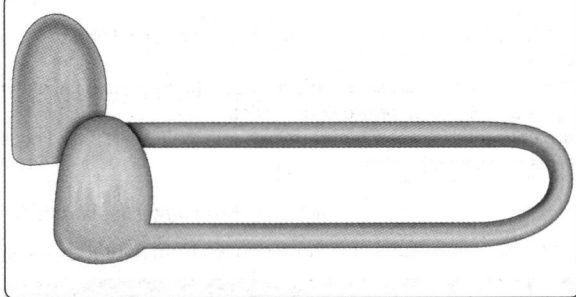

Fig. 15.6: Thudichum's nasal speculum

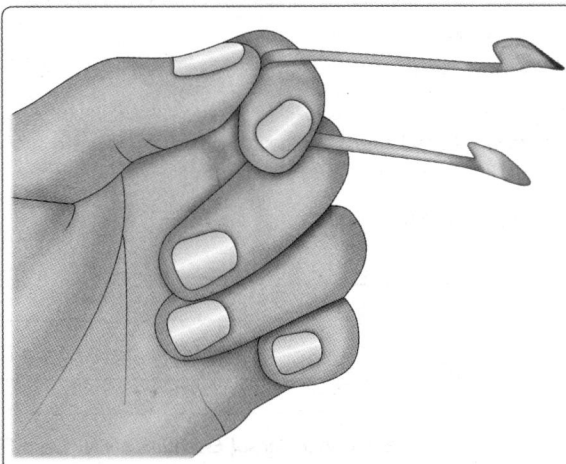

Fig. 15.7: Correct method of holding Thudichum's nasal speculum

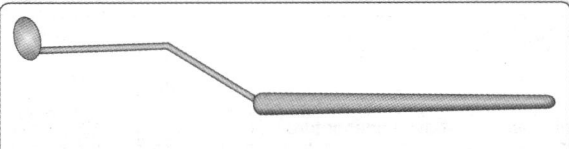

Fig. 15.8: Posterior rhinoscopy mirror

Posterior Rhinoscopy

- It consists of examining the nasopharynx and posterior part of nasal cavity by postnasal mirror
- Used to visualize posterior choanae and posterior end of inferior turbinates.

- **Structures seen on posterior rhinoscopy (Fig. 15.9):**
  - Both choanae
  - Posterior end of nasal septum
  - Opening of Eustachian tube
  - Posterior end of superior/middle and inferior turbinates
  - Fossa of Rosenmuller
  - Torus Tubarius
  - Adenoids
  - Roof and posterior wall and nasopharynx.

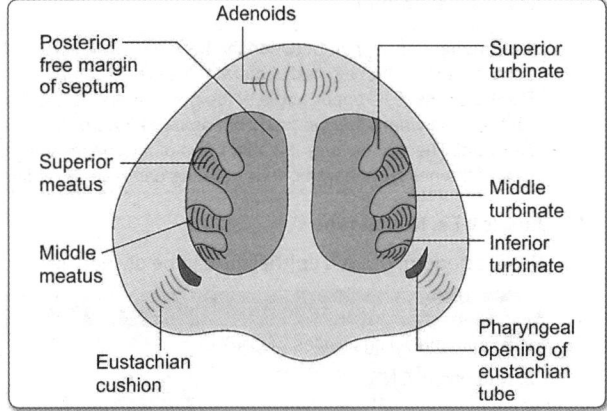

Fig. 15.9: Structures seen in posterior rhinoscopy

NEW PATTERN QUESTIONS

Q N22. Thudichum speculum is used for visualizing:
a. Posterior nasal cavity b. Posterior nares
c. Larynx d. Anterior nasal cavity

Q N23. Which is not visualized on posterior rhinoscopy?
a. Eustachian tube b. Inferior meatus
c. Middle meatus d. Superior concha

Q N24. The figure shows structure seen on posterior rhinoscopy—Identify the structure shown by 'X':

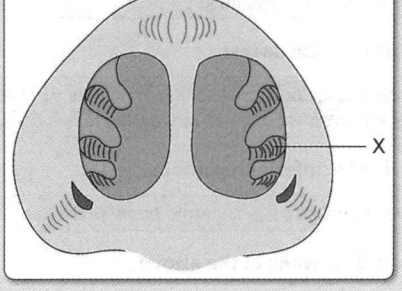

See Color Plate 11

a. Superior meatus b. Middle meatus
c. Inferior meatus d. Eustachian tube opening

Q N25. IOC for paranasal sinus:
a. CT b. MRI
c. X-ray d. Sinoscopy

Q N26. Turbinate which articulates with ethmoid is:
a. Superior b. Middle
c. Inferior d. All of the above

Explanations and References to New Pattern Questions

N1. Ans. is b i.e. Quadrilateral *Ref. Dhingra ENT 6/e, p 147*

Septal cartilage is quadrilateral in shape.

N2. Ans. is c i.e. Columella

N3. Ans. is b i.e. Rhinion *Ref. Hazarika ENT 3/e, p 231*

Columella: It is the part between the two anterior nostrils or the part between the two nasal vestibules. It forms the caudal part of nasal septum. It is formed by medial crura of the two lower lateral cartilages.
Root of nose: The upper angle of the nose where it is continuous with forehead is called as root of the nose. The deepest point at the root of nose where the two nasal bones meet the frontal bone is called as nasion, i.e. here two bones meet.
Rhinion: The point where the lower end of internasal suture, i.e suture between two nasal bones meets with the lower cartilaginous part of the nose, i.e. here bone is meeting cartilage. So rhinion is osseocartilaginous junction.

N4. Ans. is b i.e. Neural tube *Ref. Basic Histology, V Shubhadra Devi*

Neuroectoderm derived epithelium can be divided into those derived from neural tube and those derived from neural crest cells.

Neural tube derivative	Neural crest derivative
1. Ependymal lining cavities of CNS	1. Dorsal root ganglia
2. Neurons of CNS	2. Sensory ganglia of cranial nerves
3. Pineal gland	3. Adrenal medulla
4. Neurohypophysis	4. Schwann cells
5. Sensory epithelium of eye	5. Neuroglia
6. Sensory epithelium of ear	6. Sympathetic and parasympathetic ganglia
7. Sensory epithelium of nose	7. Melanocytes
	8. Pharyngeal arch cartilages

N5. Ans. is a i.e. Superior turbinate

See the text for explanation.

N6. Ans. is c i.e. Upper lateral cartilage *Ref. Dhingra ENT 6/e, p 135*

See the text for explanation.

N7. Ans. is c i.e. Cottle test *Ref. Mohan Bansal, Essentials of ENT 1/e, p 188*

Cottle test is done for checking the patency of nasal valve. The cheek is drawn laterally and patient breathes quietly. If there is subjective improvement in nasal airway, the test is considered positive and indicats nasal valve compromise.

N8. Ans. is c i.e. Inferior turbinate *Ref. Dhingra ENT 6/e, p135*

Inferior turbinate is a separate bone, rest all are a part of ethmoidal labyrinth.

N9. Ans. is d i.e. None of the above *Ref. Dhingra ENT 6/e, p 138*

Supreme turbinate is the fourth turbinate which is sometimes present. It is seen above superior turbinate.

N10. Ans. is b i.e. Middle turbinate *Ref. Hazarika ENT 3/e, p 233*

The posterior end of middle turbinate points to the opening of sphenopalatine foramen.
Also know-Sphenopalatine foramen is a route of communication between nasal cavity and pterygopalatine fossa.
Major structures passing through the foramen are:
1. Sphenopalatine branch of maxillary artery
2. Nasopalatine branch of maxillary nerve
3. Superior nasal branch of maxillary nerve.

Chapter 15: Anatomy and Physiology of Nose

N11. Ans. is c i.e. Osteomeatal complex

The plate shows region of osteomeatal complex.

N12. Ans. is d i.e. Nasolacrimal duct *Ref. Dhingra ENT 6/e, p 135*

Nasolacrimal duct opens in inferior meatus, rest all structures open in middle meatus.

N13. Ans. is c i.e. A III B II C I D IV

See the text for explanation.

N14. Ans. is d i.e. Ophthalmic artery *Ref. Dhingra 6/e, p 176*

Anterior and posterior ethmoidal arteries are branches of ophthalmic artery which is a branch of internal carotid artery.

N15. Ans. is b i.e. Air pressure control *Ref. Dhingra 6/e, p 141*

Read the text for explanation.

N16. Ans. is c i.e. 5–10 mm/min

The cilia of nasal mucosa beat constantly at speed of **5–10 mm/minutes**.

N17. Ans. is a i.e. Perversion of smell sensation *Ref. Dhingra 5/e, p 157; 6/e, p 142*

Disorders of smell
Anosmia: Total loss of sense of smell
Hyposmia: Partial loss of sense of smell
Parosmia: Perversion of smell (seen in recovery phase of post influenzal anosmia; intracranial tumors).

N18. Ans. is b i.e. Every 2-4 hours *Ref. Dhingra 6/e, p 140; Mohan Basal 1/e, p 40*

Nasal cycle: The alternate opening and closing of each side of nose is called nasal cycle
Kayser first described nasal cycle in 1895
There is rhythmic cyclical congestion and decongestion of nasal mucosa
Nasal cycle varies every 2½-4 hrs and is characteristic of an individual.

N19. Ans. is c i.e. Traps the pathogenic organisms in inspired air *Ref. Dhingra 6/e, p 141, 142*

Nasal mucosa contains goblet cells for secretion of mucus, which forms a mucus blanket. The inspired bacteria, viruses and dust particles are entrapped on this viscous mucus blanket. Hence mucociliary action is protective.

N20. Ans. is a i.e. Mucociliary action *Ref. Dhingra 6/e, p 141, 142*

As discussed in previous Question - movement of mucus in nose is mainly by mucociliary action.

N21. Ans. is a i.e. Olfactory epithelium *Ref. Dhingra 6/e, p 142*

Odor receptors are present in olfactory epithelium lining the olfactory region of nose.

N22. Ans is d i.e. Anterior nasal cavity *Ref. Tuli1/e, p 538; 2/e, p 503; Mohan Bansal p 281*

Thudichum speculum or vienna type speculum is used to visualize anterior nasal cavity (examination is called anterior rhinoscopy).

 Note: Posterior nares can be visualized during posterior rhinoscopy using posterior nasal mirror.

N23. Ans. is b i.e. Inferior meatus *Ref. Maqbool 11/e, p 164*
Posterior rhinoscopy:
- It is method of examination of the posterior aspect of nose and pharynx.
- Structures seen during rhinoscopy are shown in Figure 15.9 in the text.

N24. Ans. is b i.e. Middle meatus

See Figure 15.9 in the text.

N25. Ans. is a i.e. CT

IOC for visualising the sinus is CT scan.

N26. Ans. is c i.e. Inferior

Inferior turbinate is a separate bone whereas middle turbinate and superior turbinates are parts of ethmoidal bone. Inferior turbinate articulates with the uncinate process of ethmoid bone (via ethmoidal process) and lacrimal bone (via lacrimal process).

QUESTIONS

1. **Frontonasal duct opens into:** [PGI 98]
   a. Inferior meatus
   b. Middle meatus
   c. Superior meatus
   d. Inferior turbinate

2. **Frontal sinus drain into:** [PGI 97, 98]
   a. Superior meatus
   b. Inferior meatus
   c. Middle meatus
   d. Ethmoid recess

3. **Paranasal sinus opening in middle meatus:** [PGI 03, 98]
   a. Maxillary
   b. Anterior ethmoid
   c. Posterior ethmoid
   d. Frontal
   e. Sphenoid

4. **The maxillary sinus opens into middle meatus at the level of:** (DNB 02)
   a. Hiatus semilunaris
   b. Bulla ethmoidalis
   c. Infundibulum
   d. None of the above

5. **All drains into middle meatus** *except*: [DNB 02]
   a. Lacrimal duct
   b. Maxillary sinus
   c. Frontal sinus
   d. Ethmoidal sinus

6. **Hiatus semilunaris is present in:** [CUPGEE 02]
   a. Superior meatus
   b. Middle meatus
   c. Inferior meatus
   d. Spenoethmoidal recess

7. **Bulla ethmoidalis is seen in:** [AIIMS 92]
   a. Superior meatus
   b. Inferior meatus
   c. Middle meatus
   d. Sphenoethmoidal recess

8. **Opening of posterior ethmoid sinus is in:** [Jharkhand 06]
   a. Sphenoethmoid recess
   b. Superior meatus
   c. Inferior meatus
   d. Middle meatus

9. **Sphenoidal sinus opens into:** [Kerala 98]
   a. Inferior meatus
   b. Middle meatus
   c. Superior meatus
   d. Sphenoethmoidal recess

10. **Nasolacrimal duct opens into:** [MAHE 05]
    a. Superior meatus
    b. Middle meatus
    c. Inferior meatus
    d. Sphenopalatine recess

11. **Inferior turbinate is a:** [JIPMER 04]
    a. Part of maxilla
    b. Part of sphenoid
    c. Separate bone
    d. Part of ethmoid

12. **Ethmoid bone forms A/E:** [Bihar 05]
    a. Superior turbinate
    b. Middle turbinate
    c. Interior turbinate
    d. Uncinate process

13. **Which of the following is known as fourth turbinate?** [UP 01]
    a. Superior turbinate
    b. Aggernasi
    c. Supreme turbinate
    d. Bulous turbinate

14. **Turbinate that articulates with ethmoid is:** [AP 02]
    a. Superior
    b. Middle
    c. Inferior
    d. All of the above

15. **External nose is formed from:** [AP 96]
    a. 3 paired + 3 unpaired cartilages
    b. 3 paired + 1 unpaired cartilages
    c. 3 paired + 4 unpaired
    d. 1 paired + 1 unpaired

16. **Choana is:** [TN 03]
    a. Anterior nares
    b. Posterior nares
    c. Tonsils
    d. Larynx

17. **Direction of nasolacrimal duct is:** [AI 99]
    a. Downward, backward and medially
    b. Downward, backward and laterally
    c. Downward, forward and medially
    d. Downward, forward and laterally

18. **Which of the following bones do not contribute the nasal septum?** [AI 03]
    a. Sphenoid
    b. Lacrimal
    c. Palatine
    d. Ethmoid

19. **Quadrilateral cartilage is attached to all** *except*: [DNB 01]
    a. Ethmoid
    b. Vomer
    c. Sphenoid
    d. Maxilla

20. **All these structures are found in the lateral nasal wall** *except*: [MP 07]
    a. Superior turbinate
    b. Vomer
    c. Agger nasi
    d. Hasner's vale

21. **Nasal valve is formed by all** *except*: [MP 08]
    a. Septum
    b. Middle turbinate
    c. Lower end of upper lateral cartilage
    d. Inferior turbinate

22. **Onodi cells and Haller cells are seen in relation to:**
    a. Optic nerve and floor of orbit [AIIMS Nov 09]
    b. Optic nerve and frontal sinus
    c. Optic nerve and ethmoidal air cells
    d. Orbital chiasma and nasolacrimal duct

23. **Osteomeatal complex (OMC) connects:** [MH 02]
    a. Nasal cavity with maxillary sinus
    b. Nasal cavity with sphenoid sinus
    c. The two nasal cavities
    d. Ethmoidal sinus with ethmoidal bulla

24. **Nasal mucosa is supplied by:** [AI 92]
    a. Only external carotid artery
    b. Only internal carotid
    c. Mainly external carotid artery
    d. Mainly internal carotid artery

25. **During inspiration the main current of airflow in a normal nasal cavity is through:** [AI 07]
    a. Middle part of the cavity in middle meatus in a parabolic curve
    b. Lower part of the cavity in the inferior meatus in a parabolic curve
    c. Superior part of the cavity in the superior meatus
    d. Through olfactory area

Chapter 15: Anatomy and Physiology of Nose

26. **Function of mucociliary action of upper respiratory tract is:** [Kerala 94]
    a. Protective
    b. Increase the velocity of inspired air
    c. Traps the pathogenic organisms in inspired air
    d. Has no physiological role

27. **Veins not involved in spreading infection to cavernous sinus from danger area of face:**
    a. Lingual vein
    b. Pterygoid plexus
    c. Facial vein
    d. Ophthalmic vein
    e. Cephalic vein

Explanations and References

1. **Ans. is b i.e. Middle meatus** *Ref. Turner 10/e, p 379; Dhingra 5/e, p 178; 6/e, 136,137; TB of Mohan Bansal, p 34,35,37*
2. **Ans. is c i.e. Middle meatus**
3. **Ans. is a, b and d i.e. Maxillary; Anterior ethmoid; and Frontal**
4. **Ans. is a i.e. Hiatus semilunaris**
5. **Ans. is a i.e. Lacrimal duct**
6. **Ans. is b i.e. Middle meatus**
7. **Ans. is c i.e. Middle meatus** *Ref. Dhingra 5/e, p 152,153; Tuli 1/e, p 135, 136; Logan Turner 10/e, p 379; TB of Mohan Bansal, p 34*
8. **Ans. is b i.e. Superior meatus** *Ref. Dhingra 5/e, 153; 6/e, p138*

   Middle meatus lies between the middle and inferior turbinates and is important because of the presence of osteomeatal complex in this area.

Part of lateral nasal wall	Openings
Inferior meatus	Nasolacrimal duct
Middle meatus	Frontal sinus (which opens via fronto nasal duct) Maxillary sinus, Anterior ethmoidal sinus
Superior meatus	Posterior ethmoidal sinus
Sphenoethmoidal recess	Sphenoid sinus

9. **Ans. is d i.e. sphenoethmoidal recess** *Ref. Dhingra 5/e, p 153; 6/e, p 138; TB of Mohan Bansal, p 38*

   Sphenoethmoid recess is situated above the superior turbinate and receives opening of sphenoidal sinus.

10. **Ans. is c i.e. Inferior meatus** *Ref. Dhingra 5/e, p 150; 6/e, p 135*
    - Nasolacrimal duct opens into inferior meatus below the level of inferior turbinate[Q]
    - Nasolacrimal duct is guarded at its temporal end by a mucosal valve k/a Hasner's valve
    - Frontonasal duct opens into middle meatus.

11. **Ans. is c i.e. Separate bone** *Ref. Dhingra 5/e, p 150; 6/e, p 135; Tuli 1/e, p 135; 2/e, p 140*
12. **Ans. is c i.e. Inferior turbinate** *Ref. Dhingra 6/e, p 12; Tuli 1/e, p 135; 2/e, p 140*

    "The inferior turbinate is a separate bone, while rest of the turbinates are a part of ethmoidal labyrinth."

13. **Ans. is c i.e Supreme turbinate** (Agger nasi)

    Friends – I haven't been able to get a reference for this answer – but I am pretty sure about the answer itself.

14. **Ans. is c i.e. Inferior** *Ref. Scotts Brown 7/e, Vol 2, p 1329; Dhingra 6/e, p 136*

    Friends here it is important to read the question – the question is asking about articulation with ethmoid.
    Its discussed in previous questions:
    Middle turbinate and superior turbinate are a part of the ethmoidal bone whereas inferior turbinate is an independant bone which articulates with the ethmoid bone, completing the medial wall of nasolacrimal duct.

15. **Ans. is b i.e. 3 paired + 1 unpaired cartilages** *Ref. Dhingra 5/e, p 149, 150; 6/e, p 134; TB of Mohan Bansal, p 30*

    External nose is made up of bony framework which forms upper third part and cartilaginous forms lower two-thirds part framework.
    Cartilages of nose:
    - Paired upper lateral nasal cartilages
    - Paired lower nasal cartilages

- Lesser alar (sesamoid) cartilages – 2 or more in number
- Unpaired septal cartilage.

16. **Ans. is b i.e. Posterior nares** *Ref. Turner 10/e, p 4; Dhingra 5/e, p 150; 6/e, p 135*

    Nasal cavity

    "Nasal fossae are two irregular cavities extending from the mucocutaneous junction with the nasal vestibule in front (the anterior nares) to the junction with the nasopharynx behind (posterior nares or choanae)." *Ref. Turner 10/e, p 4*

    "Each nasal cavity communicates with the external through naris or nares and with nasopharynx through posterior nasal aperture or choana." *Ref. Dhingra 6/e, p 135*

17. **Ans. is b i.e. Downward, backward and laterally** *TB of Mohan Bansal 1/e, p 42*

    Nasolacrimal duct: It is a membranous passage which begins at the lower end of the lacrimal sac. It runs downward, backward and laterally and opens in the inferior meatus of the nose. A fold of mucous membrane called the valve of Hasner forms an imperfect value at the lower end of the duct.

18. **Ans. is b i.e. Lacrimal** *Ref. BDC 4/e, Vol 3 p 228-229; Dhingra 5/e, p 162, 6/e, p 147*

    Nasal septum is the osseocartilagenous partition between the two halves of nasal cavity.

    Its constituents are (Fig. 15.10):

    (i) Osseous part
    - The vomer
    - Perpendicular plate of ethmoid
    - Nasal crest of nasal bone
    - Nasal spine of frontal bone
    - Nasal crest of palatine bone
    - Nasal crest of maxillary bone
    - Rostrum of sphenoid bone.

    (ii) Cartilaginous part

    Septal (Qudrilateral) cartilage.

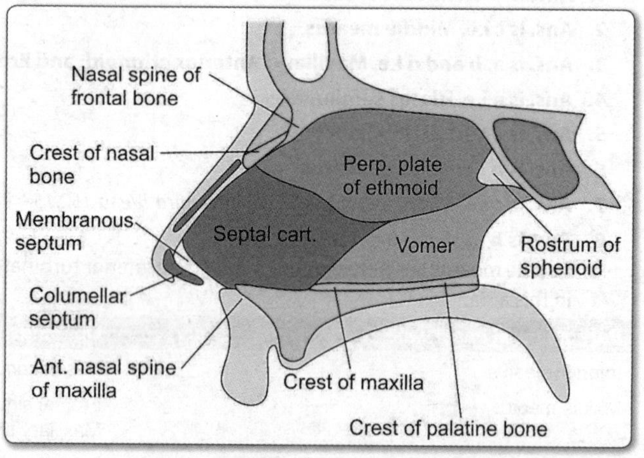

    Fig. 15.10: Anatomy of nasal septum

19. **Ans. is c i.e. Sphenoid** *Ref. Scott Brown 7/e, Vol 2, p 1326; Dhingra 6/e, p 147.*

    Quadrilateral cartilage or septal cartilage forms the nasal septum. As seen in above figure the arterior side of this cartilage forms the dorsum of external nose. It comes in contact with perpendicular plate of ethmoid, vomer and arterior nasal spine.

20. **Ans. is b i.e. Vomer** *Ref. Scott Brown 7/e, Vol 2, p 1329, 1330; Dhingra 5/e, p 150-153; 6/e, p 134-138*

    The lateral nasal wall is composed of three turbinates:
    - Superior turbinate
    - Middle turbinate
    - Inferior turbinate

    Below each turbinate is the respective meatus:
    - Inferior meatus
    - Middle meatus
    - Superior meatus
    - Above the superior turbinate lies the sphenoethmoid recess.
    - Just anterior to the middle meatus, is a small crest/mound on the lateral wall called as Agger nasi.
      - In the inferior meatus – opens the nasolacrimal duct guarded at its terminal end by a mucosal valve k/a Hasner's valve.

     Note: Vomer is an independent bone which forms the posterio inferior part of nasal septum (i.e. medial wall of nose).

21. **Ans. is b i.e. Middle turbinate** *Ref. Scotts Brown 7/e, Vol 2, p 1358; Dhingra 5/e, p 150; 6/e, p 138; TB of Mohan Bansal, p 287*

    Anterior Nasal Valve/Internal Nasal Valve
    - This is the narrowest part of nose and is less well-defined physiologically than anatomically.
    - It is formed by the lower edge of the upper lateral cartilages (limen nasi), the anterior end of the inferior turbinate and the adjacent septum.

Chapter 15: Anatomy and Physiology of Nose

22. **Ans. is a i.e. Optic nerve and floor of orbit**   *Ref. Graijs 40/e, p 558; Dhingra 5/e, p 153; 6/e p 136; TB of Mohan Bansal 1/e, p 38*

    The Onodi and Haller cells are posterior ethmoidal air cells.
    The Onodi cells are related to optic nerve and internal carotid artery and Haller cells are related to orbital floor.

23. **Ans. is a i.e. Nasal cavity with maxillary sinus**   *Ref. Scott Brown 7/e, Vol 2, p 1345*

    Osteomeatal complex lies in the middle meatus. It is the final common drainage pathway for the maxillary, frontal and anterior ethmoid sinuses into the nasal cavity (so will obviously connect any of these to the nasal cavity).

24. **Ans. is c i.e. Mainly external carotid artery**   *Ref. Dhingra 5/e, p 189,190*

    Both internal carotid artery and external carotid artery supply the nose but main artery is the external carotid artery.

25. **Ans. is a i.e. Middle part of the cavity in middle meatus in parabolic curve**   *Ref. Dhingra 5/e, p 155; 6/e, p 140*

    Nose is the natural pathway for breathing.

    During quiet respiration:
    - Inspiratory air current passes through middle part of nose between the turbinates and nasal septum.
    - Very little air passes through inferior meatus or olfactory region of nose. Therefore, weak odorous substances have to be sniffed before they can reach olfactory, area.
    - During expiratorn, air current follows the same course as during inspiration, but the entire air current is not expelled directly through the nares.
    - Friction offered at limen nasi converts it into eddies under cover of inferior and middle turbinates and thus sinuses are ventilated during expiration.

26. **Ans. is c i.e. Traps the pathogenic organisms in inspired air**   *Ref. Dhingra 5/e, p 156; 6/e, p 140*

27. **Ans. is a and e i.e. Lingual vein and Cephalic vein**   *Ref. BD Chaurasia, p 62, 63; Maqbool 11/e, p 172*

    Dangerous area of face (Fig. 15.5) of the text.

    Dangerous area of face includes upper lip and anteroinferior part of nose including the vestibule. This area freely communicates with the cavernous sinus through a set of valveless veins, anterior facial vein and superior ophthalmic vein. Any infection of this area can thus travel intracranially leading to meningitis and cavernous sinus thrombosis.

Chapter 16

Diseases of External Nose and Nasal Septum

SADDLE NOSE

- Nasal dorsum is depressed (sagging of the bridge of nose).
- Depressed nasal dorsum may involve either bony, cartilaginous or both bony and cartilaginous components.
- *Most common* etiology: Nasal trauma.

Causes of Depressed Nose/Saddle Nose

Mnemonic

H = Hematoma
O = Operative, i.e. excessive removal of septum during submucous resection
T = Trauma
S = Syphilis
A = Abscess
L = Leprosy
T = Tuberculosis
HOT SALT

Management

Augmentation rhinoplasty, i.e. filling the deformity with cartilage, bone or synthetic implant.

CROOKED/DEVIATED NOSE

Humped nose: Means there is hump over nose.
Crooked nose: The dorsum is deviated but tip is in midline (C-or S-shaped).
Deviated nose: The dorsum and tip are straight but deviated to one side.

NEW PATTERN QUESTIONS

Q N1. Crooked nose is due to:
    a. Deviated ala
    b. Deviated septum
    c. Humping nasal septum
    d. Deviated dorsum and septa

Q N2. Identify the condition of nose shown in plate:

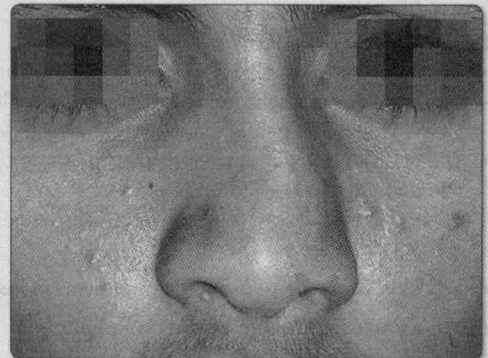

See Color Plate 12

    a. Crooked nose
    b. Deviated nose
    c. Saddle nose
    d. Humped nose

Q N3. Identify the condition of nose shown in plate:

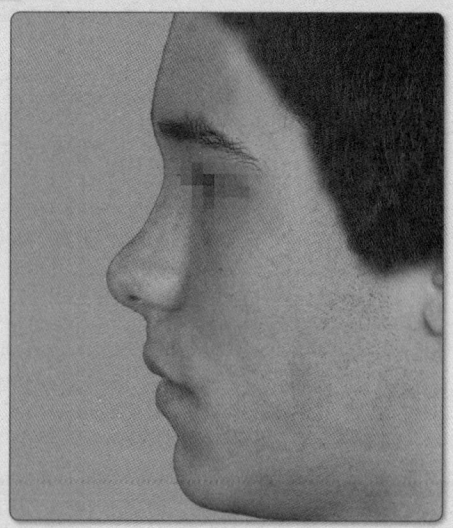

See Color Plate 13

    a. Crooked nose
    b. Deviated nose
    c. Saddle nose
    d. Humped nose

Chapter 16: Diseases of External Nose and Nasal Septum

CHOANAL ATRESIA

- Choanal atresia is a condition which results due to persistence of bucconasal membrane, which separates the primitive nose and mouth during development.^{Q}

(Right side atresia is more common than left side).^{Q}

- Unilateral atresia is more common.^{Q}
- Unilateral atresia remains undiagnosed until adult life.
- Bilateral atresia presents with respiration obstruction in newborn.
- It is more common in females.

Diagnosis

- Presence of mucoid discharge in nose.
- Absence of air bubbles in nasal discharge.
- Failure to pass a catheter from nose to pharynx.
- Putting a few drops of methylene blue dye into the nose and seeing its passage through the pharynx.
- CT scan is diagnostic - on CT choanal atresia is diagnosed if posterior choanal orifice is < 0.34 cm or if posterior vomer measures > 0.55 cm.

Treatment

In B/L choanal atresia: McGovern's technique → Placing a feeding nipple with a large hole in the mouth of the infant.
Definitive treatment: Correction of atresia by transnasal or transpalatal approach. Done at 1½ years.
Post surgery mitomycin C can be applied to decrease chances of restenosis.

> **Extra Edge**
>
> *Ref. Current Otolaryngology 2/e, p 243*
> - In utero exposure to methimazole and carbinazole can lead to choanal atresia along with other anomalies like esophageal atresia and developmental delay
> - Earlier it was said choanal atresia is bony in 90% and membranous in 10% cases. But recent studies reveal that in 29% cases, choanal atresia consists of purely bony elements and in 71% cases.
> - Choanal artresia can be associated with other malformations M/C of which is CHARGE syndrome.
> - CHARGE syndrome – The acronym CHARGE is used to describe a heterogenous group of children who exhibit atleast 4 of the following features as described below:
> - **C** = Coloboma
> - **H** = Heart defects – like TOF, PDA
> - **A** = Atresia of choara (U/L or B/L, membranous or bony)
> - **R** = Retarded growth
> - **G** = Genital anomalies
> - **E** = Ear anomalies

TUMORS OF EXTERNAL NOSE

They can be divided into three categories—Congenital, benign or malignant (Table 16.1).

Classification of Swellings of External Nose and Vestibule

Table 16.1: Classification of tumors of external nose

Congenital	Benign	Malignant
Dermoid	Rhinophyma or potato tumor	Basal cell carcinoma (rodent ulcer) Squamous cell carcinoma (epithelioma).
Encephalocele or meningoencephalocele	Papilloma hemangioma	
Glioma	Pigmented nevus	
Nasoalveolar cyst	Seborrheic keratosis Neurofibrom Tumors of sweat glands	Melanoma

Rhinophyma/Potato Tumor (Elephantiasis of Nose)

- It is a slow-growing benign tumor which occurs due to hypertrophy of the sebaceous glands of the tip of the nose.
- Seen in long standing cases of acne rosacea.
- Mostly affects men past middle age.
- Presents as a pink, lobulated mass over the nose (color is pink/red because of vascular engorgement).

Treatment

- With CO_2 laser—bulk of tumor is removed.

> **Points to Remember**
> - Basal cell carcinoma of external nose – It is the M/C malignant tumor of nose involving the nasal skin. The M/C sites on nose are, nasal tip and ala.
> - 2nd M/C malignant tumor of nose is squamous cell carcinoma.

NEW PATTERN QUESTIONS

Q N4. All are true about Rhinophyma *except*:
a. Also called as elephantiasis of nose
b. Hypertrophy of holocrine gland
c. Most commonly due to diabetes mellitus
d. Associated with acne rosacea

Q N5. Rhinophyma is associated with:
a. Hypertrophy of sebaceous gland
b. Hypertrophy of salivary gland
c. Hypertrophy of sweat gland
d. Hypertrophy of Bartholin's gland

Nasal Encephalocele

- It is a congenital condition in which there is herniation of glial tissues and meninges through a defect in the base of craniun.
- The herniation occurs during the process of development before the foramen cecum is closed. A small part of dural tissue may extend to the prenasal space through the foramen cecum. When the foramen cecum fails to close, the herniation persists leading to meningocele or meningoencephalocele in nose.
- The M/C location is occipital followed by frontal.

Clinical Feature:
- It presents as cystic polypoidal nasal mass and nasal obstruction

On Anterior Rhinoscopic examination:
- A soft, cystic bluish, compressible and translucent mass is noted
- Swelling increases in size in response to coughing
- The M/C location is occipital followed by frontal.
- The mass increases in size on drying or straining (coughing).
- Bilateral compression of internal jugular vein also leads to increase in the size of the mass called as positive **Frustenberg test**.
- IOC = MRI. First investigation = CT scan
- Thus for any polypoidal mass in nose, CT scan should be the first investigation and MRI IOC.
- **Mgt** Transnasal endoscopic excision of mass.

Nasal glioma: Glioma is not a tumor but a congenital malformation associated with hetrotopic brain tissue which presents as nasal mass. It occurs as a result of herniation of brain tissue into the nasal cavity through the foramen cecum during the intrauterine life (Fig. 16.1). Its communication gets detached due to fusion of cranial bones in late intrauterine life (that is it is similar to encelplano but with no intracranial connection).

Of the gliomas 60% are extranasal, 30% intranasal and 10% combined.

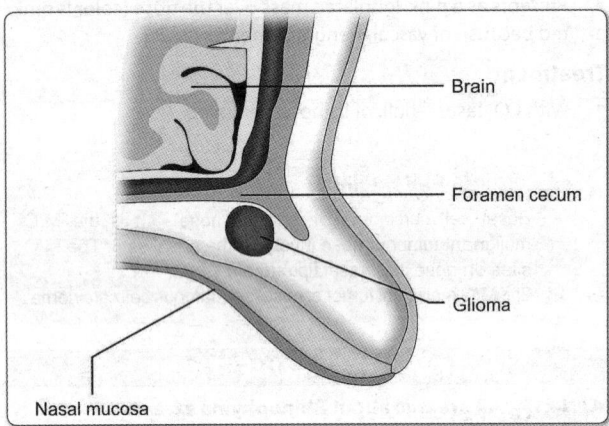

Fig. 16.1: Illustration showing formation of glioma

Clinical feature
It usually manifest in children with nasal obstruction and a bluish nasal mass. In contrast to encephalocele, gliomas are firm and noncompressible.

IOC is MRI. Frustenberg test is negative.
Management: Surgical excision.

Intranasal mass is excised by endoscopic approach. External approach is adopted, if mass is extranasal.

Dermoid:
- It is an ectodermal cyst containing epithelial lining and dermal structures.
- M/C seen over the dorsum of nose
- Always presents in midline
- C/f presents as fluctuating cystic swelling or as a nasal mass causing nasal obstruction.
  - The mass is always compressible and nonexpansible
- **Treatment:** Excision of cyst.

NEW PATTERN QUESTIONS

Q N6. A polypoidal swelling is noted in an infant near the glabella. The swelling is compressible and increases in size on coughing All of the flowing investing actions should be done *except*:
  a. Biopsy   b. CT scan
  c. MRI   d. Anterior Rhinoscopy

Q N7. Frustenberg sign is positive in:
  a. Nasal glioma   b. Nasal encephalocele
  c. Nasal dermoid   d. None of the above

Q N8. A 2 years old infant is bought to OPD by the mother with case of frequent nasal blockage. On examination a solitary polypoidal mass is seen to arise from the roof of the nose. First step in investigation is:
  a. Biopsy   b. CT scan
  c. X-ray   d. MRI

SEPTAL DEVIATIONS—DEVIATED NASAL SEPTUM

DNS is a common problem in which nasal septum is displaced.

Normally, septum lies in center therefore nasal cavities are symmetrical. In case of DNS–the cartilaginous ridge of the septum lies either toward right or left side and nasal cavities are asymmetrical.

Etiology: Septal deviation can be due to:
- **Trauma:** Birth trauma, accidental trauma and fights.
- **Developmental error:** Unequal growth between the palate and the skull base cause buckling of the nasal septum. It is seen in cleft lip and palate and in case of dental anomalies.
- **Racial factors:** Caucasians > Negroes.
- **Hereditary factors:** It runs in families.

Note: The M/C cause of DNS is birth trauma.

Types
- Anterior dislocation, i.e. anterior end of cartilaginous septum may project into one of the vestibules.
- C-shaped deformity—both cartilaginous and bony septum deviated to one side.
- S-shaped deformity—cartilaginous part deviated to one side while bony part to opposite side.
- *Spurs:* Sharp shelf like projection at the junction of the bone and the cartilage [may occur at the junction of vomer below and septal cartilage and/or ethmoid bone]

Symptoms
See Flowchart 16.1.

Points to Remember

➤ DNS is more common in males:
Cottle test:[Q]
➤ **Purpose:** To confirm whether the obstruction is in the nasal valve area, which is the narrowest part of the nasal cavity.
➤ **Method:** The patient pulls the cheeks outward and breathes quietly. If the nasal airway improves on the test side, the test is positive and indicates abnormality of the vestibular component of nasal valve

Symptoms/Pathophysiology of Septal Deviation

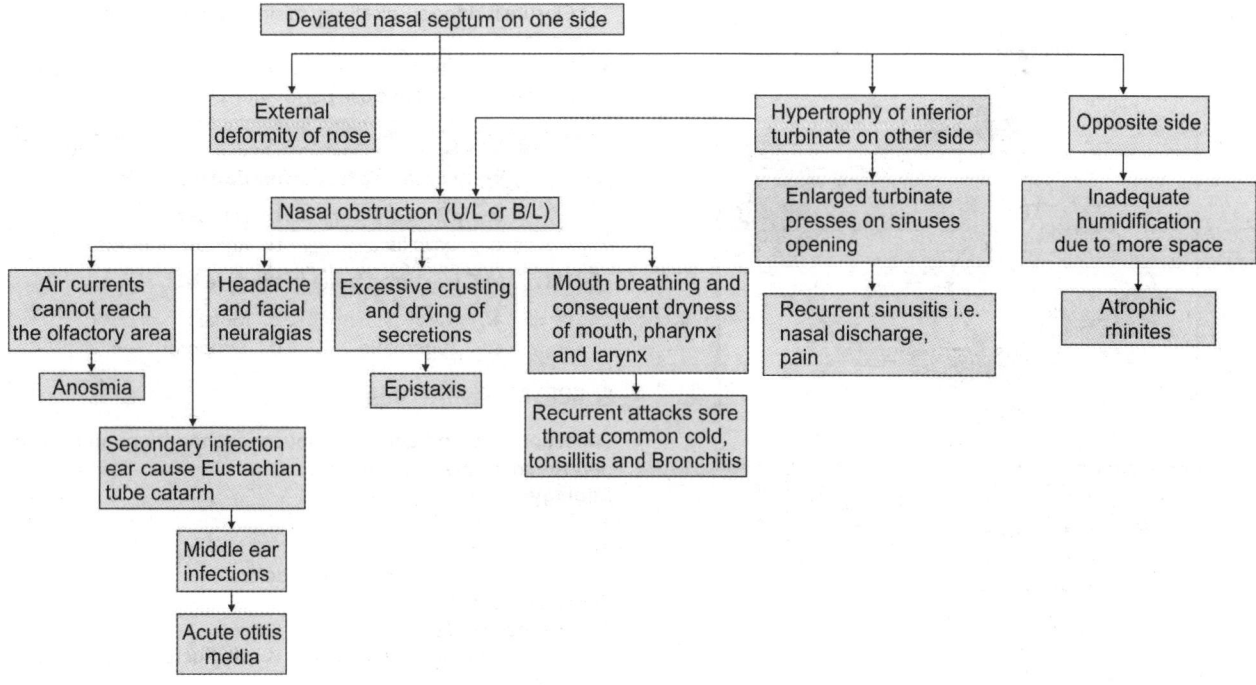

Flowchart 16.1: Symptoms of septal deviation

Treatment

- No treatment is required, if it is not causing any symptoms.
- *Surgical management is the treatment of choice.*
  - **Septoplasty:** Conservative surgery as most of the septal framework is retained. Only the most deviated parts are removed. Rest of the septal framework is corrected and reposited by plastic means. *It is the preferred operation.*
  - **Submucous Resection:** *Here apart from a thin dorsal and caudal strip, the rest of the entire septum is removed.*

Note:
- Septal surgery is usually done after the age of 17 so as not to interfere with the growth of nasal skeleton.
- Only if a child has severe septal deviation causing marked nasal obstruction, septoplasty should be done.

- The submucous resection was popularized and referred by **Killian (1904) and Freer (1902).**
- Incision given
  - **For submucous resection—Killian incision** given at 1.25 cm behind the columella at the mucocutaneous junction at the convex side of the deviation.
  - For septoplasty—Freer's hemitransfixation incision given at the caudal end of septum, on the concave side of cartilage.
- These days endoscopic septoplasty and turberoplasty are also being performed. Technique of endoscopic septoplasty and tuberoplasty was first described by Nayak et al. in 2002.
- Anesthesia used for septal surgery—surface anesthesia using 2% xylocaine and 1:50,000 adrenaline.

Important Instruments Related to Procedure

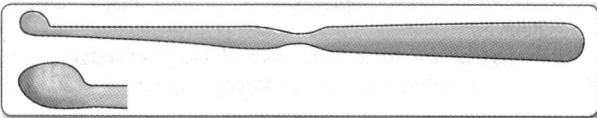

Fig. 16.2: Freer's septal knife

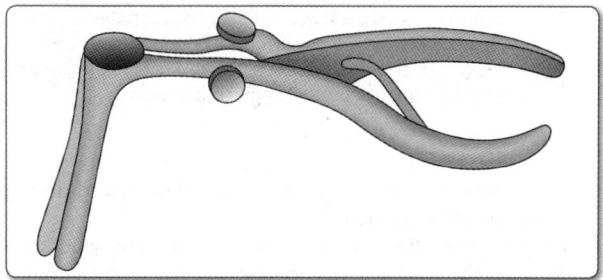

Fig. 16.3: Killian's nasal speculum

NEW PATTERN QUESTION

Q N9. Identify the incision shown in plate:

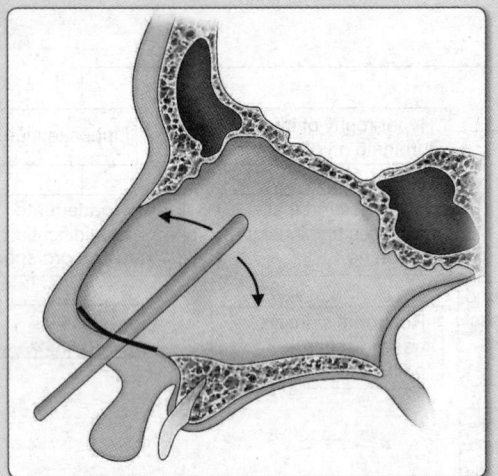

See Color Plate 14

a. Killian's incision
b. Freer's incision
c. Weber-Ferguson incision
d. Schobinger incision

SEPTAL PERFORATION

Etiology

- Trauma^Q M/C Surgical during and after submucous resection
  - Repeated cautery
  - Nose picking
  - Tight nasal packing
- Chronic inflammation [Wegener's granulomatosis, Syphilis, TB Leprosy, atrophic rhinitis]
- Nasal myiasis (maggots in nose)
- Rhinolith or neglected foreign body
- As a complication of septal abscess or hematoma, if drainage is delayed.
- Poisons (cocaine, topical steroids and decongestants)
- Tumors of septum, e.g. chondrosarcoma, granuloma
- Idiopathic

 **Note:**
- Syphilis causes perforation of the bony part while lupus, tuberculosis and leprosy involve the cartilaginous part.
- Recreational drugs like cocaine are becoming increasingly common causes of septal perforation.

Symptoms

- Small anterior perforation causes whistling sound during inspiration or expiration.
- Larger perforations result in crusts formation which can obstruct the nose and lead to excessive bleeding when it is removed.

Treatment

- If perforation is asymptomatic no treatment is required.
- Small and medium sized perforation (< 2 cm in diameter): Closure is done surgically by raising flaps and stitching on the perforation.
- Large perforation (> 2 cm in diameter): Obturators or silastic buttons are used to close perforations.

NEW PATTERN QUESTIONS

Q N10. Bony nasal septal perforation is seen in:
a. TB   b. Leprosy
c. Syphilis   d. Rhinosporidiosis

Q N11. M/C fractured bone in the face is:
a. Nasal   b. Molar
c. Zygomatic   d. Temporal

SEPTAL HEMATOMA

Collection of blood under the mucoperichondrium and mucoperiosteum of the nasal septum.

Etiology:
- Nasal trauma
- Septal surgery
- Spontaneous in bleeding disorders.

Clinical Features:
- Bilateral nasal obstruction
- Bilateral septal swelling, which is soft, fluctuant, smooth and round.

Treatment:
- **Aspiration:** Small hematoma is aspirated with a wide bore needle.
- **Incision and drainage:** Larger hematoma needs incision and drainage. It is done through a small horizontal incision that is parallel to the nasal floor. A small piece of mucosa is excised, which facilitates drainage.
- Nasal cavities are packed to prevent reaccumulation of blood.
- Systematic antibiotics prevent septal abscess.

Complications:
- **Thickened septum:** Organisation of hematoma into fibrous tissue.
- **Septal abscess:** It leads to necrosis of cartilage and depression of nasal dorsum.

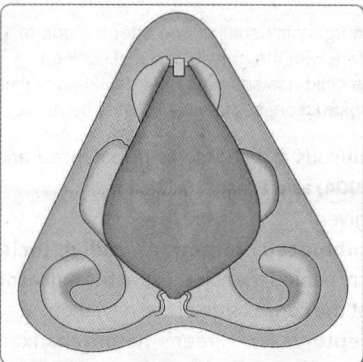

Fig. 16.4: Septal hematoma

Chapter 16: Diseases of External Nose and Nasal Septum

NEW PATTERN QUESTIONS

Q N12. What is not true about septal hematoma?
a. It can appear spontaneously
b. It resolves itself
c. Need surgical correction
d. Can cause secondary infection

Q N13. Treatment of septal hematoma is:
a. Immediate evacuation
b. Wait and watch for spontaneous regression
c. Nasal decongestants
d. Antibiotics

Q N14. Nasal septum abscess leads to:
a. Pyogenic granuloma
b. Septal perforation
c. Cutaneous fistula
d. Retropharyngeal abscess

Q N15. Identify the condition shown in the plate:

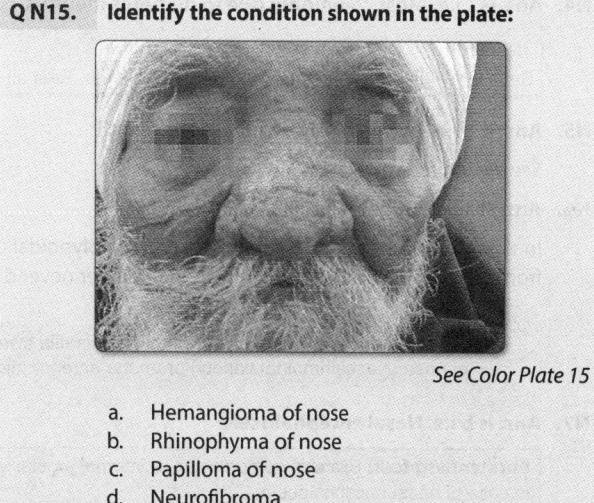

See Color Plate 15

a. Hemangioma of nose
b. Rhinophyma of nose
c. Papilloma of nose
d. Neurofibroma

Explanations and References to New Pattern Questions

N1. Ans. is d i.e. Deviated dorsum and septa *Ref. Dhingra 6/e, p 143; Essentials of ENT, Mohan Bansal, 1/e, P 197*

In crooked nose, the midline of dorsum (obviously along with septa) from frontonasal angle to the tip of nose is curved in a C- or S-shaped manner.

N2. Ans. is a i.e. Crooked nose *Ref. Essentials of ENT, Mohan Bansal, 1/e, p 223*

This is a typical presentation of crooked nose.

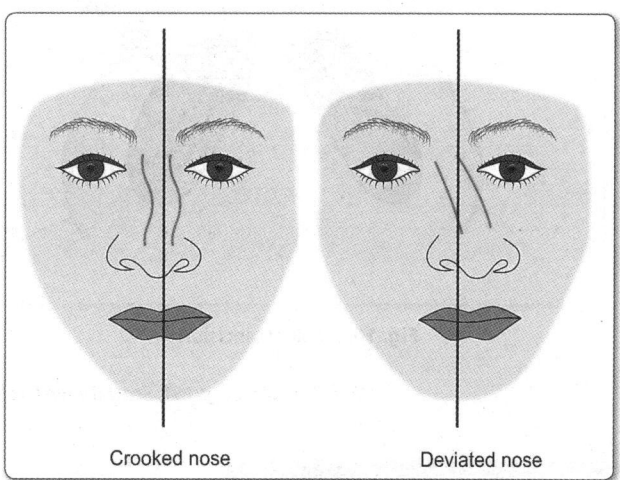

Fig. 16.5: Nasal bridge is S-shaped in crooked nose. It is straight but deviated to one side in deviated nose

N3. Ans. is c i.e. Saddle nose *Ref. Essentials of ENT, Mohan Bansal, p 213*

The deformity seen is saddle nose deformity.

N4. Ans. is c i.e. Most commonly due to diabetes mellitus   *Ref. TB of ENT, Hazarika 3/e, p 268; Dhingra 6/e, p 144*

> **Remember**
> Sebaceous glands are a variety of holocrine glands. Rest all discussed in text.

N5. Ans. is a i.e. Hypertrophy of sebaceous gland   *Ref. Dhingra 6/e, p 144*

See the text for explanation.

N6. Ans. is a i.e. Biopsy   *Ref. TB of ENT, Hazarna, 3/e, p 263*

In the question, as infant is presenting with a polypoidal compressible mass near the glabella, it should raise the suspision of a frontal encephalocele. In all such cases, remember never do a Biopsy: as it can lead to CSF Rhinorrhea.

> **Note:** An encephalocele can present as pulsatile swelling in the midline at the root of nose, glabella (nasofrontal variety), side of nose (Nasoethmoidal variety) or on the anterior middle aspect of the orbit (naso-orbital variety).

N7. Ans. is b i.e. Nasal encephalocele   *Ref. TB of ENT, Hazarika 3/e, p 263*

> **Furstenberg test:** Bilateral compression of internal jugular vein leading to increase in size of mass is positive Furstenberg test, seen in case of nasal encephalocele.
> In nasal gliomas and dermoid cyst—Furstenberg test is negative.

N8. Ans. is b i.e. CT scan

> A solitary polypoidal mass arising from roof of the nose in an infant should raise the suspicion of encephalocele.
> Remember—M/C age of presentation of encephalocele is 15-24 months of age. In such cases biopsy should never be attempted as discussed it can result in CSF rhinorrhea. First investigation done is CT scan. IOC is MRI.

N9. Ans. is b i.e. Freer's incision   *Ref. TB of ENT, Hazarika 3/e, p 284*

The incision shown in the plate is Freer's incision.

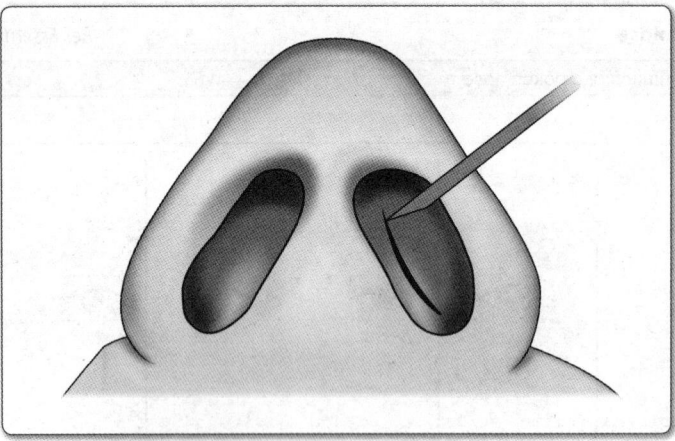

Fig. 16.6: Killian's incision

N10. Ans. is c i.e. Syphilis   *Ref. Dhingra 6/e, p 151; Scott Brown Otolaryngology 7/e, Vol 2, Ch. 124, p 1583*

Septal perforations

Bony	Cartilaginous septum	Both
Syphilis	• Lupus • Leprosy • TB	Wegners Granulomatosis

N11. Ans. is a i.e. Nasal bone   *Ref. Dhingra 6/e, p 182*

Chapter 16: Diseases of External Nose and Nasal Septum

N12. Ans. is b i.e. It resolves itself *Ref. Essentials of ENT, Mohan Bansal, p 231, 232*

> Septal hematoma should not be left to resolve spontaneously as the blood supply of septal cartilage is deprived in this case. Thus surgical management as outlined in the text should be performed as early as possible.

N13. Ans. is a i.e. Immediate evacuation *Ref. Essentials of ENT, Mohan Bansal, p 231, 232*

> See explanation of Q. N9.

N14. Ans. is b i.e. Septal perforation *Ref. Essentials of ENT, Mohan Bansal, p 232*

> **Complications of Septal Abscess**
> - **Saddle nose deformity:** The necrosis of septal cartilage causes depression of the nasal dorsum in the supratip area. It needs augmentation rhinoplasty, which is performed after 2-3 months.
> - **Septal perforation** due to necrosis of septal flaps.
> - **Meningitis.**
> - **Cavernous sinus thrombosis.**

N15. Ans. is b i.e. Rhinophyma of nose *Ref. TB of ENT, BS Tuli 2/e, p 211*

The condition shown in the plate is rhinophyma of the nose (also called as potato tumor or elephantiasis of nose).

QUESTIONS

1. **Rhinophyma is associated with:** [AI 07] [AP 96, UP 01]
   a. Hypertrophy of the sebaceous glands
   b. Hypertrophy of sweat glands
   c. Hyperplasia of endothelial cells
   d. Hyperplasia of epithelial cells

2. **True about rhinophyma:** [AI 01]
   a. Premalignant
   b. Common in alcoholics
   c. Acne rosacea
   d. Fungal etiology
   e. Treatment is shaving, dermabrasion and skin grafting

3. **Most common presentation of infant with bilateral choanal atresia:** [AIIMS 96]
   a. Difficulty in breathing
   b. Dysphagia
   c. Smiling
   d. Difficulty in walking

4. **Choanal atresia is associated with:** [PGI 08]
   a. Colobamatous blindness
   b. Heart disorder
   c. Renal anomaly
   d. Ear disorder
   e. CNS lesion

5. **True about choanal atresia:** [PGI Nov 2014]
   a. Unilateral atresia should be operated within 6-month of age
   b. Occur d/t persistence of bucconasal membrane
   c. B/l atresia usually presents with respiratory difficulties
   d. Bilateral atresia may cause cyanosis
   e. Diagnosed by failure to pass a catheter from nose to pharynx

6. **Which of the following procedure is helpful in diagnosis of choanal atresia?** [PGI May 2012]
   a. Anterior rhinoscopy
   b. Passing red rubber catheter
   c. Breath sounds by stethoscope
   d. Endoscopy of nose
   e. Acoustic rhinometry

7. **All are true about nasolabial cysts except:** [AIIMS Nov 08]
   a. They are B/L
   b. They present in adults
   c. Derived from odontogenic epithelium
   d. Strong female predilection

8. **Depressed bridge of the nose may be due to any of the following except:** [DNB 03]
   a. Leprosy
   b. Syphilis
   c. Thalassemia
   d. Acromegaly

9. **A crooked nose is due to:** [PAL 2000]
   a. Deviated dorsum but tip midline
   b. Depressed dorsum
   c. Humped dorsum
   d. Deviated dorsum and tip

10. **Percentage of newborns with deviation of nasal septum:**
    a. 2%
    b. 10% [PGI 93]
    c. 20%
    d. 60%

11. **Features associated with DNS include all of the following except:** [AI 98]
    a. Epistaxis
    b. Atrophy of turbinate
    c. Hypertrophy of turbinate
    d. Recurrent sinusitis

12. **DNS may be associated with all the following except:**
    a. Recurrent sphenoiditis
    b. Acute otitis media
    c. Hypertrophy of the inferior turbinate
    d. Recurrent maxillary sinusitis

13. **For deviated nasal septum, surgery is required for:**
    a. Septal spur with epistaxis [PGI 01]
    b. Marked septal deviation
    c. Persistent rhinorrhea
    d. Recurrent sinusitis
    e. Prolonged DNS

14. **All of the following true of septoplasty operation for DNS except:** [UPSC]
    a. Indicated in septal deviation
    b. Mucoperichondrium is removed
    c. Preferably done after 16 years of age
    d. Done in some cases of epistaxis

15. **Alternative for SMR:** [DNB 01]
    a. Tympanoplasty
    b. Septoplasty
    c. Caldwell-Luc operation
    d. Turboplasty

16. **Killian's incision is used for:** [TN 04]
    a. Submucous resection of nasal septum
    b. Intranasal antrostomy
    c. Caldwell-Luc operation
    d. Myringoplasty

17. **Which is not done in septoplasty?** [St. Johns 02]
    a. Elective hypotension
    b. Throat pack
    c. Nasal preparation with 10% cocaine
    d. None of the above

18. **Which of the following surgery is not contraindicated below 12 years of age?** [MH 03]
    a. Rhinoplasty
    b. FESS
    c. SMR
    d. Septoplasty

19. **To prevent synachiae formation after nasal surgery, which one of the following packings is the most useful?**
    a. Mitomycin [AIIMS Nov 04]
    b. Ribbon gauze
    c. Ribbon gauza with liquid paraffin
    d. Ribbon gauza steroids

20. **True about septal hematoma is:** [PGI 02]
    a. Occurs due to trauma
    b. Can lead to saddle-nose deformity
    c. Conservative treatment
    d. May lead to abscess formation

21. **Septal perforation is not seen in:** [DNB 02]
    a. Septal abscess
    b. Leprosy
    c. Rhinophyma
    d. Trauma

Chapter 16: Diseases of External Nose and Nasal Septum

22. **Perforation of palate is/are seen with:** [PGI Nov 2012]
    a. Minor aphthous ulcers
    b. Major aphthous ulcers
    c. Tertiary syphilis
    d. Cocaine abuse
23. **The etiology of anterior ethmoidal neuralgia is:** [AIIMS 03]
    a. Inferior turbinate pressing on the nasal septum
    b. Middle turbinate pressing on the nasal septum
    c. Superior turbinate pressing on the nasal septum
    d. Causing obstruction of sphenoid opening
24. **Cottle's test tests the patency of the nares in:** [JIPMER]
    a. Atrophic rhinitis
    b. Rhinosporidiosis
    c. Deviated nasal septum
    d. Hypertrophied inferior turbinate
25. **Most common location of nasal hemangioma:**
    a. Nasal septum [PGI May 2013]
    b. Inferior turbinate
    c. Vestibule
    d. Uncinate process
    e. Nasopharynx
26. **After laproscopic appendicectomy, patient had fall from bed on her nose after which she had swelling in nose and difficulty in breathing. Next step in management:**
    a. I/V antibiotics for 7–10 days [AIIMS May 2013, 07]
    b. Observation in hospital
    c. Surgical drainage
    d. Discharge after 2 days and follow up of the patient after 8 weeks
27. **A 2-year-old child is brought to the hospital with a compressible swelling at the root of nose, most likely diagnosis is:** [AIIMS 1999]
    a. A V malformation
    b. Lacrimal sac cyst
    c. Ethmoid sinus cyst
    d. Meningoencephalocele

Explanations and References

1. **Ans. is a i.e. Hypertrophy of the sebaceous glands**
   TB of Mohan Bansal, p 292
2. **Ans. is c and e i.e. Acne rosacea; and Treatment is shaving, dermabrasion and skin grafting**
   Ref. Dhingra 6/e, p 144; TB of Mohan Bansal 1/e, p 292
   - Rhinophyma is a slow-growing benign tumor which occurs due to hypertrophy of the sebaceous glands^Q of the tip of the nose.
   - Seen in long standing cases of acne rosacea.^{Q}
   - Mostly affects men past middle age.
   - Presents as a pink, lobulated mass over the nose.

   Treatment
   - Paring down the bulk of the tumor with a sharp knife, or carbon dioxide laser or scalpel (dermabraions), and the area is allowed to re-epithelize.
   - Sometimes tumor is completely excised and the raw area is covered with skin graft.
3. **Ans. is a i.e. Difficulty in breathing** *Ref. Turner 10/e, p 379; Dhingra 6/e, p 163; TB of Mohan Bansal, p 337*
   - Choanal atresia is usually U/L.
     If it occurs bilaterally the neonate presents with difficulty in breathing as infant is a nose breather and does not breathe from mouth. The neonate may have asphyxia and bilateral blockage of nose that also makes suckling difficult.
   - U/L atresia presents with nasal obstruction including snoring but goes unidentified till adult life.
4. **Ans. is a, b, d and e i.e. Colobamatous blindness; Heart disorder; Ear disorders; and CNS lesion**
   Ref. Scott Brown 7/e, Vol 1, p 1071; Dhingra 6/e, p 163; OP Ghai 6 and 7/e, p 336,337

   > - Choanal atresia is associated with CHARGE syndrome: **C**loboma of eye, **H**eart defects, Choanal **A**tresia, **R**etarded growth, **G**enital defects and **E**ar defects.

5. **Ans. is b, c, d and e i.e. Occurs d/t persistence of bucconasal membrane; B/l atresia usually presents with respiratory difficulties; Bilateral atresia may cause cyanosis; and Diagnosed by failure to pass a catheter from nose to pharynx**
   Ref. OP Ghai 7/e, p 336, 337; Logan Turner 10/e, p 377-380

6. **Ans is b, c, d and e i.e. Passing red rubber catheter, Breath sounds by stethoscope, Endoscopy of nose and Acoustic rhinometry**
   "Structure normally seen on posterior rhinoscopy are choanal polyp or atresia"   *Dhingra 5/e, p 385*
   "Choanal atresia: Posterior rhinoscopy may be undertaken in older children and will show the occlusion."
   Turner 10/e, p 380

   Thus posterior rhinoscopy and not anterior rhinoscopy are useful in the diagnosis of choanal atresia.
   "Acoustic rhinometry is a new technique which evaluates nasal obstruction by analysing reflections of a sound pulse introduced via the nostrils. The technique is rapid, reproducible, non-invasive and requires minimal cooperation from the subject. A graph of nasal cross-sectional area as a function of distance from the nostril is produced, from which several area and volume estimates of the nasal cavity can be derived. The role of acoustic rhinometry in diagnosis is somewhat limited compared to nasal endoscopy, but it is useful for nasal challenge and for quantifying nasal obstruction. It is helpful in evaluating childhood nasal obstruction, as it is well tolerated by children as young as 3 years old-a group of patients to whom objective tests have hitherto been difficult to apply."
   Ref: www.ncbi.nim.nih.gov/.../PMC 129

Section 2: Nose and Paranasal Sinuses

7. **Ans. is c i.e. Derived from odontogenic epithelium**

   Ref. http://www.maxillofacialcentre.com./Bondbook/softissue/nasolabialcyst.html#introduction;
   Scott Brown 7/e, Vol 2, p 1320; Textbook of ENT, Hazarika, p 367

   Nasolabial Cysts/Nasoalveolar Cyst/Klestadt's Cyst
   - It is a rare **non odontogenic cyst** which occurs in the region of nasolabial fold. It may arise from epithelial entrapment in the line of fusion between medial and lateral nasal process during the development of nose and cheek (hence also called epithelial inclusion cyst) or may arise as epithelial remnants of nasolacrimal duct.
   - Female >Male
   - Bilateral in approximately 10% of all cases.
   - Usually present in 4th and 5th decades of life.
   - It presents as a smooth and soft bulge in the region of nasolabial fold.
   - Large cyst obliterates the nasolabial sulcus.
   - Treatment is by surgical excision using sublabial approach.

8. **Ans. is d i.e. Acromegaly** *Ref. Dhingra 6/e, p143*

   Depressed nasal bridge results from sagging of the bridge of nose either due to injury or infection of osseous or cartilaginous part of the bridge of nose

   ```
   Causes of depressed nose/saddle nose are:
   H = Hematoma
   O = Operative, i.e. excessive removal of septum during submucous resection
   T = Trauma
   S = Syphilis
   A = Abscess
   L = Leprosy
   T = Tuberculosis
   (Mnemonic – HOT SALT)
   ```

9. **Ans. is a i.e. Deviated dorsum but tip midline** *Ref. Dhingra 6/e, p 143; Textbook of Mohan Bansal, p 291*
   - In *crooked nose* (Fig. 16.1), the dorsum of nose is deviated but tip is in midline.
   - In a *deviated nose*, both dorsum and tip are deviated.
   - *Saddle nose* is depressed nasal dorsum which may involve only cartilaginous or both bony and cartilaginous components.
   - *Humped nose*, there is a presence of hump on nose.

    Note: Both crooked nose and saddle nose are managed by septorhinoplasty whereas humped nose is managed by reduction rhinoplasty.

10. **Ans. is d i.e. 60%** *Ref. Turner 10/e, p 21*
    - Around 60% of children are born with some degree of nasal deviation.

11. **Ans. is b i.e. Atrophy of turbinate** *Ref. Dhingra 6/e, p 149; Tuli 1/e, p 153; Textbook of Mohan Bansal 1/e, p 334,335*

12. **Ans. is a i.e. Recurrent sphenoiditis**

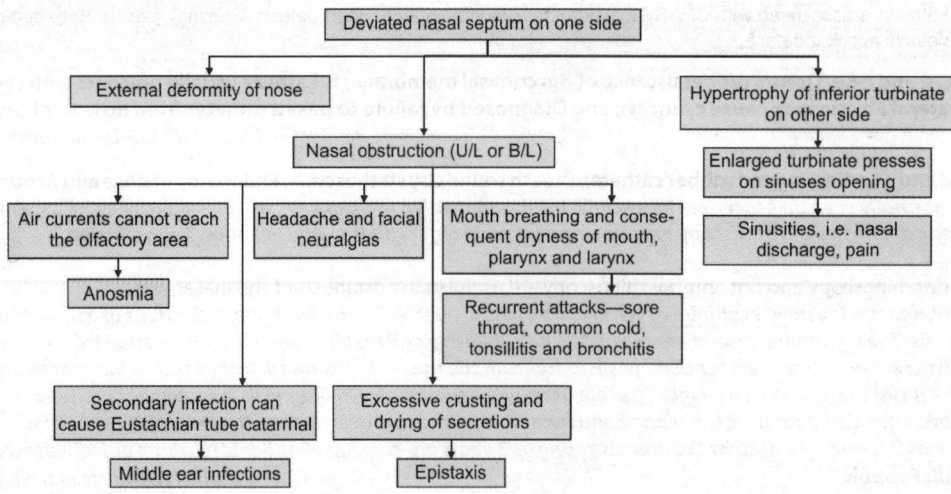

Chapter 16: Diseases of External Nose and Nasal Septum

Note:
- In deviated nasal septum, the nasal chamber on the concave side of the nasal septum is wide and shows compensatory hypertrophy of turbinates and not atrophy.
- The sphenoid sinus opens in the sphenoethmoid recess near the roof of nasal cavity and this opening is not affected by DNS.

13. **Ans. is a, b, c and d i.e. Septal spur with epistaxis; Marked septal deviation; Persistent rhinorrhea; and Recurrent sinusitis**
    Ref. Dhingra 6/e, p 413, 415; Tuli 1/e, p 507; 2/e, p 516

Indications for Surgery in DNS
- **Persistent unilateral nasal obstruction and recurrent headaches**
- Deviation causing recurrent sinusitis or otitis media
- Recurrent epistaxis from septal spur
- Access for operation in polypectomy with DNS
- As a part of septorhinoplasty for cosmetic correction of external nasal deformities.
- As a approach to hypophysectomy

Note: If instead of marked septal deviation, the option could have been only 'septal deviation' then remember minor degree of septal deviation not causing any symptoms does not require any treatment.

14. **Ans. is b i.e. Mucoperichondrim is removed** *Ref. Dhingra 6/e, p 413*
15. **Ans. is b i.e. Septoplasty**
16. **Ans. is a i.e. Submucous resection of nasal septum**
17. **Ans. is d i.e. None of the above**
    - As discussed in the text, septoplasty is a conservative procedure with less complications.
    - Hence it is the preferred surgery these days. Here only the deviated part of cartilaginous septum is removed (where as in SMR – which is a radical procedure, entire cartilaginous septum is removed). Incision used for septoplasty is Freer incision. For SMR – is done Killian Incision.

> ### Intranasal Operations
> ➢ "Intranasal operations are polypectomy, septoplasty, rhinoplasty and functional endoscopic sinus surgery. Either a laryngeal mask or a cuffed endotracheal tube may be used with a **throat pack**, depending on the anesthetist's confidence, the surgeon, the amount of blood loss and the duration of surgery. A flexible laryngeal mask or south-facing preformed tube allows the airway to be secured away from the nose.
> ➢ Topical nasal vasoconstriction is extremely useful and may be applied by the anesthetist or surgeon. Commonly used vasoconstrictors include **5–10% cocaine**, cocaine paste, xylometazoline or ephedrine drops or spray, Moffett's solution, or dental cartridge injection of local anesthetic with epinephrine (adrenaline) 1:80,000. Vasocontstriction by block of the sphenopalatine ganglion, which carries the vasodilator fibers to the nasal blood vessels, has also been described.
> ➢ **Surgery is easier with controlled hypotension**. Profuse bleeding may cause the operation to be abandoned."
> *Ref. Lees Synopsis of Anaesthesia 13/e, p 734,735*
>
> ### Intraoperative and Postoperative Considerations
> ➢ "The most important consideration of nasal surgery is achieving profound vasoconstriction in the nares to minimize and control bleeding. This vasoconstriction can be achieved with **cocaine packs**, local anesthetics, and epinephrine infiltration. Since these drugs have a profound effect on the cardiovascular system, a careful monitoring of the patients cardiovascular functioning is essential, especially for older patients or patients with known cardiac disease. A vasoconstrictor can also precipitate dysrhythmias.
> ➢ **A moderate degree of controlled hypotension** combined with head elevation decreases bleeding in the surgical site. Blood may passively enter the stomach. Placing an oropharyngeal pack or suctioning the stomach at the conclusion of surgery may attenuate postoperative retching and vomiting."
> *Current Otolaryngology 2/e, p 175*
> ➢ Thus in any nasal surgery:
>   - Elective hypotension
>   - Throat pack   } all can be done
>   - Nasal preparation with 10% cociane

18. **Ans. is b i.e. FESS**
    - Amongst all options, FESS is the only surgery which can be performed before 17 years. Remember ideally none of the forms of septal surgery can be performed before 17 years. Still in rarest circumstances, septal surgery has to performed in children septoplasty is done and never SMR.

19. **Ans. is a i.e. Mitomycin** *Ref. Journal of Laryngology and Otology 06, Vol 120, p 921-923*
    - **After Nasal surgery** it has been seen that mitomycin drops applied over nasal mucosa decrease nasal synechiae formation.
    - This is the newer approach and several trials are being done on it ... but our standard textbooks have not yet included it.
    - *"The nasal cavities are packed with ribbon gauze impregnated with Vaseline or liquid paraffin to prevent its sticking to nasal mucosa."*
    - *"Ribbon gauze impregnated with petroleum jelly or bismuth iodoform paraffin paste (BIPP) is inserted in the entire length of the nasal cavity in an attempt to tamponade the bleeding."* *Ref. Scott Brown 7/e, p 1602*

20. **Ans. is a, b and d i.e. Occurs due to trauma; Can lead to saddle-nose deformity; and May lead to abscess formation**
    See text for explanation.

21. **Ans. is c i.e. Rhinophyma**

22. **Ans. is c and d i.e. Tertiary syphilis and Cocaine abuse**
    Ref. Dhingra 6/e, p 151; Scott Brown, Otolaryngology 7/e, Vol 2, Ch. 124, p 1583

    Cause of Perforation of:

Bony septum	Cartilaginous septum	Whole septum
Syphilis	• Lupus • Leprosy • Tuberculosis	Wegner's granuloma (which includes bony septum also)

23. **Ans. is b i.e. Middle turbinate pressing on the nasal septum** *Ref. Turner 10/e, p 66; Dhingra, 6/e, p 449*

    Sluder's neuralgia or the anterior ethmoidal syndrome is pain around the bridge of the nose radiating into the forehead. It is said to originate from the middle turbinate (part of ethmoid bone) pressing on the deviated septum. This is a rare cause of headache and also k/a contact point headache.

24. **Ans. is c i.e. Deviated nasal septum** *Ref. Dhingra 6/e, p 149; TB of Mohan Bansal, p 287*

    Cottle test: It is used to test nasal obstruction due to abnormality of nasal valve as in case of deviated nasal septum.
    In this test, cheek is drawn laterally while the patient breathes quietly. If the nasal airway improves on the test side, the test is positive, and indicates abnormality of the vestibular component of nasal valve.

25. **Ans. is a i.e. Nasal septum** *Ref. Textbook of ENT, Hazarika 3/e, p 371*

    Nasal Hemagiomas:
    - Hemangioma and angioma are common in nasal septum.
    - It can also arise from turbinates, nasopharynx and rarely external nose (nasal tip is M/C site in external nose).
    - M/C features – Nasal obstruction and epistaxis.
    - Management – Laser excision.

26. **Ans. is c i.e. Surgical drainage** *Ref. Dhingra 6/e, p 150*

    She has possibly developed septal hematoma. A septal hematoma has to be drained as early as possible (Generally within 72 hrs) or else it can lead to necrosis of septal cartilage and loss of support of dorsum leading to sadding of nose. It can also get infected and lead to formation of septal abscess.

27. **Ans. is d i.e. is Meningoencephalocele**

    Two year child with compressible swelling at the root of nose is most likely a Meningoencephalocele.
    Lacrimal sac cyst occurs as a compressible swelling near the medial canthus and not root of nose.
    Ethmoid cyst (mucocele) presents as a swelling at the medial quadrant of orbit pushing the orbit forwards and laterally.
    AV malformation is a congenital abnormal connection between arteries and veins, bypassing the capillary system. These are largely found in internal organs and is rare at this site.

Chapter 17

Granulomatous Disorders of Nose, Nasal Polyps and Foreign Body in Nose

GRANULOMATOUS DISEASES OF THE NOSE

Bacterial	Fungal	Unspecified/Causes
• Syphilis	• Rhinosporidiosis	• Wegener's granulomatosis
• Tuberculosis	• Aspergillosis	
• Lupus	• Mucormycosis	• Non-healing midline granuloma
• Rhinoscleroma	• Candidiasis	• Sarcoidosis
• Leprosy	• Histoplasmosis	
	• Blastomycosis	

BACTERIAL INFECTIONS

LUPUS VULGARIS

- It is an indolent and chronic form of tuberculous infection.
- Female: Male ratio is 2:1
- *Most common* site is the **mucocutaneous junction of the nasal** septum, the nasal vestibule and the ala.
- Characteristic feature is the presence of *apple-jelly nodules* (Brown gelatinous nodules) in skin.
- Cutaneous lesion involving external nose has a typical **butterfly appearance**.
- *Lupus can cause perforation of cartilaginous part of nasal septum*
- Confirmation is by biopsy.
- T/t = ATT.

SYPHILIS (FLOWCHART 17.1)

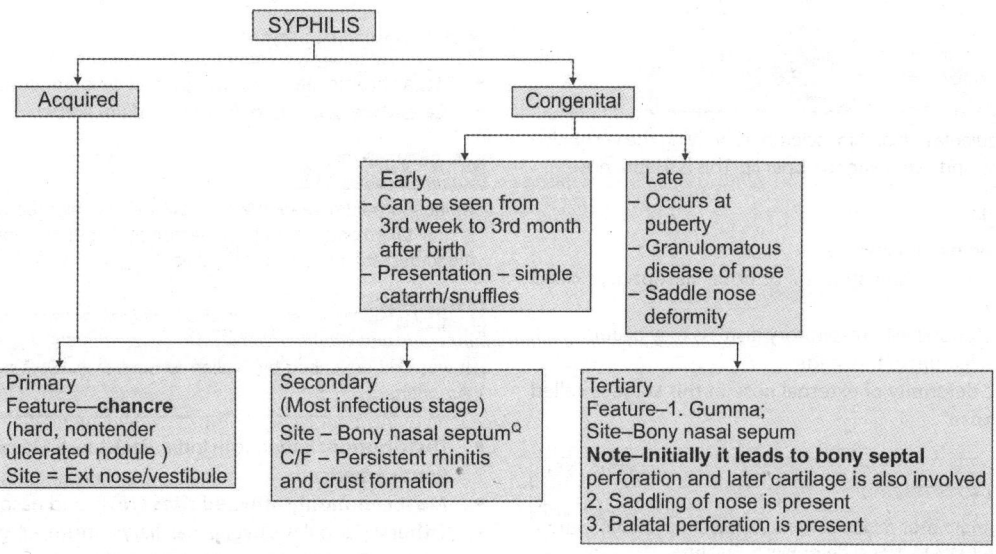

Flowchart 17.1: Types and clinical feature of syphilis

RHINOSCLEROMA (MIKULCIZ DISEASE)

It is chronic, progressive granulomatous disease commencing in the nose and extending into the nasopharynx oropharynx, larynx (subglottic area), trachea and bronchi.

Organism

Klebsiella rhinoscleromatis (Gram-negative Frisch bacillus).

Features

- Scleroma can occur at any age and in either sex.
- The disease has following stages.

Atrophic Stage

Resembles atrophic rhinitis and is characterized by foul smelling purulent nasal discharge and crusting.

Granulomatous Stage

- Proliferative stage
- The stage is characterized by granulomatous reactions and presence of *'Mikulicz cells'*
- Painless nodules are formed in nasal mucosa.
- Subdermal infiltration occurs in lower part of external nose and upper lip giving a *woody feel*.
- Severe cases may lead to broadening of nose due to thickening of the skin with characteristic **"Hebra-nose"**.

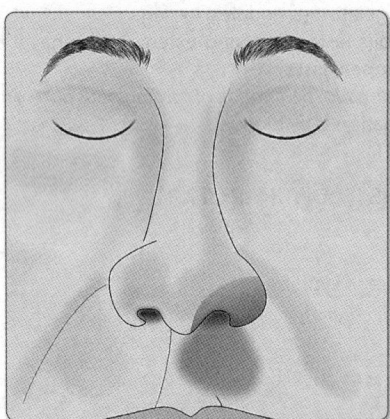

Fig. 17.1: Nodular lesion of rhinoscleroma involving the vestibulo external nose and extending to upper lip. This is "Hebra nose"

Cicatricial Stage

It is characterized by formation of:
- Adhesions fibrosis and stenosis of nose, nasopharynx and oropharynx.
- Subglottic stenosis with respiratory distress may occur.
- Pain is not a feature of this stage
- The fibrotic deformity of external nose in this stage is called as **"Taper nose"**.

Point to Remember

➤ M/C symptom of rhinoscleroma is nasal obstruction and crusting (94%) > Nasal deformity > Epistaxis.

Diagnosis

- Biopsy shows submucosal infiltrates of plasma cells, lymphocytes, eosinophils, *mikulicz cells and russell* bodies.
- **Mikulicz Cells:** are large foam cells with a central nucleus and vacuolated cytoplasm containing the bacilli).
- **Russell Bodies:** are homogenous eosinophilic inclusion bodies found in plasma cells.
- Both of them are characteristic features of rhinoscleroma.

Treatment

- Streptomycin (2 g/day) + Tetracycline (2 g/day) for a minimum of 4–6 weeks (till 2 consecutive samples are negative).
- Surgical dilatation of the cicatricial areas with polythene tubes for 6–8 weeks.

LEPROSY

- M/C in lepromatous leprosy
- **M/C affected parts:** Nasal septum (anterior part) and inferior turbinate

Feature

Leads to perforation of nasal septum and saddle nose deformity.

Treatment

Dapsone, Isoniazid and Rifampin.

NEW PATTERN QUESTION	
Q N1.	Tapir nose is seen in:
	a. Leprosy
	b. Syphilis
	c. Rhinoscleroma
	d. Lupus vulgaris

FUNGAL INFECTIONS

RHINOSPORIDIOSIS

- It is a chronic granulomatous infection of mucous membranes
- **Causative organism:** *Rhinosporidium seeberi*

Latest Concept

Rhinosporodium seeberi was previously considered as fungus. It is now taken as an aquatic protestan protozoa. It belongs to class mesomycetozoea and is unicellular.

History

It was first described by Guillermo Seeber in 1900 in a patient in Argentina.

- **Distribution:** Endemic in India, Pakistan, Sri Lanka, Africa and South America
- **Most commonly affected sites:** Nose and nasopharynx
- **Others:** Lip, palate, uvula, maxillary antrum, epiglottis, larynx, trachea, bronchi, ear, scalp, penis, vulva, vagina.

- **Mode of affection:** Through contaminated water of pond (M/C route). It is common in farmers and people bathing in ponds. The spores get deposited in traumatized part of nose and completes its life cycle there (Fig. 17.2).

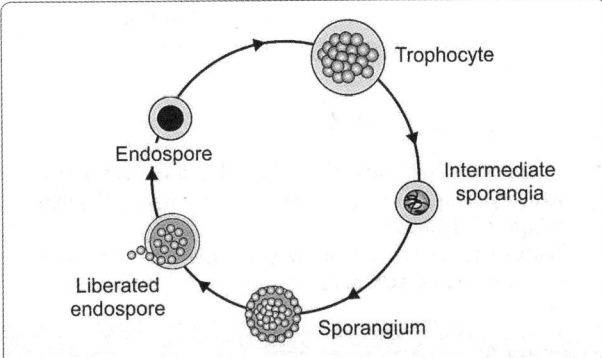

Fig. 17.2: Life cycle of R. seeberi

Features
- Young males are more affected (15-40 years).
- Lesions are polypoid and papillomatous friable masses which bleed easily on touch.
- **They are strawberry** (pink to purple) colored and studded with white dot's representing the sporangia.
- Patients complain of nasal discharge which is blood tinged. Sometimes frank epistaxis is the only presenting complaint.

Diagnosis
It is made by biopsy which shows several sporangia and spores.

Treatment
- Endoscopic excision of the mass followed by cauterization of its base.
- Recurrence may occur after surgery.
- Medical management with dapsone decrease the recurrence rate. Injection corticosteroid and amphotericin can also be used.

ASPERGILLOSIS

- *Aspergillosis is the commonest fungal infection of the nose and sinuses.*
- **Causative organism:** *A. fumigatus* (90%) > *A. niger* and *A. flavus*
- **Spread:** air-borne

Features
- It can affect any age group.
- Black or grayish membrane seen on nasal mucosa.
- Maxillary sinus shows a fungal ball

Treatment
Surgical debridement and antifungal drugs.

MUCORMYCOSIS

It is an aggressive opportunistic fungal infection.

Predisposing Factors
- Immunosuppressed patients
- Uncontrolled diabeties

Features
- Mucormycosis differs from other fungi as it has a remarkable affinity for blood vessels and arteries leading to extensive endothelial damage and thrombosis.
- The disease begins in the nose and paranasal sinus and spreads to orbit, cribiform plate, meninges and brain.
- *Typical finding:* Black necrotic mass seen filling the entire nasal cavity.
- Erosion of the nasal septum and the hard palate may be seen.

Investigations
- Sinus radiographs show thickened sinus walls and spotty destruction of the bony walls.
- MRI detects early vascular and intracranial invasion.

Treatment
- Systemic - Amphotericin B
- Surgical debridement of the affected tissues
- *Orbital exenteration* is mandatory in case of ophthalmoplegia and loss of vision.

Points to Remember
- Syphilis affects the bone, while tuberculosis affects the cartilagenous framework of nose.
- Rhinoscleroma is caused by Frisch bacillus, i.e. *Klebsiella rhinoscleromatis*. Mikulicz cells and Russel bodies are typical of the histopathological examination.
- Sarcoidosis resembles tuberculosis except for caseation, and Kveim test and biopsy are diagnostic.

NEW PATTERN QUESTIONS

Q N2. Nasal polypoidal mass with subcutaneous nodules on skin are seen in:

a. Zygomycosis   b. Rhinosporidiosis
c. Sporotrichosis   d. Aspergillosis

Q N3. Ideal treatment of rhinosporodiosis is:

a. Rifampicin
b. Excision with cautery at base
c. Tetracycline
d. Laser

Q N4. Strawberry skin appearance of nasal mucosa is seen in:

a. Wegener's granulomatosis
b. Sarcoidosis
c. Kawasaki disease
d. Rhinosporidiosis

Q N5. Mulberry shaped polypoidal mass is seen in:
a. Rhinosporidiosis b. Rhinoscleroma
c. Rhinophyma d. Inferior turbinate hypertrophy

Q N6. Aspergillosis is M/c caused by:
a. A. fumigatus b. A. niger
c. A. flavus d. None of these

Q N7. Which of the following is a lethal midline granuloma of nose?
a. Wegener's granuloma
b. Rhinosporidium
c. Lupus
d. Stewarts granuloma

Q N8. Mikulicz cells and Russell bodies are seen in:
a. Rhinoscleroma b. Rhinosporidiasis
c. Scleroderma d. Lupus vulgaris

Q N9. Mitral cells are seen in:
a. Rhinoscleroma b. Olfactory tract
c. Rhinosporidiosis d. Optic nerve

NASAL POLYPS

- Polyps are non-neoplastic pedunculated masses which are sparsely cellular and are covered by normal epithelium, i.e. columnar ciliated epithelium.
- **Features:** They are soft, fleshy, pale, *insensitive to pain and do not shrink with the use of vasoconstrictors.*

Table 17.1: Types of nasal polyp

Ethmoidal polyps	Antrochoanal polyps (Killians polyp)
Age group = 30–60 years **Sex** = Male > Female **M/C Site**: Ethmoid sinus (can also arise from middle turbinate and middle meatus). **Etiology:** Allergy (M/C). **On examination**: *B/L* Multiple, smooth, glistening sessile or pedunculated polyps Lining epithelium initially is columnar, later due to trauma it undergoes squamous metaplasia. **Symptoms** Presenting symptom B/L nasal blockage.	• Seen in children and young adults (male > female) • Maxillary antrum (floor and medial wall) **Etiology** = Allergy + Infection **On examination** – U/L, pale, white, translucent It has 3 parts: • Antral • Choanal • Nasal **Symptoms—** U/L nasal blockage (which can become bilateral when polyp grows into nasopharynx and obstructs opposite choana) • Hyponasal voice • Nasal discharge • Conductive deafness due to (blockage of Eustachian tube)
Others • Partial/complete loss of smell • Pain over nasal bridge forehead/cheek • Postnasal drip Broadening of nose (frog face deformity) **Note:** Polyps do not present with epistaxis/bleeding **O/E** • **Anterior rhinoscopy**—multiple, smooth, bluish gray grape-like masses. • On probing – All polyps are insensitive to probing and donot bleed. **Investigation**– X-ray of PNS **IOC:** NCCT of nose and paranasal sinus. **Treatment** Surgical • Effective only in 50% cases Drug used – Intranasal corticosteroids Medical T/t – Not done as it is recurrent. **Surgery** • *Simple polypectomy:* Indicated in case of one/two polyps • Intransal ethmoidectomy: Done when polyps are multiple and sessile. Since it is a blind procedure it can give rise to orbital complications • *Extranasal ethmoidectomy:* Indicated when polyps recurr after intranasal procedures [Howarth's incision (Incision given medial to the inner canthus of the eye)] • *Horgans transantral ethmoidectomy:* When polypoidal changes are also seen in the maxillary antrum. • *Endoscopic sinus surgery:* It is the latest procedure for removal of small polyps under good illumination using 0° and 30° sinoscope, i.e. Functional endoscopic sinus surgery (**FESS**).	**Anterior rhinoscopy:** It is not visualized as they are posterior. *Posterior rhinoscopy* – Smooth, white spherical masses seen in choana **IOC:** NCCT nose and paranasal sinus. Treatment 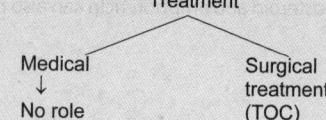 *Surgical Management* • Intranasal polypectomy: Indicated in - young patients with incomplete dentition. • Caldwell-Luc operation (i.e. opening the maxillary artrum through canine fossa by sublabial approach). It is done, if there is recurrence and age of patient is more than 17 years. • Nowadays antrochoanal polyp is being treated by FESS

- They do not bleed on touch and are insensitive to probing and never present with epistaxis or bleeding from nose.
- Types of nasal polyp are described in Table 17.1.

Point to Remember
➢ Samters triad – It is a triad of asthma, aspirin intolerance and nasal polyps.

Relation of Polyp to Bernoulli's Phenomenon

Bernoulli's theorem states that as velocity of air increases, lateral pressure decreases. More the velocity, more is the drop in lateral pressure. When air passes through nasal valve area—narrowest part, the velocity of air increases, which leads to drop in pressure such that negative pressure occurs. This negative pressure facilitates accumulation of edematous fluid in the submucosa leading to polyp formation.

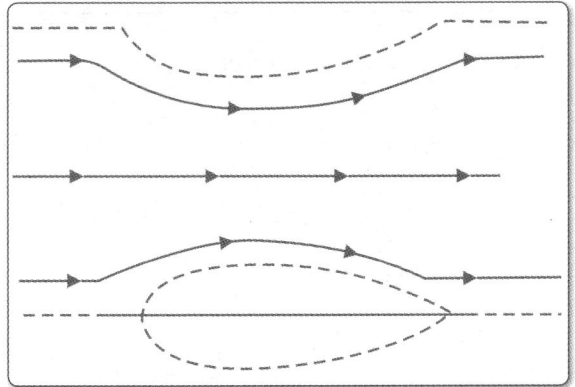

Fig. 17.3: Bernoulli's phenomenon—Negative pressure seen at the stenotic site, facilitates accumulation of fluid in the submucosa

Points to Remember

Some important points to remember in a case of nasal polyp
1. If a polypus is red and fleshy, friable and has granular surface, especially in older patients, think of malignancy.
2. Simple nasal polyp may masquerade a malignancy underneath. Hence all polypi should be subjected to histology.
3. A simple polyp in a child may be a glioma, an encephalocele or a meningoencephalocele. It shold always be aspirated and fluid examined for CSF. Careless removal of such polyp would result in CSF rhinorrhoea and meningitis.
4. Multiple nasal polypi in children may be assoicated with mucoviscidosis.
5. Expistaxis and orbital symptoms associated with a polyp should always arouse the suspicion of malignancy.

NEW PATTERN QUESTIONS

Q N10. Frog face deformity is seen in:
a. Nasal polyp
b. Syphilis of nose
c. Wegner's granulomatosis
d. TB of nose

Q N11. Samter's triad includes:
a. Nasal polyps
b. Aspirin sensitivity
c. Bronchiectasis
d. Bronchial asthma
e. Immunodeficiency

Q N12. Most common nasal mass:
a. Polyp
b. Papilloma
c. Angiofibroma
d. None of these

Q N13. Antrochoanal polyp arises from:
a. Maxillary sinus
b. Frontal sinus
c. Ethmoidal sinus
d. Sphenoidal sinus

FOREIGN BODIES IN NOSE

May be organic or inorganic and are mostly seen in children.^{Q}

Clinical Features

Unilateral foul smelling discharge in a child is pathognomic of a foreign body.^{Q}

Treatment

- Removal under LA/GA.^{Q}
- In children use of oral positive pressure technique called as **'Parent's Kiss'** technique is being practiced for removal of anterior nasal foreign body *(Scott Brown)*.

Complications

- Nasal infection (vestibulitis) and sinusitis
- Rhinolith formation.
- Inhalation into the tracheobronchial tree

■ RHINOLITH

- It is stone formation in the nasal cavity.
- Rhinolith forms around the nucleus of a small exogenous foreign body or blood clot when calcium, magnesium and phosphate deposit around it.

Clinical Features

- More common in adults.
  Presents as unilateral nasal obstruction and foul smelling discharge (often blood stained)
- Ulceration of the surrounding mucosa may lead to frank epistaxis and neuralgic pain.

Treatment

Removal under GA. Some hard and irregular rhinolitis may require lateral rhinotomy

■ NASAL MYIASIS (MAGGOTS IN NOSE)

- It results from the prescence of ova of flies particularly Chrysomyia species in the nose which produce ulceration and destruction of nasal structure.

- Mostly seen in atrophic rhinitis when the mucosa becomes insensitive to flies laying eggs inside

Clinical features

Initial
- 3–4 days maggots produce
- Intense irritation
  Sneezing
- Lacrimation
- Headache
- Thin blood stained discharge

Later

Maggots may crawl out of nose and there is foul smell.

Complications
- Destruction of nose, sinuses, soft tissues of face, palate and eyeball.
- Fistulae in nose and palate
- Death occurs due to meningitis

Treatment

Instillation of chloroform water and oil in nose and plugging the nose, so that maggots do not crawl out.
- Patient should be isolated

ALSO KNOW

For undergraduate students:

> **VIVA for UG**
> **Causes of unilateral blood stained nasal discharge in a child**
> - Foreign body in nose
> - Rhinolith
> - Nasal diphtheria
> - Nasal myiasis
> - Acute/Chronic unilateral sinusitis.

Chapter 17: Granulomatous Disorders of Nose, Nasal Polyps and Foreign Body in Nose

Explanations and References to New Pattern Questions

N1. Ans is c i.e. Rhinoscleroma   *Ref. Textbook of ENT, Hazarika 3/e, p 308*

Tapir nose and Hebra nose are seen in rhinoscleroma.

N2. Ans is b i.e. Rhinosporidiosis   *Ref. Dhingra 6/e, p 158,159*

In Rhinosporiodiosis leafy, polypoidal mass of pink-purple color is seen attached to nasal septum or lateral wall. Subcutaneous nodules may be seen on skin.

N3. Ans is b i.e. Excision with cautery at base   *Ref. Dhingra 6/e, p 159*

Read the preceeding text.

N4. Ans is b i.e. Sarcoidosis   *Ref. Dhingra 6/e, p 160*

Strawberry skin appearance of nasal mucosa is seen in sarcoidosis.

N5. Ans is a i.e. Rhinosporidiosis

Mulberry shaped polypoidal mass of nose indicates rhinosporidiosis.

N6. Ans is a i.e. A. fumigatus

- A. fumigatus > A. niger is the M/c cause of aspergillosis (90%) of nose.
- Aspergillosis is the commonest fungal infection of nose.

N7. Ans is d i.e. Stewarts granuloma   *Ref. Textbook of ENT, Hazarika, 3/e, p 313*

Midline nonhealing granulomas of nose are:
1. Wegners granuloma
2. Stewarts granuloma

Stewarts granuloma is also called as lethal midline granuloma or midfacial lymphoma. It is a rare T-cell lymphoma which gradually ulcerates the cartilage and bone of the nose and midface. It is strongly associated with Epstein Barr virus.

N8. Ans is a i.e. Rhinoscleroma   *Ref. Dhingra 6/e, p 156*

See text for explanation.

N9. Ans is b i.e. Olfactory tract   *Ref. Essentials of ENT, Mohan Bansal, p 181*

Mitral cells are present in olfactory bulb of the olfactory tract.

N10. Ans is a i.e. Nasal polyp   *Ref. Textbook of ENT, Hazarika 3/e, p 344*

Frog face deformity is seen in ethmoidal polyp. There is widening of the intercanthal distance with frog face deformity in extensive ethmoidal polyposis.

N11. Ans. is a, b and d i.e. Nasal polyps; Aspirin sensitivity; and Bronchial asthma

Ref. Scott Brown 7th/ed, Vol 2, p 1472; Internet search – wikipedia.org; Textbook of Mohan Bansal, p 307

Samter's triad is a medical condition consisting of asthma, aspirin sensitivity, and nasal/ethmoidal polyposis. It occurs in middle age *(twenties and thirties are the most common onset times)* and may not include any allergies.
- *Most commonly, the first symptom is* rhinitis.
- The disorder typically progresses to asthma, then polyposis, with aspirin sensitivity coming last.
- The aspirin reaction can be severe, including an asthma attack, anaphylaxis, and urticaria in some cases. Patients typically react to other NSAIDs such as ibuprofen, although paracetamol is generally considered safe.
- Anosmia (lack of smell) is also typical, as the inflammation reaches the olfactory receptors in the nose.

N12. Ans is a i.e. Polyp

> **Remember**
> M/C Nasal masses are polyps.

N13. Ans is a i.e. Maxillary sinus   *Ref. Dhingra 6/e, p 175*

Antrochoanal polyp arises from the mucosa of maxillary sinus near accessory ostium.

QUESTIONS

1. A 68-year-old Chandu is a diabetic and presented with black, foul smelling discharge from the nose. Examination revealed blackish discoloration of the inferior turbinate. The diagnosis is: [AIIMS 99]
   a. Mucormycosis
   b. Aspergillosis
   c. Infarct of inferior turbinate
   d. Foreign body

2. IDDM patient presents with septal perforation of nose with brownish black discharge probable diagnosis is: [AI 97; RJ 06]
   a. Rhinosporidiosis
   b. Aspergillus
   c. Leprosy
   d. Mucormycosis

3. Rhinosporidiosis is caused by: [PGI 99; UP 00]
   a. Fungus
   b. Virus
   c. Bacteria
   d. Protozoa

4. True statement about Rhinosporidiosis is: [AI 99]
   a. Most common organism is klebsiella rhinoscleromatis
   b. Seen only in immunocompromised patients
   c. Presents as a nasal polyp
   d. Can be diagnosed by isolation of organism

5. In rhinosporidiosis, the following is true: [PGI 99]
   a. Fungal granuloma
   b. Grayish mass
   c. Surgery is the treatment
   d. Radiotherapy is treatment

6. Ideal treatment of rhinosporidiosis is: [AIIMS 97]
   a. Rifampicin
   b. Excision with cautery at base
   c. Dapsone
   d. Laser

7. Rhinoscleromatis is caused by: [PGI 99]
   a. Klebseilla
   b. Autoimmune
   c. Spirochetes
   d. Rhinosporidium

8. Mikulicz cell and russel bodies are characterisitc of: [JIPMER 02; Bihar 06]
   a. Rhinoscleroma
   b. Rhinosporidiosis
   c. Plasma cell disorder
   d. Lethal midline granuloma

9. Which of the following feature (s) of rhinoscleroma is/are true except: [PGI Nov 2014]
   a. Atrophy of nasal mucosa
   b. Caused by fungus
   c. Treatment by antifungal drug
   d. Caused by bacteria
   e. Causative organism may be cultured from biopsy material

10. Atrophic dry nasal mucosa, extensive encrustations with woody' hard external nose is suggestive of [MH 05]
    a. Rhinosporidiosis
    b. Rhinoscleroma
    c. Atrophic rhinitis
    d. Carcinoma of nose

11. Apple-jelly nodules on the nasal septum are found in case of: [MP 05]
    a. Tuberculosis
    b. Syphilis
    c. Lupus vulgaris
    d. Rhinoscleroma

12. About nasal syphilis the following is true: [PGI 02]
    a. Perforation occurs in septum
    b. Saddle nose deformity may occur
    c. In newborn, it presents as snuffles
    d. Atrophic rhinitis is a complication
    e. Secondary syphilis is the common association

13. Killian term is used for which of the following polyp?
    a. Ethmoidal
    b. Antrochoanal [UP 05]
    c. Tonsillar cyst
    d. Tonsillolith

14. All the following are true of antrochoanal polyp except: [AI 94]
    a. Common in children
    b. Single and unilateral
    c. Bleeds on touch
    d. Treatment involves avulsion

15. All of the following are true about antrochonal polyp, except: [TN 07]
    a. Single
    b. Unilateral
    c. Premalignant
    d. Arises from maxillary antrum

16. Antrochoanal polyp is characterized by: [PGI Dec 03]
    a. Usually bilateral
    b. It is of allergic origin
    c. It arises from maxillary antrum
    d. Caldwell-Luc operation is treatment of choice in recurrent cases
    e. Recurrence is common

17. True about antrochoanal polyp: [PGI Nov 2016]
    a. Starts as edema of maxillary sinus mucosa
    b. Suppressed by steroids
    c. Comes out via accessory ostium and grows in the choana and nasal cavity
    d. More common in adults than children
    e. Commonly presents as unilateral nasal obstruction

18. The most appropriate management for antrochoanal polyp in children is: [AIIMS 02]
    a. Caldwell-Luc operation
    b. Intranasal polypectomy
    c. Corticosteroids
    d. Wait and watch

19. A patient presents with antrochoanal polyp arising from the medial wall of the maxilla. Which of the following would be the best management for the patient?
    a. FESS with polypectomy [AIIMS May 2014]
    b. Medial maxillectomy (TEMM)
    c. Caldwell-Luc procedure
    d. Intranasal polypectomy

20. Treatment for recurrent atrochoanal polyp: [MP 2007]
    a. Caldwell-Luc operation
    b. FESS
    c. Simple polypectomy
    d. Both a and b

21. The current treatment of choice for a large antrochoanal polyp in a 10-year-old is: *[AIIMS Nov 2005, 2002, May 2014]*
    a. Intranasal polypectomy
    b. Caldwell-Luc operation
    c. FESS
    d. Lateral rhinotomy and excision
22. The current treatment of choice for a large antrochoanal polyp in a 30-year-old man is: *[AIIMS Nov 05]*
    a. Intranasal polypectomy
    b. Caldwell-Luc operation
    c. Functional endoscopic sinus surgery (FESS)
    d. Lateral rhinotomy and excision
23. Which of the following statements is not correct for Ethmoidal polyp? *[AIIMS 02]*
    a. Allergy is an etiological factor
    b. Occur in the first decade of life
    c. Are bilateral
    d. Are often associated with bronchial asthma
24. Regarding ethmoidal polyp, which one of the following is true? *[Kolkata 05]*
    a. Epistaxis
    b. Unilateral
    c. <10 years
    d. Associated with bronchial asthma
25. Recurrent polyps are seen in: *[UP 07]*
    a. Antrochoanal polyp   b. Ethmoidal polyp
    c. Nasal polyp   d. Hypertrophic turbinate
26. In a patient with multiple bilateral nasal polyps with X-ray showing opacity in the paranasal sinuses. The treatment consists of all of the following *except*: *[AIIMS 02]*
    a. Epinephrine   b. Corticosteroids
    c. Amphoterecin B   d. Antihistamines
27. Patient with ethmoidal polyp undergoes polypectomy. Presents 6 months later with ethmoidal polyp. Correct Rx: *[AIIMS 95]*
    a. Intranasal ethmoidectomy
    b. Extranasal ethmoidectomy
    c. Caldwell-Luc procedure
    d. Polypectomy
28. "Bernoulli's theorem" explains: *[UP 07]*
    a. Nasal polyp   b. Thyroglossal cyst
    c. Zenker's diverticulum   d. Laryngomalacia
29. Topical steroids are not recommended post-surgery for: *[AIIMS November 2014]*
    a. Allergic fungal sinusitis   b. Chronic rhinosinusitis
    c. Antrochoanal polyp   d. Ethmoidal polyps
    e. Lingual nerve
30. In Caldwell-Luc operation the nasoantral window is made through: *[TN 04]*
    a. Superior meatus   b. Inferior meatus
    c. Middle meatus   d. None of the above
31. Most common complication of Caldwell-Luc operation is: *[AP 00]*
    a. Oroantral fistula   b. Infraorbital nerve palsy
    c. Hemorrhage   d. Orbital cellulitis
32. Multiple nasal polyp in children should guide the clinician to search for underlying: *[AP PG 2012]*
    a. Mucoviscidosis   b. Celiac disease
    c. Hirschsprung's disease   d. Sturge-Weber syndrome
33. A Rapidly destructive infection of nose and paranasal sinuses in diabetics is:
    a. Histoplasmosis   b. Sporotrichosis
    c. Mucormycosis   d. Sarcoidosis
34. Frish bacillus causes:
    a. Rhinosleroma   b. Rhinosporidiosis
    c. Rhinophyma   d. Lupus vulgaris
35. About foreign body in a child true statement is:
    a. Unilateral fetid discharge   *[PGI June 03]*
    b. Presents with unilateral nasal obstruction
    c. Has torrential epistaxis
    d. Inanimate is more common than animate
    e. Always removed under GA
36. Most common cause of U/L mucopurulent rhinorrhea in a child is: *[Kolkata 01/FMGE 2013]*
    a. Foreign body
    b. Adenoids which are blocking the airways
    c. Deviated nasal septum
    d. Inadequately treated acute frontal sinusitis
37. A child has retained disc battery in the nose. What is the most important consideration in the management? *[AIIMS Nov 14]*
    a. Battery substance leaks and cause tissue damage
    b. It can lead to tetanus
    c. Refer the child to a specialist for removal of battery
    d. Instill nasal drops
38. What is a Rhinolith: *[AI 91]*
    a. Foreign body in nose
    b. Stone in nose
    c. Deposition of calcium around foreign body in nose
    d. Misnomer
39. Maggots in the nose are best treated by: *[AI 98; 96]*
    a. Chloroform diluted with water
    b. Liquid paraffin
    c. Systemic antibiotics
    d. Lignocaine spray
40. Feature of granulomatosis with polyangiitis: *[PGI May 2015]*
    a. Nasal polyp   b. Perforated nasal septum
    c. Persistent sinus   d. Crusting of nasal mucosa
    e. Collapse of nasal bridge
41. The combination of nasal polyps, bronchial asthma and aspirin sensitivity is referred to as: *[APPG 2016]*
    a. Santer's triad   b. Saint's triad
    c. Virchow's triad   d. Trotter's triad
42. Deformities occurring in leprosy patients is/are:
    a. Facies leonina   b. Low set ear   *[PGI May 17]*
    c. Saddle nose   d. Lagophthalmos
    e. Micrognathia

Explanations and References

1. **Ans. is a i.e. Mucormycosis**
2. **Ans. is d i.e. Mucormycosis**   *Ref. Dhingra 6/e, p 159; TB of Mohan Bansal, p 317*
   - **Mucormycosis** is fungal infection of nose and paranasal sinuses which may prove rapidly fatal if untreated.
   - It is seen in uncontrolled diabetes or in those taking immunosuppressive drugs.
   - It presents as black necrotic mass filling the nasal cavity and eroding the septum and hard palate.
   - **Treatment** is by amphotericin B^Q and surgical debridement.

    Note: Most common fungal infection of nose is Aspergillosis.^{Q}

3. **Ans. is d i.e. Protozoa**
4. **Ans. is c i.e. Presents as a nasal polyp**
5. **Ans. is a and c i.e. Fungal granuloma; and Surgery is the treatment**
6. **Ans. is b i.e. Excision with cautery at base**   *Ref. Dhingra 6/e, p 158,159; TB of Mohan Bansal, p 316, 317*
   Rhinosporodiosis is a Granuloma^Q caused by *Rhinosporidium seeberi* which is now taken as a protozoa not fungus.
   Rest all is given in preceeding text.
7. **Ans. is a i.e. Klebsiella**
8. **Ans. is a i.e. Rhinoscleroma**
9. **Ans. is b and c i.e. Caused by fungus and treatment by antifungal drugs**
10. **Ans. is b i.e. Rhinoscleroma**   *Ref. Dhingra 6/e, p 156; Scott Brown's 7/e, Vol 2, Chapter 115, p 1462,1463; TB of Mohan Bansal, p 315*

Rhinoscleroma

- It is a chronic granulamatous disease caused by gram-negative Frisch bacteria *Klebsiella rhinoscleromatis*.

Pathologically

- **Mikulicz cells or foam cells and Russell bodies are its characteristic features.**
- Russell bodies are homogenous eosinophilic inclusion bodies found in plasma cells.
- In a patient presenting with atrophic dry nasal mucosa, extensive crusting and woody hard external nose:
  - Rhinoscleroma should be suspected.
- **In Q 10 for option (e) "Causative organism can be cultured from biopsy material."** Read the following lines from Essentials of ENT by Mohan Bansal. *"Culture of infected tissue: The causative organisms are cultured and that is diagnostic.."......Essentials of ENT, Mohan Bansal, p 217*

11. **Ans. is c i.e. Lupus vulgaris**   *Ref. Dhingra 6/e, p 157; Scott Brown's Otolaryngology 7/e, Vol 2, Chapter 115, p 1456; Current Otorhinology 2/e, p 261; TB of Mohan Bansal, p 316*
    - Lupus vulgaris is the chronic and more common form of tubercular infection affecting the skin and mucous membrane of nose
    - Apple-jelly appearances are brown gelatinous nodules and are typical skin lesions of lupus.

12. **Ans. is e i.e. Secondary syphilis is the common association**   *Ref. Dhingra 6/e, p 157*
    Nasal syphilis may be:
    - **Acquired:**   – Primary, e.g. chancre in vestibule
      - Secondary, e.g. simple rhinitis, crusting and fissuring leading to atrophic rhinitis
      - Tertiary, e.g. Gumma leads to septal perforation and saddle nose deformity (due to collapse of nasal bridge)
    - **Congenital:**   – Early (first 3 months): Presenting as snuffles, purulent nasal discharge, fissuring excoriation.
      - late (around puberty): Gumma in septum and other stigmatas.
    - Teritary syphilis is a common association: primary and secondary syphilis are rare association in nasal syphilitis.
    - Septal perforation occurs in bony part in case of syphilis.

13. **Ans. is b i.e. Antrochoanal**   *Ref. Internet search*
    Killian's polyp is the name given to antrochoanal polyp based on Gustain Killians.
14. **Ans. is c i.e. Bleeds on touch**
15. **Ans. is c i.e. Premalignant**

Chapter 17: Granulomatous Disorders of Nose, Nasal Polyps and Foreign Body in Nose

16. **Ans. is c and d i.e. It arises from maxillary antrum; Caldwell-Luc operation is treatment of choice in recurrent cases**
    Ref. Dhingra 6/e, p 174, 175; Scott Brown 7/e, Vol 2, Chapter 121, p 1554; TB of Mohan Bansal, p 308,309
    - Nasal polyps are non-neoplastic masses[Q] of edematous nasal or sinus mucosa. They do not bleed on touch and are insensitive to probing and never present with epistaxis or bleeding from nose.
    - Recurrence is uncommon in case of antrochoanal polyp.
    - Antrochoanal polyps arise from maxillary artrum and then grow into choana and nasal cavity.

    [For details of Antrochoanal polyps see text]

17. **Ans. is a, c and e i.e. Starts as edema of maxillary sinus mucosa, comes out via accessory antrum and grows in the choana and nasal cavity and commonly presents as unilateral nasal obstruction.** *Ref. Dhingra 6/e pg 173*

    Antro choanal polyp

    The polyp arises from mucosa of maxillary antrum near its accessory ostium, comes out of it and grows in the choana and nasal cavity (*Ref. Dhingra 6/e pg 173*) (options a and c are correct).
    Usually seen in children and young adult (*Ref. Dhingra 6/e pg 173*) (option d is incorrect)
    Unilateral nasal obstruction is presenting symptom (option e is correct)
    Management is surgery, not steroids (option b is incorrect).

18. **Ans. b i.e. Intranasal polypectomy**
    A patient presents with antrochoanal polyp arising from the medial wall of the maxilla. FESS with polypectomy would be the best management for the patient.
    Functional Endoscopic Sinus Surgery (FESS):
    - **Current treatment of choice of antrochoanal polyp is endoscopic sinus surgery,** which has **superseded other modes of polyp removal.**
    - In this procedure, **all polyps are removed under endoscopic control** especially from the the key area of the osteomeatal complex. This procedure helps to **preserve the normal function of the sinuses. FESS can be done under local anesthesia** although **general anesthesia is preferred.**

19. **Ans. a i.e. FEES with polypectomy**
20. **Ans. is b i.e. FESS** *Ref. Dhingra 6/e, 175; 2/e, p 182, 183; Tuli 1/e, p 175; 2/e, p182,183; Turner 10/e, p 55*
21. **Ans. is c i.e. FESS**
22. **Ans. is c i.e. Functional endoscopic sinus surgery (FESS)** *Ref. Dhingra 6/e, p 175; Maqbool 11/e, p 206*
    - Current treatment of choice of antrochoanal polyp is endoscopic sinus surgery which has superceded other modes of polyp removal in all age groups.
    - In this procedure all polyps are removed under endoscopic control especially from the key area of the osteomeatal complex. This procedure helps to preserve the normal function of the sinuses. FESS can be done under local anesthesia although general anesthesia is preferred
    - **Caldwell-Luc** operation is avoided these days.
23. **Ans. is b i.e. Occurs in the first decade of life** *TB of Mohan Bansal, p 310*
24. **Ans. is d i.e. Associated with bronchial asthma**
    Ref. Scott Brown 7/e, Vol 2, Chapter 121, p 1550; Dhingra 6/e, p 172; Turner 10/e, p 373; TB of Mohan Bansal, p 310
25. **Ans. is b i.e. Ethmoidal polyp** *Mohan Bansal, p 308*

    Ethmoidal Polyps
    - **They are *mostly seen in adults*.**[Q]
    - *Etiology—usual cause of ethmoidal polyps is allergy*[Q]
    - **"Allergic nasal polyps are rarely, if ever seen in childhood. They are only seen in childhood in association with mucoviscoidosis."** *Turner 10/e, p 373*
    - Ethmoidal polyps are also associated with:
        – Bronchial asthma
        – Aspirin intolerance
        – Cystic fibrosis
        – Nasal mastocystosis
        – Syndromes like: *Kartageners/Young syndrome/Churg-Strauss syndrome*

Ethmoidal Polyps – Features

Mnemonic

Adult B M R
Adult – It is seen in adults
- B = Bilateral
- M = Multiple
- R = Recurrence is common

26. Ans. is c i.e. Amphotericin B
Ref. Dhingra 6/e, p 173; Turner 10/e, p 52, 54
- This patient is having ethmoidal polyp (because polyps are multiple and bilateral)
- Main etiology of polyps is allergy.
- Medical treatment of polyps is the same as that for allergic rhinitis which consists of:
  - Antihistaminics
  - Steroids—helpful in patients who cannot tolerate antihistamine or have asthma along with polyps. It is also useful to prevent recurrence after surgery
  - Decongestants such as epinephrine, phenylephrine, xylometazoline, etc.
- Antifungals (e.g. Amphotericin B) have no role in treatment of polyps.

27. Ans. is b i.e Extranasal ethmoidectomy
Ref. Dhingra 6/e, p 173

Treatment of ethmoidal polyp
- *Simple polypectomy:* When there are one or two pedunculated polyps.
- *Intranasal ethmoidectomy:* Indicated when polyps are multiple and sessile.
- *Extranasal ethmoidectomy:* This is indicated when polyps recur after intranasal procedures.
- *Transantral ethmoidectomy:* Indicated when infection and polypoidal changes are also seen in the maxillary antrum. In this case antrum is opened by Caldwell-Luc approach and the ethmoidal air cells approached through the medial wall of the antrum.

Note: These days, ethmoidal polypi are removed by endoscopic sinus surgery (FESS) which is the TOC.

28. Ans. is a i.e. Nasal polyp
Ref. Textbook of ENT, Hazarika 3/e, p 343
See text for explanation.

29. Ans. is c i.e. Antrochoanal polyp
Ref. Scott-Brown 7/e, p 1553; Turner 10/e, p 55
Topical steroids are not recommended in post surgery for antrochoanal polyps.

> For antrochoanal polyps, cause is infection and not the allergy. Antrochoanal polyps are single, unilateral and rarely recur. Topical steroids are rarely recommended.

30. Ans is b i.e. Inferior meatus
Ref. Dhingra 6/e, p 411, 412; Tuli 1/e, p 495; 2/e, p 459; Scott Brown 7/e, Vol 2, p 1491,1492

Surgery	Done through
1. Caldwell-Luc operation	Inferior meatus
2. Antral puncture	Inferior meatus
3. Dacryocystorhinostomy	Middle meatus

31. Ans. is b i.e. Infraorbital nerve palsy
Ref. Scott Brown 7/e, Vol 2, p 1494
M/C Complication of Caldwell-Luc operation is injury to infraorbital nerve which occurs is 21% cases.

32. Ans. is a i.e. Mucoviscidosis
Ref. Dhingra 6/e, p 175
"Multile nasal polypi in children may be associated with mucoviscidosis."
Ref: Dhindra 6/e, p175

33. Ans. is c i.e. Mucormycosis
Ref. Dhingra 6/e, p 159

Mucormycosis

- It is a furgal infection of nose and paranasal sinuses which may prove rapidly fatal
- It is seen in uncontrolled diabetes or in those taking immunosuppressive drugs
  For more details—refer to preceding text.

Chapter 17: Granulomatous Disorders of Nose, Nasal Polyps and Foreign Body in Nose

34. **Ans. is a i.e. Rhinoscleroma** *Ref. Dhingra 6/e, p 156*
    Rhinoscleroma is a chronic granulomatous disease caused by Gram negative bacillus called *Klebsiella rhinoscleromates* or Frisch bacillus
35. **Ans. is a, b and d i.e. Unilateral fetid discharge; Presents with unilateral nasal obstruction; and Inanimates is more common than animate**
    Ref. Dhingra 6/e, p 161; Turner 10/e, p 62; Scott Brown 7/e, Vol 1, p 1186

Foreign Bodies in Children can be

Animate	Inanimate
• Examples are screwworms, larvae, maggots and black carpet beetles	• These are more common • Examples are *peas, beans, dried pulses, nuts, paper*, cotton wool and pieces of pencil

Clinical Features
- Unilateral foul smelling discharge in a child is pathognomic of a foreign body
- It can lead to vestibulitis

Treatment
- Removal with forceps or blunt hook under LA

Indications of giving GA in Nasal Foreign Body Removal
- Uncooperative or very apprehensive child
- Troublesome bleeding, if the foreign body is firmly embedded in granulation tissue
- Posteriorly placed foreign body.
- If a foreign body is strongly suspected but can't be found.

36. **Ans. is a i.e. Foreign body** *Ref. Dhingra 6/e, p 161; Turner 10/e, p 63*
    "A unilateral nasal discharge is nearly always due to a foreign body and if discharge has an unpleasant smell, it is pathognomic."
    Ref. Turner 10/e, p 63
    "If a child presents with unilateral, foul smelling nasal discharge, foreign body must be excluded." *Ref. Dhingra 6/e, p 161*
37. **Ans. is a i.e. Battery substance leaks and cause tissue damage** *Ref: Dhingra 6/e, p 161; Scott-Brown 7/e, p 1186; Turner 10/e, p 62*
    Most important consideration in the management of retained disc battery in the nose of a child is the leakage of battery substance leading to tissue damage.

    "If the FB is a small button battery, moisture within the cavity may lead to tissue damage. Irrigation or nasal wash should not be used. If the battery leaks, there may be liquefactive necrosis and organ injury. It should be removed immediately."—http://www.patient.co.uk/doctor/nasal-injury-and-nasal-foreign-bodies Professional Reference

38. **Ans. is c i.e. Deposition of calcium around foreign body in nose** *Ref. Dhingra 6/e, p 161; Tuli 1/e, p 149; Scott-Brown 7/e, Vol 1, p 1186; Textbook of Mohan Bansal, p 349*
    Rhinoliths are calcareous masses which result due to deposition of salts-like calcium and magnesium carbonates and phosphates around the nucleus of a foreign body.
    For more details, see text part.
39. **Ans. is a i.e. Chloroform diluted with water** *Ref. Dhingra 6/e, p 162*
    Chloroform water or vapor must be instilled in order to anesthetize or kill the maggots and so release their grip from the skin.
    - Maggots are larval forms of flies, particularly of the genus chrysomyia.[Q]
    - Patient may present as a simple case of epistaxis.[Q]
    - Maggots cause extensive destruction of nose, sinuses, soft tissues to face, palate or around the nose.[Q]
    - Death may occur from meningitis.[Q]
40. **Ans. is b, c, d and e i.e. Perforated nasal septum, Persistent sinus, Crusting of nasal mucosa, Collapse of nasal bridge**
    Ref. Dhingra 6/e, p 159-60; Logan Turner 10/e, p 60

    ### Wegener's Granulomatosis
    - It is a systemic disorder
    - Early symptoms include clear or blood-stained nasal discharge which later become purulent. The patient often complains of **persistent cold or** sinus (option c correct)
    - Nasal findings include crusting, granulations **septal** perforation and a saddle **nose** (option b and e correct)

> "The nose and paranasal sinuses are involved in over 90% of cases of Wegener granulomatosis. It is often not realized that involement at these sites is more common than involvement of lungs or kidneys. Examination shows **bloodstained crusts and friable mucosa**"
> —CMDT 2015/222.

Wegener's granulomatosis is not mentioned as aetiology of nasal polyp—Dhingra 6/e, p 172, 173.

41. **Ans. is a i.e. Santer's triad**
42. **Ans. is a, c and e i.e. facies leonina, saddle nose and lagophthalmos**

Face deformities in leprosy

• Mask faces	• Loss of eyebrows (superciliary madonosis)
• Faces leonina	• Loss of eyelashes (ciliary madarosis)
• Sagging face	• Depressed nose—saddle nose
• Lagophthalmos	• Perforated nasal septum

Chapter 18

Inflammatory Disorders of Nasal Cavity

RHINITIS

Classification (Table 18.1)

Table 18.1: Classification of rhinitis

Acute inflammation	Chronic inflammation
• Acute Rhinitis • Acute nasal diphtheria	*Specific:* • Nasal syphilis, tuberculosis • Lupus and leprosy • Rhinoscleroma • Rhinosporidiosis • Sarcoidosis *Nonspecific:* • Atrophic rhinitis • Rhinitis sicca • Rhinitis caseosa *Allergic:* • Seasonal allergic rhinitis • Perennial allergic rhinitis • Vasomotor rhinitis

ACUTE INFLAMMATORY CONDITION

ACUTE RHINITIS/CORYZA

- Frequently referred to as *common cold*.
- Seen in adults and school going children.
- Caused by viruses specially rhinovirus, (M/C cause), influenza and parainfluenza virus, ECHO virus, adenoviruses and retroviruses
- Secondary invaders are Streptococci, Staphylococci, Pneumococci, *H. influenza* and *M. catarrhalis*.

Clinical Features

- There is burning/tickling sensation at the back of the nose followed by nasal stuffiness, rhinorrhea and sneezing.
- Low-grade fever.
- Initially discharge is watery and profuse but becomes mucopurulent later due to secondary bacterial invasion.
- Dry cough due to post nasal drip.

Treatment

- Bed rest
- Vitamin C
- Antihistaminics and anti-inflammatory drugs
- Antibiotics if secondary infection occurs.

CHRONIC INFLAMMATORY CONDITIONS

- Nasal syphilis
- Tuberculosis of nose
- Lupus vulgaris ⎫
- Leprosy ⎬ Details discussed in chapter on granulomatous disease of the nose
- Rhinoscleroma
- Rhinosporidiosis ⎭

HYPERTROPHIC RHINITIS

The condition occurs a sequelae of simple rhinitis if not treated properly.

It is characterized by thickening of mucosa, submucosa, seromucinous glands, periosteum and bone.

Symptoms

- Nasal obstruction
- Thick and sticky nasal discharge.

Signs

- Hypertrophy of turbinates: especially inferior turbinates.
- Mulberry like appearance of nasal mucosa seen.[Q]

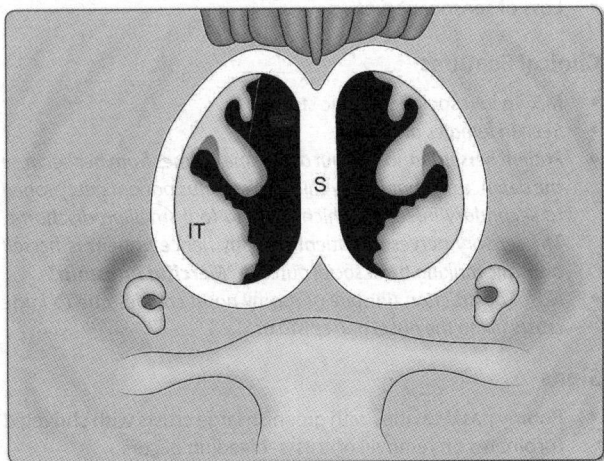

Fig. 18.1: Features of hypertrophic rhinitis—hypertrophied inferior turbinate and mulberry mucosa

- Does not pit on pressure.
- Shows very little shrinkage with vasoconstrictor drugs.

Treatment

To relieve nasal obstruction by reducing the size of turbinates by doing turbinectomy. Turbinectomy can be performed by:
- Laser
- Submucosal diathermy
- Cryosurgery or by
- Submucous resection of turbinate bone

ATROPHIC RHINITIS/OZAENA

In contrast to hypertrophic rhinitis, atrophic chronic inflammatory disease is characterized by progressive atrophy of the nasal mucosa and the underlying bone of the turbinates. There is associated **excessive crusting** which leads to nasal obstruction in spite of abnormal patency of nasal passages.

Etiology

Hereditary
Endocrinal pathology such as estrogen deficiency as it starts at puberty. Stops after menopause
Racial factors—seen more in Whites and Yellow races
Nutritional deficiency: Deficiency of vitamin A, D, E and iron may be responsible for it
Infective: *Klebsiella ozanae, Diphtheriods P. cocobacillus ozaola.* (Because of this atrophic rhinitis is also called as ozanae).
Autoimmune process—causing destruction of nasal, neurovascular and glandular elements may be the cause

Pathology

- Everything in nose atrophies.
- *Ciliated columnar epithelium is lost and is replaced by stratified squamous type.*
- Atrophy of seromucinous glands.
- Turbinates are resorbed leading to widening of nasal chambers.
- Loss of sensory nerves.

Clinical Features

- M/C in low socioeconomic status.
- *Seen in females at puberty.*
- Patient herself is anosmic but a foul smell comes from her because the defence mechanism by cilia are lost, thus patient gets proned to secondary infection which leads to foul smelling discharge. The sensory nerves of patient atrophy hence patient is herself anosmic making her a social outcast-**"Merciful Anosmia".**
- Nasal obstruction (in spite of roomy nasal cavities due to large crusts filling the nose) and epistaxis.

Signs

- Roomy nasal cavities with greenish large crusts with shriveled turbinates on removal of crusts–bleeding occurs.
- Nasal mucosa appears pale due to atrophy of feeding arteries (obliterative endarteritis)
- Septal perforation may be present.
- Nose may show saddle deformity.
- Atrophic changes may be seen in the pharyngeal mucosa.
- Atrophic changes may be seen in the larynx - *Atrophic laryngitis (laryngitis sicca)*
- Eustachian tube obstruction can lead to hearing loss.

Investigations

X-ray PNS (Water's view)—Thickening of the walls of the sinuses

Treatment

Medical

- **Warm nasal alkaline solution:** 280 ml warm water + 1 part of the following powder:
  - Sodium bicarbonate (28.4 g) + Sodium biborate (28.4 g) + 2 parts of Sodium chloride (56.7 g) (**Remember—BBC**)
  - The purpose of the solution is to loosen and remove the crusts and the thick tenacious secretions.
- **25% glucose in glycerin:**
  - Following removal of the crust the nose is painted with 25% glucose in glycerin.
  - Glucose on fermentation produces lactic and which inhibits proteolytic organisms, Glycerine—is a hygroscopic agent (absorbs water from atmosphere & moisture mucosa).
- **Other local antibiotics:** *Kemicetine antiozaena solution:* 1 ml contains chloramphenicol(90 mg), oestradiol dipropionate (0.64 mg), Vit D2 (900 IU) and propylene glycol
- **Potassium iodide:** by mouth to increase the nasal secretion
- **Human placental extract** is given in the form of submucosal injection, it increases the blood supply nasal mucosa
- **Other drugs:**
  Rifampicin, Streptomycin to decrease the odor and crusts.
  Estradiol spray to increase vascularity of nasal mucosa
  Placental extract injected submucosally.

Surgical

Aim: To reduce the size of roomy nasal cavities
- **Young's operation^Q:**
  - Closure of both the nostril following elevation of the nasal vestibular folds. They are opened after 6 months.
- **Modified Young's operation:**
  - Partial closure of the nostril leaving behind a 3 mm hole.
  - This remains for a period of 2 years.

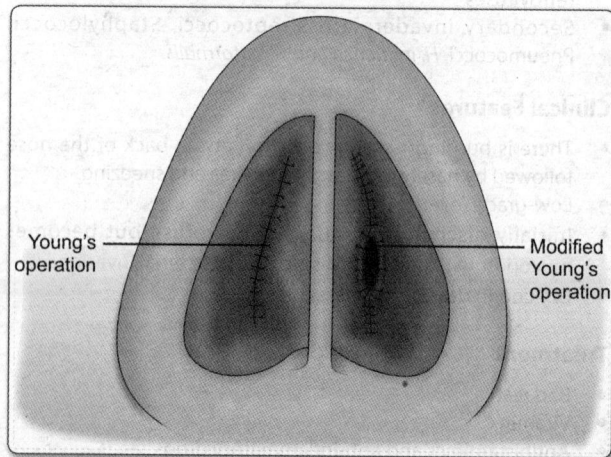

Fig. 18.2: Young's operation and modified Young's operation

- Narrowing of the nasal cavity by - **(Lautenslager's operation)**
  - Submucosal injection of teflon paste
  - Insertion of fat, cartilage, bone or teflon strips under the mucoperiosteum of floor and lateral wall of nose
  - Section and medial displacement of lateral wall of nose

NEW PATTERN QUESTIONS

Q N1. Merciful anosmia is seen in: [FMGE 2013]
  a. Atrophic rhinitis
  b. Allergic rhinitis
  c. Ethmoidal polyposis
  d. Wegener's granulomatosis

Q N2. Ozaena is another name for:
  a. Hypertrophic rhinitis b. Allergic rhinitis
  c. Rhinitis sicca d. Atrophic rhinitis

Q N3. Young's operation is indicated for:
  a. Vasomotor rhinitis b. Atrophic rhinitis
  c. Rhinitis sicca d. Rhinitis caseosa

RHINITIS SICCA

- Seen in patients working in hot, dry and dusty surroundings are iron smith & bakery workers.
- The respiratory ciliated columnar epithelium of anterior part of nose undergoes squamous metaplasia with atrophy of seromucinous glands.

The condition is similar to atrophic rhinitis, but with a difference that only anterior 1/3rd of nose is affected.

Treatment
- Correction of occupational surroundings
- Antibiotic and steroid ointment
- Nasal douching.

NEW PATTERN QUESTION

Q N4. Rhinitis sicca is characterized by:
  a. Drying of anterior 1/3 of nasal cavity
  b. Drying of middle 1/3 of nasal cavity
  c. Drying of posterior 1/3 of nasal cavity
  d. Drying of entire nasal cavity

ALLERGIC RHINITIS

- It is an immunoglobin E (IgE) mediated Type I hypersensitive reaction of nasal mucosa to airborne allergens.
- Clinically allergic rhinitis is of 2 types (Table 18.2).

Table 18.2: Types of allergic rhinitis

Seasonal	Perennial
Symptoms appear in and around a particular season generally March-May or August-September.	Symptoms are present throughout the year

Contd...

Seasonal	Perennial
It is because of pollens of some particular grass or flowers which act as allergen	In this case-house dust, perfumes, sprays, drugs, tobacco, smoke, chemical, fumes, etc. act as allergen
In morning symptoms are usually worse and are aggravated by dry windy condition	Symptoms are not as severe as in seasonal type

Clinical Features
- No age or sex predilection
- Onset is at 12–16 years of age (i.e. adolescence). Peak prevalence is during third and fourth decade.
- Patients present with itching of eyes and nose, sneezing, profuse watery discharge, postnasal drip, concomittant coughing and wheezing, nasal obstruction.

Signs
- **Nose:**
  - Nasal mucosa is pale, boggy, hypertrophic and may appear bluish.
  - Transverse crease is present on the nose due to upward rubbing of nose **(allergic salute)**.
  - Turbinates are swollen.
- **Ear:** Otitis media with effusion due to blockage of Eustachian tube is a possibility in children
- **Pharynx:** Granular pharyngitis.
- **Larynx:** Edema of the vocal cords and hoarseness of voice.
- **Eyes:** Dark circles, i.e. *allergic shiners* are seen under the eyes and creases are seen in lower eyelid skin (Dennis morgan lines).

Investigations
All tests of allergy are positive.
- **Blood tests:** ↑TLC, ↑DLC (eosinophilia)
- **Nasal smear:** Eosinophils seen
- **Skin tests:** Are done to identify the allergen:
  - Prick test
  - Scratch test
  - Intradermal test

 Point to Remember

Note: Prick test is preferred over the others since the other two are less reproducible, more dangerous and may give false positive result.

- **RAST (Radioallergosorbent Test):** Serum IgE measurement is done *in vitro*. (not done now)

Treatment
- Avoidance of allergens.
- **Antihistaminics:** They are frequently used as a **first-line therapy** because most of them are available without a prescription

- **Corticosteroids:** They act on the late phase reaction and prevent a significant influx of inflammatory cells. Corticosteroids can be given either intranasally or systemically (in severe cases)
- **Decongestants**

Act on adrenergic receptors of nasal mucosa and respiratory tract

↓

Vaso constriction

↓

Decrease turbinate congestion

↓   ↓

No effect on rhinorrhea or sneezing   Improved nasal patency

Note: Intranasal decongestant, i.e. oxymetazoline can cause rebound nasal congestion and dependency if used for more than 3–4 days (rhinitis medicamentosa)[Q]

- Immunotherapy can be tried

Point to Remember

Contraindications to Immunotherapy
➢ Coexistent asthma
➢ Patients taking β-blocker
➢ Other medical / Immunological disease
➢ Age < 5 year
➢ Pregnancy.

Surgery

Ref: Scott Brown 7th/ed Vol 2 pp 1400,1401

- Nasal surgery may be required when there is a marked septal deviation or bony turbinate enlargement (Grade D), which makes topical nasal sprays usage difficult.
- It is never the first line of treatment.
- Mucosal hypertrophy (Grade C) is preferably dealt medically, since after surgery the problem tends to recur within months.

VASOMOTOR RHINITIS (NON ALLERGIC RHINITIS)

It is a non allergic rhinitis which occurs due to parasympathetic overactivity. The parasympathetic overactivity leads to congestion and vasodilatation.

Symptoms

- More common in emotionally unstable persons especially in women of 20–40 years.
- Paroxymal sneezing—just after getting out of bed in morning.
- Nasal obstruction.
- Excessive clear rhinorrhea.
- Postnasal drip.

Signs

- Nasal mucosa appears to be normal and shining.
- Hypertrophic turbinates.
- No eye symptoms seen.

Treatment (Table 18.3)

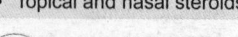

Table 18.3: Treatment of vasomotor rhinitis	
Medical	Surgical
• Avoidance of provoking symptoms	• Treatment of complications
• Oral/nasal decongestants like phenylephrine & nasal xylometazoline	• Vidian neurectomy (sectioning of parasympathetic fibers)
• Topical and nasal steroids	

Note: For undergraduate students—**saline irrigation** is an important adjuvant to treatment as it helps to avert intranasal stasis and reduces crusting. Its use not only increases the efficacy of intranasal topical medications but also improves ciliary function.

Other Drugs which can be Used

- Anticholenergics like ipratropium bromide as they block parasympathetic input and so decrease rhinorrhea. It should be avoided in patients of narrow angle glaucoma, BPH or bladder neck obstruction.
- Azelastine spray – It works in case of vasomotor rhinitis but has a bitter taste which precludes its frequent use.

RHINITIS CASEOSA/NASAL CHOLESTEATOMA

It is a chronic inflammation of the nose characterized by accumulation of offensive cheesy material resembling cholesteatoma.

Features

- Usually U/L and is M/C in males.
- The nose gets filled with whitish offensive debris with invasion of the bony structures and the soft tissues of the face.

Treatment

- Removal of debris by scooping it out
- Repeated irrigation

Point to Remember

Rhinitis medicamentosa[Q]
➢ Caused by excessive use of topical decongestant nasal drops.[Q]

Thus nasal decongestants should not be given continuously for more than 5 days.

Management: Withdrawl of offending drug and short course of systemic and local steroids.

Chapter 18: Inflammatory Disorders of Nasal Cavity

NEW PATTERN QUESTIONS

Q N5. Vidian neurectomy is done in:
a. Allergic rhinitis b. Atrophic rhinitis
c. Vasomotor rhinitis d. Rhinitis sicca

Q N6. Rhinitis medimentosa is due to:
a. Nasal decongestants
b. Steroid
c. Antihistaminics
d. Surgery

Q N7. Allergic rhinitis treatment includes all *except*:
a. Antibiotics b. Avoiding allergen
c. Corticosteroids d. Surgery

Q N8. All of the following drugs can lead to rhinitis *except*:
a. ACE inhibitors b. Methyldopa
c. Reserpine d. Oxymetazoline

Q N9. Allergic salute is seen in:
a. Acute rhinitis
b. Allergic rhinitis
c. Hypertrophic rhinitis
d. Atrophic rhinitis

Q N10. TOC of vasomotor rhinitis is:
a. Vidian neurectomy b. Steroids
c. Antibiotics d. Surgery

Explanations and References to New Pattern Questions

N1. Ans. is a i.e. Atrophic rhinitis   *Ref. Dhingra 6/e, p 154*
In atrophic rhinitis, there is foul smell from the nose, making the patient a social outcast though the patient himself is unaware of the smell due to marked anosmia which accompanies the degenerative changes. This is called as **merciful anosmia**.

N2. Ans. is d i.e. Atrophic rhinitis   *Ref. Dhingra 6/e, p 153*
See text for explanation

N3. Ans. is b i.e. Atrophic rhinitis
Young's operation i.e. closure of both the nostrils following elevation of both the nasal vestibular folds is done in atrophic rhinitis. Modified Young's operation is partial closure of both the nostrils.

N4. Ans. is a i.e. Drying of anterior 1/3 of nasal cavity   *Ref. Dhingra 6/e, p 155*
In rhinitis sicca — condition is confined to the anterior third of nose.

N5. Ans. is c i.e. Vasomotor rhinitis   *Ref. Dhingra 6/e, p 170*
Excessive rhinorrhea of vasomotor rhinitis which is not corrected by medical therapy and is bothersome to the patient, can be relieved by sectioning of parasympathetic secretomotor fibers to nose (vidian neurectomy).

Indications of vidian neurectomy
1. Vasomotor rhinitis
2. Intrinsic rhinitis
3. Crocodile tears

N6. Ans. is a i.e. Nasal decongestants   *Ref. Textbook of ENT Mohan Bansal 1/e, p 331*
Rhinitis medicamentosa: The long term use of cocaine and topical nasal decongestants (cause rebound congestion) leads to rhinits medicamentosa's

N7. Ans. is a Antibiotics   *Ref. Dhingra 6/e, p 168, 169; Textbook of ENT Mohan Bansal 1/e, p 327-30*
Now Friends, you actually donot need any reference or explanation to answer this question as it is obvious antibiotics do not have any role in treating allergy.
Rest all options–avoiding allergens, corticosteroids and surgery can be used as management options for allergic rhinitis for more details see the preceding text.

N8. Ans. is d i.e. Oxymetazoline   *Ref. Dhingra 6/e, p 170*

Drug induced rhinitis
• Antihypertensive drug—reserpine, guanethidine, methyldopa, propranolol, ACE inhibitor
• Neostigmine
• Contraceptive drugs

N9. Ans. is b i.e. Allergic rhinitis
Allergic salute is a transverse crease present on the nose due to upward rubbing of nose.

N10. Ans. is a i.e. Vidian neurectomy

QUESTIONS

1. **Common cold is caused primarily by:** [Karnatka 94]
   a. Viruses
   b. Bacteria
   c. Fungi
   d. Allergy

2. **Early mediators of allergic rhinitis are:** [PGI 03]
   a. Leukotriene
   b. IL-4
   c. IL-5
   d. Bradykinin
   e. PAF

3. **In Allergic rhinitis nasal mucosa is:** [MP 03]
   a. Pale and swollen
   b. Pink and swollen
   c. Atrophied
   d. Bluish and atrophied

4. **All of the following surgical procedures are used for allergic rhinitis except:** [AIIMS 04]
   a. Radiofrequency ablation of the inferior turbinate
   b. Laser ablation of the inferior turbinate
   c. Submucosal placement of silastic in inferior turbinate
   d. Inferior turbinectomy

5. **All are implicated in etiology of atrophic rhinitis except:** [DNB 02]
   a. Chronic sinusitis
   b. Nasal deformity
   c. DNS
   d. Strong hereditary factors

6. **Which of the following organisms is known to cause Atrophic Rhinitis?** [MP 07]
   a. *Klebsiella pneumoniae*
   b. *Klebsiella ozaenae*
   c. *Streptococcus pneumoniae*
   d. *Streptococcus foetidis*

7. **Cause of nasal obstruction in atrophic rhinitis:** [PGI 00, 97]
   a. Crusting
   b. Polyp
   c. Secretions
   d. DNS

8. **All are true regarding atrophic rhinitis except:** [AP 04]
   a. More common in males
   b. Crusts are seen
   c. Anosmia is noticed
   d. Young's operation is useful

9. **All are true about ozaenae except:** [UP 03]
   a. Common in female
   b. It is usually unilateral
   c. Nasal cavity is filled with greenish crusts
   d. Atrophic pharyngitis

10. **Alkaline douche solution of nose does not contain:**
    a. NaCl
    b. Na biborate
    c. $NaHCO_3$
    d. Glucose

11. **Young's operation is done for:** [JIPMER 02] [Jharkhand 06, MP 03] [FMGE 13]
    a. Allergic rhinitis
    b. Atropic rhinitis
    c. Vasomotor rhinitis
    d. Idiopathic rhinitis

12. **Vidian neurectomy is done in:** [CUPGEE 97]
    a. Vasomotor rhinitis
    b. Rhinitis sicca
    c. Allergic sinusitis
    d. Epistaxis

13. **Mulberry appearance of nasal mucosal membrane is seen in:** [MP 06]
    a. Coryza
    b. Atrophic rhinitis
    c. Maxillary sinusitis
    d. Chronic hypertrophic rhinitis

14. **True about Vasomotor rhinitis:** [PGI May 2015]
    a. It is a type of allergic reaction
    b. Clinically simulate nasal allergy
    c. Nasal mucosa generally congested and hypertrophic
    d. Hypertrophy of inferior turbinate is commonly present
    e. Anti-histaminics and oral nasal decongestant are used in treatment

Chapter 18: Inflammatory Disorders of Nasal Cavity

Explanations and References

1. **Ans. is a i.e. Viruses**
   Ref. Dhingra 6/e, p 152; TB of Mohan Bansal, p 299
   Common cold/coryza/Acute Rhinitis is primarily caused by viruses, e.g. Adenovirus, Picorna virus, Rhinovirus, Coxsackie and ECHO viruses. Secondary Invasion by bacteria occurs later.

   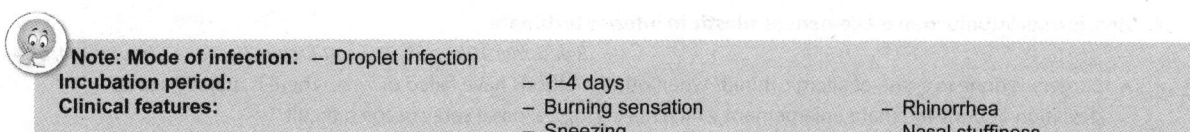

   Note: Mode of infection: – Droplet infection
   Incubation period: – 1–4 days
   Clinical features: – Burning sensation   – Rhinorrhea
                        – Sneezing   – Nasal stuffiness

2. **Ans. is a, b, c, d and e i.e. Leukotriene; IL-4, IL-5, Bradykinin; and PAF**
   Ref. Robbin's 7/e, p 208,209; Current Otolaryngology 2/e, p 267,268; Dhingra 6/e, p 167
   Allergic rhinitis is Type 1 hypersensitivity reaction

Pathology

In individuals who have genetic predisposition to allergy
↓

Allergen exposure
↓ leads to

IgE antibody production
↓
Attaches to mast cell (by Fc end)

On subsequent exposure to the same allergen
↓
It attaches itself to IgE antibody (which in turn is attached to mast cell) by its F_{ab} end
↓
Degranulation of mast cell
↓
Release of mediators
Like histamine^Q, leukotriene^Q, cytokines^Q
Prostaglandins^Q, Platelet activating factor^Q
↓

Called as Early phase/Humoral reaction

- Early phase occurs within 10–15 mins (max 30 mins) of allergen exposure
- It is due to release of mediators viz. histamine, cytokine, Prostaglandins, leukotrienes, platelet activating factor
- Release of histamine causes symptoms like – sneezing, rhinorrhea, itching, vascular permeability, vasodilatation, glandular secretion

↓
Release of cytokines and leukotrienes in the early phase causes influx of inflammatory cells (eosinophils)
↓

Called as later phase of cellular reaction
↓

- Occurs 2–8 hours after initial sensitization
- Causes symptoms like Nasal congestion and postnasal drip

3. Ans. is a i.e Pale and swollen
Ref. Scott Brown 7/e, Vol 2 Chapter 109, p 1393; Dhingra 6/e, p 167

Appearance of mucosa	Condition
• Nasal mucosa pale, boggy, swollen and bluish	• Allergic rhinitis
• Nasal mucosa congested and swollen (Hypertrophic)	• Vasomotor rhinitis
• Mulberry appearance	• Chronic hypertrophic rhinitis
• Pale and atrophied nasal mucosa	• Atrophic rhinitis

4. Ans. is c i.e. Submucosal placement of silastic in inferior turbinate
Ref. Turner 10/e, p 39,53; Scott Brown 7/e, Vol 2, Chapter 104, p 1400,1401

- Surgery is done in a case of allergic rhinitis when other methods have failed or when there is marked septal deviation or bony turbinate enlargement which makes topical nasal spray usage difficult
- It should never be used as first line of treatment.

Surgery

To relieve nasal obstruction	To relieve rhinorrhea
To relieve obstruction, **turbinate reduction** or turbinate resection is done by either diathermy— to fibrose, the vascular spaces of inferior turbinates, Cryosurgery, **Laser cautery, Radiofrequency ablation** or turbinectomy	• **Ovidian neurectomy** is done to relieve rhinorrhoea: a. Excision of vidian nerve b. Diathermy/division of vidian nerve

Note: Submucosal injection of teflon or placement of silastic is the treatment option for Atrophic rhinitis. Where we need to make nasal cavity more roomy.

5. Ans. is c i.e. DNS
Ref. Dhingra 6/e, p 153

Atrophic Rhinitis

Primary	Secondary

The exact etiology is not known
It can be due to:
H = **Hereditary factors**
E = **Endocrinal disturbance** because it starts at puberty and cease after menopause. Female > Male. Therefore endocrinal cause is possibility.
R = **Racial factors** –White and Yellow races are susceptible
N = **Nutritional deficiency** of Vit A, D and iron
I = **Infective** (organisms like Klebsiella ozaenae, diphtheroids, *P. vulgaris, E. coli, Staphylocci, Streptococci*)
A = **Autoimmune** process
	Secondary rhinitis can be due to:
	• Specific infections like:
	  – Syphilis
	  – Leprosy
	  – Rhinoscleroma
	• **Longstanding purulent sinusitis**
	• Radiotherapy to nose
	• Surgical removal of turbinates

Note: DNS can lead to unilateral atrophic rhinitis on the wider side.[Q]

6. Ans. is a i.e. *Klebsiella pneumoniae*
Ref. Scott Brown 7/e, Vol 2 Chapter 115, p 1465; Dhingra 6/e, p 154; TB of Mohan Bansal, p 313

Organism known to cause Atrophic rhinitis are:
- *Coccobacillus ozaenae*
- *Diphtheroid bacillus*
- *Klebsiella ozaenae* — *Ref. Scott Brown 7/e, Vol 2, p 1465*
- *Bordettela bronchiseptica*
- *Pasteurella multocida*
- *P. vulgaris*
- *E. coli*
- *Staphylococcus* — *Ref. Dhingra 6/e, p 154*
- *Streptococcus*

Chapter 18: Inflammatory Disorders of Nasal Cavity

7. **Ans. is a i.e. Crusting** *Ref. Turner 10/e, p 40; Dhingra 6/e, p 152,154; TB of Mohan Bansal, p 313*
8. **Ans. is a i.e. More common in males** *Ref. Dhingra 6/e, p 152,154*
9. **Ans. is b i.e. It is usually unilateral** *Ref. Scott Brown 7/d Vol 2 Chapter 115, p 1465, Dhingra 6/e, p 153, 164*
10. **Ans. is d i.e. Glucose** *Ref. Dhingra 6/e, p 154*
11. **Ans. is b i.e. Atrophic rhinitis**
    Ref. Dhingra 6/e, p 152; Scott Brown 7/e, Vol 2, Chapter 155, p 1466; TB of Mohan Bansal, p 314

    Atrophic rhinitis: We have done in detail in text. Here just remember.
    - It is more **common in females.**ᵠ
    - **Age**—Usually starts at puberty and ceases after menopause.ᵠ
    - It is always **bilateral**ᵠ except in case of DNS where atrophic rhinitis is seen on the wider side. For other details read the text.

12. **Ans. is a i.e. Vasomotor rhinitis** *Ref. Dhingra 6/e, p 170; Scott Brown 7/e, Vol 2, p 1412*

    Excessive rhinorrhea in vasomotor rhinitis not corrected by medical therapy and bothersome to the patient, is relieved by sectioning the parasympathetic secretomotor fibers to nose, i.e. vidian neurectomy.

    Note: The parasympathetic/secretomotor supply of the nose comes through the vidian nerve (also called the nerve of pterygoid canal). It is formed by greater superficial petrosal branch of facial nerve joining deep petrosal nerve derived from plexus around internal carotid artery (sympathetic nerve supply).

13. **Ans. is d i.e. Chronic hypertrophic rhinitis** *Ref. Dhingra 6/e, p 153; Mohan Bansal p 337*

    Mulberry like appearance of nasal mucosa is seen in chronic hypertrophic rhinitis.
    [For details kindly see the preceding text]

14. **Ans. is b, c, d and e i.e clinically simulate nasal allergy, nasal mucosa is generally congested and hypertrophic, hypertrophy of inferior turbinate is commonly present and anti-histamines and oral nasal decongestant are used in treatment.**
    Ref. Dhingra 6/e,pgs170; Logan Turner 10/e,pgs373

    Vasomotor Rhinitis (VMR)
    - It is **nonallergic** rhinitis but clinically simulating nasal allergy with symptom of nasal obstruction, rhinorrhoea & sneezing
    - The **tests of nasal allergy are negative.** (i.e. option a is incorrect)
    - Sign: **Nasal mucosa over the turbinates is generally congested & hypertrophic.** In some, it may be normal
    - Complication: Long standing cases develop nasal, **polyphypertrophic rhinitis** & sinusitis
    - Medical treatment: Avoidance of physical factor which provoke symptoms; anti-histaminics & oral nasal decongestant; systemic steroid (i.e. option e is correct)

    M/C turbinate to undergo hypertrophy in vasomotor rhinitis is inferior turbinate (i.e. option d is correct)

Chapter 19

Epistaxis

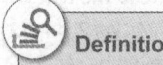
Definition
Epistaxis is bleeding from inside the nose.

AREAS OF NASAL BLEED

Little's Area
- Most common site for epistaxis in children and young adults.
- **Location:** Anteroinferior part of the nasal septum[Q]
- **Arteries contributing:** (Fig. 19.1)
  - Sphenopalatine artery[Q] (also called as **artery of epistaxis**)
  - Anterior ethmoidal
  - Septal branch of *greater palatine*[Q] *artery*
  - Septal branch of superior labial[Q] artery (branch of Facial artery)
- These arteries form the **Kiesselbach's plexus.**[Q]
- Thus epistaxis is mainly arterial.

History
> This area is called as **Little's area** as it was identified by **James Little in 1879**. It is also called as **locus valsalvae** and is the confluence of internal and external carotid artery. This vascular area is the most common site of nose bleed in children and young adults. It gets dried due to the effect of inspiratory current and easily traumatised due to frequent picking (fingering) of nose.

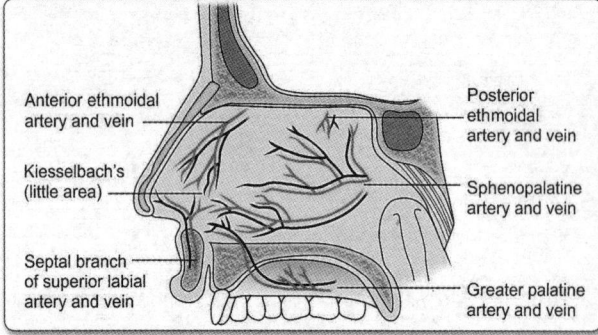

Fig. 19.1: Blood supply of nasal septum

Retrocolumellar Vein
Location: Just behind the columella at the anterior edge of the Little's area.
- The retrocolumellar vein of this area then runs along the floor of the nose to anastomise with the various plexus of the lateral wall of the nose.

- **Common site of venous** *bleeding* in young people (<35 yrs).

Woodruff's Plexus
- **Location:** Found in the lateral nasal wall inferior to the posterior end of inferior turbinate.
- **Contributing vessels:** Anastomosis between sphenopalatine artery and posterior pharyngeal artery.
- **Browne's area:** Located at the part end of nasal septum.
- **Features:**
  - It is a venous plexus
  - Common cause of posterior epistaxis.

CLASSIFICATION OF EPISTAXIS

Classification I
According to *Scott Brown 7th/ed Vol 2 p 1600*

Anterior epistaxis: Bleeding from a source anterior to the plane of the piriform aperture. This includes bleeding from the anterior septum and rare bleeds from the vestibular skin and mucocutaneous junction.
Posterior epistaxis: Bleeding from a vessel situated posterior to the piriform aperture. This allows further subdivision into lateral wall, septal and nasal floor bleeding.

 Note: For undergraduate students nobody can challenge above definition but in case a short note is asked an anterior and posterior epistaxis then the following Table 19.1, given on next page of the guide from Dhingra should also be reproduced.

Classification II
Epistaxis can also be classified as:
- **Childhood epistaxis:** i.e. if it occurs in age < 16 years
- **Adult epistaxis:** i.e. if it occurs in age > 16 years

Classification III
Primary

Between 70% and 80% of all cases of epistaxis are idiopathic, spontaneous bleeds without any proven precipitant or causal factor. This is called as primary epistaxis.

Secondary

Those cases where the cause of epistaxis is defined like trauma, surgery or anticoagulant overdose.

Chapter 19: Epistaxis

Table 19.1: Types of epistaxis and their features

	Anterior Epistaxis	Posterior Epistaxis
	Blood flows out from the front of nose	Blood flows back into the throat
Incidence	More common	Less common
Site	Mostly from Little's area or anterior part of lateral wall	Mostly from posterosuperior part of nasal cavity; often difficult to localise the bleeding point
Age	Mostly occurs in children or young adults	After 40 years of age
Cause	Mostly trauma	Spontaneous; often due to hypertension or arteriosclerosis
Bleeding	Usually mild, can be easily controlled by local pressure or anterior pack	Bleeding is severe, requires hospitalization; postnasal packing often required

EPISTAXIS IN CHILDREN

Scott Brown 7th/ed Vol 1 p 1064

- Epistaxis is common and usually innocuous event in childhood
- It is rare in children < 2 years
- Peak prevalence is in **3–8 years of age**.
- There is a seasonal variation with a higher prevalence in the winter months, due to greater frequency of upper respiratory tract infections or to the drying effect of inspired air of modern central heating systems.

- **M/C site of origin of bleed**—Anterior part of nasal septum (because this part of nasal mucosa is thin and is exposed to dry air currents).
- **M/C site of bleeding**—Little's area
- **M/C cause of Epistaxis**—Idiopathic
- **2nd M/C cause:** Digital trauma/Nose pricking in little's area which is due to crusting which occurs because of URTI.
- In any child with unilateral epistaxis, foreign body should be ruled out.

Cause of Recurrent Epistaxis in Children

- Allergic rhinitis
- Retained nasal foreign body
- Use of nasal sprays as intranasal steroid sprays
- Hemorrhagic disease as in – ITPP, Von Willebrand disease
- Vascular abnormalities – A/V malformations, hemangioma
- Angiofibroma (Suspected in adolescent boys)
- Nasal parasitosis/Nasal mycosis.

ADULT RECURRENT EPISTAXIS

When recurrent bleeds occur in adults, secondary epistaxis is most likely therefore the causes listed below are the same for **Recurrent/secondary Epistaxis**.
- Coagulopathy secondary to liver disease, kidney disease, leukemia or myelosuppression
- Trauma
- **Post surgery:** As after inferior turbinectomy, iatrogenic damage to anterior ethmoidal artery during endoscopic sinus surgery or damage to internal carotid artery during posterior ethmoid or sphenoid sinus surgery
- Patients on warfarin
- Hereditary hemorrhagic telangiectasia
- Tumors–Juvenile nasopharyngeal angiofibroma hemangiopericytoma.

- **M/C cause of epistaxis in adults:** Hypertension
- **M/c site in adults:** Woodruff plexus
- Any young male with profuse and recurrent epistaxis should be investigated for angiofibroma.

MANAGEMENT OF NOSE BLEED

First-aid Methods

- Nasal pinching (called as **Trotter's method**)
- Applying ice cold water to head or face or give ice packs to dorsum of nose
- **Trotter's method:** Old fashioned method of controlling epistaxis. Make the patient sit up with a cork between his teeth and allow him to bleed till he becomes hypotensive.

Treatment in Hospital

Sedation

- Pethidine is given to allay the fear and anxiety of the patient.

Anterior Nasal Packing

- If bleeding continues, nose should be packed with a ribbon gauze soaked in neosporin antiseptic cream for 24 to 48 hours. Merocel packs can be used as an alternative to ribbon gauze packing (although costly but gives less discomfort to the patient).

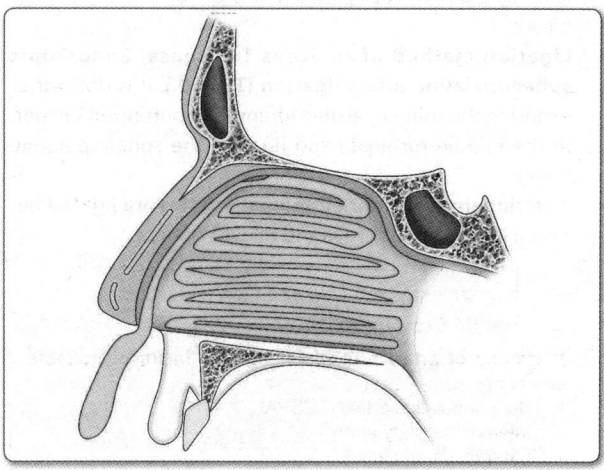

Fig. 19.2: Anterior nasal packing

- A balloon tamponade may be used as an alternative to nasal packing. It is less traumatic.

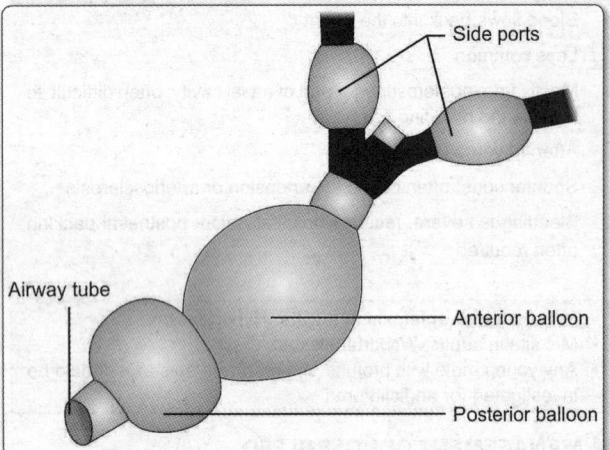

Fig. 19.3: Showing a balloon tamponade

Posterior Nasal Packing

- If bleeding does not stop by anterior nasal packing, it indicates posterior bleeding, and postnasal packing should be done. Posterior nasal packing can cause cardiovascular complications like pulmonary hypertension and corpulmonale since it leads to sleep apnea.

VESSEL LIGATION IN UNCONTROLLABLE BLEEDS

- **External carotid artery ligations:** Operation of choice in Elderly and debilitated patients in anterior epistaxis.
  - **Indication:** bleeding from the external carotid artery system when all conservative methods have failed
  - **Site for ligation:** above the origin of superior thyroid artery.
- **Maxillary artery ligation:** Performed in the pterygopalatine fossa by Caldwell-Luc approach. It is performed in posterior bleeds.
- **Ligation method of choice is Transnasal Endoscopic sphenopalatine artery ligation (TESPAL).** It is done after exposing the sphenopalatine foramen by putting an incision in the middle turbinate and ligating the sphenopalatine artery.
- **Anterior and posterior ethmoidal arteries are ligated** between inner canthus of eye and midline of nose.

Points to Remember

Hierarchy of arteries used for ligation in uncontrollable epistaxis:
- Sphenopalatine artery (TESPAL)
- Internal maxillary artery
- External carotid artery
- Anterior/posterior ethmoidal artery.

Extra Edge

Hereditary hemorrhagic telangiectasia or Esler-Weber Rendu disease:
Hereditary hemorrhagic telangiectasia involves the anterior part of nasal septum and causes recurrent episodes of profuse bleeding. It is managed by KTP or Nd Yag Laser or by septodermoplasty

NEW PATTERN QUESTIONS

Q N1. Location of Woodruff plexus is:
a. Posterior end of middle turbinate
b. Anterior end of septum
c. Posterior end of inferior turbinate
d. Posterior end of superior turbinate

Q N2. M/C cause of epistaxis in children is:
a. Nose picking   b. Tumor
c. Hypertension   d. Adenoid

Q N3. Causes of epistaxis are all *except*:
a. Allergic rhinitis
b. Foreign body
c. Tumor
d. Hypertension

Q N4. Most common site of nose bleed in child:
a. Woodruff area   b. Brown area
c. Little's area   d. None

Q N5. Posterior epistaxis is commonly seen in:
a. Children with ethmoidal polyps
b. Foreign bodies of the nose
c. Hypertension
d. Nose picking

Q N6. A child with unilateral nasal obstruction along with a mass in cheek and profuse and recurrent epistaxis:
a. Glomus tumor
b. Antrochoanal polyp
c. Juvenile nasal angiofibroma
d. Rhinolith

Q N7. Which is known as artery of epistaxis?
a. Anterior ethmoidal artery
b. Sphenopalatine artery
c. Greater palatine artery
d. Septal branch of superior labial artery

Q N8. Which of the following is not a cause of epistaxis?
a. Alcohol
b. Environment
c. NSAID's
d. Antrochoanal polyps

Chapter 19: Epistaxis

Explanations and References to New Pattern Questions

N1. Ans. is c i.e. Posterior end of inferior turbinate *Ref. Dhingra ENT 6/e, p 176*

> Woodruff's plexus is a plexus of veins situated inferior to posterior end of inferior turbinate. It is the site of posterior epistaxis in adults.

N2. Ans. a i.e. Nose picking *Ref. Scott Brown 7/e, Vol. 1, p 1064*

> M/C cause of epistaxis in children — Idiopathic
> 2nd M/C cause of epistaxis in children—
>
> Infection/Trauma
> ↓
> Development of crusts
> ↓
> Nasal picking/Digital trauma
> ↓
> Nasal bleed

N3. Ans. is a i.e. Allergic rhinitis *Ref. Dhingra 6/e, p 176,167; TB of Mohan Bansal 1/e, p 294*

Amongst the options given, foreign body, tumor, hypertension all can lead to epistaxis.

> **Remember**
> Many nasal problems can lead to epistaxis viz nasal trauma, viral rhinitis, chronic infections of nose (which lead to crust formation like atrophic rhinitis, rhinits sicca, TB of nose), foreign bodies in nose (maggots and non living), DNS, neoplasms (hemangioma, papilloma, carcinoma or sarcoma).

Two nasal conditions which do not lead to epistaxis:
- Nasal polyps
- Allergic rhinitis

Pharyngeal conditions which lead to epistaxis:
- Adenoiditis
- Juvenile angiofibroma
- Malignant tumors

N4. Ans. is c i.e. Little's area *Ref. TB of Mohan Bansal 1/e, p 294*

"The most common site of bleeding in children and young people is Little's area."

N5. Ans. is c i.e. Hypertension *Ref. Dhingra 6/e, p 178, Table 33.1; TB of Mohan Bansal 1/e, p 294*

M/C cause of epistaxis in adults is hypertension
- M/C site – Woodruff area
- Causes posterior epistaxis

N6. Ans. is c i.e. Juvenile nasal angiofibroma *Ref. Dhingra 6/e, p 246*

A child presenting with unilateral nasal obstruction along with mass in cheek and profuse and recurrent epistaxis should immediately raise the suspicion for Juvenile angiofibroma, details of which are dealt in chapter on 'Tumors of pharynx'.

N7. Ans. is b i.e. Sphenopalatine artery *Ref. internet search*

The sphenopalatine artery (nasopalatine artery), a branch of maxillary artery and is commonly known as Artery of Epistaxis.

N8. Ans. is d i.e. Antrochoanal polyps *Ref. Scotts Brown 7/e Vol 2 Pg 1605*

Alcohol can lead to liver disease, hence it can be a cause of epistaxis. Environment and NSAID's can cause epistaxis. Polyps are a rare cause of epistaxis.

QUESTIONS

1. **Common site of bleeding:** [PGI 08]
   a. Woodruff's plexus   b. Brown' area
   c. Little's area   d. Vestibular area
2. **Woodruff's plexus is seen at:** [AP 95; TN 99; AP 03]
   a. Anteroinferior part of superior turbinate
   b. Middle turbinate
   c. Posterior part of inferior turbinate
   d. Anterior part of inferior turbinate
3. **Little's area is situated in nasal cavity in:**
   a. Anteroinferior   b. Anterosuperior
   c. Posteroinfesion   d. Posterosuperior
4. **Main vascular supply of Little's area is all except:**
   a. Septal branch of superior labial artery
   b. Nasal branch of sphenopalatine artery
   c. Anterior ethmoidal artery
   d. Palatal branch of sphenopalatine artery
5. **Which artery does not contribute to Little's area?** [PGI 98]
   a. Anterior ethmoidal artery
   b. Septal branch of facial artery
   c. Sphenopalatine artery
   d. Posterior ethmoidal artery
6. **Which of the following arteries of the Kiesselbach's plexus is not a branch of External carotid artery:**
   a. Sphenopalatine artery   [AIIMS Nov 17]
   b. Greater palatine artery
   c. Anterior and middle ethmoid arteries
   d. Septal branch of the superior labial artery
7. **Most common cause for nose bleeding is:** [AIIMS 95]
   a. Trauma to Little's area
   b. AV aneurysm
   c. Posterosuperior part of nasal septum
   d. Hiatus semilunaris
8. **M/C cause of epistaxis in 3-year-old child:** [PGI 98]
   a. Nasal polyp
   b. Foreign body
   c. Upper respiratory catarrh
   d. Atrophic rhinitis
9. **In a 5-year-old child, most common cause of unilateral epistaxis is:** [PGI 97]
   a. Foreign body   b. Polyp
   c. Atrophic rhinitis   d. Maggot's
10. **Recurrent epistaxis in a 15-year-old female the most common cause is:** [JIPMER 90]
    a. Juvenile nasopharyngeal fibroma
    b. Rhinosporiodiosis
    c. Foreign body
    d. Hematopoietic disorder
11. **Diagnosis in a 10-year-old boy with recurrent epistaxis and a unilateral nasal mass is:** [SGPGI 05]
    a. Antrochoanal polyp   b. Hemangioma
    c. Angiofibroma   d. Rhinolith
12. **Epistaxis in elderly person is common in:** [AI 04]
    a. Foreign body
    b. Allergic rhinitis
    c. Hypertension
    d. Nasopharyngeal carcinoma
13. **Systemic causes of epistaxis are all except:** [UP 02]
    a. Hypertension
    b. Anticoagulant treatment
    c. Hereditary telangiectasia
    d. Hemophilia
14. **Which of the following is/are true about posterior epistaxis:** [PGI Nov 14]
    a. Posterior packing is done
    b. Often due to chronic hypertension
    c. Persistent case-ligation of anterior ethmoidal artery
    d. Severe bleeding in comparison with anterior epistaxis
    e. More commonly occur in elderly
15. **A 70-year-aged patient with epistaxis, hypertensive with BP = 200/100 mm Hg. On examination no active bleeding noted, next step of management is:**
    a. Observation
    b. Internal maxillary artery ligation
    c. Anterior and posterior nasal pack
    d. Anterior nasal pack
16. **Source of epistaxis after ligation of external carotid artery is:** [AIIMS 93]
    a. Maxillary artery
    b. Greater palatine artery
    c. Superior labial artery
    d. Ethmoidal artery
17. **If posterior epistaxis cannot be controlled, which artery is ligated:** [Kolkata 00]
    a. Posterior ethmoidal artery
    b. Maxillary artery
    c. Sphenopalatine artery
    d. External carotid artery
18. **In case of uncontrolled epistaxis, ligation of internal maxillary artery is to be done in the:** [Kolkata 01]
    a. Maxillary antrum
    b. Pterygopalatine fossa
    c. At the neck
    d. Medial wall of orbit
19. **Treatment of choice in recurrent epistaxis in a patient with hereditary hemotelangiectasis:** [Kolkata 05]
    a. Anterior ethmoidal artery ligation
    b. Septal dermoplasty
    c. External carotid artery ligation
    d. Internal carotid artery ligation

20. **Kiesselbach's plexus is situated on the:** [DNB 2005, 11]
    a. Medial wall of the middle ear
    b. Lateral wall of the nasopharynx
    c. Medial wall of the nasal cavity
    d. Laryngeal aspect of epiglottis
21. **Posterior epistaxis occurs from:** [Kerala 2010]
    a. Woodruff's plexus   b. Kiesselbach's plexus
    c. Atherosclerosis   d. Little's area
22. **All are true about epistaxis except:** [PGI Nov 2016]
    a. Kiesselbach plexus is source in 90% cases
    b. If anterior packing is left in nose for more than 48 hours, antibiotics should be given
    c. Anterior packing is easy to insert and less traumatic than balloon tamponade
    d. Trotter method is a first aid method
    e. Cauterization is done in refractory cases under GA
23. **In intractable epistaxis, following vessels can be ligated except:** [PGI May 2016]
    a. Internal carotid artery   b. External carotid artery
    c. Maxillary artery   d. Anterior ethmoidal artery

Explanations and References

1. **Ans. is a, b and c i.e. Woodruff's plexus, Brown's area; and Little's area**
2. **Ans. is c i.e. Posterior part of inferior turbinate** *Ref. TB of Mohan Bansal, p 297*
3. **Ans. is a i.e. Anteroinferior**
4. **Ans. is d i.e. Palatal branch of sphenopalatine artery**
5. **Ans. is d i.e. Posterior ethmoidal artery** *Ref. Dhingra 6/e, p 176; Scott Brown 7/e, Vol 2, p 1597; TB of Mohan Bansal, p 293*

Common Sites of Bleeding

Site	Located	Formed by	Characteristic
Little's area (M/C site of epistaxis)	Anteroinferior part of nasal septum	• Anterior ethmoidal artery • Septal branch of superior labial artery • Septal branch of sphenopalatine artery • Greater palatine artery	M/C site of bleeding
Woodruff's area	Under the posterior end of inferior turbinate	• Sphenopalatine artery • Posterior pharyngeal artery	• It is a venous plexus • Common cause of posterior epistaxis
Retrocolumellar vein	Behind the columella at the anterior edge of little's area		• M/C site of venous bleeding in children
Brown's area	Posterior part of septum	• Posterior part of septum	• Site for hypertensive posterior epistaxis

6. **Ans. is c i.e. Anterior and middle ethmoid arteries**

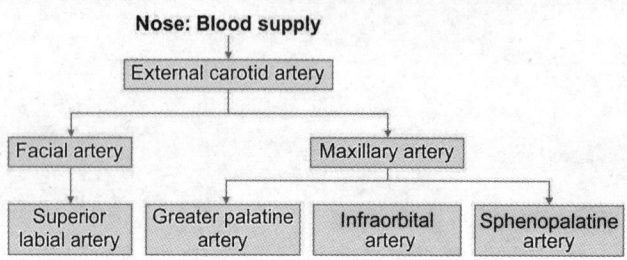

 Note: Anterior and Middle ethmoidal artery are branches of ophthalmic artery which is a branch of internal carotid artery.

7. **Ans. is a i.e Trauma to the little's area** *Ref. Dhingra 6/e, p 176; TB of Mohan Bansal, p 293*
   - Little area *(also called as Kiesselbach's plexus)* is a highly vascular area in the anteroinferior part of nasal septum just above the vestibule
   - It is the most common site for nasal bleeding as this area is exposed to the drying effect of inspiratory current and to finger nail trauma.

8. **Ans. is c i.e. Upper respiratory catarrh** *Ref. Scott Brown 7/e, Vol 1, p 1064*
   - Friends – I know some of you must be thinking foreign body as the answer but it is not the most common cause.
   - **M/C** *cause of epistaxis in children is idiopathic.*

   2nd M/C cause of epistaxis in children is

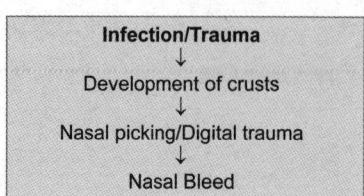

Still if you have doubt read the following lines of Scotts Brown:
"Epistaxis – Children are especially susceptible to nose bleeds due to extensive vascular supply to nasal mucosa and the frequency with which they develop upper respiratory tract infections." *Ref. Scott Brown 7/e, Vol 1, p 1063*

Chapter 19: Epistaxis

"Epistaxis is more common in children with upper respiratory allergies." Ref. Scott Brown 7/e, Vol 1, p 1063
"There is a seasonal variation with a higher prevalence in the winter months perhaps due to the greater frequency of upper respiratory tract infections." Ref. Scott Brown 7/e, Vol 1, p 1063

9. **Ans. is a i.e. Foreign body** Ref. Dhingra 6/e, 161; SK De 5/e, p 245

   Most common cause of unilateral epistaxis in children is **Foreign body.**
   In case of Foreign Body of Nose *"The child presents with unilateral nasal discharge which is often foul smelling and occasionally blood-stained."* Ref. Dhingra 6/e, p 161

10. **Ans. is d i.e. Hematopoietic disorder** Ref. Read Below

    As such this answer is not given anywhere but we can come to the correct answer by exclusion.
    Option "a" is Juvenile nasopharyngeal fibroma.
    It is seen in adolescent males and is therefore the most common cause of recurrent epistaxis in males and not in females.
    Ref. Dhingra 6/e, p 346
    Option "b" is Rhinosporidiosis is a cause of epistaxis but usually occurs in young males from India. Ref. Turner 10/e, p 61
    Option "c" is Foreign body which is a cause of epistaxis in children and is not commonly seen in 15 years of age.
    So we are left with hematopoietic disorder which can be seen in a 15-year-old female. Ref. Dhingra 6/e, p161

11. **Ans. is c i.e. Angiofibroma** Ref. Dhingra 6/e, p 246

    Recurrent epistaxis in a 10-year-old boy with **unilateral nasal mass** is diagnostic of juvenile nasopharyngeal fibroma.
    For details, see chapter on Pharyngeal Tumor.

12. **Ans. is c i.e. Hypertension** Ref. Maqbool 11/e, p 180; Textbook of Mohan Bansal, p 295

    According to Scott Brown 7th/ed Vol 2 p 1600 – **M/C cause of adult epistaxis is idiopathic** though a number of factors increase its chances like use of NSAIDs and alcohol. It further says there is no proven association between hypertension and adult Epistaxis, but still
    "Elevated blood pressure is observed in almost all epistaxis admissions. This apparent hypertension in acute admissions may be a result of anxiety associated with hospital admission and the invasive techniques used to control the bleeding."
    Ref. Dhingra 6/e, p167

    But still the answer to this question is hypertension by ruling out other options:
    - **Option a** – foreign body – is a cause of epistaxis in children and not in elderly age group
    - **Option b** – allergic rhinitis – does not lead to epistaxis Ref. Dhingra 5/e, p 181
    - Nasopharyngeal carcinoma does cause epistaxis and is seen in elderly age group but is not the most common cause as in itself nasopharyngeal carcinoma is not common.

    "Nasal tumors seldom present as epistaxis in isolation Juvenile nasopharyngeal angiofibroma and hemangiopericytoma are rare vascular tumors which can present with severe or recurrent epitaxis in association with nasal obstruction."
    Ref. Dhingra 5/e, p 263

    - Hence our answer by exclusion is hypertension.
    - The answer is further supported by Maqbool 11th/ed p 180 which says:
    "Hypertension is a very common disease and causes epistaxis frequently in elderly patients."

13. **Ans. is d i.e. Hemophilia** Ref. Scott Brown 7/e, Vol 2, p 1605

    Epistaxis in Adult

Primary	Secondary
No cause is identified but may be due to:	Cause is identified and it is due to:
• Use of NSAIDs	• Coagulopathy secondary to liver disease/kidney disease/leukemia or myelosuppression
• Use of alcohol	• Trauma
• Hypertension (role not proven)	• Post surgery like inferior turbinectomy, Endoscopic sinus surgery
	• Warfarin intake (anticoagulant treatment)
	• Hereditary hemorrhagic telangiectasia

    Hemophilia is a Secondary Cause of Epistaxis in Children Ref. Scott Brown 7/e, Vol 1, p 1065
    Hence the answer is d i.e. hemophilia which is not a cause of secondary epistaxis but is implicated in the etiology of primary epistaxis though its role is doubted there also.

14. **Ans. is a, b, d and e i.e. posterior packing done, often due to chronic hypertension, severe bleeding in comparison with anterior expistaxis and more commonly occur in elderly** Ref. Dhingra 6/e,pgs177-180
    Posterior Epistaxis
    - Mainly the blood flows back into the throat
    - Posterior nasal packing is required for the patient bleeding posteriorly into the throat

- Ligation of maxillary artery is done in uncontrollable posterior epistaxis. Approach is via Caldwell-Luc operation. This procedure is now superceded by transnasal endoscopic sphenopalatine artery ligation
- Woodruff's area: It is a plexus of veins situated inferior to posterior end of inferior turbinate. It is the site of posterior epistaxis "A posterior pack may be used if the bleeding is predominantly in this area"- Logan Turner 10th/32

Feature	Anterior epistaxis	Posterior epistaxis
Incidence	More common	Less common
Site	Mostly from Little's area or anterior part of lateral wall	Mostly from posterosuperior part of nasal cavity; often difficult to localize the bleeding point
Age	Mostly occurs in children or young adults	After 40 years of age
Cause	Mostly trauma	Spontaneous; often due to hypertension or arteriosclerosis
Bleeding	Usually mild, can be easily controlled by local pressure or anterior pack	Bleeding is severe, require hospitalization; postnasal pack often required

15. Ans. is a i.e. Observation *Ref. Scott Brown 7/e, Vol 1, p 1065*
- We do not need any reference to answer this particular question as the answer is hidden in the question only.
- The question itself says that no active bleeding is seen—so no need to do anything just observe the patient and because his BP is 200/100 mm Hg which is quite high, give him antihypertensive drugs.

ALSO KNOW

Management strategy for adult primary epistaxis

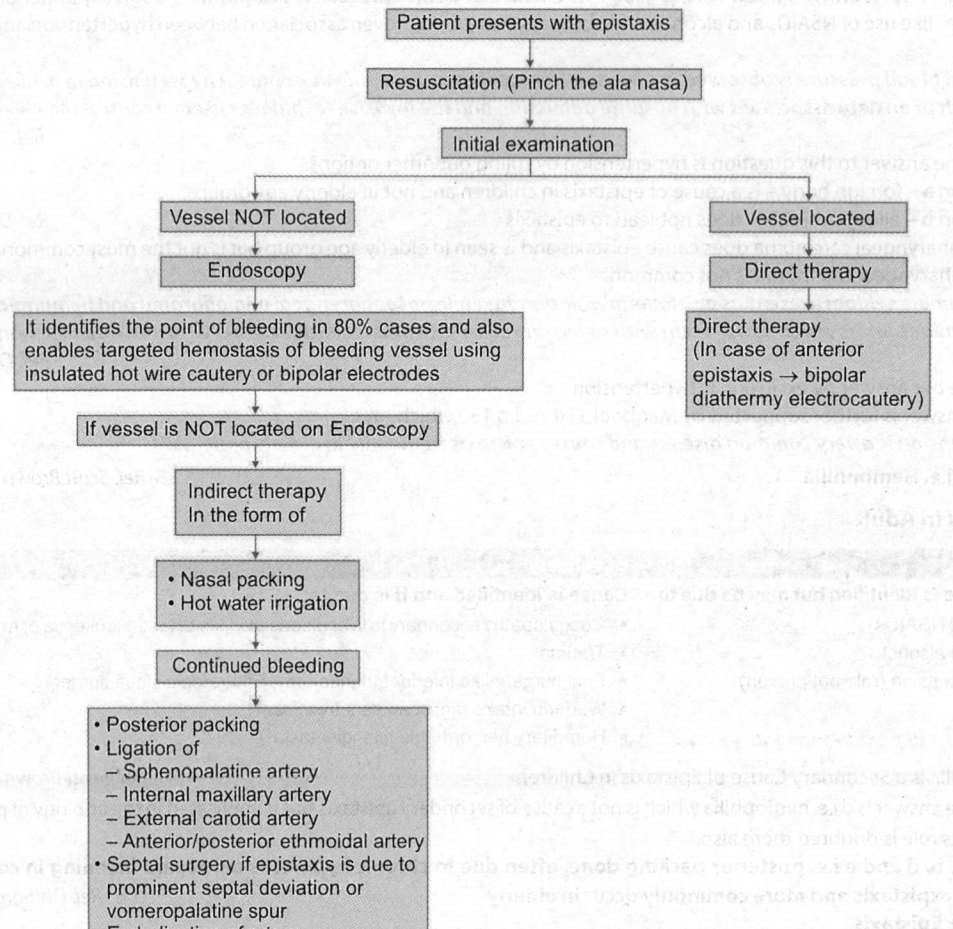

Chapter 19: Epistaxis

16. Ans. is d i.e. Ethmoidal artery *Ref. Dhingra 6/e, p 178; TB of Mohan Bansal 1/e, p 35; Scott Brown 7/e Vol 2, p 1599*
Both: Internal carotid artery and external carotid artery

Nose is supplied by both internal and external carotid artery.

Internal carotid artery	External carotid artery
• Anterior ethmoidal artery • Posterior ethmoidal artery	**Facial Artery** • Superior labial artery **Maxillary Artery** • Greater palatine artery • Branches of sphenopalatine artery (nasopalatine, post nasal septal branches and posterior lateral nasal branches • Anterior superior dental artery

In the Question
- Greater palatine artery
- Superior labial artery
- Maxillary artery

Are all branches of external carotid artery.
If external carotid artery is ligated, the source of epistaxis will be **ethmoidal artery** which is a branch of **Internal carotid artery.**

17. Ans. is c i.e. Sphenopalatine artery *Ref. Scott Brown 7/e, Vol 2, p 1603,1606*
Ligation technique is reserved for intractable bleeding where the source cannot be located or controlled by other techniques.

The hierarchy of arteries used for ligation is:
• Sphenopalatine artery • Internal maxillary artery • External carotid artery • Anterior/posterior ethmoidal artery

> Earlier the most common artery ligated was maxillary artery but now endonasal sphenopalatine artery ligation (ESPAL) is the ligation of choice.

"ESPAL is the current ligation of choice controlling bleeding in over 90% of cases with a low complication rate."
Ref. Scott Brown 7/e, Vol 2, p 1606

Transnasal Endonasal Sphenopalatine Ligation (TESPAL or ESPAL)
• It is the most popular procedure for ligation and has replaced internal maxillary artery ligation. • Can be done under LA/GA • Incision is given 8 mm anterior and under the posterior end of middle turbinate • Sphenopalatine artery is ligated in **the sphenopalatine foramen**^Q • Success rate ~100% • Complications very rare – rebleeding, infection and nasal adhesions

Internal Maxillary Artery Ligation

Earlier it was the ligation procedure of choice for uncontrolled bleeding:
- Internal maxillary artery is ligated in the pterygopalatine fossa using a Caldwell-Luc approach (3rd part of the artery is ligated)^Q
- Success rate – 89%
- Complications – Sinusitis, damage to infraorbital nerve, oroantral fistula, dental damage and anesthesia, and rarely ophthalmoplegia and blindness.

External carotid artery ligation and anterior and posterior ethmoidal artery ligation is not commonly done.

18. Ans. is b i.e. Pterygopalatine fossa *Ref. Scott Brown 7/e, Vol 2, p 1603; Textbook of Mohan Bansal, p 296*

Ligation of	Site
• Sphenopalatine artery	Sphenopalatine foramen
• Internal maxillary artery	Pterygopalatine fossa
• External carotid artery	Above the origin of superior thyroid artery
• Ethmoidal arteries	Between inner canthus of eye and midline of nose

19. **Ans. is b i.e. Septal dermoplasty**

    Ref. Dhingra 6/e, p 180; Scott Brown 7/e, Vol 2, p 1605; Textbook of Mohan Bansal 1/e, p 297

    - Hereditary hemotelangiectasia (HHT) or Osler-Weber-Rendu disease is an autosomal dominant condition affecting blood vessels in the skin, mucous membranes and viscera
    - The genetic abnormality is located to chromosome 9 and 12
    - *Classical features:*
        - Telangiectasia
        - A/V malformations
        - Aneurysms
        - Recurrent epistaxis (seen in 93% cases)

    Management

    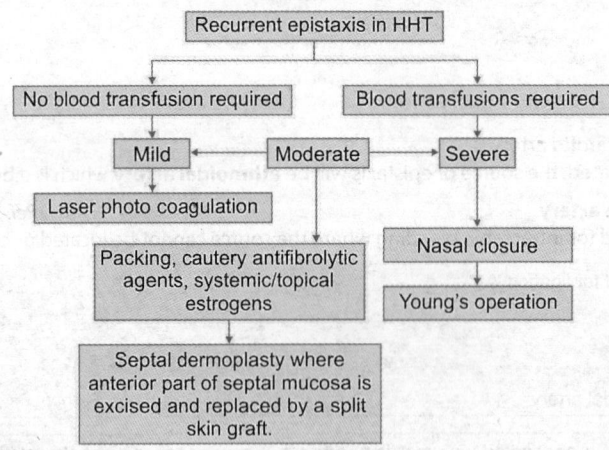

20. **Ans. is c i.e. Medial wall of nasal cavity**

    Ref. Dhingra 6/e, p 176

    Kiesselbach's plexus is situated in the anterior inferior part of nasal septum (which forms the medral wall of nose) just above the vestibule.

21. **Ans. is a i.e. Woodruff's pleux**

    Ref. Dhingra 6/e, p 450

    Explanation: Repeat

22. **Ans. is None**

    All the options given in the question are correct
    - Kiesslebach plexus is source of epistaxis in 90% cases
    - Trotters method: It is the gold standard first aid method – Also called as Hippocratic method

    > - Set with head forward
    > - Pinch the fleshy part of nose firmly
    > - Hold nose for 20 minutes
    > - Put some ice packs on forehead or nape of neck
    > - Spit out any blood in the mouth

    - Option C – Anterior packing is easy to insert and is less traumatic than balloon tamponade (True)
    - True Balloon tamponade is used for controlling posterior epistaxis and is invasive procedure whereas anterior packing is done is all those cases of (active) anterior epistaxis where cauterization failed. It is less traumatic than Balloon tamponade
    - If anterior packing is left in place for more than 48 hours then antibiotic coverage should be given (True)
    - Cauterization is done is refractory cases under GA (True)

23. **Ans. is a i.e. internal carotid artery**

    (Ref: Dingra 6/e pg 179-180)

    The arteries which are ligated in case of epistaxis in sequence:
    1. Sphenopalatine artery (TESPAL)
    2. Internal maxillary artery
    3. External carotid artery
    4. Anterior/Posterior ethmoidal artery

Chapter 20A

Diseases of Paranasal Sinus—Sinusitis

SINUSITIS

ANATOMY AND PHYSIOLOGY OF PARANASAL SINUSES

Paranasal sinuses are a group of air containing spaces that surround the nasal cavity.

Development

- 1st sinus to develop—Maxillary sinus
- Maxillary and ethmoid sinuses are present at birth, while sphenoid sinus is rudimentary at birth and frontal sinus is recognizable at 6 years of age and is fully developed by puberty.

Mnemonic

Order of development of sinuses:
Miss Eshani So Friendly
Maxillary > **E**thmoid > **S**phenoid > **F**rontal

Maxillary sinus	Frontal sinus
- Well developed at birth - 1st sinus develop - Reaches adult size by 15 years - *Most common* site of bacterial sinusitis - *Most common* site of noninvasive fungal sinusitis - On X-ray: visible at 4–5 months after birth - Completely developed by 9 year of age (at the time of second dentition) - Largest sinus in the body - Floor of maxillary sinus is related to 2nd premolar and 1st molar - Also called as **antrum of high more**	- Last sinus to develop - Develops 2 years after birth (Not present at birth) - Characteristic feature—Pott's puffy tumor - Mucocele - Ivory osteoma - X-ray visible at 6 years of age[Q] - Maximum size achieved by puberty[Q]
Ethmoidal sinus	**Sphenoidal sinus**

- Well developed at birth
- Reaches adult size by 12 years
- Most pneumatised at birth hence M/C sinusitis in children
- Clinically ethmoid cells are divided by the basal lamina into anterior ethmoid group which opens into middle meatus and posterior ethmoid group which opens into superior meatus
   – Ant group includes cells : (a) Agger nassi cells (b) Ethmoidal bulla (c) Supraorbital cells (d) Fronto-ethmoid cells (e) Haller cells
   – The posterior group includes onodi cells
- Leads to orbital cellulitis
- Adenocarcioma seen mostly in wood worker
- X-ray: visible at 1st year of age and complete by puberty
- **Most common cause of acute sinusitis in children.**[Q]
	- Not present at birth
	- Reaches full size by 15 years of age
	- Least common sinusitis
	- Major cause of cavernous sinus thrombophlebitis
	- **X-ray:** appears by 4 year of age[Q].
	- Bones of Bertin also called sphenoidal turbinates initially cover the anterior wall of sinus, but after 10 years, fuse with it.
	- The roof of sphenoid sinus is related to pituitary gland and lateral walls are related to optic nerve, internal carotid A, cavernous sinus and cranial nerves 3, 4, 5 and 6.

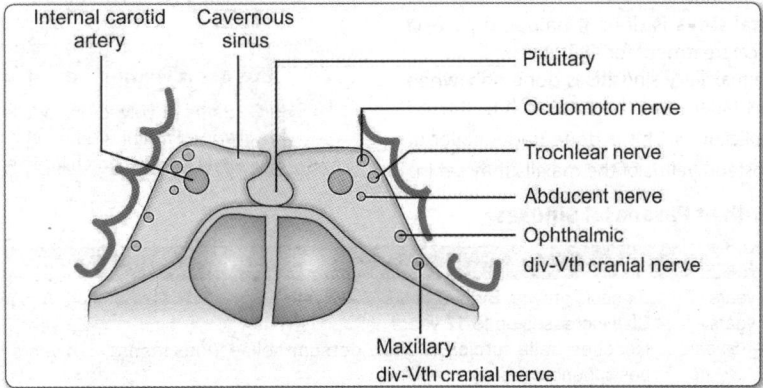

Fig. 20A.1: Relations of sphenoid sinus

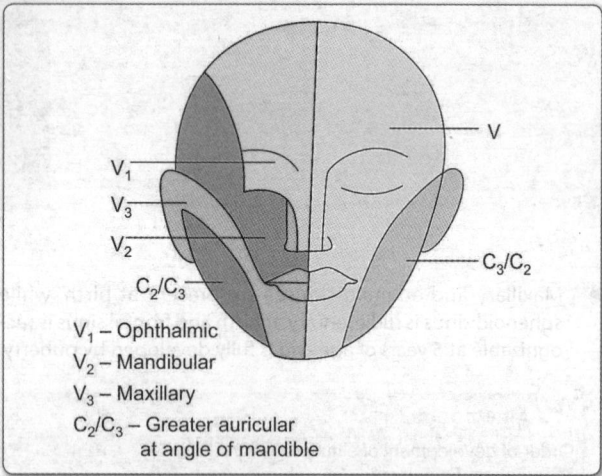

Fig. 20A.2: Anterior view of face: showing segmental innervation

- V_1 – Ophthalmic
- V_2 – Mandibular
- V_3 – Maxillary
- C_2/C_3 – Greater auricular at angle of mandible

Nerve Supply of Paranasal Sinuses

Nerve supply of various sinuses

Maxillary: Maxillary nerve (Infraorbital and alveolar nerves)
Frontal: Ophthalmia nerve (vi) (Sphenoidal branch)
Ethmoidal: Ophthalmia nerve (vi) (Nasociliary branch) and maxillary (from sphenopalatine fossa)
Sphenoidal: Ophthalmia nerve (vi) (Nasociliary branch) and maxillary (V_2).

Points to Remember

- Ethmoidal sinuses are well-developed at birth, hence infants and children below 3 years of age are more likely to have acute ethmoiditis; but above this age, maxillary sinusitis is more commonly seen:
- Foramina of Breschet are venous drainage channels located in the posterior wall of Frontal sinus.

Clinical Correlation

- **Periodicity is a characteristic feature of frontal sinus infections** in which the pain increases gradually on waking up and becomes maximum by midday, starts diminishing by evening, hence also called office headache.
- **Trephination of frontal sinus** is done if pain and pyrexia persist despite of medical treatment for 48 hours.
- **Antral lavage** in acute maxillary sinusitis is done only when medical treatment has failed and the patient has started showing signs of complications. This is done under cover of antibiotics, otherwise osteomyelitis of the maxilla may set in.

Development and Growth of Paranasal Sinuses

Sinus	At birth	Adult size	Growth	Radiological appearance (Age)
Maxillary	Present	15 years	Biphasic growth: Birth–3 years, 7–12 year	4–5 months
Ethmoid	Present	12 years	Size increases up to 12 years	1 year
Sphenoid	Absent	10–15 years	Reaches sella turcica (7 yrs), dorsum sellae (late teens), basisphenoid (adult)	4 years
Frontal	Absent	20 years	Invades frontal bone (2–4 yrs), size increases until teens	6 years

- **Dental infections** are important cause of maxillary sinusitis because of relation of roots of molars and premolars with the floor of maxillary sinus.

NEW PATTERN QUESTIONS

Q N1. Antrum of Highmore is:
a. Maxillary sinus b. Frontal sinus
c. Ethmoid sinus d. Sphenoid sinus

Q N2. Sinus which is not present at birth?
a. Maxillary b. Frontal
c. Ethmoid d. Sphenoid

Q N3. First paranasal sinus to develop at birth is:
a. Maxillary b. Ethmoidal
c. Frontal d. Sphenoidal

Q N4. The sinus which is most superior in face is?
a. Maxillary b. Frontal
c. Ethmoid d. Sphenoid

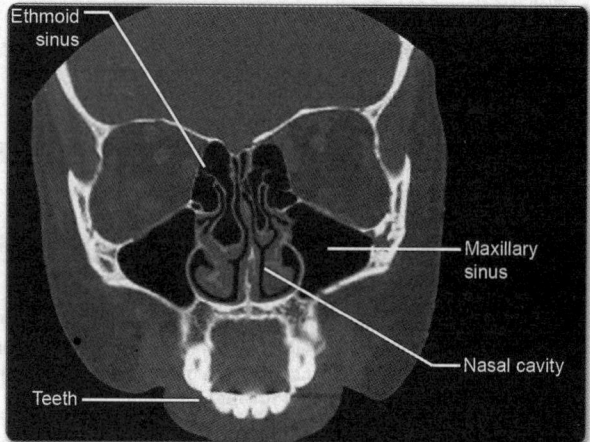

Fig. 20A.3: CT of PNS

ACUTE SINUSITIS

- It is acute inflammation of the paranasal sinuses of > 7 days and less than 4 weeks duration.

Points to Remember

- M/C Sinus involved in adults in order of frequency: Maxillary > Frontal > Ethmoid > Sphenoid
- M/C sinus involved in children = Ethmoidal sinus

Etiology

Secondary bacterial infection following viral rhinitis.

> **Points to Remember**
>
> **Causative organisms**
> - M/C—*Streptococcus pneumoniae*
> - 2nd M/C—*H. influenzae*
> - Others—Moraxella

> **Clinical Features**
>
> **As per Rhinosinusitis Task Force definition:**
> - **Major symptoms of sinusitis** include facial pain, pressure, congestion, nasal obstruction, nasal/postnasal discharge, hyposmia, and fever.
> - **Minor symptoms** are headaches, halitosis, and dental pain.
> - **Diagnosis** requires *two major criteria* or *one major and two minor criteria*.

- **Maxillary sinusitis**
  - **Pain site:** upper jaw with radiation to the gums and teeth. It is aggravated by coughing and stooping.
  - Headache in Frontal region.
  - **Tenderness:** Over the cheeks (Fig. 20A.4).
  - Postnasal drip.
- **Frontal sinusitis**
  - **Headache:** Over the frontal sinus area in the forehead.
  - Pain is typically periodical in nature.^Q
  - *Often called as Office Headache.*^Q As maximum pain occurs by midday and decreases by evening
    - **Tenderness:** Along the frontal sinus floor just above the medial canthus (Fig. 20A.5).
    - Edema of upper eyelid.
- **Ethmoid sinusitis**
  - More often involved in infants and young children.^Q
  - **Pain:** Over the nasal bridge and inner canthus of eye and is referred to parietal eminence.
  - **Tenderness** is along inner canthus (Fig. 20A.6).
  - Edema of the upper and lower eyelids.
- **Sphenoiditis**
  - Rare entity on its own.
  - Occurs subsequent to ethmoiditis/pansinusitis.
  - Severe occipital or vertical headache and is sometimes referred to mastoid process.^Q
  - **Pain** may be felt retroorbitally due to close proximity with Vth nerve.
  - Postnasal drip seen on posterior rhinoscopy.

Note: Vertical headache with postnatal discharge is suggestive of sphenoid sinusitis.

Methods of eliciting tenderness of various sinuses.

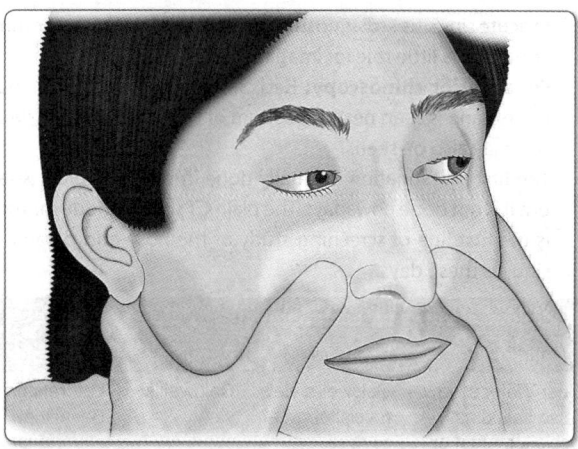

Fig. 20A.4: Eliciting the maxillary sinus tenderness

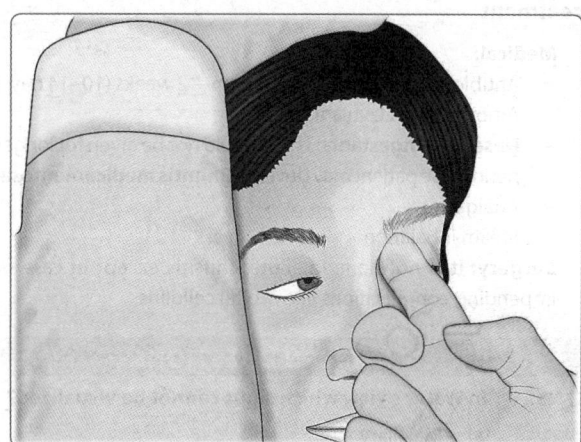

Fig. 20A.5: Eliciting the frontal sinus tenderness

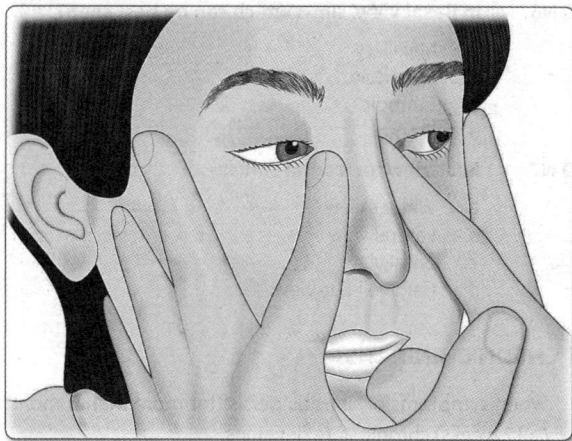

Fig. 20A.6: Eliciting the tenderness of ethmoidal sinuses

Diagnosis

- In acute sinusitis—diagnosis is mainly made on clinical ground and there is little role for imaging.
- **On anterior rhinoscopy:** Red, shiny and swollen mucous membrane is seen near the ostium of the sinus, and trickle of pus may also be seen.
- The first investigation is usually done in past was plain X-ray but it is not done nowadays. The plain CT scan without contrast is the first line of screening study of the nose and paranasal sinuses these days.

Radiological Views for Each Sinus			
Maxillary	Frontal	Ethmoids	Sphenoid
Best-Water's view (also called as occipitomental or nose chin position) and basal view	Caldwell's view (occipitofrontal or nose forehead view)	Caldwell's view	Lateral and Basal view

Treatment

- **Medical:**
  - Antibiotics are given for minimum—2 weeks (10–14 days) Amoxicillin + clavulanic acid.
  - **Nasal decongestants:** They should not be given for longer period else patient may develop **Rhinitis medicamentosa**.
  - Analgesics
  - Steam inhalation
- **Surgery:** It is not done in acute sinusitis except in case of impending complications like orbital cellulitis.

NEW PATTERN QUESTIONS

Q N5. In Water's view which sinus cannot be visualized?
  a. Maxillary
  b. Frontal
  c. Sphenoid
  d. Ethmoid

Q N6. In Basal view, sinus which can be best seen?
  a. Maxillary
  b. Sphenoid
  c. Ethmoid
  d. Frontal

Q N7. Best view for frontal sinus:
  a. Water's view
  b. Lateral view
  c. Basal view
  d. Caldwell-Luc view

CHRONIC SINUSITIS

- When symptoms of sinusitis persist for more than 3 months (≥ 12 weeks) chronic state develops.
- **Organisms:** Mixed aerobic and anaerobic.

Note: Maxillary sinus is most commonly involved in chronic sinusitis.

Diagnosis

Diagnosis is done by nasal endoscopy (1st investigation done) If any pathology is seen on endoscopy, then NCCT nose and PNS is done.

Note: NCCT has replaced X-ray PNS practically nowadays.

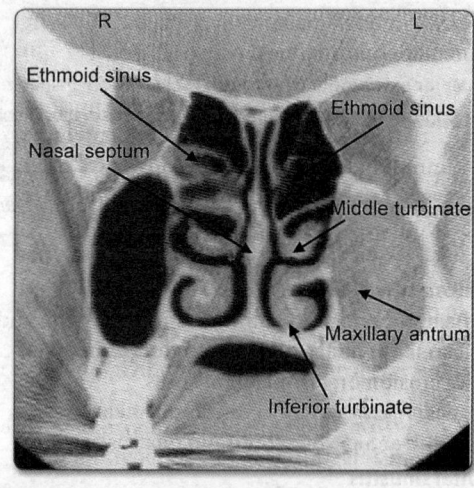

Fig. 20A.7: CT paranasal sinuses with left maxillary sinus hazy
Courtesy: BS Tuli TB of ENT, Jaypee Brothers Medical Publishers Pvt. Ltd., 2/e, p 202

Also Know

D/D of opaque maxillary sinus
1. Traumatic (collection of blood/edema)
2. Infective cause, allergic
3. Neoplasm
4. Miscellaneous - fibrous dysplasia, Dentigerous cyst

Treatment

Medical

- Antibiotics, mucolytics, nasal irrigation, cortcosteroids to reduce mucosal swelling associated with the inflammatory response.

Surgical

- **Indication:** If medical treatment given for a period of 3–4 weeks fail.

Surgeries for Chronic Sinusitis

(a) For Chronic Maxillary Sinusitis:
(i) *Antral lavage*: Done by performing antral puncture in inferior meatus[Q] with the help of Tilley Lichtwitz trocar and cannula.

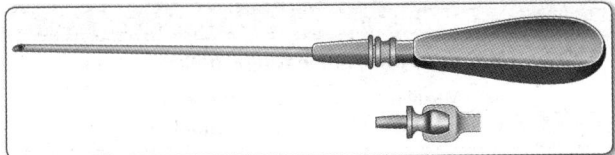

Fig. 20A.8: Lichtwitz trocar and cannula used for proof puncture. Puncture is done in inferior meatus[Q]

(ii) *Intranasal antrostomy*: Done by making a window in inferior meatus to facilitate drainage through gravity.

(iii) *Caldwell-Luc operation*: Discussed later.

(iv) *FESS*: These days all sinus surgeries have been replaced by FESS—discussed later

(b) Chronic Frontal Sinusitis:

(i) *Trephination of frontal sinus*: Done in acute frontal sinusitis if pain persists or exacerbates or there is fever inspite of antibiotic treatment for 48 hrs. Also done in chronic frontal sinusitis.

A 2 cm long horizontal incision is made in superomedial part of eye to expose frontal sinus. A hole is made and pus drained.

(ii) *External frontal ethmoidectomy (Howarth's or Lynch operation)*: Frontal sinus is entered via inner margin of the orbit.

(iii) *Other surgeries*: Paterson operation, osteoplastic flap operation.

These surgeries are seldom done now and are replaced by FESS.

- Recently, endoscopic sinus surgery is replacing radical operations on the sinuses and provides good drainage and ventilation. It also avoids external incisions.

Points to Remember
- Acute sinusitis = Symptoms for < 4 weeks
- Subacute sinusitis = Symptoms for 4–12 weeks
- Chronic sinusitis = Symptoms for > 12 weeks
- Recurrent sinusitis = 4 or more episodes of sinusites each year, lasting for more than 7–10 days.

NEW PATTERN QUESTIONS

Q N8. Howarth procedure is related to:
a. External frontonasal ethmoidectomy
b. Frontal sinus trephine
c. Endoscopic sinus surgery
d. Maxillary antrostomy

Q N9. Antral puncture (proof puncture) is done through:
a. Superior meatus   b. Inferior meatus
c. Middle meatus   d. None

Q N10. Sudden death in case of maxillary wash is due to:
a. Hemorrhage   b. Meningitis
c. Air embolism   d. Thrombus of maxillary artery

Q N11. Proof puncture is done in:
a. Ethmoid sinusitis   b. Sphenoid sinusitis
c. Maxillary sinusitis   d. Frontal sinusitis

Q N12. Infundibulotomy is done for:
a. Approaching nasolacrimal duct
b. Approaching middle meatus
c. Rhinoplasty
d. Choanal atresia repair

FUNGAL SINUSITIS

- Fungal infection occurs mostly in traumatic cases with compound fractures, in uncontrolled diabetics, debilitated patients, such as carcinoma, and in patients on immunosuppressants, antibiotics or steroids.
- Most common fungal species are *Aspergillus* (M/C), *Actinomyces*, *Mucor*, *Rhizopus* or *Absidia* species of fungus.
- May occur in noninvasive or invasive form.
- Commonest organisim involved in non invasive form is *Aspergillus fumigatus* followed by *Dematiaceous* species (Bipolaris, Curvularia, Alternaria).
- Noninvasive form may either persent as a fungal ball or allergic fungal rhinosinusitis (AFRS) and usually affect immunocompetent individuals.

Fungus Ball

- Fungus ball occurs in adult females
- **M/C agent:** Aspergillus
- Most common sinus involved – Maxillary > sphenoid sinus
- M/C involved sinus is ethmoid sinus
- M/C symptom – unilateral postnasal discharge
- Most important investigation—CT scan
- Fungus ball is the main fungal rhinosinusitis in an immunocompetent patient.

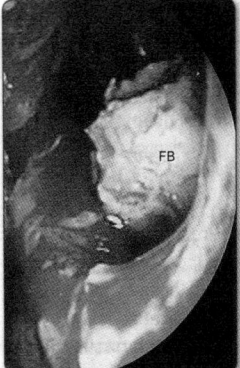

Fig. 20A.9: Fungal ball (FB) in maxillary sinus
Courtesy: BS Tuli TB of ENT, Jaypee Brothers Medical Publishers Pvt. Ltd., 2/e, p 200

Investigation

CT scan: Majority of sinuses show near complete opacification. On unenhanced CT, the sinuses are typically opacified by centrally hyperdense material with peripheral rim of hypodense mucosa.

- Surgery (FESS) is the most effective treatment for fungal ball.

Allergic Fungal Rhinosinusitis

- AFS is a noninvasive fungal rhonosinusistis.
- *Dermatiaceous* species are the fungal agents mostly responsible for AFRs.
- Seen in immunocompetent hosts with allergy to fungus.
- M/C involved sinus is ethmoid sinus
- **The sinus mucosa is hyperplastic and hypertrophic but there is no evidence of invasion**
- **Criteria for diagnosis of allergic fungal rhinosinusitis as proposed by Bent and Kuhn includes 5 criteria**: (1) nasal polyps, (2) hypersensitivity type I for fungus, (3) eosinophilic mucin demonstrated visually or histopathologically without invasion, (4) positive fungal stain or culture, and (5) characteristic CT findings.
- CT findings demonstrate unilateral or asymmetric involvement of the sinuses. Due to the allergic mucin, heterogeneous opacities are seen on CT. These opacitites are due to accumalation of iron and manganese in the mucin (not due to hemosiderin as was earlier thought).
- Treatment = Antifungals.

Chronic or Indolent Invasive Fungal Rhinosinusitis

- Chronic invasive fungal rhinosinusitis is a rare pathology occurring mostly in immunocompetent patients.
- Aspergillus is the most frequent agent isolated in this pathology.

Acute Fulminant Fungal Rhinosinusitis

- Fulminant invasive fungal rhinosinusitis occurs in immunocompromised patients (HIV, diabetes, chemotherapy)
- Early diagnosis and control of primary immunological disorders is essential for the prognosis.

Complications of Paranasal Sinus Infection	

Local	• Mucocele/Mucopyocele
	• Mucous retention cyst
	• Osteomyelitis
	  – Frontal bone *(more common)*
	  – Maxilla

Orbital	• Preseptal inflammatory edema of lids • Subperiosteal abscess • Orbital cellulitis • Orbital abscess • Superior orbital fissure syndrome
Intracranial	• Meningitis • Extradural abscess (M/c) • Subdural abscess (2nd M/c) • Brain abscess (M/c site-borstal lobe) • Cavernous sinus thrombosis
Descending infections	• Otitis media • Pharyngitis • Tonsillitis • Laryngitis

NEW PATTERN QUESTIONS

Q N13. M/C sinus involved in fungal ball:
 a. Maxillary b. Sphenoid
 c. Frontal   d. Ethmoid

Q N14. M/C sinus involved in allergic fungal rhinosinusitis:
 a. Maxillary b. Sphenoid
 c. Frontal   d. Ethmoid

ORBITAL COMPLICATIONS

- M/C complication of sinusitis
- Mostly seen in children

Point to Remember
➤ The orbital complication of sinusitis are mainly due to ethmoiditis.

- Patients complain of high fever, with pain in eye on the side of lesion, chemosis, proptosis and diplopia. Vision may be diminished.

Superior Orbital Fissure Syndrome

- Occurs subsequent to sphenoiditis.

Points to Remember
Features
➤ Deep orbital pain
➤ Frontal headache
➤ Progressive paralysis of III, IV and VI nerve (first nerve to get involved) cranial nerve.

Orbital Apex Syndrome

Superior orbital fissure syndrome with involvement of optic nerve and maxillary nerve.

Treatment

- Antibiotics, analgesics and nasal decongestants.
- Surgical decompression in case of visual loss.

CAVERNOUS SINUS THROMBOSIS

Usually results from infection of ethmoid and sphenoid sinuses.
- **Clinical features:**
  - *Onset is abrupt with fever chills and rigor*
  - Swelling of one eye initially followed by both eyes with in 12–24 hours
  - *Involvement of IIIrd, IVth, Vth and VIth cranial nerve* (1st nerve to be involved)
  - **Since 1st nerve involved is VIth nerve** hence it leads to paralysis of lateral rectus muscle, **i.e. lateral gaze palsy**. Later on complete ophthalmoplegia occurs due to involvement of other cranial nerves
  - *Chemosis of conjunctiva*

- **Proptosis**
  - Pupils are dilated and fixed (due to involvement of sympathetic plexus around carotid artery).
  - *Decreased vision* (due to optic nerve damage).
  - *Decreased sensation in distribution of Vth nerve (ophthalmic division)* and engorgement of retinal vessels.
- **Treatment:** Antibiotics in high doses for 4–6 weeks and drainage of involved sinus.

Note: Cavernous sinus thrombosis can be differentiated from other orbital complications as their is B/L involvement in cavernous sinus thrombosis and VIth nerve is first to be involved, whereas in orbital cellulitis cranial nerve III, IV and VI are concurrently involved.

OSTEOMYELITIS

Osteomyelitis is infection of the bone marrow.

Organism Causing
- Staphylococcus
- Streptococcus
- Anaerobes

Osteomyelitis of the Frontal Bone is Most Common as:
- It is a diploic bone and the lesion is essentially thrombophlebitis of diploic bone.
- It follows infection of frontal sinus.
- It is common in adults since this sinus is not developed in infants and children.

Clinical Features
- Fever, malaise, headache.
- Puffy swelling under the periosteum of frontal bone **(Pott's puffy tumor).**

Treatment
- Broad spectrum antibiotics for 4–6 weeks.
- Surgical drainage of the sinus through frontonasal duct.

Osteomyelitis of the Maxilla
More often in infants and children because of the presence of spongy bone in the anterior wall of the Maxilla.

DENTAL COMPLICATIONS
- Second premolar and the first molar are directly in relation to the floor of the Maxillary sinus.
  Therefore, acute sinusitis may produce dental pain.

SYSTEMIC COMPLICATIONS
- **Toxic shock syndrome:** Is rare, but potentially fatal.
  - **Organism:** *Staphylococcus aureus.*
  - **Symptoms:** Fever, hypotension, rash with desquamation and multisystem failure.

CHRONIC COMPLICATIONS

Mucoceles/Pyoceles

Definition
It is an epithelial-lined; mucus-containing sac completely filling the sinus. It occurs due to obstruction of the ostia of sinus and subsequent sinus infection or inflammation. Secretions are usually sterile and if it gets infected it forms a pyocele.

Features
- **Common in patients:** 40–70 years.
- Males = Females.

Point to Remember
- Sinuses affected in order of frequency: Frontal > ethmoid > maxillary > sphenoid.

Frontal Sinus Mucocele
- Presents as a firm, nontender swelling in superomedial quadrant of the orbit.
- Displacement of the eyeball—Forward, downward and lateral, i.e. proptosis.
- Dull, mild headache in frontal region.

Mucocele of Ethmoid
Presents as a retention cyst, pushing orbit forward and laterally.

Treatment
Frontoethmoidal Mucoceles: Radical frontoethmoidectomy using an external modified Lynch-Howarth's incision with free drainage of frontal sinus into the middle meatus. Some can be removed endoscopically.

NEW PATTERN QUESTIONS	
Q N15.	**Bilateral proptosis and bilateral 6th nerve palsy in seen is:**
	a. Cavernous sinus thrombosis
	b. Meaningitis
	c. Hydrocephalus
	d. Orbital cellulitis
Q N16.	**Orbital cellulitis most commonly occurs after which sinus infection?**
	a. Maxillary b. Frontal
	c. Ethmoidal d. Sphenoidal
Q N17.	**Which of the following is not a complication of sinusitis?**
	a. Cavernous sinus thrombosis
	b. Nasal furunculosis
	c. Preseptal cellulitis
	d. Osteomyelitis

SURGERIES FOR SINUSITIS

Indications of Nasal Endoscopic Surgery (FESS)

A. Nasal conditions:
Indian = **In**flammation of sinus (sinusitis - chronic and fungal)
Prime = **P**olyp removal
Munister = **Mu**cocelea of frontal and ethmoid sinus
Chan = **Ch**oanal atresia repair
Sepeak = **Se**ptoplasty
Foluent = **Fo**reign body removal
Epnglish = **Ep**istaxis

B. Other conditions
Note
Nose is related to orbit, anterior cranial fossa and pituitary. Hence FESS can be used in:
- **Orbital conditions**
  - Orbital decompression
  - Optic nerve decompression
  - Blow out of orbit
  - Drainage of periorbital abscess
  - Dacryocystorhinostomy
- CSF leak
- Pituitary surgery like trans-sphenoid hypophysectomy

FUNCTIONAL ENDOSCOPIC SINUS SURGERY (FESS)

It is the surgery of choice in most sinusitis. It uses nasal endoscopes of varying angulation (0°, 30°, 45°, 70°) to gain access to the outflow tracts and ostia of sinuses, employing atraumatic surgical techniques with mucosal preservation to improve sinus ventilation and mucociliary clearance.

 Note: A 0.4 mm Hopkins rod telescope is mostly used.

History
- The term functional endoscopic sinus surgery was introduced by David Kennedy
- Hirschmann attempted endoscopic examination of sinonasal cavity in 1901, but populated by Messer clinger 171978.
- Reichert performed first endoscopic sinus surgery with a 7 mm edoscope in 1910.

FESS is Based on 3 Principles
- Site of pathogenesis in sinusitis (OMC) is osteomeatal complex.
- Mucociliary clearance of the sinuses is always directed toward the natural ostium.
- The mucosal pathology in sinuses reverts back to normal once the sinus ventilation and mucociliary clearance is improved.

 Note: In FESS = Opening is made via middle meatus.

The Basic Steps of FESS (Messerklinger's Technique)

In FESS, the osteomeatal complex (OMC) is to be approached moving from anterior to posterior.

1. First step is removal of uncinate process (uncinectomy) using Blakesleyx forceps. By doing **uncinectomy**, the ethmoidal infundibulum gets exposed, hence it is called as **infundibulotomy**.
2. Next step is clearance of anterior ethmoid disease by exenteration of anterior and posterior ethmoidal cells **(i.e, anterior ethmoidectomy and posterior ethmoidectomy)** after removing bulla ethmoidalis.
3. This step is followed by **widening the ostea of maxillary sinus** (i.e. middle meatal antrostomy).

The endoscopic sinus surgery removes the cause of the disease process as well as treats the sinusitis by facilitating natural drainage of the sinus through its antism. It normalizes the mucosal changes by providing adequate ventilation, hence called as **functional endoscopic surgery**.

 Note: Another technique of FESS is when it is approached from posterior to anterior called as **Wigands technique**. This technique is useful in extensive polyps when surgical landmarks are not visible.

Contraindications
- Intracranial complications following acute sinusitis like meningitis, epidural abscess, etc.
- Involvement of lateral wall and floor of maxillary antrum.
- Pathology localized to lateral recesses of frontal sinus.

Complications of FESS

Major complications can be orbital (Periorbital ecchymosis, Emphysema, Optic nerve injury) and intracranial injury (CSF leak), carotid artery injury, injury to cranial nerves III, IV, V and VI.

Other complications include major hemorrhage from sphenopalatine and ethmoidal arteries, injury to nasolacrimal duct, rhinorrhea anosmia, and synechiae formation.

 Note: Optic nerve injury occurs in posterior ethmoidal and sphenoidal sinus surgeries, while carotid artery injury occurs in surgeries of the sphenoid sinus.

OTHER PROCEDURES TO APPROACH SINUS

CALDWELL-LUC'S SURGERY

The operation was described by George Caldwell of New York (1983) and Herry Luc of Paris (1897)

In this procedure *Maxillary antrum is entered through* an opening in its anterior wall by giving a *the sublabial incision through Canine fossa. After entering the maxillary antrum, the pathology is removed. Later on the antrum is connected to the nose through a nasoantral window made via the inferior meatus.*

Indications (Present)

- Foreign bodies in the antrum
- Dental cyst
- Oroantral fistula
- Fractures of maxilla
- As an approach to pterygopalatine fossa (maxillary artery ligation/Vidian neurectomy) and ethmoids (transantral ethmoidectomy).

Note: With advent of FESS, Caldwell-Luc is not done for sinusitis and polyp removal.

Can you Take Biopsy by this Approach in Maxillary Carcinoma?
Note: No. Biopsy via Caldwell-Luc's is a contraindication in malignancy maxilla as it leads to spread of the neoplasm to the cheek.

M/C Complication

- Facial swelling (M/C complication)
- Infra-orbital anesthesia/neuralgia due to traction on the nerve is the 2nd M/C complication.

Instruments used in Caldwell-Luc surgery

Tilley's Harpoon

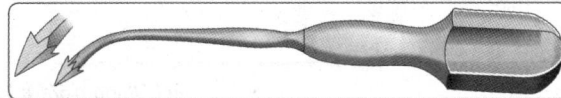

Fig. 20A.10: Tilley's harpoon

Tilly's antral burr: Used to enlarge and smoothen the hole made by harpoon in intranasal inferior meatal antrostomy, longer used now.

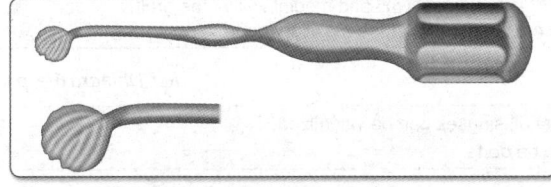

Fig. 20A.11: Tilley's antral burr

Luc's forceps: Used in Caldwell-Luc operation (to remove mucosa), submucosal resection (SMR) operation (to remove bone or cartilage) polypectomy (to grasp and avulse polyp) and to take biopsy from the nose or throat.

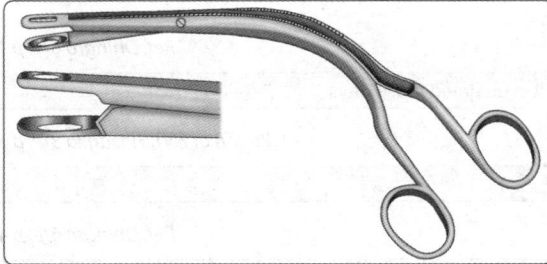

Fig. 20A.12: Luc's forceps

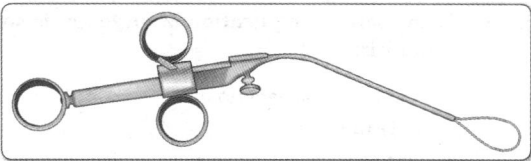

Fig. 20A.13: Krause nasal snare

> **Extra Edge**

> - **Lund-Mackay staging** is used in radiological assessment of chronic rhinosinusitis. The scoring is based on CT scan findings of the sinuses (Maxillary, frontal, sphenoid, arterior ethmoid and posterior ethmoid)
> - **Lund-Kennedy Endoscopic scores:**
>   In this staging system endoscopic appearance of nose is seen for:
>   1. Presence of polyp
>   2. Presence of discharge
>   3.. Presence of edema, scarring or adhesion and crusting.

NEW PATTERN QUESTIONS

Q N18. In Caldwell-Luc operation the nasoantral window is made through:
  a. Superior meatus
  b. Inferior meatus
  c. Middle meatus
  d. None of the above

Q N19. Commonest complication of Caldwell-Luc operations is:
  a. Oroantral fistula
  b. Infraorbital nerve injury
  c. Hemorrhage
  d. Orbital cellulitis

Q N20. Caldwell-Luc surgery approach is via.
  a. Hard palate
  b. Sublabial sulcus
  c. Inferior meatus
  d. Superior meatus

Q N21. Nerve injured in Caldwell-Luc surgery is:
  a. Lingual nerve
  b. Infraorbital nerve
  c. Optic nerve
  d. Facial nerve

Q N22. In functional endoscopic sinus surgery (FESS) opening is made through:
  a. Sphenoethmoidal recess
  b. Osteomeatal complex
  c. Inferior turbinate
  d. Middle turbinate

Section 2: Nose and Paranasal Sinuses

Q N23. Most feared complication of endoscopic sinus surgery is:
a. Retro-orbital hematoma
b. CSF rhinorrhea
c. Internal carotid injury
d. Nasolacrimal duct injury

Q N24. In nasal endoscopy, eustachian tube is examined at:
a. 1st pass
b. 2nd pass
c. 3rd pass
d. 4th pass

Q N25. Endoscopic surgery through intranasal approach is used for surgery of all organs except:
a. Lacrimal gland
b. Cerebellum
c. Pituitary gland
d. Optic nerve

Explanations and References to New Pattern Questions

N1. Ans. is a i.e. Maxillary sinus *Ref. Dhingra ENT 6/e, p 187*

Maxillary Sinus is called as Antrum of Highmore.

N2. Ans. is b i.e. Frontal *Ref. Dhingra ENT 6/e, p 189, TB of ENT, Hazarika 3/e, p 238*

Both sphenoid and Frontal sinus are absent at birth, but the last to develop is frontal sinus, hence we are taking it as correct option.

> **Remember**
> 1st sinus to develop: Maxillary sinus
> Last sinus to appear: Frontal sinus
> Sinus not present at birth: Frontal and sphenoid
> Well pneumatized sinus in infant: Ethmoidal sinus.

N3. Ans. is a i.e. Maxillary *Ref. Dhingra 6/e, p 187*

Maxillary sinus is the first sinus to develop after birth

N4. Ans. is b i.e. Frontal sinus *Ref. Dhingra 6/e, p 187*

- The superior most sinus is frontal sinus—as it is located between the inner and outer table of frontal bone, above and deep to supraorbital margin.
- This is followed by ethmoid sinus situated between the upper third of lateral nasal wall and medial wall of the orbit.
- Next is sphenoid sinus in the body of sphenoid and most inferior is maxillary sinus in the maxillary bone.

N5. Ans. is c i.e. Sphenoid sinus *Ref. Dhingra 6/e, p 433*

- Sphenoid sinus cannot be visualized with normal Water's view. Rest all sinuses can be visualized.
- To visualize sphenoid sinus—Water's view with mouth open should be done.

N6. Ans. is b i.e. Sphenoid sinus *Ref. Dhingra 6/e, p 434*

Sphenoid > post-ethmoid > maxillary sinus
This is the order of the sinuses, best seen in basal view.

N7. Ans. is d i.e. Caldwell-Luc view *Ref. Dhingra 6/e, p 434*

Best view for frontal sinus is Caldwell-Luc view

N8. Ans. is a i.e. External frontonasal ethmoidectomy. *Ref. Dhingra 6/e, p 196*

Howarth's or Lynch operation is external frontonasal ethmoidectomy. It is outdated these days.

N9. Ans. is b i.e. Inferior meatus *Ref. TB of ENT, Hazarika 3/e, p 311*

See text for explanation.

N10. Ans. is c i.e. Air embolism *Ref. Dhingra 6/e, p 409*

Air embolism is a rare, fatal complication of antral lavage (maxillary wash).

Chapter 20A: Diseases of Paranasal Sinus—Sinusitis

N11. Ans. is c i.e. Maxillary sinusitis   *Ref. Dhingra 6/e, p 408*

In antral puncture or proof puncture medial wall of maxillary sinus is punctured in the region of inferior meatus for antral lavage.

> Indications of proof puncture (Antral lavage)
> 1. Chronic and subacute maxillary sinusitis for confirming diagnosis and washing out pus.
> 2. To collect specimen in case of suspected malignancy.

N12. Ans. is b i.e. Approaching middle meatus   *Ref. TB of ENT Hazarika 3/e, p 332*

> Infundibulotomy—the uncinate process is removed to open the ethmoidal infundibulum. This is done to approach middle meatus.

N13. Ans. is a i.e. Maxillary

N14. Ans. is b i.e. Sphenoid   *Ref. www.ncbi library*

> M/C: – Sinus involved in fungal ball: – Maxillary sinus
> M/C: – Sinus involved in allergic fungal rhinosinusitis: – Sphenoid

N15. Ans. is a i.e. Cavernous sinus thrombosis   *Ref. Dhingra 6th/e, p 204*

Friends alway remember in cavernous sinus thrombosis there is bilateral orbital involvement whereas in orbital cellulitisit, it is unilateral.

Differences between orbital cellulitis and cavernous sinus thrombosis

	Orbital cellulitis	Cavernous sinus thrombosis
Source	Commonly ethmoid sinuses	Nose, sinuses, orbit, ear and pharynx
Onset end progress	Slow	Abrupt
Crania nerve involvement	Involved concurrently with complete ophthalmoplegia	Involved individually and progressively
Side	Usually involve affected side eye	Involves both eyes
Toxemia	Absent	Present
Fever	Present	High temperature with chills
Mortality	Less	Very high

N16. Ans. is c i.e. Ethmoidal

> Orbital cellulitis occurs most commonly after ethmoid sinusitis as the ethmoid is separated from the orbit by a thin papery bone, the lamina papyracea.

N17. Ans. is b i.e. Nasal furunculosis   *Ref. Dhingra 6/e, p 198 (Table 38.1)*

> See the text for explanation.

N18. Ans. is b i.e. Inferior meatus   *Ref. Dhingra 6/e, p 411*

N19. Ans. is b i.e. Infraorbital nerve injury   *Ref. Dhingra 6/e, p 411*

N20. Ans. is b i.e. Sublabial sulcus

N21. Ans. is b i.e. Infraorbital N

> See the text for explanation.

N22. Ans. is b i.e. Osteomeatal complex

> See the text for explanation.

N23. Ans. is c i.e. Internal carotid injury   *Ref. Operative Otolaryngology H/N Surgery 2/e, chap. 20*

> The most feared complication of FESS is internal carotid A injury. This is followed by orbital complications.

N24. Ans. is a i.e. 1st pass   *Ref. Dhingra 6/e, p 417*

Nasal endoscopy for diagnostic purpose—consists of passing a 4 mm 30° endoscope through three passes:
1. **1st pass—to examine through the nasopharynx**
    a. Opening of eustachian tube
    b. Walls of nasopharynx
    c. Upper surface of self palate and uvula
    d. Opening of eustachian tube of opposite side
2. **2nd pass—It is passed medial to middle turbinate to examine**
    a. Sphenoethmoid recess
    b. Superior meatus
    c. Opening of sphenoid sinus
    d. Posterior ethmoidal
3. **3rd pass**—Endoscopic is passed to middle meatus to visualize structures of middle meatus in detail.

N25. Ans. is b i.e. Cerebellum

As discussed in the text, FESS is endoscopic sinus surgery but is also used in case of surgery of orbit, anterior cranial fossa and pituitary gland as nose is related to these organs.

Chapter 20A: Diseases of Paranasal Sinus—Sinusitis

QUESTIONS

1. Which sinus is NOT a part of paranasal sinus? [MP 09]
   a. Frontal b. Ethmoid
   c. Sphenoid d. Pyriform
2. True about sphenoid sinus: [PGI May 2010]
   a. Lined by stratified squamous epithelium
   b. Duct open in middle meatus
   c. Open in sphenoethmoid recess
   d. Present at birth
   e. Present in greater wing of sphenoid
3. All are pneumatization patterns of sphenoid sinus except:
   a. Pre sellar b. Post sellar
   c. Concha bullosa d. Conchal
4. Sinus not present at birth is: [Maharashtra 02]
   a. Ethmoid b. Maxillary
   c. Sphenoid d. Frontal
5. Which facial sinus continues to grow even in adulthood?:
   [AIMS Nov 2017]
   a. Frontal b. Maxillary
   c. Ethmoid d. Sphenoid
6. True about ethmoidal sinus: [PGI Nov 2014]
   a. Fully developed by 25 yr
   b. Consists of 3–18 sinus on each side
   c. Absent at birth
   d. Lamina papyracea separate it from orbit
   e. Anterior ethmoidal group cells—open into superior meatus
7. Pain sensations from the ethmoidal sinus are carried by: [Ai 2011]
   a. Supraorbital nerve
   b. Lacrimal nerve
   c. Nasociliary nerve
   d. Infraorbital nerve
8. Maxillary sinus achieves maximum size at: [Manipal 06]
   a. At birth b. At primary dentition
   c. At secondary dentition d. At puberty
9. Which among the following sinuses is most commonly affected in a child? [PGI 99]
   a. Sphenoid b. Frontal
   c. Ethmoid d. Maxillary
10. In acute sinusitis, the sinus most often involved in children is: [UPSC 07]
    a. Maxillary b. Sphenoid
    c. Ethmoid d. Frontal
11. Sinus least involved in sinusitis is: [UP 08]
    a. Maxillary b. Ethmoid
    c. Frontal d. Sphenoid
12. Common organisms causing sinusitis: [AI 01]
    a. Pseudomonas
    b. Moraxella catarrhalis
    c. Streptococcus pneumoniae
    d. Staphylococcus epidermidis
    e. H. influenzae
13. Which of the following is the most common etiological agent in paranasal sinus mycoses? [AIIMS May 06]
    a. Aspergillus sp b. Histoplasma
    c. Conidiobolus coronatus d. Candida albicans
14. Which among the following is true regarding fungal sinusitis? [PGI 01]
    a. Surgery is required for treatment
    b. Most common organism is Aspergillus niger
    c. Amphoterecin B IV is used for invasive fungal sinusitis
    d. Hazy appearance on X-ray with radiopaque density
    e. Seen only in immunodeficient conditions
15. True about allergic fungal sinusitis: [PGI May 2015]
    a. Fungal hyphae is present in allergic mucin which is pathological hallmark
    b. Invasion of the sinus mucosa with fungus
    c. Allergic reaction to fungus
    d. Antifungal treatment lead to improvement of symptom
    e. Surgical clearance is mainstay of treatment
16. All of the following are diagnostic criteria of allergic fungal sinusitis (AFS) except: [AI 08]
    a. Areas of High attenuation on CT scan
    b. Orbital invasion
    c. Allergic eosinophilic mucin
    d. Type 1 Hypersensitivity
17. Periodicity is a characteristic feature in which sinus infection: [COMED 06]
    a. Maxillary sinus infection b. Frontal sinus infection
    c. Sphenoid sinus infection d. Ethmoid sinus infection
18. Sphenoid sinusitis pain is referred most commonly to: [AP 2005]
    a. Occiput b. Cost of nose
    c. Frontal d. Temporal region
19. Best view for frontal sinus: [AIIMS Nov 2010]
    a. Caldwell b. Towne
    c. Water's d. Lateral view
20. Caldwell view is done for [AIIMS 2011]
    a. Sphenoid sinus b. Maxillary sinus
    c. Ethmoid sinus d. Frontal sinus
21. For viewing superior orbital fissure-best view is: [AIIMS 97]
    a. Plain AP view b. Caldwell view
    c. Towne view d. Basal view
22. Complications of acute sinusitis: [PGI 03]
    a. Orbital cellulitis b. Pott's puffy tumor
    c. Conjunctival chemosis d. Subdural abscess
    e. Pyocele
23. Complication of sinus disease include: [AIIMS 93]
    a. Retrobulbar neuritis
    b. Orbital cellulitis
    c. Cavernous sinus thrombosis
    d. Superior orbital fissure syndrome
    e. All of the above

24. **Orbital cellulites is a complication of:** [MP 09]
    a. Parasinusitis
    b. Faciomaxillary trauma
    c. Endoscopic sinus surgery
    d. All of these

25. **Angular vein infection commonly causes thrombosis of:** [TN]
    a. Cavernous sinus
    b. Sphenoidal sinus
    c. Petrosal sinus
    d. Sigmoid sinus

26. **A patient with sinus infection develops chemosis, B/L proptosis and fever, the diagnosis goes in favor of:**
    a. Lateral sinus thrombosis [PGI 99]
    b. Frontal lobe abscess
    c. Cavernous sinus thrombosis
    d. Meningtitis

27. **Most definitive diagnosis of sinusitis is:** [AIIMS 92]
    a. X-ray PNS
    b. Proof puncture
    c. Sinoscopy
    d. Transillumination test

28. **Pathognomic feature of maxillary sinusitis is:** [UP 07]
    a. Mucopus in the middle meatus
    b. Inferior turbinate hypertrophy
    c. Purulent nasal discharge
    d. Atrophic sinusitis

29. **Frontal mucocele presents as:** [PGI 96]
    a. Swelling above medial canthus, below the floor of frontal sinus
    b. Swelling above eyebrow lateral to grabella
    c. External proptosis
    d. Intianasal swelling

30. **Mucocele is commonly seen in sinus:** [DNB 07]
    a. Frontal
    b. Maxillary
    c. Ethmoid
    d. Sphenoid

31. **Most common site for osteoma is:** [MP 08]
    a. Maxillary sinus
    b. Ethmoid sinus
    c. Frontal sinus
    d. Sphenoid sinus

32. **A 2-year-old child with purulent nasal discharge, fever and pain since 2 months. His fever is 102–103°C, and leucocyte count is 12000 cu/mm. X-ray PNS showed opacification of left ethmoidal air cells. The culture of the eye discharge was negative. Which of the following would be most useful further step in evaluation of this patient?** [AI 10]
    a. CT scan
    b. Urine culture
    c. Blood culture
    d. Repeat culture of the eye discharge

33. **A 24-year-old female with long standing history of sinusitis present with fevers, headache (recent origin) and personality changes; Fundus examination revealed papilledema. Most likely diagnosis is:**
    a. Frontal lobe abscess
    b. Meningitis
    c. Encephalitis
    d. Frontal bone osteomyelitis

34. **Cavernous sinus thrombosis following sinusitis results in all of the following signs except:** [PGI]
    a. Constricted pupil in response to light
    b. Engorgement of retinal veins upon ophthalmoscopic examination
    c. Ptosis of eyelid
    d. Ophthalmoplegia

35. **All are true about mucormycosis, except:** [PGI]
    a. Lymph invasion
    b. Angio invasion
    c. Long-term deferoxanine therepy
    d. Septate hyphae
    e. May lead to blindness

36. **The best surgical treatment for chronic maxillary sinusitis is:** [MP 02]
    a. Repeated antral washout
    b. Fiberoptic endoscopic sinus surgery
    c. Caldwell-Luc's operation
    d. Horgan's operation

37. **FESS means:** [Mahara 02]
    a. Factual endoscopic sinus surgey
    b. Functional endonasal sinus surgery
    c. Factual endonasal sinus surgery
    d. Functionl endoscopic sinus surgery

38. **Endoscopic nasal surgery is indicated in:** [Manipal 04]
    a. Chronic sinusitis
    b. Epistaxis
    c. Both
    d. None

39. **Indications of FESS:** [PGI Nov 2010]
    a. Inverted papilloma
    b. Orbital abscess
    c. Nasal polyposis
    d. Optic nerve decompression
    e. CSF rhinorrhea

Explanations and References

1. **Ans. is d i.e. Pyriform** *Ref. 6/e, p 187; TB of Mohan Bansal, p 37*
   Paranasal sinuses are air containing cavities in certain bones of skull. They are four on each side. Clinically, paranasal sinuses have been divided into two groups.

Anterior group	Posterior group
It includes:	**It includes:**
• Maxillary sinus	• Posterior ethmoidal sinus (opens in superior meatus)
• Frontal sinus	
• Anterior ethmoidal sinus	• Sphenoid sinus (opens in sphenoethmoidal recess)

    Note: All of Anterior group sinuses open in the middle meatus^Q

2. **Ans. is c i.e. Open in sphenoethmoid recess** *Ref. Dhingra 6/e, p 188*
   - All paranasal sinuses are lined by respiratory epithelium (**i.e. ciliated pseudo-stratified columnar epithilium**) **i.e. option a is incorrect**.

   Sphenoid sinus: Important points
   - It is not present at birth
   - It occupies the body of sphenoid
   - Ostrum of sphenoid sinus is situated in the upper part of anterior wall and drains into sphenoethmoidal recess.
   - On x ray: Sphenoid sinus is visible by 4 years of age.

3. **Ans. is c i.e. Concha bullosa (Read below)**
   Three types of sphenoid sinus pneumatization patterns have been found. Pneumatization patterns depend on the position of the sinus in relation to the sella turcica (over the body of sphenoid:)
   a. **Conchal**; no pneumatization occurs below the sella. There is a solid block of bone beneath the sella.
   b. **Pre sellar**; pneumatization does not extend beyond the anterior border of sella turcica.
   c. **Sellar/Post sellar**; In this case pneumatization occurs both below and posterior to the sella turcica. **This is the most common type of sphenoid pneumatization** seen among individuals

4. **Ans. is d i.e. Frontal** *Ref. Scott Brown 7/e, Vol 2, p 1320; TB of Mohan Bansal 1/e, p 39*
5. **Ans. is a i.e. Frontal**
   Development and grwoth of paranasal sinuses

Sinus	At birth	Adult size	Growth	Radiological appearance (age)
Maxillary	Present	15 years	Biphasic growth: Birth–3 years, 7–12 year	4–5 months
Ethmoid	Present	12 years	Size increases up to 12 years	1 year
Sphenoid	Absent	15 years	Reaches sella turcica (7 yrs), dorsum sellae (late teens), basisphenoid (adult)	6 years
Frontal	Absent	20 years	Invades frontal bone (2–4 yrs), size increases until teens	4 years

   Thus the last sinus to develop is frontal sinus and its pneumatization continues till adolescence

6. **Ans. b and d, i.e. Consists of 3-18 sinus on each side and lamina papyracea separate it from orbit** *Ref. BDC 4/e, Vol. III p 234*
   Ethmoidal sinus
   - Clinically, ethmoidal cells are divided into **anterior ethmoidal group which** opens **into the middle meatus** and posterior ethmoidal group, which opens into the superior meatus and sphenoethmoidal recess
   - Their number varies from 3 to 18
   - The thin paper like lamina of bone (**lamina papyracea**) **separating air cells from** the **orbit** can be easily destroyed leading to spread of ethmoidal infections into orbit
   - Ethmoidal sinus are present at birth & reach adult size by 12 years

7. **Ans. is c i.e. Nasociliary nerve**
   As discussed in preceding text, nasociliary nerve-branch of ophthalmic division of trigeminal nerve carries pain sensation from ethmoid sinus.

8. **Ans. is c i.e. At secondary dentition** *Ref. Maqbool 11/e, p 148; Turner 10/e, p 9*
   - Maxillary sinus is the first sinus to develop at birth.
   - It is completely developed by 9 years of age, i.e. approximately at the time of secondary dentition.

9. **Ans. is c i.e. Ethmoid**
10. **Ans. is c i.e. Ethmoid** *Ref. Tuli 1/e, p 190; Dhingra 6/e, p 193*

> Most common sinusitis in children is Ethmoid.
> Most common sinusitis in adults is Maxillary.

"Ethmoidal sinuses are well developed at birth, hence infants and children below 3 years of age are more likely to have acute ethmoiditis; but after this age, maxillary antral infections are more commonly seen." *Ref. Tuli 1/e, p 190*
"Ethmoid sinuses are more often involved in infants and young children." *Ref. Dhingra 6/e, p 193*

11. **Ans is d i.e. Sphenoid** *Ref. Dhingra 6/e, p 193; Turner 10/e, p 48*

"Isolated involvement of sphenoid sinus is rare. It is often a part of pansinusitis or is associated with infection of posterior ethmoidal sinus." *Ref. Dhingra 6/e, p 193*
"The sphenoid sinus is rarely affected on its own" *Ref. Turner 10/e, p 48*
The reason for sphenoid sinus to be least affected is that it opens high up in the sphenoethmoid recess which is not affected by most of the conditions of nose

In Nutshell remember:

> M/c sinus affected in adults—Maxillary
> M/c sinus affected in children—Ethmoid
> Sinus which is least affected—Sphenoid

12. **Ans. is c and e i.e. *Streptococcus pneumoniae*; and *H. influenzae***
Ref. Harrison 17/e, p 205; Scott Brown 7/e, Vol 2, p 1441; TB of Mohan Bansal, p 299

According to Harrison 17/e, p 205
"Among community-acquired cases, S. pneumoniae and nontypable Haemophilus influenzae are the most common pathogens, accounting for 50–60% of cases. Moraxella catarrhalis causes disease in a signigicant percentage (20%) of children but less often in adults. Other streptococcal species and Staphylococcus aureus cause only a small percentage of cases, although there is increasing concern about community strains of methicillin – resistant S. aureus (MRSA) as an emerging cause."

According to Nelson 18th/ed, pp 1749,1750
"The bacterial pathogens causing acute bacterial sinusitis in children and adolescents include Streptococcus pneumoniae (= 30%), nontypable Haemophilus influenzae (=20%)."

According to scotts Brown 7th/ed, p 1441
M/C Organism causing sinusitis in adults is also Streptococcus pneumoniae followed by H. influenza.
In children:
M/C is Streptococcus pneumoniae (30–43%) followed by both H. influenza and Moraxella catarrhalis (20–28% each)

13. **Ans. is a i.e. *Aspergillus sp*** *Ref. Maqbool 11/e, p 225; Scott Brown 7/e, Vol 1 and 2, p 1452; TB of Mohan Bansal, p 317*
Most common type of fungal infection of nose and paranasal sinuses are due to *Aspergillus*.
A. fumigatus > A. niger > A. flavus are the most frequent offenders.

14. **Ans. is a, c and e i.e. Surgery is required for treatment; Amphoterecin B IV is used for invasive fungal sinusitis; and Seen only in immunodeficient conditions** *Ref. Maqbool 11/e, p 225; Scott Brown 7/e, Vol 2, p 1455; TB of Mohan Bansal, p 317, 318*

Fungal Sinusitis

Most common cause: *Aspergillus*
Most common species: *A. fumigatus* (90%) > *A. niger* > *A. flavus*. *Ref. Maqbool 11/e, p 225*
Other offenders are: Mucor, Rhizopus, Alternaria
- **Fungal infection can be of following types:**
    i. Fungus ball
    ii. Allergic fungal rhinosinusitis
    iii. Chronic or indolent invasive fungal sinusitis
    iv. Acute fulminant fungal rhinosinusitis

Option – a – Surgery is required for treatment – (correct) as in all forms of fungal sinusitis – some or the other form of surgery is required.
Option – b – M/c organism is *Aspergillus niger*.
Incorrect – M/c is *A. fumigatus* (Maqbool 11/e, p 228)
Option – c – Amphotericin IV is used for invasive fungal sinusitis
Correct – *Ref. Dhingra 5/e, p 210, 6/e, p 196*
Option – d – Hazy appearance on X-ray with radiopaque density
Correct – Sinusitis gives hazy appearance on X-ray

Option – e – Seen only in immunodeficient condition
Incorrect – only the acute fulminant form is more common in immunodeficient state whereas others are seen in immnocompetent hosts.

15. **Ans. is a, c and e i.e. Fungal hyphae is present in allergic mucin which is pathological hallmark, Allergic reaction to fungus and Surgical clearance is mainstay of treatment.** *Ref. P.L. Dhingra 6/e, p 196; Logan Turner 10/e, pgs 51-52; Ballenger's Otorhinolaryngology 16/e, p 764,770*

Allergic Fungal Sinusitis
- It is an **allergic reaction** to the causative fungus and presents with sinunasal polyposis and mucin. The latter contains eosinophils, Charcot-Leyden crystals and fungal hyphae
- There is **no invasion of the sinus mucosa with fungus**
- Usually more than one sinus are involved on one or both sides
- CT scan shows **mucosal thickening with hyperdense areas**
- There may be expansion of the sinus or bone erosion due to pressure, **but no fungal invasion**
- Treatment is endoscopic surgical clearance of the sinuses with provision of drainage and ventilation. This is combined with pre and postoperative systemic steroids.

16. **Ans. is b i.e. Orbital invasion** *Ref. www.ncbi.nlm.nih.gov.*
Ref. Current Diagnosis and Treatment in Otorhinology 2/e, p 276; Scott Brown 7th/ed Vol 2, p 1452-1454; Ear Nose and Throat Histopathology 2/e, p 152; Patterson's Allergic Disease 6/e, p 778; Allergy and Immunology: An Otolaryngic Approach (2001), p 239

Bent and Kuhn Diagnostic Criteria

Major criteria	Minor criteria
1. Type I hypersensitivity	Asthma
2. Nasal polyposis	Unilateral disease
3. Characteristic CT findings	Bone erosion
4. Eosinophilic mucin without invasion	Fungal cultures
5. Positive fungal stain	Charcot Leyden crystals
	Serum eosinophilia

Note: Patients must meet all the major criteria for diagnosis. Minor criteria are to support the diagnosis, not for making the diagnosis. Bony erosion seen is due to expansive nature of the mucin and not caused by true fungal invasion. M/C bony erosions occur in orbit, followed by anterior, middle and posterior cranial fossa (Option b is also correct but then it is not a major diagnostic criteria).

17. **Ans. is b i.e. Frontal sinus infection** *Ref. Dhingra 6/e, p 192, 193*
Pain of frontal sinusitis shows **characteristic periodicity,** i.e. comes upon waking, gradually increases and reaches its peak by midday and then starts subsiding. It is also called *"office headache"* as it is present only during office hours.

18. **Ans. is a i.e. Occiput** *Ref. Dhingra Turner 10/e, p 35; Maqbool 11/e, p 208; Tuli 1/e, p 188*
- **Acute sphenoditis:** *'Headache – usually localized to the occiput or vertex. Pain may also be referred to the mastoid region.'*
Ref. Dhingra 6/e, p 194

Also Know

Sinus	Pain felt in area
Maxillary sinus	Along the infraorbital margin and referred to upper teeth or gums on affected side (along the distribution of superior orbital nerve) Pain is aggravated on stooping or coughing.
Frontal sinus	Pain localized over forehead. It has a characteristic periodicity
Ethmoid sinus	Pain localized over the nasal bridge, inner canthus and behind the ear.

19. **Ans. is a i.e Caldwell view**

20. **Ans is d i.e. Frontal sinus**
"Lateral view is best for the sphenoid sinus."
Caldwell view is the occipito frontal view. The frontal sinuses are seen clearly in this view.

View	Structure seen
• Waters view (with mouth open)	• All four sinuses
• Schuller's view	• Mastoid

View	Structure seen
• Towne's view	• Petrous pyramid
• Lateral view	• Sphenoid sinus

21. Ans. is b i.e. Caldwell view *Ref. Dhingra 6/e, p 434*
- Superior orbital fissure can be seen by caldwell view and water's view.

22. Ans. is a, b, c and d i.e. Orbital cellulitis; Pott's puffy tumor; Conjunctival chemosis; and Subdural abscess
Ref. Scotts Brown 7/e, Vol 2, p 1539,1540; TB of Mohan Bansal, p 305

Complications of Sinusitis—Acute Sinusitis

Local (due to local spread)	Systemic (due to hematogenous spread)

• **Frontal sinusitis** can cause
    – **Subperiosteal abscess**/or pott's puffy tumor
    – **Osteomyelitis**
• **Ethmoid sinusitis** can cause
    – **Orbital cellulites**
The stages of orbital cellulitis are:
    – **Preseptal cellulitis** (infection anterior to orbital septum)
    – **Postseptal cellulitis** or orbital cellulitis without abscess (i.e. infection posterior to orbital septum)
    – **Subperiosteal abscess** (pus collects beneath the periosteum)
    – **Orbital abscess** (pus collects in orbit)
    – **Cavernous sinus thrombosis**/abscess (includes chemosis)
• **Maxillary sinusitis** – no acute complications
• **Sphenoid sinusitis** can lead to
    – **Cavernous sinus thrombosis**
    – **Intracranial complications**
	• **Brain abscess** (can occur as a result of local spread as well hematogenous spread secondary to maxillary sinusitis associated with dental disease)
	• **Meningitis**
	• **Toxic shock syndrome**

Note:
1. Mucocele, Pyocele and pneumatocele are complications of Chronic Sinusitis
2. If infection in the frontal sinus spreads to the marrow of frontal bone, localized osteomyelitis with bone destruction can result in a doughy swelling of forehead, classically called as **'Pott's Puffy Tumor'**. Surgical drainage and debridement should be done in this case.

23. Ans. is e i.e. All of the above *Ref. Tuli 1/e, p 196; Scott Brown 7/e, Vol 2, p 1539,1540; TB of Mohan Bansal, p 305*

As Discussed in Previous Question:
- There is no confusion regarding orbital cellulitis, and cavernous sinus thrombosis being the complications of sinusitis.
- *Dhingra* does not mention Retrobulbar neuritis as one of the complications of sinusitis but according to. Posterior *Ref. Tuli 1st/ed, p 196* group of sinuses can lead to neuritis with impaired vision.

Complications of Posterior Group of Sinuses
- Superior orbital fissure syndrome/orbital apex syndrome.
- Cavernous sinus thrombosis.
- Neuritis with impaired vision.
- Oroantral fistula/sublabial fistula.

24. Ans. is d i.e. All of these *Ref. Scott Brown 7/e, Vol 2, p 1485; Parson Disease of Eye 20/e, p 457*
Orbital cellulitis can occur as a complication of sinusitis and injuries. As far as endoscopic sinus surgery is concerned, it can lead to orbital and intracranial complications so orbital cellulitis can occur in it also.

25. Ans. is a i.e. Cavernous sinus *Ref. Dhingra 6/e, p 201; TB of Mohan Bansal, p 307*

26. Ans. is c i.e. Cavernous sinus thrombosis
Angular vein which begins from medial angle of eye, continues as the facial vein. The facial vein communicates with the cavernous sinus through the deep facial vein and pterygoid plexus of veins.
B/L proptosis, fever and chemosis point towards cavernous sinus thrombosis.

27. Ans. is c i.e. Sinoscopy *Ref. Scott Brown 7/e, Vol 2, p 1442; Current Otolaryngology 2/e, p 277; Turner 10/e, p 43*
According to *Scott Brown's 7/e, Vol 2, p 1142—*

"There are many possible methods to make diagnosis of rhinosinusitis but there is much debate related to best method. It has become increasingly clear that the diagnosis of ABRS (acute bacterial rhinosinusitis) is best made on clinical grounds and criteria."
But this option is not given.
Scott Brown's further says:
"At this time, a maxillary sinus tap with cultures, revealing pathogenic organism remains the gold standard for the diagnosis of ABRS, although there is increasing interest in the role of endoscopic-guided middle meatal cultures, in lieu of maxillary sinus tap. It has even been suggested that endoscopically guided cultures may be a preferred culture technique to maxillary sinus taps, as they can identify patients with ethmoid infection."
Ref. Scott Brown 7/e, Vol 2, p 1442

> **Remember**
> - The 1st investigation to be done in chronic sinusitis is nasal endoscopy (to visualize the nasal mucosa, meatuses etc) If any pathology is found then NCCT of nose & PNS is done.
> - Best Investigation for chronic sinusitis – NCCT nose & PNS

28. **Ans. is a i.e. Mucopus in the middle meatus** *Ref. Dhingra 5/e, p 205*
    - **Characteristic finding of maxillary sinusitis on Rhinoscopy** is pus or mucopus in the middle meatus.
    - Mucosa and turbinates may appear red and swollen.

> **Remember**
> Dental infections are an important source of maxillary sinusitis.

29. **Ans. is a i.e. Swelling above medial canthus, below the floor of frontal sinus**

30. **Ans. is a i.e. Frontal** *Ref. Dhingra 6/e, p 198; Tuli 1/e, p 196; Scott Brown 7/e, Vol 2, p 1531*
    A **mucocele** is an epithelial lined, mucus containing sac completely filling the sinus and capable of expansion:
    - Mucocele are *most commonly* formed in Frontal sinus followed by ethmoid sinus and rarely in maxillary sinuses and sphenoid.
    - Mucocele of frontal sinus presents as a swelling in the floor of frontal sinus above the inner (medial) canthus. It displaces the eyeball forward, downward and laterally.
    IOC = CT scan
    TOC = Endoscopic sinus surgery

    ### According to Dhingra, 6th/ed p 198—
    - Least common sinus assopciated with Mucocele formation is sphenoid.
    - But Scott Brown 7th/ed Vol 2 p 1531 says:
      – Most of the cases of mucocele of sphenoid sinus are referred to neurosurgeons. Therefore, it seems it is less common but actually the sinus least involved by mucocele is maxilla.

31. **Ans. is c i.e. Frontal sinus** *Ref. Scott Brown 7/e, Vol 2, p 1521*
    - Craniofacial osteomas are benign tumors often originating in the paranasal sinuses
    - The frontal sinus is the most frequent location followed by the ethmoid, maxillary and sphenoid sinus, respectively
    - Age of presentation = second to fifth decade with a male–femate ratio – 3:1.
    - *Presentation:*
      – Generally they are an incidental finding on radiography
      – It may produce symptoms like –
      – Visual impairment
      – Intracranial neurological complications like meningitis or pneumocephalus with seizure.

    Management
    Removal by endoscopic sinus surgery.

32. **Ans. is a i.e. CT scan** *Ref. Dhingra 5/e, p 208-213*
    The child is presenting with fever and purulent nasal discharge with X-ray PNS showing opacification of ethmoidal sinus, i.e. probably the child is having chronic sinusitis (as it is present for the past 2 months) with an acute exacerbation. Now the most dreaded complication of ethmoidal sinusitis is orbital complication.
    "Orbital complication – most of the complications, follow infection of ethmoids as they are separated from the orbit only by a thin lamina of bone – lamina papyracea. Infection travels from these sinuses either by ostitis or a thrombophlebitic process of ethmoidal veins."
    Ref. Dhingra 5/e, p 213

    The best method to assess the status of ethmoidal air cells and its complications is CT scan.
    "CT is particularly useful in ethmoid and sphenoid sinus infections and has replaced studies with contrast material."
    Ref. Dhingra 5/e, p 209

33. **Ans. is a i.e. Frontal lobe abscess** *Ref. Read below*
    - Patient is presenting with fever, headache and personality changes which is typical of frontal lobe abscess (which is a complication of chronics sinusitis). In meningitis and encephalitis although patient presents with fever and headache, but personality changes are not seen.
    - Frontal bone osteomyelitis (Pott's puffy tumor) presents as doughy swelling on forehead.

34. **Ans. is a i.e. Constricted pupil in response to light** *Ref. Dhingra 5/e, p 214*
    Ptosis and ophthalmoplegia occur in cavernous sinus thrombosis due to involvement of III, IV and V cranial nerves. Retinal vessels are also engorged but pupils are fixed and dilated (not constricted), due to involvement of III nerve and sympathetic plexus.

35. **Ans. is b, c and d i.e. Angio invasion, Long-term deferoxamine therapy and Septate hyphae** *Ref. Current Otolaryngology 3/e, p 295*
    - Mucormycosis is caused by Rhizopus species, Rhizomucus and Absidia species.
    - Intitially, the disease runs a subtle course with only fever and rhinorrhea. Latter on, it invades the orbit and intracranial cavity with rapid loss of vision, meningitis, cavernous sinus thrombosis and multiple cranial nerve palsies.
    - It has marked predilection for vascular invasion leading to widespread thrombosis, tissue necrosis, and gangrene.
    - Characteristic nasal finding is a dark necrotic turbinate surrounded by pale mucosa blackish discharge and crusts.
    - M/C site is middle turbinate followed by middle meatus and septum.
    - Investigation of choice is MRI, while biopsy is confirmatory.
    Treatment: Includes amphotericin–B, heparin, hyperbaric oxygen, and debridement.

36. **Ans. is b i.e. Fiberoptic endoscopic sinus surgery** *Ref. Current Otolaryngology 2/e, p 279,280; Dhingra 5/e, p 205, 209*

Discussed in text

37. **Ans. is d i.e. Functional endoscopic sinus surgery**

38. **Ans. is c i.e. Both** *Ref. Dhingra 6/e, p 419; Head and Neck surgery, DeSouza, p 127; Scott Brown 7/e, Vol 2, p 1481*

39. **Ans. is All**

Indications of Functional Endoscopic Surgery (FESS)

A. **Nasal conditions:**
   Indian = **In**flammation of sinus (sinusitis - chronic and fungal)
   Prime = **P**olyp removal
   Minister = **Mu**cocelea of frontal and ethmoid sinus
   Can = **Cho**anal atresia repair
   Speak = **Se**ptoplasty
   Fluent = **F**oreign body removal
   English = **Ep**istaxis

B. **Other conditions:** Nose is related to orbit, anterior cranial fossa and pituitary. Hence FESS can be used in:
   - **Orbital conditions**
     – Orbital decompression
     – Optic nerve decompression
     – Blow out of orbit
     – Drainage of periorbital abscess
     – Dacryocystorhinostomy
   - CSF leak
   - Pituitary surgery like trans sphenoid hypophysectomy.

Chapter 20B

Diseases of Paranasal Sinus—Sinonasal Tumor

SINONASAL TUMOR

PREDISPOSING FACTORS

- Nickel with duration of exposure (approximately 18–36 years) predisposes to squamous cell carcinoma and anaplastic carcinoma.
- Hardwood and softwood predisposes to Adenocarcinoma of ethmoidal sinus.

Other Agents

- Hydrocarbons
- Mustard gas
- Radium dial workers: Soft tissue sarcoma
- Welding/soldering
- **Age at presentation:** 5th decade
- **Sex:** Male:Female = 2:1

1. M/C malignancy of nasal skin = Basal cell carcinoma
2. M/C benign tumor of nose = Capillary hemangioma (arises from nasal septum)
3. M/C benign tumor of paranasal sinus = Osteoma (M/C site frontal sinus)
4. M/C malignant tumor of a nose and PNS = Squamous cell carcinoma followed by adenocarcinoma.

Papilloma

- **Site:** Skin of the nasal vestibule and the anterior part of the septum.
- **Treatment:** Cautery/cryotherapy.

Inverted Papilloma/Transitional Cell Papilloma/Schneiderian Papilloma/Ringertz Tumor

- **Age:** 40–70 years (≈ 50 years)
- **Sex:** Male > Female
- **Site:** Lateral nasal wall in middle meatus rarely on the septum
- It is associated with *human papilloma virus*[Q]
- **Features:**
  - **It shows finger-like** epithelial invasions into the underlying stroma of the epithelium rather than on surface so-called as inverted papilloma
  - It is usually unilateral and is a locally aggressive tumor.
  - Patients complain of U/L nasal obstruction rhinorrhea and unilateral epistaxis
  - In 10–15% cases there may be associated squamous cell carcinoma (i.e. Premalignant condition).

- **Treatment:** Maxillectomy is the treatment of choice. It can be performed by lateral rhinotomy or sub labial degloving approach. These days endoscopic approach is preferred.
- They have a tendency to recur after surgical removal (as it is multicentric).

MALIGNANT TUMORS OF NOSE

Squamous Cell Carcinoma is the Most Common Histological Type of Tumor

- Also known as **nose pickers cancer**.
- **Site:** Lateral wall of nose is most commonly involved.
- Nasal cancer may be an extension from maxillary or ethmoid cancer.
- Metastasis is rare.
- **Age:** Seen in men > 50 years of age
- **Treatment:** Radiotherapy and surgery.

Malignant Melanoma

- **Age:** > 50 year
- **Gross:** Bluish-black polypoidal mass.
- **Most common site:** Anterior part of nasal septum
- **Treatment:** Wide surgical excision.

Olfactory Neuroblastoma (Esthesioneuroblastoma)

- Neuroendocrine tumor
- **Age:** Two peaks—one at 11–20 years and second one at 50–60 years
- It is M/C in females
- **Site:** Upper part (upper third) of the nasal cavity. It can spread intracranially; requires anterior craniofacial resection followed by RT/CT.

Adenoid Cystic Carcinoma

- **Site:** Antrum and Nose
- **On microscopic examination:** Swiss - cheese pattern is seen.
- Has a potential of perineural spread

Basal Cell Carcinoma

- Usually seen in middle age and above (40–80 years)
- M/C in Males.
- Main etiology is UV exposure.
- Usually seen above a line joining angle of mouth and ear lobule.
- Commonest site is inner canthus of eye.

- Commonest variety is Nodular (painless shiny nodule). Later it forms an ulcer with hard raised edges.
- **It is a locally infiltrating tumor which may erode surrounding tissue. Hence also known as *Rodent ulcer*.**
- No lymphatic/bloodstream spread.
- Diagnostic procedure of choice is Wedge biopsy.
- Treatment of choice is wide surgical excision.
- Chemotherapy in the form of topical 5% imiquimod, topical 5 fluorouracil is also being used.
- In patients > 60 years = Radiotherapy is the treatment.

Note—Moh's Surgery is being done in Basal Cell Cacrinoma

It involves sequential excision of the tumor under frozen section control with 100% evaluation of tumor margins. Specimens are evaluated on a horizontal basis (normal frozen sections give us only 10% tumor margin and specimen is evaluated on a vertical basis).

Moh's surgery is useful for basal cell carcinoma arising in difficult areas like inner canthus where wide excision may not be practical and for recurrent tumors. It has the best cure rate for basal cell carcinoma.

NEW PATTERN QUESTION

Q N1. Moh's surgery is done in:
a. Squamous cell CA of nose
b. Laryngeal cancer
c. Basal cell CA of nose
d. Dermoid cyst of nose

PARANASAL SINUS TUMOR

Benign Neoplasms

Osteoma

Most common benign slow growing tumor of paranasal sinus.
- **Most common sinus involved** is Frontal > Ethmoids > Maxillary sinus
- **Features**
  - Most of them are clinically silent
  - If close to the ostium, it can lead to formation of mucocele.
  - It can cause headache, diplopia

On X-ray and CT: Osteomas appears as dense mass and gives a **ground glass appearance.**

Treatment
- Excision
- Frontal and sphenoid osteomas are removed by external fronto-ethmoidectomy (**Lynch Howarth approach**).

Fibrous Dysplasia:
- It is a tumor like lesion of bone. Here the medullary bone is replaced by fibro-osseous tissue. The condition is self limiting and not encapsulated.
- Age- M/C is 5-15 years.
- M/C in females.
- No specific racial predilection.
- Presents as painless swelling of bone which can lead to cosmetic or functional disability.
- More common in maxilla than mandible.
- M/C site in maxilla is canine fossa area or zygomatic area.
- X-ray PNS and CT scan shows ground glass appearance.
- Mgt = Surgery.
- Radiotherapy is not done as it can promote malignant transformation.

Extra Edge

➤ McCune-Albright syndrome—is a combination of polyostotic fibrous dysplasia, skin hyperpigmentation and endocrine disease.

NEW PATTERN QUESTIONS

Q N2. M/C site of osteomas among paranasal sinuses is:
a. Maxillary   b. Frontal
c. Ethmoidal   d. Sphenoid

Q N3. M/C site for fibrous dysplasia is:
a. Maxillary   b. Frontal
c. Sphenoid   d. Ethmoid

Malignant Tumors of Paranasal Sinus

Etiology

Seen more commonly in people working in:
- **Hardwood furniture industry leads to adenocarcinoma of ethmoid and upper nasal cavity** (called as wood workers carcinoma)
- Nickel refining leads to squamous cell Ca and anaplastic carcinoma.
- Leather industry
- Manufacture of mustard gas

Note: While hardwood is a carcinogen for sinonasal adenocarcinoma, softwood exposure increases risk of squamous cell carcinoma.

Histology

- **80% are sqamous cell Ca^Q**
- **Others:** Adenocarcinoma, Adenoid cystic carcinoma, Melanoma and sarcomas
- **Site:** M/C Maxillary antrum followed by ethmoid sinus, frontal and sphenoid series
- **Age:** Seventh decade of life
- **Sex:** Male > Female
- **Symptoms:** Silent for longtime.

Early features	Late features depend on the spread
• Nasal stuffiness • U/L Epistaxis • Facial paraesthesia or pain • Epiphora • Dental pain leading to frequent change of dentures	• Medial – Nasal cavity, ethmoids • Anterior – Cheek • Inferior – alveolus leading to Malocclusion, loose teeth • Superior – Orbit leading to Diplopia, Proptosis loss of vision • Posterior – Pterygoid plates leading to tresmus Intracranial spread can also occur

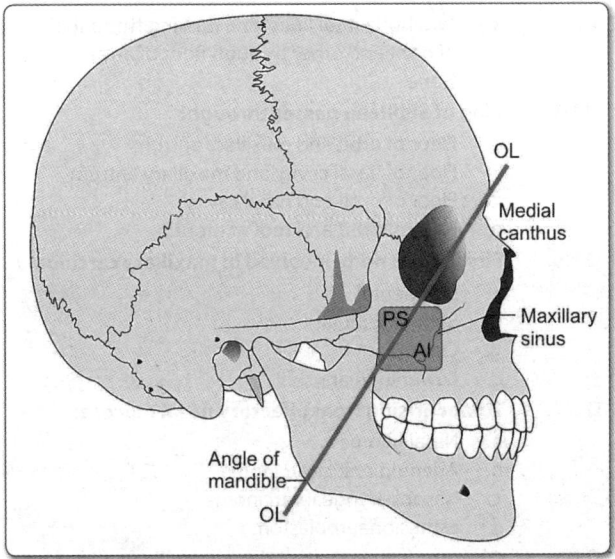

Fig. 20B.1: Ohngren's classification. Ohngren's line is an imaginary line (OL), which extends between medial canthus and the angle of mandible, divides the maxilla into two regions anteroinferior (AI) and posterosuperior (PS). AI growths are easy to manage and have better prognosis than PS tumors

Courtesy: Textbook of Diseases of Ear, Nose and Throat, Mohan Bansal, Jaypee Brothers Medical Publishers Pvt. Ltd., p 357

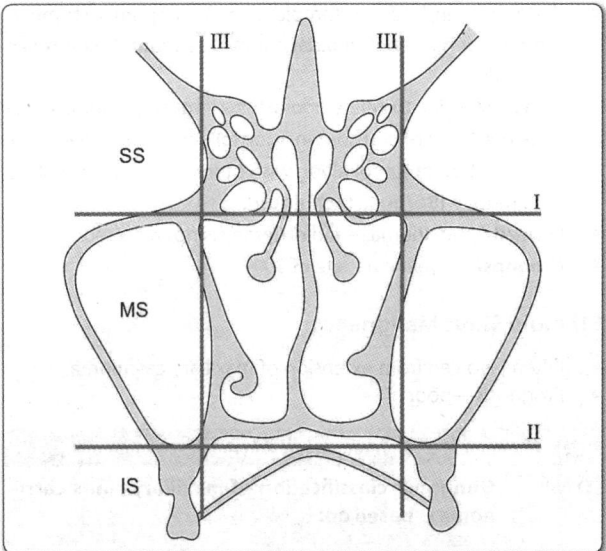

Fig. 20B.2: Lederman's classification. Two horizontal lines of Sebileau, one passing through the orbit floors (I) and other through antral floors (II), divide the area into three regions: Suprastructure (SS), mesostructure (MS), and Infrastructure (IS). The vertical line (III) at the plane of medial wall of orbit separates ethmoid sinuses and nasal fossa from the maxillary sinuses

Courtesy: Textbook of Diseases of Ear, Nose and Throat, Mohan Bansal, Jaypee Brothers Medical Publishers Pvt. Ltd., p 357

Lymphatic Spread

- Nodal metastases are uncommon
- Earliest metastasis occurs to Retropharyngeal lymph node
- Commonest LN involved is submandibular lymph node.

Diagnosis

- Biopsy
- CECT of Nose and PNS (Best investigation)

Classification

1. **Ohngren's classification:**
   - An imaginary plane drawn extending between medial canthus of eye and angle of mandible.
   - Growths above this plane have poorer prognosis than those below it (Fig. 20B.1).
2. **TNM Classification and Stage groupings of the paranasal sinuses. This classification is not important from PG Entrance point of view.**
3. **Lederman's classification (Fig. 20B.2):**

   Two horizontal 'lines of Sebileau' are drawn:
   One – Passing through floors of orbit
   Other – Through floor of antrum

Thus Dividing this Area into

- *Suprastructure* – ethmoid, sphenoid, frontal sinus
- *Mesostructure* – maxillary sinus and respiratory area of nose
- *Infrastructure* – alveolar process

Treatment

- For squamous cell carcinoma—surgery followed by radiotherapy.
- Surgery—Total or partial maxillectomy
- **Incision Used: Weber-Ferguson incision**

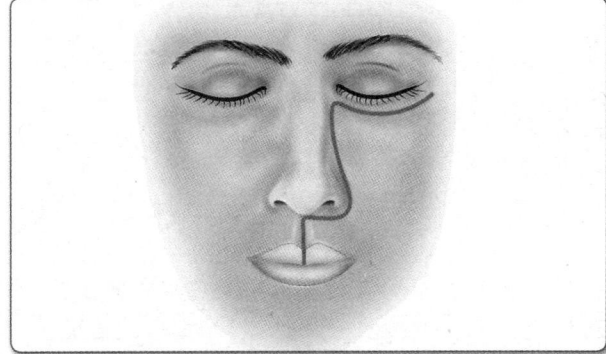

Fig. 20B.3: Weber-Ferguson's incision for maxillectomy starts at the upper lip philtrum on the operative side and goes up to the columella. It continues round the margin of the ala and up the lateral border of the nose. Near the medial canthus of eye it turns laterally in a rounded fashion to go 5 mm below the lower lid margin

Courtesy: Essential of ENT, Mohan Bansal
Jaypee Brothers Medical Publishers Pvt. Ltd., p 251

- If tumor extends to the ethmoid or in case of primary tumor of ethmoid or maxilloethmoidal complex; a **craniofacial resection** is done.
- Tumor extension to infratemporal fossa is managed surgically by extended Weber-Ferguson's incision followed by condylectomy and resection of tumor along with pterygoid plate and pterygoid muscle **(Barbosa technique)**.
- In small T_1 carcinomas – radiotherapy is not required.
- **Prognosis**: 5-year cure rate of 30%.

Ethmoid Sinus Malignancy

- Often involved from extension of maxillary carcinoma.
- Prognosis—poor

NEW PATTERN QUESTIONS

Q N4. Ohngren's classification of maxillary sinus carcinoma is based on:
   a. Imaginary plane between the medical canthus of eye and angle of mandible
   b. Imaginary plane between lateral canthus of eye and angle of mandible
   c. Two horizontal lines, one passing through floor of orbit and other through floor of antrum
   d. None

Q N5. Line of Sebileau passes through:
   a. Floor of orbit and maxillary antrum
   b. Floor of nasal cavity and maxillary antrum
   c. Floor of orbit and nasal cavity
   d. Floor of orbit and roof of mouth

Q N6. First lymph node involved in maxillary carcinoma:
   a. Submental
   b. Submandibular
   c. Clavicular
   d. Lower jugular

Q N7. Tumor arising from olfactory nasal mucosa:
   a. Nasal glioma
   b. Adenoid cystic carcinoma
   c. Nasopharyngeal carcinoma
   d. Esthesioneuroblastoma

Q N8. Ohngren's line that divides maxillary sinus into superolateral and inferomedial zone is related to:
   a. Maxillary sinusitis   b. Maxillary carcinoma
   c. Maxillary osteoma   d. Infratemporal carcinoma

Chapter 20B: Diseases of Paranasal Sinus—Sinonasal Tumor

Explanations and References to New Pattern Questions

N1. Ans. is c i.e. Basal cell CA of nose

See text for explanation.

N2. Ans. is b i.e. Frontal *Ref. TB of ENT, Hazarika 3/e, P 370*

M/C sinus to develop osteoma is frontal sinus
M/C sinus to develop malignancy is maxillary sinus
M/C sinus to develop mucocele is frontal sinus

N3. Ans. is a i.e. Maxillary *Ref. TB of ENT, Hazarika 3/e, P 371*

M/C bone involved is maxilla. The fibrous tissue can expand to fill the maxillary sinus also.

N4. Ans. is a i.e. Imaginary plane between the medial canthus of eye and angle of mandible

See text for explanation.

N5. Ans. is a i.e. Floor of orbit and maxillary antrum

See text for explanation.

N6. Ans. is b i.e. Submandibular *Ref. Dhingra 6/e, p 207*
In paranasal sinus tumors

- *Lymphatic spread:* Nodal metastases are uncommon and occur only in the late stages of disease. Submandibular and upper jugular nodes are enlarged. Maxillary and ethmoid sinuses drain primarily into retropharyngeal nodes, but these nodes are inaccessible to palpation.
- *Systemic metastases* are rare. May be seen in the lungs (most commonly) and occasionally in bone.
- *Intracranial spread* can occur through ethmoids, cribriform plate or foramen lacerum.

N7. Ans. is d i.e. Esthesioneuroblastoma *Ref. Dhingra 6/e, p 204*

Also called as olfactory placode tumor as it arises from olfactory epithelium in the upper third of nose. Bimodal peak of incidence at 10-20 and 50-60 years.

N8. Ans. is b i.e. Maxillary carcinoma

See text for explanation.

QUESTIONS

1. **Inverted papilloma arises from:** [AI 2006]
   a. Roof of nasal cavity   b. Medial wall of nose
   c. Lateral wall of nose   d. None
2. **Inverted papilloma:** [PGI 02; PGI Nov 09]
   a. Is common in children   b. Arises from lateral wall
   c. Always benign   d. Can be premalignant
   e. Causes epistaxis   f. Recurrence is rare
3. **True about inverted papilloma:** [PGI Dec 08]
   a. Arises mainly from nasal septum
   b. Common in children
   c. Risk of malignancy
   d. Postoperative radiotherapy useful
   e. Also known as Scheiderian papilloma
4. **Inverted papilloma is characterized by all *except*:**
   a. Also called as Schneiderian papilloma [MP 06]
   b. Seen more often in females
   c. Presents with epistaxis and nasal obstruction
   d. Originates from lateral wall of nose
5. **True about tumors of PNS and Nasal Ca:** [PGI Dec 06]
   a. Squamous cell Ca is the most common type
   b. Adenocarcinoma can occur
   c. Melanoma is most common
   d. Adenoid cystic Ca is most common
6. **Most common malignancy in maxillary antrum is:** [PGI 93]
   a. Mucoepidermoid Carcinoma
   b. Adeno cystic Ca
   c. Adenocarcinoma   d. Squamous cell Ca
7. **Wood workers are associated with sinus Ca:** [PGI Dec 06]
   a. Adeno Ca   b. Squamous cell Ca
   c. Anaplastic Ca   d. Melanoma
8. **Adenocarcinoma of ethmoid sinus occurs commonly in:** [PGI Dec 2006]
   a. Fire workers   b. Chimney workers
   c. Watch makers   d. Wood workers
9. **Early maxillary carcinom presents as:** [PGI 90]
   a. Bleeding per nose
   b. Supraclavicular lymph node
   c. Proptosis
   d. Nasal discharge
10. **Ca maxillary sinus stage III (T3 N0 M0), treatment of choice is/Ca maxillary sinus is treated by:**
    a. Radiotherapy   [TN 06; AP 05; AIIMS 01, AIIMS 97]
    b. Surgery + Radiotherapy
    c. Chemotherapy
    d. Chemotherapy + Surgery
11. **True about basal cell carcinoma:** [PGI 04]
    a. Equal incidence in male and female
    b. Commoner on the trunk
    c. Radiation is the only treatment
    d. Commonly metastasize
    e. Chemotherapy can be given
12. **Which of the following nasal tumors originates from the olfactory mucosa?** [AI 12]
    a. Neuroblastoma   b. Nasal glioma
    c. Esthesioneuroblastoma   d. Antrochoanal polyp
13. **Most common site for osteoma is:** [MP 2008, DNB 12]
    a. Maxillary sinus   b. Ethmoid sinus
    c. Frontal sinus   d. Sphenoid sinus
14. **Commonest site of Ivory osteoma:** [DPG 2006]
    a. Frontal-Ethmoidal region   b. Mandible
    c. Maxilla   d. Sphenoid
15. **Ground glass appearance of maxillary sinus on CT scan is seen on:** [DPG 2007]
    a. Maxillary sinusitis   b. Maxillary carcinoma
    c. Maxillary polyp   d. Maxillary fibrous dysplasia
16. **Identify the line marked on face in the picture below?** [AIIMS May 2017]
    a. Ohngren's line   b. Kasami line
    c. Frankfurt's line   d. Donaldson line

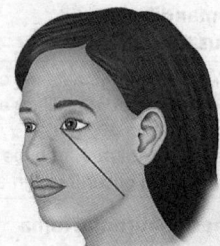
See Color Plate 16

17. **Which of the following is/are true about the T-stage of maxillary sinus carcinoma:** [PGI May 2017]
    a. Stage T4a- Frontal sinus involvement
    b. Stage T3- Ethmoid sinus involvement
    c. Stage T2- Sphenoid sinus involvement
    d. Stage T2- Bone of the posterior wall of maxillary sinus
18. **The patient came with an ulcer on the side of the nose as shown, which bleeds on itching. What is the diagnosis?**
    a. Squamous cells carcinoma   [AIIMS Nov 2017]
    b. Basal cell carcinoma
    c. Marjolin's ulcer
    d. Nevus

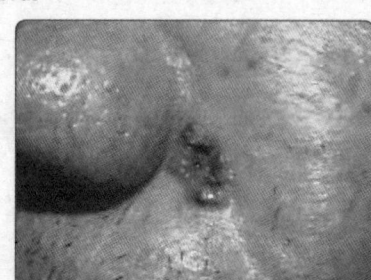
See Color Plate 17

Explanations and References

1. **Ans. is c i.e. Lateral wall of nose**
2. **Ans. is b, d and e i.e. Arises from lateral wall; Can be premalignant; and Causes epistaxis**
3. **Ans. is c and e i.e. Risk of malignancy; and Also known as Schneiderian papilloma**
4. **Ans. is b i.e. Seen more often in females**
   Ref. Dhingra 5/e, p 216; Turner 10/e, p 56; Current Otolaryngology 2/e, p 289, 6/e, p 202; TB of Mohan Bansal, p 354
   Read the text for explanation.
5. **Ans. is a and b i.e. Squamous cell Ca is the most common type; and Adenocarcinoma can occur** *Ref. Dhingra 6/e, p 205*
6. **Ans. is d i.e. Squamous cell Ca** *Ref. Dhingra 6/e, p 205*
   - More than 80% of the malignant tumors of paranasal sinus and of nose are of squamous cell variety. Rest are Adenocarcinoma, Adenoid cystic carcinoma, Melanoma and various types of sarcomas.
   - **Maxillary sinus is the most frequently involved sinus.** Other sites in decreasing order are nasal cavity, ethmoid sinuses, frontal and sphenoid sinus.
7. **Ans. is a i.e. Adeno Ca** *Ref. Dhingra 6/e, p 205*
8. **Ans. is d i.e. Wood workers**
   - Workers of furniture industry develop adenocarcinoma of the Ethmoids and upper nasal cavity. While those engaged in Nickel refining get squamous cell and Anaplastic carcinoma.
9. **Ans. is a and d i.e. Bleeding per nose; and Nasal discharge**
   Ref. Current Otolaryngology 3/e, p 312; Scott Brown 7/e Vol 2, p 2424; TB of Mohan Bansal, p 358
   Read the preceeding text for explanation.
10. **Ans. is b i.e. Surgery + Radiotherapy** *Ref. Dhingra 6/e, p 205; Current Otolaryngology 2/e, p 290; TB of Mohan Bansal, p 358*
    Read the preceeding text for explanation.
11. **Ans. is e i.e. Chemotherapy can be given** *Ref. Current Otolaryngology 3/e, p 238,239; Scott Brown 7/e, Vol 2, p 1705,1706*
    Read the preceeding text for explanation.
12. **Ans. is c i.e. Esthesioneuroblastoma** *Ref. Dhingra 6/e, p 204; Current Otolaryngology 3/e, p 313*

Esthesioneuroblastoma

Esthesioneuroblastoma (ENB), also known as olfactory neuroblastoma, is a rare neoplasm originating from olfactory neuroepithelium superior to middle turbinate. They are initially unilateral and can grow into the adjacent sinuses, contralateral nasal cavity and they can spread to orbit and brain. It can cause paraneoplastic syndrome by secreting vasoactive peptides. Since it can spread intracranially craniofacial resection is the surgery of choice. Combination therapy (Surgery + RT + CT) is used in management.

 Note: Contrary to other nasal malignancies it is M/C in females

13. **Ans. is c i.e. Frontal sinus** *Ref. Dhingra 6/e, p 205*
14. **Ans. is a i.e. Fronto-Ethmoid region**
    Ivory osteomas are most commonly seen in frontal sinus followed by ethmoid and maxillary sinus.
15. **Ans. is d i.e. Maxillary fibrous dysplasia** *Ref. Internet search*
16. **Ans. is a i.e. Ohngren's line** *Ref. Dhingra 6/e, p207*
    Ohngren's line extends from medial canthus of eye to angle of mandible. Growths anterior inferior to this plane (infra structural) have a better prognosis than those postero superior (supra structural)
17. **Ans. is a & b i.e. stage T_4a – frontal sinus involvement; stage T_3 - ethmoid sinus involvement**
    T staging of maxillary sinus carcinoma
    T_1 = Limited to maxillary sinus (No bone destruction or erosion)
    T_2 = Maxillary sinus involved + bone destruction extending to pterygoid plates
    T_3 = Maxillary sinus + ethmoid sinus involved
    T_4a = Maxillary sinus + sphenoid or frontal sinus involved
    T_4b = Tumor invades any of the following – orbit, brain, middle cranial fossa, cranial nerves, naso phaynx etc.

18. **Ans. is b i.e. Basal cell carcinoma**

    Basal cell carcinoma (BCC) is a slow-growing epithelial malignancy that arises from the basal layer of the epidermis it is invasive and locally destructive. BCC accounts for almost 80% of newly diagnosed malignancies in the United States and is the most common malignancy in humans around the world.

    Risk factors for BCC are similar to all nonmelanoma skin cancers, with excessive UV exposure the primary driving force.

    Clinically, BCC can be identified by its nodular, pearly opalescence and prominent telangiectasia. It has a raised, rolled border with central ulceration and may be pruritic. Some subtypes occur as a sacrlike lesion in an area that has nerver been injured or in an area of normal-appearing skin that repeatedly ulcerates and heals.

    Microscopically, BCC shows nests of uniform, extremely dark basaloid cells with oval nuclei and scarce cytoplasm. Distinct islands and cords of these cells often show a palisading border. **A picket fence"** arrangement of cells is common, similar to the basal layer of the skin.

    BCC almost universally arises in hair-bearing; skin and is dependent on the surrounding dermal stroma for growth.

SECTION 3

Oral Cavity

Section Outline

21. Oral Cavity

Chapter 21

Oral Cavity

ANATOMY OF NOSE

SUBMUCOUS FIBROSIS

- Chronic insidious process characterized by fibrosis in **submucosal layers of oral cavity**.
- Joshi in 1953 first described this condition in India.

Etiology

- **Prolonged local irritation:** Due to mechanical and chemical irritation caused by chewing betel nut, areca nut, tobacco, etc.
- **Dietary deficiency:** Vitamin A, Zinc and antioxidants.
- Localized collagen disease.
- **Racial:** Mainly affects Indians.
- In India it is *more common* in poor socioeconomic status.

Pathology

- Epithelial atrophy and submucosal fibroelastic transformation leading to trismus and difficulty in protruding the tongue.
- It is a premalignant condition.
- Leukoplakia and squamous cell carcinoma may be associated with it (malignant transformation = 3 to 7.6%).

Clinical Features

- *Most common* in ages between 20 and 40 years.
- Intolerance to spicy food.
- Soreness of mouth with constant burning sensation.
- Redness and repeated vesicular eruptions on palate and pillars.
- Difficulty in opening mouth fully and protruding the tongue.

> **Point to Remember**
>
> Blanching of mucosa over **soft palate**, **facial pillars** and **buccal mucosa** (the three most common sites for submucous fibrosis).

Treatment

Medical

- Avoid irritant factors.
- Treat anemia and vitamin deficiencies.
- Topical injection of steroids combined with hyalase.

Surgical

- Indicated in advanced cases to relieve trismus.
- Includes release of fibrosis followed by skin grafting or use of flaps.

TUMORS OF ORAL CAVITY

- Carcinoma of the oral cavity is overall the most common carcinoma in India in males
- Most common cancer of oral cavity in World: **Ca tongue (lateral border of the tongue).**
- Most common cancer of oral cavity in India: **Buccal mucosa (Lip) > Anterior tongue**
- *Most common* type of oral cancer: **Squamous cell carcinoma.**
  —*Bailey and Love 24th/ed p 704*
- 98% cancer of lip occurs in lower lip. Only 2% occur in upper lip
- In upper lip the M/C variety of cancer is basal cell carcinoma (not squamous cell carcinoma).

Etiology and Risk Factors for Tumor of Oral Cavity

> **Mnemonic**
>
> **6 (s)**
> - Smoking/tobacco chewing
> - Spirit (alcohol)
> - Sharp jagged tooth and ill-fitting dentures
> - Sepsis
> - Syndrome of Plummer-Vinson (iron deficiency anemia)
> - Syphilitic glossitis

- **Premalignant conditions**
  - Leukoplakia (most common)
  - Erythroplakia (maximum risk)
  - Chronic hyperplastic candidiasis
- **Conditions increasing risk**
  - Oral submucosa fibrosis
  - Syphilitic glossitis
  - Sideropenic dysphagia
- **Risk is doubtful**
  - Oral lichen planus
  - Discoid lupus erythematosus
  - Dyskeratosis congenita.

Points to Remember

Oral cavity cancer with
- Best prognosis: Ca lip
- Worst prognosis: Ca floor of mouth
- Highest incidence of lymph node metastasis: Ca tongue followed by Ca floor of mouth
- Sunlight exposure as predisposing factor: Ca lip

LN metastasis is most common in: CA tongue > floor of mouth > Lower alveolus ≥ Buccal mucosa > upper alveolus > Hard palate.

Extra Edge
- Verrucous CA (Ackerman's tumor) is a less virulent form of squamous cell CA thought to be caused by HPV.

Investigation
- Edge biopsy is recommended for diagnosis in all cases.
- Fine-needle aspiration cytology (FNAC) is done for lump in neck especially suspicious lymph nodes.
- Magnetic resonance imaging (MRI), when available, is investigation of choice, for staging of head and neck malignancies.

NEW PATTERN QUESTIONS	
Q N1.	Areas of carcinoma of oral mucosa can be identified by Staining with:
	a. 1% zinc chloride
	b. 2% silver nitrate
	c. Gentian violet
	d. 2% toluidine blue
Q N2.	The most common site of oral cancer among Indian population is:
	a. Tongue
	b. Floor of mouth
	c. Alveobuccal complex
	d. Lip

Staging

Irrespective of site same staging is recommended for all oral cavity tumors.

T Stage	CSDT 11/e, p 286
T1	Tumor ≤ 2 cm
T2	Tumor more than 2 cm but less than 4 cm
T3	Tumor more than 4 cm
T4	Tumor invades adjacent structures like lateral pterygoid muscle
N Stage	
N0	No regional lymph node metastasis

Contd...

Contd...

N1	Metastasis in a **single ipsilateral node, 3 cm** or less in size.
N2	*Metastasis in*
N2a	**Single ipsilateral lymph node 3 to 6 cm** in size
N2b	**Multiple ipsilateral** lymph nodes, none more than **6 cm** in greatest dimension
N2c	**Bilateral or contralateral lymph nodes**, none more than **6 cm** in greatest dimension
N3	**Metastasis in a lymph node** more than **6 cm** in greatest dimension
M Stage	
M0	No distant metastasis
M1	Distant metastasis

Most common site for

Carcinoma	Most common site
Lip carcinoma	Vermilion of lower lip
Tongue carcinoma	Lateral border
Cheek carcinoma	Angle of mouth
Larynx carcinoma	Glottis
Nasopharynx carcinoma	Fossa of Rosenmuller
Ranula	Floor of mouth beneath the tongue
Epulis	Root of teeth

Treatment

(Ref. Current Otolaryngology 3/e, p 380 onward

Squamous cell cancers of oral cavity are primarily treated surgically, while those of oropharynx are primarily treated with radiotherapy.

Carcinoma Lip
- **M/C site** of CA lip: **Vermillion of lower lip**^{Q}
- Typically seen in **males of 40–70 years**^{Q}
- There is definite correlation between **CA lip** and **exposure to sunlight** (UV radiations^Q)
- **M/C presentation: Non-healing** ulcer or growth^Q
- LN metastasis is **rare** and **develops late,** mainly to **submental** and **submandibular** LNs^Q
- **Bilateral lymphatic spread** is seen in **CA lower lip**^{Q}

Treatment of Carcinoma Lip^Q	
T1 and T2	• Surgery is TOC^Q (excision and repair)
	– If 1/3rd or less of lip is involved: 'V' or 'W' shaped **full thickness** excision with lateral margin of 5 mm + **Primary closure**^{Q}
	– If more than 1/3rd of lip is involved: Flap reconstruction (**Abbe Estlander's** flap or Gilles flap)
	• **Radiotherapy** can also be done
T3 and T4	Combined **radiation** and **surgery**^{Q} (exicision and neck dissection)

Prognosis
- CA lip has the best prognosis^Q in CA oral cavity.

Note:
- When 1/3 to 2/3 of lip is involved-Abbe Estlander flap is best
- When > 2/3 of lip involved-Gilles flap is best

Chapter 21: Oral Cavity

NEW PATTERN QUESTIONS

Q N3. Abbe-Estlander flap is used for:
a. Lip
b. Tongue
c. Eyelid
d. Ears

Q N4. Abbe-Estlander flap is based on:
a. Lingual artery
b. Facial artery
c. Labial artery
d. Internal maxillary artery

Q N5. Stain used to detect premalignant lesion of lip is:
a. Crystal violet
b. Giemsa
c. Toluidine blue
d. Silver nitrate

CARCINOMA BUCCAL MUCOSA (CHEEK)

- **M/C site of CA oral cavity in India: Buccal mucosa**[Q]
- Related to chewing a combination of **tobacco mixed with betel leaves, areca nut** and **lime sheel**[Q]
- Most malignant tumors are **low grade SCC**[Q]
- Frequently appearing on background of leukoplakia
- **Lymphatic spread** is first to **level** I and II **LNs**[Q].

Clinical Features
- **Pain is minimal,** obstruction of Stenson's duct can lead to parotid enlargement.

Treatment
- **T1: Excision** with primary closure[Q]
- **T2: Surgery ± Radiotherapy**[Q]
- **T3: and T4: Surgery + Radiotherapy or chemoradiation**[Q]

NEW PATTERN QUESTIONS

Q N6. M/C site of metastasis of CA of buccal mucosa is:
a. Regional lymph nodes
b. Liver
c. Brain
d. Heart

Q N7. In the reconstruction following excision of previously irradiated cheek, the flap will be:
a. Tongue
b. Cervical
c. Forehead
d. Pectoralis major myocutaneous

CARCINOMA TONGUE

- **M/C site** is **middle of lateral** border[Q] or ventral aspect of the tongue
- **M/C histological type** is squamous cell carcinoma[Q].

- **M/C associated risk factors** are tobacco and alcohol[Q].
- **M/C variety** is **ulcerative**[Q].
- **30% patients** presents with **cervical node metastasis**[Q]. M/C = **superior deep Jugular nodes**
- Presents as **painless mass** or **ulcer** that **fails to heal** after minor trauma[Q]
- **M/C site: Lateral border** of the **junction of middle** and **posterior third**[Q].
- **Primary site** for **cervical metastasis** is **superior deep jugular nodes (Level II)**[Q].
- For diagnosis, **wedge biopsy** is taken from the edge of ulcer but in **proliferative growth, punch biopsy** is taken[Q].
- Tongue has a rich lymphatic drainage, hence in all stages of cancer tongue concurrent treatment to neck nodes should be given.

Treatment of Carcinoma Oral Tongue–Lateral border

T1	**Partial glossectomy** with primary closure[Q] or **Brachy therapy (Interstitial irradiation)**
T2	**Hemiglossectomy** for **small well-circumscribed** and **well differentiated lesion**[Q]
	Radiotherapy – external beam RT. for large, poorly differentiated lesion[Q]
T3	**Total glossectomy** followed by **radiation**[Q]
T4	**Surgery** (Total glossectomy, mandibulectomy, laryngectomy) + Postoperative radiation[Q]

Management of Recurrence

- **Most recurrences** occur within **2 years.**
- **Radiation failure** is managed by **glossectomy**[Q].
- **Surgical failure** is managed by **radiation**[Q].
- If recurrence is **limited to mucosa,** it is best managed by **surgery**
- If recurrence is in the **soft tissue** of the **neck, palliation** is indicated.

Carcinoma of posterior third or base of tongue

- **Remains asymptomatic for long** time and patient **present with metastasis in cervical nodes**[Q].
- **First node involved** is **superior deep jugular nodes (Level II),** spread is then along the jugular chain to the mid-jugular (Level III and lower jugular (Level IV)[Q].

Clinical Features
- Early symptoms: Sore throat, feeling of lump in throat, and slight discomfort on swallowing
- Because many **lesions** are **silent,** level III neck mass is often the **first sign**[Q].

Note:
- Management – For all stages Chemoradiation.

NEW PATTERN QUESTIONS

Q N8. Commando's operation is for:
a. Mandible
b. Oral Cancer
c. Maxillary CA
d. Nasal CA

Q N9. M/C site for cancer of tongue is:
  a. Lateral border
  b. Dorsum
  c. Posterior 1/3
  d. Tip of tongue

NEW PATTERN QUESTION

Q N10. Orodental fistula is most common after extraction of:
  a. 2nd incisor   b. 1st premolar
  c. 2nd premolar   d. 1st molar

■ DENTIGEROUS (FOLLICULAR CYST)

- Dentigerous is a cyst which envelops the whole or part of the crown of the unerupted **permanent tooth.**
- **Seen in:** 3rd – 4th decade.
- **Most common site: Mandibular 3rd molar tooth**
- **Most common type: Central type,** i.e. the cyst surrounds the crown of the tooth
- **Cyst lining:** Non-keratinizing stratified squamous epithelium. The fluid inside is cholesterol rich
- **Radiography:** Unilocular cyst or soap bubble appearance
- **Treatment:** Enucleation with the removal of the associated tooth.

■ DENTAL CYST

- Dental cyst (radicular cyst, periodontal cyst) are inflammatory cysts which occur as a result of pulp death i.e. caries. Especially in the permanent tooth.
- It is the most common cystic lesion in the jaw
- **Peak incidence:** - 4th decade
- 60% found in the maxilla
- **Egg-shell crackling:** May be elicitable due to cortical thinning
- **Content:** Straw-colored fluid, rich in cholesterol
- **Radiograph:** The cysts are round/ovoid radiolucencies with sclerotic margin is a normally erupted toots.

■ SIALOLITHIASIS (STONE IN SALIVARY GLAND)

- 80–90% of calculi develop in Wharton's duct of submandibular gland. Stenson's duct of parotid constitutes 10–20% and sublingual only 1%.
- 80% submandibular stones are radiopaque while parotid stones are radiolucent.
- **Treatment:** It depends on site:
  – If stone is lying within the submandibular duct; anterior to the crossing of lingual nerve, stone can be removed by longitudinal incison over the duct. Duct should be left open.
  – If stone is distal to lingual nerve, it should be treated with simultaneous excision of submandibular gland.
- Parotid stones are removed surgically by exposing the duct and stone is released.

■ SALIVARY GLAND TUMORS (TABLE 21.1)

- Major salivary gland tumor are mostly benign.
- Minor salivary gland tumor are mostly malignant.
- In children >50% salivary gland tumors are malignant.
- *Most common* tumor of major salivary glands/most common benign salivary gland tumor—pleomorphic adenoma.
- *Most common* malignant tumor of major salivary glands – Mucoepidermoid carcinoma.
- *Most common* malignant tumor of minor salivary galnds – Adenoid cystic carcinoma.

Table 21.1: Summary of salivary gland tumor

Tumor type	Most common site	Important feature	Management
Pleomorphic adenoma (Mixed Tumor)	Parotid gland tail (superficial lobe)	• M/C benign salivary gland tumor^Q • M/C tumor of major salivary gland^Q • Affects women around 40 years^Q • In pleomorphic adenoma of sub-mandibular gland M/C age affected is 60 yrs^Q • 80% of parotid pleomorphic adenomas arise in superficial lobe^Q • Encapsulated but sends pseudopods into surrounding glands (so enucleation is not done as treatment) • Malignant transformation occurs in 3–5% of cases • Facial nerve infiltration indicates carcinomatous change	• Superficial parotidectomy **(Patey's operation)**
Warthin's tumor/ Adenolymphoma	Parotid gland exclusively (M/c site being lower part of parotid overlying angle of mandible)	• It is the second M/C benign tumor of salivary glands • Can also arise from cervical nodes • Smoking its risk • It never involves facial nerve • It shows hot spot in 99Tcm scan which is diagnostic	• Superficial parotidectomy

Contd...

Chapter 21: Oral Cavity

Contd...

Tumor type	Most common site	Important feature	Management
Adenoid cystic minor salivary gland carcinoma (Cylindroma)	Minor salivary gland	• It is the only salivary gland tumor which is more common in men • M/C cancer of minor salivary gland followed by adenocarcinoma and mucoepidermoid carcinoma • Invades perineural space and lymphatics • M/C head and neck cancer associated with perineural invasion • Unlike other salivary gland tumors it is more radiosenstive	• Radical parotidectomy followed by postoperative radiotherapy if margins are positive
Mucoepidermoid carcinoma	Parotid gland	• M/C malignant salivary gland tumor in children • M/C malignant tumor of parotid • M/C **radiation induced** neoplasm of salivary gland carcinoma • Consists of mixture of squamous cells, mucous-secreting cells, intermediate cells and clear or hydropic cells • Mucin producing tumor is low-grade type; squamous cell T/m is high grade type	• Superficial/Total parotidectomy + radical neck dissection
Acinic cell adeno carcinoma	Exclusively parotid gland affecting women mostly	• Rare tumor with low-grade malignancy • Tends to involve the regional lymph nodes	• Treatment is radical excision • Only tumor which responds to radiotherapy so, irradiation
Squamous cell carcinoma therapy is useful	Submandibular gland	• Arises from squamous metaplasia of the lining epithelium of the ducts	

- *Most common* site of minor salivary glands tumor – Hard palate.
- *Malignancy varies inversely* with the *size of gland* (90% of minor salivary gland tumors are malignant).
- All salivary gland tumors are mostly present in parotid gland except adenoid cystic carcinoma which is seen most commonly in minor salivary glands and squamous cell carcinoma which is seen most commonly submandibular gland.
- *Most common Benign tumor/overall tumor of salivary glands in children is* hemangioma — *Scott'-Brown's 7th/ed*
- *Most common* malignant salivary gland tumor in children – Mucoepidermoid — *vol 1, p 1248*
- 2nd *most common* malignant tumor in children—Acinic cell cancer.
- For most tumor types there is a slight female preponderance
- Most common etiological agent for salivary gland tumor is exposure to radiation
- Most salivary gland tumors are insidious in onset and grow slowly. Pain is extremely uncommon
- ***Most helpful*** imaging technique for salivary gland tumor are contrast enhanced computed tomography (CT) and Gadolinium MRI (is preferred)
- ***Open surgical biopsy is contraindicated*** in salivary gland tumors as it seeds the tumor to the surrouding tissue.
- ***Investigation of choice*** for salivary gland swellings – FNAC. as MRI cannot distinguish between benign and malignant lesions
- Treatment is exicision not enucleation as tumor has microscopic extensions outside the capsule.
- Majority of salivary gland tumors are radioresistant.

NEW PATTERN QUESTIONS

Q N11. Parasympathetic fibers of the sublingual salivary gland are found in:
   a. Facial N   b. Glossopharyngeal N
   c. Vagus N   d. Hypoglossal N

Q N12. Perineural invasion is seen in:
   a. Adeno CA
   b. Adenoid cystic carcinoma
   c. Basal cell carcinoma
   d. Squamous cell CA

Q N13. Percentage of submaxillary calculi that can be visualized by X-ray:
   a. 20%   b. 50%
   c. 60%   d. 80%
   e. 100%

CERVICAL SWELLING

Midline swelling of neck (from above downward) is k/a cervical swelling

Mnemonic

Lymph	**L**udwig's angina
Node	**E**nlarged submental lymph nodes
Sublingual	**S**ublingual dermoid
Likes	**L**ipoma
The	**T**hyroglossal cyst
Sweet	**S**ubhyoid bursitis
Girl	**G**oiter
Living (in)	**L**ipoma
Retro	**R**etrosternal goiter
Thymus	**T**hymic swelling

Mnemonic
(Though a little weird but is very helpful) Lymph Nodes Sublingual Likes The Sweet Girl Living (in) Retro Thymus.

BRANCHIAL CYST AND BRANCHIAL FISTULA

- Remnants of the brachial apparatus, present in fetal life
- Branchial cysts are characteristically found anterior and deep to the upper third of the sternocleidomastoid muscle.
- Branchial fistulas are those derived from 2nd branchial cleft and open externally in the lower third of neck, near the anterior border of sternocleidomastoid. Its internal orifice is located in the tonsillar fossa.

Features

- Cysts and sinuses are lined by **stratified squamous epithelium.**
- **Content:** Straw-colored fluid rich in cholesterol.
- **Branchial cysts:** Present in the third decade.
- **Branchial sinus:** Present since birth.
- **Male:** Female = 3:2.
- 60% of them are present on left side.

> - Sites of occurrence of the cyst:
>   – Upper neck (most common)
>   – Lower neck
>   – Parotid gland
>   – Pharynx and posterior triangle

Treatment
Excision of the cyst and fistula.

THYROGLOSSAL CYST

It is a cystic swelling which arises from the remnant of thyroglossal duct.

Development of Thyroglossal Cyst (Fig. 21.1)

- Thyroglossal tract passes down from foramen cecum of the tongue between genioglossi muscle in front, passing behind the hyoid bone to the upper border of thyroid cartilage ultimately ending in the pyramidal lobe of thyroid gland.

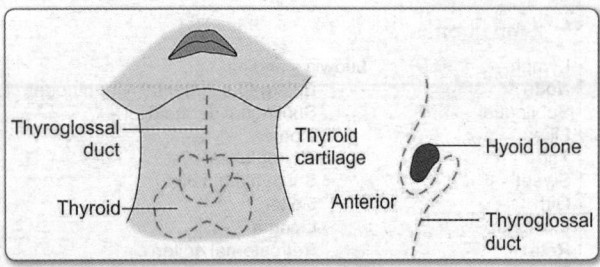

Fig. 21.1: Sites of thyroglossal duct cyst

- Normally this tract disappears by the 5th – 10th week except in the lower part forming isthmus of thyroid.
- Sometimes, a part of it may remain patent giving rise to a cystic swelling due to retention of secretions resulting in thyroglossal cyst.
- **Epithelial lining:** Pseudostratified ciliated/columnar squamous.
- **Importance:** Squamous carcinoma may arises in the cyst.

Clinical Features

- **Age:** Although congenital can be seen at any age from birth up to 70 years. (Mostly present between 15 and 30 years).
- **Position:** Midline in 90% cases.
  In 10% cases, it occurs an one side in which 95% are on left side and 5% on right side.
- **Clinically:** Swelling moves sideways only. On protruding the tongue or on deglutition—it moves upward.

Treatment

Sistrunk's operation (stepladder surgery) in which tract is completely excised along with middle of hyoid bone.

Note:
- If body of hyoid is *not* removed recurrence occurs in 85% cases.
- Recurrence after removal of hyoid = 2–8%
- In cases of infected thyroglossal cyst: abscess should be incised and drained.
- After complete subsidence of inflammatory reaction (approximately 6 weeks) thyroglossal cyst and its epithelial tract should be excised
- Carcinoma arising in the thyroglossal cyst are:
  – Papillary adenocarcinoma (85%)
  – Follicular adenocarcinoma (15%)
  – Adenocarcinoma
  – Squamous carcinoma

Differences between Thyroglossal Cyst and Thyroglossal Fistula

Thyroglossal cyst	Thyroglossal fistula
Congenital	Never congenital, always acquired following infection/inadequate cyst removal
Present anywhere along thyroglossal tract	
Most common site subhyoid	Median fistula of neck
Moves upward on protrusion of tongue as well as on swallowing	Moves upward on protrusion of tongue

FRACTURE OF THE NOSE

It is the *most common* facial bone to get fractured.[Q]

Chapter 21: Oral Cavity

Classification of Nasal Fracture (Table 21.2)

Table 21.2: Classification of nasal fracture

Class 1 fracture	Class 2 fracture	Class 3 fracture
Chevallet fracture	**Jarjavay fracture**	**Naso-orbito-ethmoid fracture**
• Depressed nasal fracture • Fracture line runs parallel to the dorsum and the nasomaxillary suture line • Nasal septum is not involved generally in this injury • It is involved only in severe cases • **Features:** Does not cause gross deformity • **Treatment:** Fracture reduction done either immediately or after 5–7 days, once edema settles	• Involve the nasal bone, the frontal process of the maxilla and the **septal structures** leading to septal deviation • Ethmoidal labyrinth and the orbit are spared • It leads to significant cosmetic deformity. • **Treatment:** Closed reduction of the nasal bone fracture done after the edema subsides (5 to 7 days) with open reduction of the septal deformity (septoplasty done if the patient is more than 17 years)	• Caused by high velocity trauma • Ethmoidal labyrinth is involved • Presents with multiple fractures of the roof of ethmoid, orbit and sometimes extends as far back as the sphenoid and parasellar regions • CSF leak and pneumocranium are seen • **Treatment:** immediate treatment with open surgery

Note:
- Distal part of the nasal bone is very thin and therefore more susceptible to injury.
- Untreated nasal bone fractures lasting for more than 21 days require **open reduction**
- Any cerebrospinal fluid (CSF) leak persisting for more than 2 weeks have to be considered for repair.
- Forceps used in:
  - Reduction of nasal bone – **Walsham forcep**
  - Reduction of septal facture – **Asch forcep**

NEW PATTERN QUESTIONS

Q N14. Chevallet fracture of nasal septum is:
a. Horizontal backwards
b. Vertically backwards
c. Transverse backwards
d. Oblique backwards

Q N15. In Jarjavay fracture of nasal bone, the fracture line is:
a. Oblique
b. Comminuted
c. Vertical
d. Horizontal

Symptoms of Nasal Fracture
- **Most common symptom:** Epistaxis
- External nasal deformity
- Nasal obstruction due to blood clot
- **Palpation:**
  - Tenderness present
  - Crepts present
- Watery nasal discharge indicates CSF leak due to fracture of cribriform plate in roof of nose.

■ FRACTURE OF MAXILLA

Le Fort classified fracture of maxilla into three types (Table 21.3)

Table 21.3: Classification of Le Fort type fracture

Le Fort type 1 fractures	Type 2 (Pyramidal fracture)	Type 3 (Craniofacial dysostosis)
• **Type 1 (transverse Guerin fracture)** separates the palate from midface and on X-ray or CT it appears as **floating palate or teeth**	This fracture involves the pterygoid plates, fronto-nasal maxillary buttress and often the skull base via the ethmoid bone On X-ray it appears as **floating maxilla**	In this fracture the facial skeleton separates from the cranial base

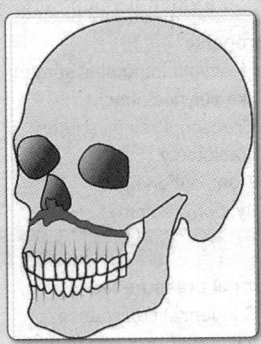

(a) Le Fort 1 (Guerin)

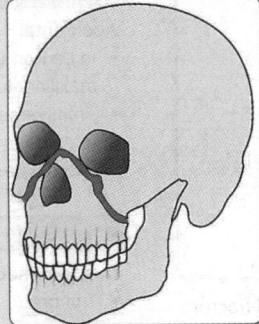

(b) Le Fort 2 (Pyramidal)

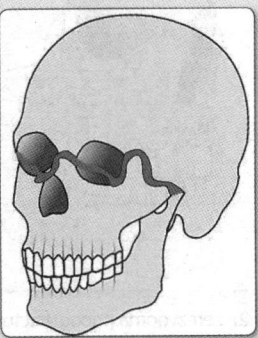

(c) Le Fort 3 (Craniofacial dysjunction)

Le Fort fractures

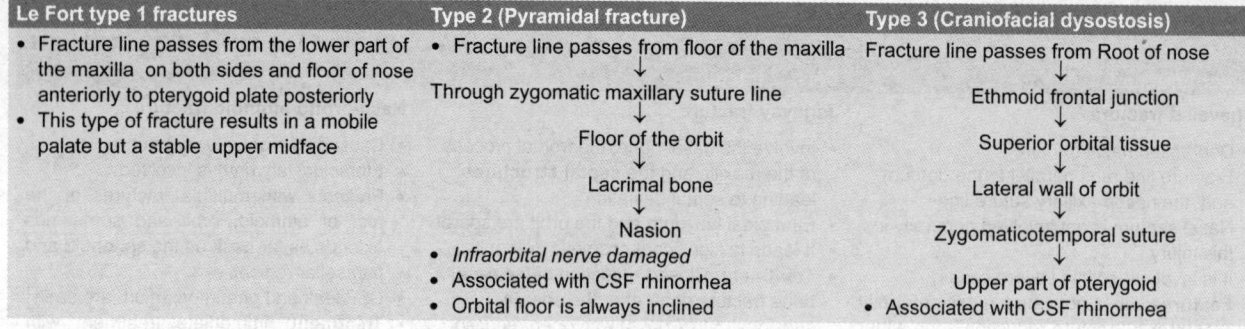

Le Fort type 1 fractures	Type 2 (Pyramidal fracture)	Type 3 (Craniofacial dysostosis)
• Fracture line passes from the lower part of the maxilla on both sides and floor of nose anteriorly to pterygoid plate posteriorly • This type of fracture results in a mobile palate but a stable upper midface	• Fracture line passes from floor of the maxilla ↓ Through zygomatic maxillary suture line ↓ Floor of the orbit ↓ Lacrimal bone ↓ Nasion • *Infraorbital nerve damaged* • Associated with CSF rhinorrhea • Orbital floor is always inclined	Fracture line passes from Root of nose ↓ Ethmoid frontal junction ↓ Superior orbital tissue ↓ Lateral wall of orbit ↓ Zygomaticotemporal suture ↓ Upper part of pterygoid • Associated with CSF rhinorrhea

ZYGOMATIC FRACTURE (TRIPOD FRACTURE)

Zygomatic fracture is the second M/C facial fracture (after nasal bone).
- **Commonly called Tripod Fracture Since the Bone Breaks at three Places**
  1. Zygomaticofrontal or Frontozygomatic suture
  2. Zygomaticotemporal suture
  3. Infraorbital rim (Fig. 21.2)

Clinical Features
- Orbital features
  - Ecchymosis of periorbital region within 2 hours of injury is pathognomic
  - Step—deformity at the infraorbital margin
  - Restricted ocular movement
  - Periorbital emphysema
  - Diplopia
- Other features
  - Flattening of the malar prominence
  - Anesthesia in the distribution of the infraorbital nerve
  - Trismus (Due to zygoma impinging on coronoid process of mandible)

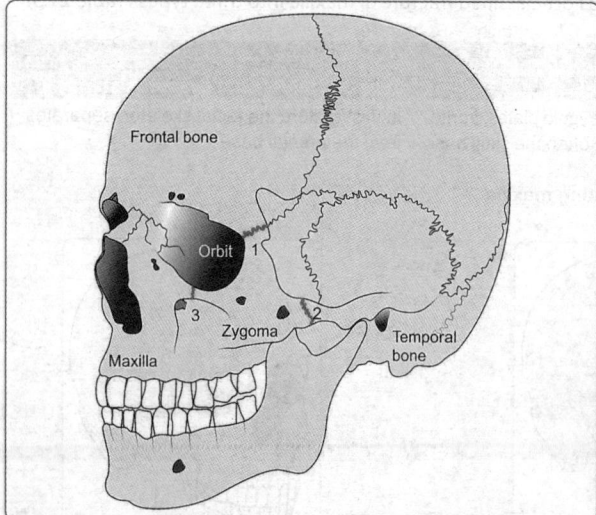

Fig. 21.2: Left zygoma (tripod) fracture showing three sites of fracture. (1) Zygomaticofrontal; (2) Zygomaticotemporal; (3) Infraorbital

Courtesy: Textbook of Diseases of Ear, Nose and Throat, Mohan Bansal. Jaypee Brothers Medical Publishers Pvt. Ltd., p 344

Diagnosis
- Water's view and exaggerated Water's view X-ray
- CT scan (orbit)

Treatment
- Only displaced fractures are to be treated
- Open reduction and internal wire fixation is carried out.

NEW PATTERN QUESTION

Q N16. **Tripod fracture is seen in:**
   a. Mandible
   b. Maxilla
   c. Nasal bone
   d. Zygoma

CEREBROSPINAL FLUID RHINORRHEA

(Scott Brown 7/e, vol 2 p 1636-1639)

- It is the flow of CSF from nose (due to leakage of CSF from the subarachnoid space into nasal cavity).
- Usual sites of CSF leak are cribriform plate that forms the roof of ethmoid sinus > frontal sinus (posterior walls) > floor of the anterior cranial fossa.

Etiology

Traumatic (Immediate/delayed–within 3 months of injury)	
Accidental	**Iatrogenic**
• In Le Fort II and Le Fort III maxillary fracture • Transverse fracture of temporal bone • Class 3 nasal fracture	• Headlight Intranasal surgery like polypectomy • Endoscopic sinus surgery craniotomy • Trans-sphenoidal hypophysectomy
Atraumatic	
Due to raised ICT	**Normal pressure leaks**
• Tumors • Hydrocephalus • Destructive bony lesions like granuloma	• Congenital dehiscence of nasal roof • Focal atrophy • Osteomyelitic erosion

Note: Historically the M/C cause of CSF rhinorrhea was head injury with involvent of cribriform plate of ethmoid but now M/C cause is Iatrogenic trauma surgery.

CSF can escape from following routes:
- Middle/posterior fossa via mastoid cavity, sphenoid sinus
- Anterior cranial fossa via:
  - Frontal, Ethmoid Sphenoid sinus
  - Cribriform plate
  - From middle ear via Eustachian tube

Clinical Features
Unilateral, clear watery discharge dripping on looking down, which increases on coughing, sneezing or exertion.

Diagnosis

On Examination
- **Reservoir sign:** (Done to elicit CSF rhinorrhea) After being supine → the patient is made to sit up in the upright position with the neck flexed. If there is sudden rush of clear fluid, it indicates CSF rhinorrhea.
- **Handkerchief test:** Stiffening of the handkerchief occurs with rhinitis *(due to presence of mucus)* but not in CSF rhinorrhea.
- **Double ring** sign, **halo sign** or double target sign is seen in blood stained CSF fluid. A drop when collected on a piece of filter paper, produces a central red spot (due to blood) and a peripheral lighter halo around the blood circle (if CSF is present).
- **Nasal endoscopy:** With/without fluorescein—can help in diagnosis.

Biochemical Examination
- **Glucose and chloride concentration:** Glucose level of > 30 mg% is confirmatory for CSF.
- **β₂ transferrin on electrophoresis:** Presence of β_2 transferrin is pathognomic for CSF rhinorrhea. This is the only test which should be used to confirm CSF rhinorrhea. Besides CSF, β_2 transferrin is present in perilymph and aqueous humor.
- Another protein called the **beta trace protein** is also specific for CSF and is widely used in Europe. It is secreted by meninges and choroid plexus. Facilities to test these proteins are not easily available everywhere.
- **Imaging modality of choice:** To diagnose the site of leak—T2 weighted MRI.

Treatment
Early cases of post-traumatic CSF rhinorrhea can be managed by conservative measures such as bed rest, elevating the head of the bed, stool softeners, and avoidance of nose blowing, sneezing and straining. Prophylactic antibiotics can be used to prevent meningitis. Acetazolamide decreases CSF formation. These measures can be combined with lumbar drain if indicated.

In persistent cases surgical repair can be done by the following:
- **Neurosurgical intracranial approach.**
- **Extradural approaches** such as external ethmoidectomy for cribriform plate and ethmoid area, trans-septal sphenoidal approach for sphenoid and osteoplastic flap approach for frontal sinus leak.
- **Transnasal endoscopic:** With the advent of endoscopic surgery for nose and sinuses, most of the leaks from the anterior cranial fossa and sphenoid sinus can be managed endoscopically with a success rate of 90% with first attempt. Principles of repair include:
  - Defining the sites of bony defect.
  - Preparation of graft site.
  - Underlay grafting of the fascia extradurally followed by placement of mucosa (as a free graft or pedicled flap).
  - If bony defect is larger than 2 cm, it is repaired with cartilage (from nasal septum or auricular concha) followed by placement of mucosa.

Note: CSF leak from frontal sinus often requires osteoplastic flap operation and obliteration of the sinus with fat.

NEW PATTERN QUESTIONS

Q N17. CSF rhinorrhea occurs due to fracture of:
a. Roof of orbit
b. Cribriform plate of ethmoid bone
c. Frontal sinus
d. Sphenoid bone

Q N18. The pathognomic test for CSF in suspected CSF rhinorrhea is:
a. Glucose concentration
b. Handkerchief test
c. Halo sign
d. Beta-2 transferrin

Q N19. CSF rhinorrhea TOC is:
a. Putting swab in nose
b. Craniotomy
c. Advising frequent blowing of nose
d. Wait and watch for 7 days and start antibiotics

Q N20. Management of persistent cases of CSF rhinorrhea is:
a. Head low position on bed
b. Straining activities
c. Endoscopic repair
d. All of the above

BLOW OUT FRACTURE OF ORBIT

- Blunt trauma to the orbit leads to increase in intraorbital pressure and so orbit gives way through the floor and medial wall. There is herniation of the orbital contents into the maxillary antum. This is known as orbital blow out. This herniation of orbital contents into the maxillary antrum is visualized radiologically as a convex opacity bulging into the antrum from above. This is known as **tear drop sign**.
- The symptoms include enophthalmos, diplopia, restricted upward gaze and infraorbital anesthesia.
- **Forced deduction test:** Detects extraocular muscle entrapment in blowout fractures.

NEW PATTERN QUESTIONS

Q N21. A patient present with enophthalmos after a trauma to face by blunt object. There is no fever and no extraocular muscle palsy. Diagnosis is:
- a. Fracture maxilla
- b. Fracture zygoma
- c. Blow out fracture
- d. Fracture ethmoid

Q N22. Grayish white membrane in throat may be seen in all of the following infections except:
- a. Streptococcal tonsilitis
- b. Diphtheria
- c. Adenovirus
- d. Ludwig's angina

Q N23. Black color patch in the mouth is seen in:
- a. Acute tonsilitis
- b. Peritonsillar abscess
- c. Vincent's angina
- d. Leukemia

Q N24. Trench mouth is:
- a. Submucosal fibrosis
- b. Tumor at uveal angle
- c. Ulcerative lesion of the tonsil
- d. Retension cyst of the tonsil

Q N25. The typical characteristic of diphtheric membrane is:
- a. Loosely attached
- b. Pearly white in color
- c. Firmly attached and bleeds on removal
- d. Fast component occasionally

FRACTURE OF MANDIBLE

Fracture of mandible is classified by **Dingmans classification** depending on location.

Condylar fractures (35%) are most common followed by those of angle (20%), body (20%) and symphysis (15%) of mandible.

Management
- Open reduction–preferred treatment
- Close reduction–not preferred as it needs immobilization of the joint for three weeks which can lead to ankylosis of the TM joint.

LEVELS OF LYMPH NODES IN NECK

- **Level 1** Includes submental and submandibular lymph nodes.
- **Level 2** Nodes lie along the upper one-third of IJV between base of skull and hyoid bone
- **Level 3** Nodes along the middle third of IJV between hyoid bone and upper border of cricoid cartilage.
- **Level 4** Nodes along the lower third of JJV between cricoid cartilage and clavicle.
- **Level 5** These nodes lie in posterior triangle of neck including transverse cervical and supraclavicular nodes.
- **Level 6** These are nodes in anterior compartment including prelaryngeal, pretracheal and paratracheal groups.
- **Level 7** Includes nodes of upper mediastinum below suprasternal notch.

Clinical Vignettes to Remember

1. Vestibule is seen in ear (in inner ear bony labyrinth), nose (skin lined portion of nose), larynx (part above ventricular bands) and oral cavity.
2. L:N of tongue is jugulo-omohyoid LN (as from all parts of tongue, lymphatics finally drain into jugulo-omohyoid LN).
3. M/C lymph node enlarged in tongue malignancy = Submandibular LN (as M/C site for Ca tongue = lateral aspect which drains into submandibular LN)
4. In XII nerve paralysis deviates to paralyzed side on protusion due to action of unaffected genioglossus muscle on opposite side.
5. For lip reconstruction Abbe-Estlander flap (Fig. 21.3) is used which is based on labial artery. Other flaps which could be used are Karapandzic flap, Gillie's fan flap.
6. To delineate the area from which biopsy should be taken in oral leisons–supravital staining with toluidine blue dye is used.
7. A 40-year-old chronic cigratte smoker presents with reddish shiny plaques in the floor of mouth. Most common D/D is–Erythroplakia.
8. A 42-year-old male who is a sale's manager in a leading firm presents with grayish atropic area in the lower lip due to long-standing sunlight exposure. The most important D/D is actinic chelosis. (Note: Actinic chelosis is common in males $\geq$ 40 years and can lead to squamous cell carcinoma).

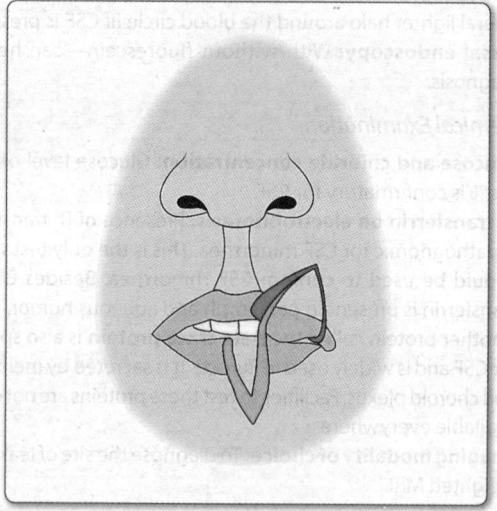

Fig. 21.3: Abbe-Estlander flap

9. M/C site for mandibular fracture = condylar fracture.
10. Pneumocephalus can be seen in fracture of frontal sinus.
11. 1st/Most important step in management of faciomaxillary trauma – Airway management
12. Palatal myoclonus is seen in multiple sclerosis.
13. A 14-year-old boy presents with fever, sore-throat ulcers and cervical lymph node enlargement. Throat-swab is positive for beta hemolytic Streptococcus and was put on penicillin but he developed rubelliform rash and symptoms worsened– Diagnosis is – Infectious mononucleosis (also k/a glandular

fever). Caused by EBV. Gold standard test for diagnosing this condition – EBV antibodies. Management–steroids.
14. In a case of recurrent edema of uvula and laryngeal edema – always suspect hereditary angioneurotic edema (HANE). Paitents may also have edema of gut. It is caused due to deficiency of enzyme C1 esterase inhibitor.
15. Behcet's syndrome – is oculo-oro-genital syndrome characterized by a triad of—
    - Aphthous like ulcers in oral cavity. The edge of the ulcer is characteristically punched out.
    - Genital ulceration
    - Uveitis
16. Taste buds are highest in circumvallate papillae > Foliate papillae > Fungiform papillae.
    There are practically no buds in felliform papillae.

Clinical Condition	Seen in
Black membrane in mouth	Vincent argina
Grayish white membrane on tonsils + B/L cervical lymphadenitis in a febrile patient	Diphtheria
Cystic translucent swelling in the floor of mouth	Ranula
Opaque swelling in midline in the floor of mouth	Dermoid cyst
Black hairy tongue	Chronics smokers, Drugs like lansoprazole, antibiotic use.
Fissured tongue	Syphilis, Vit B deficiency, Anemia
Wickham's striae	Lichen planus

NEW PATTERN QUESTIONS

Q N26. Battle sign is:
  a. Periorbital ecchymosis
  b. Ecchymosis around mastoid area
  c. Facial congestion and cyanosis
  d. Pulsatile ear discharge

Q N27. Battle sign is associated with:
  a. Fracture zygoma
  b. Fracture of anterior cranial fossa
  c. Fracture of middle cranial fossa
  d. Nasoethmoid fracture

Q N28. Identify the condition shown in the plate:

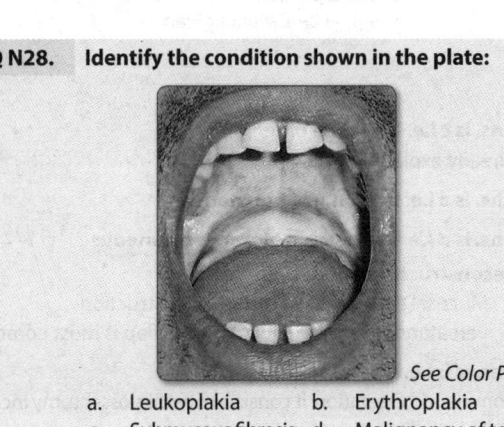

See Color Plate 18

  a. Leukoplakia   b. Erythroplakia
  c. Submucous fibrosis   d. Malignancy of tongue

Explanations and References to New Pattern Questions

N1. Ans. is d i.e 2% Toluidine blue   *Ref. Internet Search*
Toluidine blue is a metachromatic dye which can efficiently detect the mitotic figures in sections of paraffin embedded human tissue especially in oral cavity.

N2. Ans. is c i.e. Alveobuccal complex
M/C site of oral cancer in India is alveobuccal complex.

N3. Ans. is a i.e. Lip   *Ref. Bailey 26/e, p 712-713, Devita 9/e, p 744-745*

N4. Ans. is c i.e. Labial artery
Abbe-Estlander flap is used for reconstruction of upper or lower lip. It is based on Labial artery.

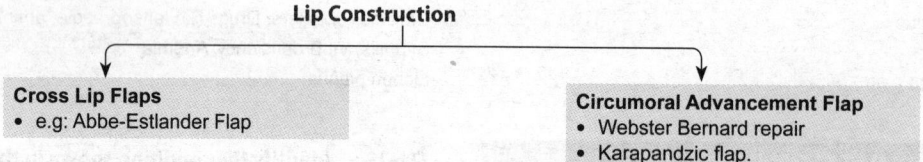

N5. Ans. is c i.e. Toluidine blue   *Ref. Internet Search*
Already explained

N6. Ans. is a i.e. Regional lymph nodes

N7. Ans. is d i.e. Pectoralis major myocutaneous   *Ref. Bailey 26/e, p 716, Devita 9/e, p 749*
Reconstruction of Cheek
- Mucosal flaps are used in flap reconstruction.
- Percutaneous major myocutaneous flap is most commonly used flap for head and neck reconstruction.

N8. Ans. is b i.e. Oral cancer   *Ref. Dhingra 6/e, p 228*
Commando Operation: It consists of hemiglossectomy including a portion of the floor of mouth, segmental or hemimandibulectomy and block dissection of neck nodes.

N9. Ans. is a i.e. Lateral border   *Ref. Dhingra 6/e, p 227*
Read the text for explanation

N10. Ans. is d i.e. 1st molar   *Ref. Dhingra 5/e, p 200*
Read the text for explanation

N11. Ans. is a i.e. Facial N
The submandibular and sublingual glands receive their parasympathetic input from facial nerve via the submandibular ganglion. The parotid gland receives its parasympathetic input from the glossopharyngeal nerve via the otic ganglion.

N12. Ans. is b i.e. Adenoid cystic carcinoma.
Adenoid cystic carcinoma is the M/C cancer of minor salivary glands. It invades the perineural space, i.e. it is associated with perineural invasion.

N13. Ans. is d i.e 80%   *Ref. Bailey and Love 24/e, p 723; 25/e, p 755*
80% of all salivary stones occur in the submanidbular glands because their secretions are highly viscous. 80% of submandibular stones are radiopaque and can be identified on plain radiograph.

N14. Ans. is b i.e. Vertically backwards   *Ref. Logan Turne 10/e, p 21*

N15. Ans. is d i.e. Horizontal
Chevallet fracture of nasal septum
- Due to a blow from below.
- Runs vertically from anterior nasal spine of maxilla upwards to the junction of bony and cartilaginous dorsum of nose.
- Jarjavay fracture: The fracture line is horizontal

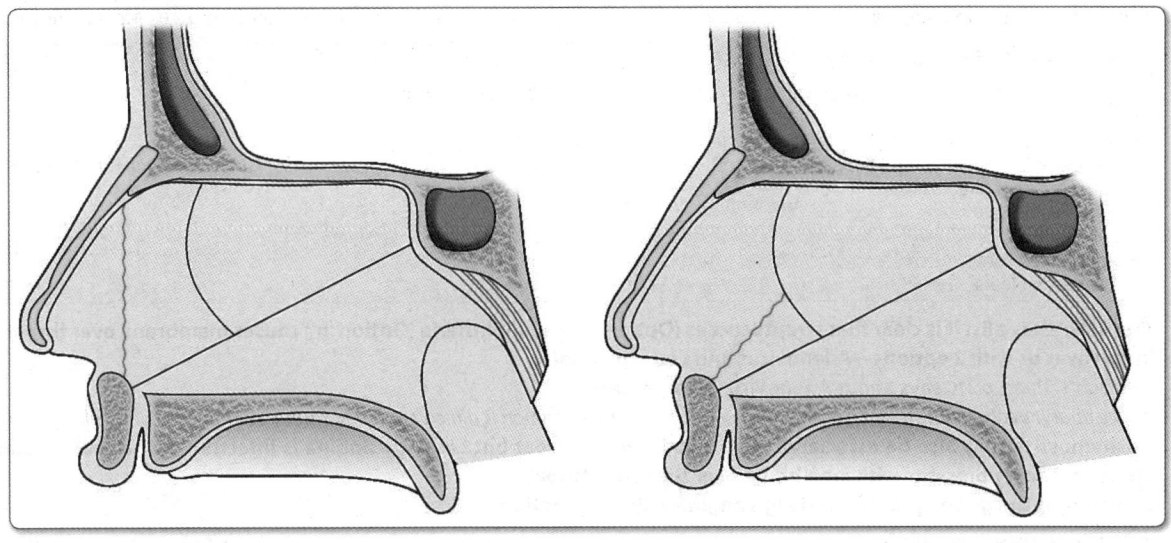

Chevallet fracture   Jarjavay fracture

N16. Ans. is d i.e. Zygoma *Ref. Dhingra 6/e, p 183*

Fracture of zygoma is called as **tripod fracture** as when the bone fractures, it is separated at its three processes viz zygomatico-frontal, zygomatico temporal and infraorbital.

N17. Ans. is b i.e. Cribriform plate of ethmoid sinus.

Read the text for explanation.

N18. Ans. is d i.e. Beta-2 transferrin

Tests for detecting CSF rhinorrhea
- Reservoir sign
- Handkerchief test
- Most sensitive lab test is to look for **Beta-2 transferrin** in the nasal secretion
- Best test to detect CSF leak — **intrathecal radionucleotide test**.

N19. Ans. is d i.e. Wait and watch for 7 days and then start antibiotics.

See the text for explanation.

N20. Ans. is c i.e. Endoscopic repair *Ref. Dhingra 6/e, p 164*

As discussed is preceeding text. CSF rhinorrhea can be managed by

Conservative approach
- Bed rest
- Elevating head of bed
  (Not lowering it, as given in options)
- Stool softeners
- Avoidance of sneezing/straining activities
  (Not performing, as given in option)

Surgical repair: In persistent cases surgical repair is performed by
- Neurosurgical intracranial approach
- Endoscopic repair
- Extradural approach

N21. Ans is c i.e. Blow out fracture *Ref. Dhingra 6/e, p 184*

Blow out fracture is isolated fracture of orbital floor, when a large blunt object strikes the globe.

It presents with:
- Ecchymosis of lid, conjunctiva and sclera
- Enophthalmos
- Diplopia due to displacement of eyeball
- Anesthesia of cheek and upper lip, if infraorbital nerve is involved.

N22. Ans. is d. i.e. Ludwig's angina *Ref. Dhingra 5/e, p 274; Harrison 17/e, p 210; Mohan Bansal p 544*

> **Membrane in Throat is Caused by**
> - Pyogenic organisms viz. Streptococci, Staphylococci causing membranous tonsillitis
> - Diphtheria
> - Vincent's angina *(Caused by fusiform bacilli and spirochetes: Borrelia vincentii)*
> - Candidiasis/monoliasis/oral thrush   —Maqbool 11th/ed p 280
> - Infectious mononucleosis
> - Agranulocytosis
> - Leukemia
> - Aphthous ulcers
> - Traumatic ulcers

From the above list it is clear that streptococcus (Option 'a') and diphtheria (Option 'b') causes membrane over throat. This leaves us with 2 options—Adenovirus and Ludwig's angina

Harrison 17th/ed, p 210 **says about Adenovirus pharyngitis:**

"Since pharyngeal exudate may be present on examination, this condition is difficult to differentiate from streptococcal pharyngitis."

So adenovirus may also be associated with membrane in throat but Ludwig's angina is infection of the submandibular space and never presents with membrane over the tonsil/throat.

So amongst the given options—Ludwig's angina is the best option.

N23. Ans. is c i.e. Vincent's angina *Ref. Logan Turner 10/e, p 87, 88*

Vincent's Angina: (Ulcerative Gingivitis/Trench mouth)

- Was common during first world war (due to lack of oral hygiene) and is less common now.
- Caused by fusiform bacillus and spirochetes: *Borrelia vincentii*.
- It manifests as necrotizing gingivostomatitis with oropharyngeal ulcerations and dark gray membrane.

On Examination

- Membrane generally present on one tonsil but may involve the gum soft, and hard palate.
- *It appears as grayish black slough* which bleeds when it is removed.
- Ulcers are visible on tonsil after removal of membrane.
- Membrane reforms after removal.
- Characteristic smell in breath (halitosis), so also called as Trench mouth.

Treatment

- Systemic antibiotics: *Penicillin, Erythromycin, Metronidazole.*
- Warm sodium bicarbonate gargles.
- Barrier nursing of the patient as disease is infectious.

N24. Ans. is c i.e. Ulcerative lesions of tonsil *Ref. Turner 10/e, p 87, 88*

Trench mouth/Vincent's angina is ulcerative gingivostomatitis.

N25. Ans. is c i.e. Firmly attached and bleeds on removal *Ref. Dhingra 5/e, p 308, 309, 6/e, p 260*

- **In diphtheria:** membrane is dirty gray in color.
- It extends beyond the tonsils, on to the soft palate and posterior pharyngeal wall.
- It is adherent and its removal leaves a bleeding surface.
- Cervical lymph nodes particularly the jugulodigastric lymph node are enlarged and become tender, giving a bull neck appearance

N26. Ans. is b i.e. Ecchymosis over the mastoid area.

N27. Ans. is c i.e. Fracture of middle cranial fossa.

Battle sign is mastoid ecchymosis and is an indication of fracture of posterior or middle cranial fossa of the skull and may suggest underlying brain trauma. The ecchymosis is a result of extravasation of blood along the path of the posterior auricular artery.

Also know: **Raccoon eyes** — bruising around the eyes, often associated with Battle sign.

N28. Ans. is c i.e. Submucous fibrosis

The plate shows white fibrous bands involving soft palate, faucial pillars and retromolar area. It is oral submucous fibrosis.

QUESTIONS

1. **Fordyce's (Spots) Granules in oral cavity arise from:** [AIIMS 04]
   a. Mucous glands
   b. Sebaceous glands
   c. Taste buds
   d. Minor salivary glands

2. **True about aphthous ulcer:** [PGI June 05]
   a. Viral predisposition
   b. Recurrent ulcer
   c. Deep ulcers
   d. Involves the mucosa of the hard palate
   e. Steroids given as treatment

3. **Regarding Ranula all are true except:** [MAHE 05]
   a. Retention cyst
   b. Arises from submandibular gland
   c. Translucent
   d. Plunging may be a feature

4. **True regarding Ranula:** [AI 01]
   a. It is also called as epulis
   b. It is a cystic swelling in the floor of mouth.
   c. It is a type of thyroglossal cyst
   d. It is a type of mucus retention cyst

5. **Premalignant leison of oral cavity includes:** [PGI Nov 10]
   a. Erythroplakia
   b. Fordyce spots
   c. Leukoplakia
   d. Keratoacanthoma
   e. Aphthous ulcer

6. **Risk factors for oropharyngeal region carcinoma:**
   a. Sideropenic dysphagia
   b. Oral submucous fibrosis
   c. Erythroplakia
   d. Leukoplakia
   e. Chronic hypertrophic candidiasis

7. **Which of the following is premalignant condition?** [AIIMS 91]
   a. Chronic glossitis
   b. Submucous fibrosis
   c. Hypertrophic glossitis
   d. Aphthous stomatitis

8. **The most common premalignant condition of oral carcinoma is:** [AI 95, 96]
   a. Leukoplakia
   b. Erythroplakia
   c. Lichen planus
   d. Fibrosis

9. **The most common site of oral cancer among Indian population is:** [AI 04]
   a. Tongue
   b. Floor of mouth
   c. Alveobuccal complex
   d. Lip

10. **Not included in oral cavity Ca:** [PGI May 2010]
    a. Base of tongue
    b. Gingivobuccal sulcus
    c. Soft palate
    d. Hard palate
    e. Buccal mucosa

11. **Carcinoma tongue most frequently develops from:** [AI 02]
    a. Tip
    b. Lateral border
    c. Dorsal portion
    d. All portions equally

12. **A patient has carcinoma of right tongue on its lateral border of anterior 2/3rd, with lymph node of size 4 cm in level 3 on left side of the neck, stage of disease is:**
    a. N0
    b. N1   [AIIMS May 07]
    c. N2
    d. N3

13. **A patient with Ca tongue is found to have lymph nodes in the lower neck. The treatment of choice for the lymph nodes is:** [AIIMS 01]
    a. Lower cervical neck dissection
    b. Suprahyoid neck dissection
    c. Teleradiotherapy
    d. Radical neck dissection

14. **Carcinoma of buccal mucosa commonly drain to the following lymph nodes sites:** [AI 97]
    a. Submental
    b. Submandibular
    c. Supraclavicular
    d. Cervical

15. **Metastasis of carcinoma buccal mucosa goes to:**
    a. Regional lymph node
    b. Liver   [AIIMS 96]
    c. Heart
    d. Brain

16. **A patient presented with a 1×1.5 cm growth on the lateral border of the tongue. The treatment indicated would be:**
    a. Laser ablation   [AIIMS 02]
    b. Interstitial brachytherapy
    c. External beam radiotherapy
    d. Chemotherapy

17. **A 70-year-old male who has been chewing tobacco for the past 50 years present with a six months history of large, fungating, soft papillary lesions in the oral cavity. The lesion has penetrated into the mandible. Lymph nodes are not palpable. Two biopsies taken from the lesion proper show benign appearing papillomatosis with hyperkeratosis and acanthosis infiltrating the subjacent tissues. The most likely diagnosis is:** [AI 04]
    a. Squamous cell papilloma
    b. Squamous cell carcinoma
    c. Verrucous carcinoma
    d. Malignant mixed tumor

18. **An 80-year-old patient present with a midline tumor of the lower jaw, involving the alveolar margin. He is edentulous. Treatment of coice:** [AI 01]
    a. Hemimandibulectomy
    b. Commando operation
    c. Segmental mandibulectomy
    d. Marginal mandibulectomy

19. **An old man who is edentulous squamous cell carcinoma in buccal mucosa that has developed infiltrated to the alveolus. Following is not indicated in treatment:**
    a. Radiotherapy   [AI 02]
    b. Segment mandibulectomy
    c. Marginal mandibulectomy involving removal of outer table only
    d. Marginal mandibulectomy involving removal of upper half of mandible

20. **Which Ca has best prognosis:** [AIIMS 98]
    a. Carcinoma lip
    b. Carcinoma cheek
    c. Carcinoma tongue
    d. Carcinoma palate

21. **True statement about oral cancer is/are:** [PGI 04]
    a. Most common in buccal mucosa
    b. Systemic metastasis uncommon

c. Responds to radiotherapy
d. Surgery is treatment of choice
e. Syphilis and dental irridation predisposes

22. **In carcinoma of lower lip secondaries are seen in:** [AI 91]
    a. Upper cervical LN
    b. Supraclavicular LN
    c. Axillary LN
    d. Mediastinal LN

23. **Calculus is most commonly seen in which salivary gland?**
    a. Sublingual
    b. Palatal [AIIMS June 99]
    c. Parotid
    d. Submandibular

24. **The most common tumor of the salivary gland is:** [AI 02; AIIMS 98]
    a. Mucoepidermoid tumor
    b. Warthin's tumor
    c. Acinic cell tumor
    d. Pleomorphic adenoma

25. **Most common salivary gland tumor in children:** [AIIMS 99]
    a. Lymphoma
    b. Adenoid cystic Ca
    c. Pleomorphic adenoma
    d. Mucoepidermoid Ca

26. **All are true for pleomorphic adenoma except:** [PGI 99]
    a. Arises from parotid
    b. May turn into malignant
    c. Minor salivary gland can be affected
    d. None

27. **Treatment of choice for pleomorphic adenoma:** [AIIMS 96, 98, 01; AI 97; PGI 95, 99]
    a. Superficial parotidectomy
    b. Radical parotidectomy
    c. Enucleation
    d. Radiotherapy

28. **Ramavati, a 40-year-old female, presented with a progressively increasing lump in the parotid region. On oral examinations, the tonsil was pushed medially. Biopsy showed it to be pleomorphic adenoma. The appropriate treatment is:** [AIIMS 01]
    a. Superficial parotidectomy
    b. Lumpectomy
    c. Conservative total parotidectomy
    d. Enucleation

29. **Which of the following is not an indication of radiotherapy in pleomophic adenoma of parotid?** [AI 04]
    a. Involvement of deep lobe
    b. 2nd histologically benign recurrence
    c. Microscopically positive margins
    d. Malignant transformation

30. **Mixed tumors of the salivary glands are:** [AI 06]
    a. Most common in submandibular gland
    b. Usually malignant
    c. Most common in parotid gland
    d. Associated with calculi

31. **In which one of the following head and neck cancer perineural invasion is most commonly seen:** [AI 05]
    a. Adenocarcinoma
    b. Adenoid cystic carcinoma
    c. Basal cell carcinoma
    d. Squamous cell carcinoma

32. **Acinic cell carcinoma of the salivary gland arise most often in the:** [AI 06]
    a. Parotid salivary gland
    b. Minor salivry glands
    c. Submandibular salivary glands
    d. Sublinguial salivary glands

33. **A Warthin's tumor is:** [AIIMS 03, 05]
    a. An adenolymphoma of parotid gland
    b. A pleomorphic adenoma of the parotid
    c. A carcinoma of the parotid
    d. A carcinoma of submandibular salivary gland

34. **All of the following are true regarding Warthin's tumor except:** [AIIMS 02]
    a. More common in females
    b. Commonly involve the parotid glands
    c. They arise from the epithelial and the lymphoid cells
    d. 10% are bilateral

35. **Treatment of choice for Warthin's tumor is:**
    a. Superficial parotidectomy [AIIMS 01; AI 98]
    b. Enucleation
    c. Radiotherapy
    d. Injection of a sclerosing agent

36. **Mucoepidermoid carcinoma of parotid arises from:**
    a. Mucus secreting and epidermal cells [PGI 99]
    b. Excretory cells
    c. Myoepithelium cells
    d. Acinus

37. **True statement [s] about salivary gland tumors:** [PGI 04]
    a. Pleomorphic adenoma can arise in submandibular gland
    b. Warthin's tumor arises from submandibular gland
    c. Pleomorphic adenoma is most common tumor of submandibular gland
    d. Acinic cell Ca is most malignant
    e. Frey's syndrome can occur after parotid surgery

38. **In surgery of submandibular salivary gland, nerve often involved:** [PGI June 97]
    a. Hypoglossal
    b. Glossopharyngeal
    c. Facial
    d. Lingual

39. **In which of the following conditions sialography is contraindicated?** [AI 05/AI 07]
    a. Ductal calculus
    b. Chronic parotitis
    c. Parotid obstruction
    d. Acute sialadenitis

40. **Most common cause of unilateral parotid swelling in a 27 year old male is:** [AI 01]
    a. Warthin's tumor
    b. Pleomorphic adenoma
    c. Adenocarcinoma
    d. Hemangioma

41. **True about Ludwig's angina:** [PGI 07]
    a. Involves both submandibular and sublingual spaces
    b. Most common cause is dental infection
    c. Bilateral
    d. Spreads by lymphatics

42. **A patient of head injury was brought to the hospital. Patient was conscious having clear nasal discharge through right nostril. NCCT head was done which reveated non-operable injury to frontobasal area. What is the most appropriate management?** [AIIMS PGI Nov 14]
    a. Wait and watch for 4–5 days to allow spontaneous healing
    b. Do an MRI to localize the leak and control the discharge endoscopically
    c. Put a dural catheter to control CSF leak
    d. Approach transcranially to repair the damaged frontobasal region

43. **True about quinke disease:** *[PGI June 05] [June 04]*
    a. Bacterial infection   b. Peritonsillar abscess
    c. Vocal cord edema   d. Edema of uvula
44. **Le Fort's fracture does not involve:** *[Kerala 89]*
    a. Zygoma   b. Maxilla
    c. Nasal bone   d. Mandible
45. **Craniofacial dissociation is seen in:** *[SGPGI 05, TN 06]*
    a. Le Fort 1 fracture   b. Le Fort 2 fracture
    c. Le Fort 3 fracture   d. Tripod fracture
46. **Which of the following is/are true about Leforts fracture:** *[PGI May 17]*
    a. It is fracture of zygomatic bone
    b. May cause CSF rhinorrhea
    c. Type 1: complete separation of facial bones from the cranial bones
    d. Classified as types 1 to 5
47. **Tear drop sign is seen in:** *[SGPI 05]*
    a. Fracture of floor of orbit
    b. Fracture of lateral wall of nose
    c. Le Fort's fracture
    d. Fracture on zygomatic arch
48. **Clinical features of fracture zygoma is/are:** *[PGI Nov 09]*
    a. Cheek swelling   b. Trismus
    c. Nose bleeding   d. Infraorbital numbness
    e. Diplopia
49. **Fracture zygoma shows all the features except:** *[AI 97]*
    a. Diplopia   b. CSF rhinorrhea
    c. Epistaxis   d. Trismus
50. **Tripod fracture is seen in:** *[MP 08]*
    a. Mandible   b. Maxilla
    c. Nasal bone   d. Zygoma
51. **Which is not seen in fracture maxilla?** *[AIIMS 91]*
    a. CSF rhinorrhea   b. Malocclusion
    c. Anesthesia upper lip   d. Surgical emphysema
52. **CSF rhinorrhea occurs due to fracture of:** *[AIIMS 97]*
    a. Roof of orbit
    b. Cribriform plate of ethmoidal bone
    c. Frontal sinus
    d. Sphenoid bone
53. **The most common site of leak in CSF rhinorrhea is:**
    a. Ethmoid sinus   *[AI 05]*
    b. Frontal sinus
    c. Petrous part of temporal bone
    d. Sphenoid sinus
54. **CSF rhinorrhea is seen in:** *[PGI June 03]*
    a. LeFort's fracture Type I   b. Nasal fracture
    c. Nasoethmoid fracture   d. Frontozygomatic fracture
55. **True about CSF rhinorrhea is:** *[PGI 02]*
    a. Occurs due to break in cribriform plate
    b. Contains glucose
    c. Requires immediate surgery
    d. Contains less protein
56. **Target sign is seen in a blot test from nasal discharge in which of these conditions?** *[AIIMS Nov 17]*
    a. Traumatic CSF leak   b. Fracture mastoid
    c. Spontaneous CSF leak   d. Meningoencephaloccle
57. **Immediate treatment of CSF rhinorrhea requires:**
    a. Antibiotics and observation   *[AIIMS 97]*
    b. Plugging with paraffin guage
    c. Blowing of nose
    d. Craniotomy
58. **CSF rhinorrhea is diagnosed by:** *[AI 07]*
    a. Beta-2 microglobulin
    b. Beta-2 transferrin
    c. Thyroglobulin
    d. Transthyretin
59. **The pathognomonic test for CSF in suspected CSF rhinorrhea is:** *[MP 07]*
    a. Glucose concentration
    b. Handkerchief test
    c. Halo sign
    d. Beta-2 transferrin
60. **After laparoscopic appendectomy, patient had fall from bed on her nose after which she had swelling in nose and slight difficulty in breathing. Next step in management:**
    a. IV antibiotics for 7–10 days   *[AIIMS 07]*
    b. Observation in hospital
    c. Surgical drainage
    d. Discharge after 2 days and follow-up of the patient after 8 weeks
61. **Ideal time of correcting fracture of nasal bone is:**
    a. Immediately   *[Kolkata 00]*
    b. After few days
    c. After 2 weeks
    d. After 3–4 weeks
62. **Perforation of palate is/are seen with:** *[PGI Nov 2012]*
    a. Minor aphthous ulcers   b. Major aphthous ulcers
    c. Tertiary syphilis   d. Cocaine abuse
63. **Veins not involved in spreading infection to cavernous sinus from danger area of face:** *[PGI May 2013]*
    a. Lingual vein   b. Pterygoid plexus
    c. Facial vein   d. Ophthalmic vein
    e. Cephalic vein
64. **True about Andy Gump deformity:** *[PGI May 2015]*
    a. Occurs due defects of the anterior mandibular arch
    b. Hemimandibulectomy can cause it
    c. Marginal mandibulectomy can cause it
    d. Treatment is adequate reconstruction of anterior mandibular arch with plate and graft
65. **Which of the following is true regarding mandibular fracture?** *[PGI Nov 2014]*
    a. Inferior alveolar nerve damage may occur
    b. Panorex radiograph is very helpful in management
    c. Ramus is the most common site of fracture
    d. Condylar fracture heals spontaneously and require no active intervention
    e. Condylar fracture is the most common site

Explanations and References

1. **Ans. is b i.e. Sebaceous gland**

   Ref. Scott Brown's Otolaryngology 7/e, vol 2, p 1824; Harrison 17/e, p 128; Dhingra 5/e, p 205, 6/e, p 220; Turner 10/e, p 233; Mohan Bansal p 379

   ### Fordyce's Spot
   - Yellowish lesions seen in buccal and labial mucosa.
   - They are ectopic sebaceous glands and do not have any erythematous halo.
   - Seen in up to 80% of population.
   - No clinical significance.

   Points to Remember
   - **Forchhiemer spots:** seen in rubella, infectious mono nucleosis and scarlet fever.
   - **Rothe's spots:** seen in Infective endocarditis
   - **Rose spots:** seen in Typhoid fever
   - **Kopliks spot:** seen in Measles *(above the second molar).*

2. **Ans. is a, b and e i.e. Viral predisposition; Recurrent ulcer; and Steroids given as treatment**

   Ref. Dhingra 5/e, p 230, 6/e, p 218; Mohan Bansal p 381-2

   Aphthous ulcers are recurrent and superficial ulcers, usually involving movable mucosa i.e. inner surfaces of lips, buccal mucosa, tongue, floor of mouth and soft palate, while sparing mucosa of the hard palate and gingivae.

   ### Etiology
   Is unknown but may be due to:
   - Nutritional deficiency of vit. B12, folic acid and iron.
   - Viral infection
   - Hormonal changes

   ### Treatment
   - Topical steroids and cauterization with 10% silver nitrate

   Points to Remember
   - Recurrence is common in ulcers.
   - M/C cause of viral oral ulcer = Herpes simplex type I
   - Painless oral ulcers are seen in—syphilis
   - Bechet's syndrome is oral ulcers + genital ulcers + eye disease (iridocyclitis and retinal vasculitis) + vascular malformation.

3. **Ans. is b i.e. Arises from submandibular gland.**
4. **Ans. is b i.e. It is a cystic swelling in the floor of mouth.**

   Ref. Dhingra 5/e, p 237, 6/e, p 224; Surgical Short Cases 3/e, p 45,46; Mohan Bansal p 403

   ### Ranula
   - It is a thin walled bluish retention cyst.^Q
   - Seen in the floor of mouth on one side of the frenulum.^Q
   - It arises due to obstruction of duct of sublingual salivary gland.
   - It is almost always unilateral.

   #### Clinical Features
   - Seen mostly in children and young adults.
   - Only complain—swelling in the floor of mouth
   - Cyst may rupture spontaneously but recurrence is common

O/E
Bluish in color - Brilliantly translucent^Q
Lymph nodes are not enlarged

Types
Simple: Situated in floor of mouth without any cervical prolongation.
Deep/plunging: Ranula which extends to the neck through the muscles of mylohyoid.
Such prolongation appears in submandibular region.

Management
- Surgical exicision of ranula along with sublingual salivary gland is the ideal treatment.
- M/C D/D of ranula = sublingual dermoid^Q (opaque midline swelling)
- During excision of ranula = M/C nerve which can be damaged is lingual nerve.^{Q}

Note:
- Cavernous ranula is a type of lymphangioma which invades the fascial planes of neck
- Obstruction of duct of sublingual salivary gland leads to ranula formation but obstruction of parotid and submandibular gland duct leads to their atrophy. This is because sublingual gland is active throughout whereas parotid and submandibular gland secret saliva only in response to food.

5. **Ans. is a and c i.e. Erythroplakia; and Leukoplakia.**
6. **Ans. is a, b, c and d i.e. Sideropenic dysphagia, Oral submucous fibrosis, Erythroplakia and Leukoplakia.**
7. **Ans. is b i.e. Submucous fibrosis.** *Ref. Devita 7/e, p 982; Bailey and Love 25/e, p 735*

Lesions and conditions of the oral mucosa associated with an increased risk of malignancy.

Premalignant conditions	Conditions increasing risk	Risk is doubtful
- Leukoplakia - Erythroplakia - Speckled erythroplakia - Chronic hyperplastic candidiasis	- Oral submucosa fibrosis - Syphilitic glossitis - Sideropenic dysphagia (Paterson-Kelly syndrome)	- Oral lichen planus - Discoid lupus erythematosus - Dyskeratosis congenita.

... Bailey and Love 25/e, p 735

Note:
- Friends in the table 46.2 given in Bailey and Love, Leukoplakia is not included in conditions associated with increased risk but in the description just given below it – leukoplakia is specially mentioned.
- Premalignant lesion is morphologically altered tissue where cancer is more likely to occur e.g. Leukoplakia whereas premalignant condition is a generalized state where there is significantly increased risk of cancer, e.g. syphilis, submucous fibiosis.
- Plummer Vinson syndrome can lead to post-cricoid carcinoma (M/C), carcinoma of tongue, esophagus and stomach.

8. **Ans. is a i.e. Leukoplakia** *Ref. Devita 7/e, p 982; Bailey and Love 25/e, p 735; Mohan Bansal p 376-7*
"Leukoplakia is the most common premalignant oral mucosal lesion." Mohan Bansal p 377
"The malignant potential of erythroplakia is 17 times higher than in leukoplakia." Mohan Bansal p 376

Points to Remember

> Most common premalignant condition for oral cancer : ***Leukoplakia or speckled leukoplakia***
> Premalignant condition with highest risk for oral cancer : ***Erythroplakia. (M/C Site = lower alveolar margin and floor of mouth)***
> Painless oral ulcers are seen in–syphilis
> Bechet's syndrome = oral ulcers + genital ulcers + eye disease (iridocyclitis and retinal vasculitis) + vascular malformation.

Important Points on Leukoplakia

- ***Clinical white patch*** that cannot be characterized clinically or pathologically as any other disease is leukoplakia.
- Most common ***site*** is buccal mucosa and oral commissures.

- Tobacco smoking and chewing are main etiological factor.
- If patient stops smoking for 1 year, it will disappear in 60% of cases.
- Features suggestive **malignant change** in leukoplakia are induration, speckled or nodular appearance.
- Chances of malignant changes in leukoplakia increases with *increases in age of lesion and age of patient*.
- **All lesions** must be biopsied and sent for histology as it has 2–8% risk of malignancy.

Lesion	Treatment
– Hyperkeratosis	Follow-up at 4 monthly interval/chemopreventive drugs
– Dysplasia	Surgical excision or CO_2 laser exicison

> **Remember**
> **Chemopreventive drugs used in oral malignancy:**
> - Vit. A, E, C
> - Flavonoids
> - Betacarotene
> - Celecoxib

9. **Ans. is c i.e. Alveobuccal complex** *Ref. ASI 1st/ed p 348; Oncology and Surgery Journal 2004 p 161*

> **Frequencies of various cancer of oral cavity in India are :**
> - Buccal mucosa 38%
> - Anterior tongue 16%
> - Lower alveolus, floor of mouth 15%

So, *most common* site of oral cancer among Indian population is buccal mucosa or in this question alveobuccal complex (due to their predilection for pan chewing where tobacco is kept in lower gingivobuccal sulcus.

> **Remember**
> - *Most common* site of oral cancer in world: Tongue
> - *Most common* histological variety of oral cancer: Squamous cell carcinoma
> - *M/C* histological variety of lip carcinoma – Squamous cell carcinoma
> - *M/C* histological variety of upper lip carcinoma – Basal cell carcinoma
> - Oral malignancy with best prognosis = lip cancer
> - M/C site for Ca lip = lower lip
> - Oral malignancy with worst prognosis = floor of mouth.

10. **Ans. is a and c. i.e. Base of tongue and Soft palate** *Ref. Dhingra 6/e, p 226, 240*

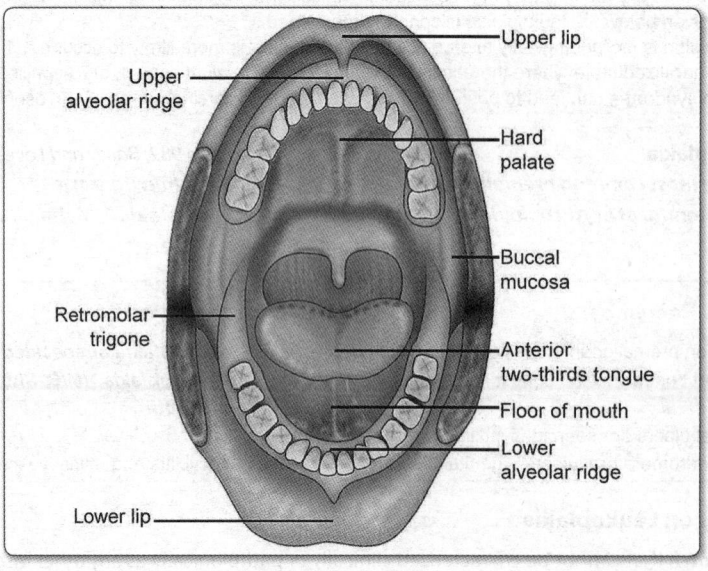

Oral cavity overview

Base of tongue (posterior 1/3rd tongue) and soft palate are parts of oropharynx and not oral cavity   *Ref. Dhingra 6/e, p 240*

Oral cavity includes	
• Lips	• Buccal mucosa
• Gums	• Retromolar trigone
• Hard palate	• Anterior 2/3rd of tongue (oral tongue)
• Floor of mouth	

11. Ans. is b i.e. Lateral border   *Ref. Dhingra 5/e, p 240, 6/e, p 227; Scott Brown 7/e, vol 2, p 2552; Mohan Bansal p 407*

"Most common site of carcinoma tongue is middle of lateral border or the ventral aspect of the tongue followed by tip and dorsum."   *Ref. Dhingra 6/e, p 227*

Cancer	Most common site
• Lip	Vermillion of lower lip
• Tongue	Lateral border
• Cheek	Angle of mouth
• Nasopharyngeal carcinoma	Fossa of Rosenmuller
• Larynx	Glottis

12. Ans. is c i.e. N2
    Ref. Schwartz 9/e, p 491; Devita Oncology 7/e, p 665, 672, 689; Dhingra 5/e, p 241, 6/e, p 228; Mohan Bansal p 406

Classification of stage of tumor of oral cavity based on size of lymph node.

≤3 cm	Between 3 cm and 6 cm	>6 cm
Stage N1	Stage N2	Stage N3

In the given question   :   Size of lymph node is 4 cm so it belong to stage N2
For detailed classification   :   See text given in the beginning.

> **Remember**
> For all head and neck cancers except the nasopharynx, the 'N' classification system is uniform.

13. Ans. is d i.e. Radical neck dissection   *Ref. Bailey and Love 25/e, p 716; Mohan Bansal p 408*

Management of Neck Nodes in Oropharyngeal Cancers

> **If the nodes are clinically negative (i.e. there is occult metastasis)**
> - Generally tongue cancers and to a lesser extent floor of mouth cancers give rise to occult metastases
> - It is always good to actively treat cervical lymph nodes in even absence of obvious disease.
>
> **In Ca tongue with no nodes**
> - Extended supraomohyoid neck dissection (i.e. removal of LN levels I, II, III and IV) in continuity with primary tumor
>
> **In Ca of floor of mouth and mandibular alveolar with no nodes**
> - Supraomohyoid neck dissection (i.e. removal of LN levels I, II and III in continuity with primary tumor)
>
> **If lymph nodes are involved–options are:**
> - Selective supraomohyoid neck dissection (for stage N1)
> - Radical neck dissection (for all other stages)

Now in the question, the size and number of nodes involved is not given but it is given that 'lymph nodes in the lower neck' are involved. So the option supraomohyoid dissection is ruled out (as it is done in case of either occult metastasis or single ipsilateral node < 3 cm) and the obvious answer is radical neck dissection.

14. Ans. is b i.e. Submandibular   *Ref. Dhingra 5/e, p 240; 6/e, p 227*
- M/C lymph node involved in any oral malignancy is Submandibular LN
- Maximum LN metastases are seen in cancer tongue followed by floor of mouth.
- Lymphatic metastasis is least in lip cancer followed by hard palate.

Lymphatic drainage of tongue, Floor of mouth and Buccal mucosa:
- Level I: Submandibular LN
- Level II: Upper deep cervical LN
- Level III: Middle deep cervical LN
- Level IV: Lower deep cervical LN

Lymphatic drainage of oropharyngeal tumors:
- Level I: Jugulodigastric LN
- Level II: Upper deep cervical LN
- Level III: Juguloomohyoid or middle deep cervical LN
- Level IV: Lower deep cervical LN

15. **Ans. is a i.e. Regional lymph node.** *Ref. Devita 7/e, p 682; Schwartz 9/e, p 494*

    "Tumors in this area have a propensity to spread locally and to metastasize to regional lymphatics"
    —*Schwartyz 9/e, p 494, 495*

16. **Ans. is b i.e. Interstitial brachytherapy.**
    As discussed in the text:

Tumor of lateral border of tongue
T1 stage (< 2 cm in size): Interstitial irradiation or excision (partial glossectomy).
T2 stage (> 2 cm) in size: External beam radiotherapy or hemiglossectomy

    In the question, the size of tumor is < 2 cm so TOC is interstitial brachytherapy.

17. **Ans. is c i.e. Verrucous carcinoma.**
    Ref. Scott Brown 7/e, vol 2, p 2561; Diagnostic Histopathology of Tumors by Fletcher 2/e, Vol I, p 211, 212

    Although M/C variety of buccal cancer is squamous cell cancer, Verrucous carcinoma is a variety of well-differentiated squamous cell carcinoma which is locally aggressive involving the bone but lymph node metastasis is uncommon. Histologically, these tumors show marked hyperkeratosis and acanthosis with dysplasia limited to deeper layers. Repeated biopsies report it as squamous papilloma.

    "Histologically verrucous carcinoma are characterized by marked acanthosis, hyperkeratosis often with broad bullous process showing central columns of keratin. There is no cytological evidence of malignancy."

18. **Ans. is c i.e. Segmental mandibulectomy**
    Ref. Devita 9/e, p 746; Cummings Otolaryngology 4/e, p 1608; Oncology and Surgery 2004 p 169
    - Surgery is the treatment of choice in mandible cancers.
    - **Radiotherapy is contraindicated as it can lead to osteoradionecrosis of mandible.**
    - Mandible is managed surgically by marginal or segmental resection.
    - Marginal (rim) resection keeps the outer/lower rim (1 cm thick mandible) intact to mantain cosmesis.
      It is indicated when there is involvement of periosteum only or with minimal alveolar/cortical involvement.
    - Segmental resection removes a full segment of mandible creating a defect which necessitates reconstruction.

Mandibulectomy	
Marginal Mandibulectomy	**Segmental Mandibulectomy**
• Conservative mandibulectomy[Q]	• Entire through and through segment of mandible is resected.
• Refers to partial excision of the superior portion of mandible in vertical phase[Q]	• Results in mandibular discontinuity[Q]
• Inner cortical surface and a prortion of underlying medullary cavity is excised[Q]	• Requires major reconstructive procedure for cosmetic and functional purposes[Q]
• Preserve mandibular continuity[Q]	• Indications:
• Indicated when tumor lies within 1 cm of the mandible or abuts the periosteum without evidence of direct bony invasion[Q]	– Invasion of the medullary space of the mandible[Q]
	– Tumor fixation to the occlusal surface of the mandible in the edentulous patient[Q]
	– Invasion of tumor into the mandible via the mandibular or mental foramen[Q]
	– Tumor fixed to the mandible[Q]

19. **Ans. is a i.e. Radiotherapy** *Ref. Read below*
    Radiotherapy is absolutely contraindicated in carcinoma mandible because it can lead to osteoradionecrosis of mandible.

20. **Ans. is a i.e. Carcinoma lip** *Ref. Cummings Otolaryngology 4/e, p 1594, 1602; Mohan Bansal p 406*

    - Oral malignancy with best prognosis is carcinoma lips.
    - Oral cancer with worst prognosis is floor of mouth carcinoma.

    5-Year Survival Rates in cancer oral cavity

Site	Lip	Tongue	Palate	Cheek
Stage I and II	90%	75%	80%	65–75%
Stage III and IV	50%	40%	40%	50% (Stage III); 30% (Stage IV)

    As is clear from above text for some stage carcinoma lip has highest 5-year survival rate or has the best prognosis.

21. **Ans. is b, c, d and e i.e. Systemic metastasis uncommon; Responds to radiotherapy; Surgery is treatment of choice; and Syphilis and dental irradiation predisposes** *Ref. Dhingra 5/e, p 238; 6/e, p 226; Bailey and Love 25/e, p 740*
    - **Most common site of oral cavity carcinoma in world** is tongue; *In India* it is buccal mucosa. (so option a is incorrect)
    - *Tumors of oral cavity are radiosensitive but because of its serious complications (Xerostomia; Mandibular necrosis) it is not indicated as primary treatment. Surgery is the treatment of choice in tumors of oral cavity.* (So option c ard d both are correct)
    - As discussed in the preceding text – etiological factors for oral cancers are:
      6S viz :
      - **Smoking**
      - **Spirit**
      - **Sharp jagged tooth**
      - **Sepsis**
      - **Syndrome of Plummer-vinson**
      - **Syphilitic glossitis (option e is correct)**
    - Thus option, i.e. syphilis and dental irradiation predispose is correct.
    - M/C method of spread of oral cancers is by local invasion and lymphatic spread.
    - Systemic metastasis is rare (i.e. option b is correct)

22. **Ans. is a i.e. Upper cervical LN** *Ref. Dhingra 5/e, p 239; 6/e, p 227*
    - As discussed earlier M/C lymph node involved in any oral malignancy is submandibular LN. In carcinoma of lips also – submental and submandibular nodes are involved first. At later stages, deep cervical group of LN's may get involved.
    - Submental and submandibular are included in upper cervical LN or level 1 lymph nodes

23. **Ans. is d i.e. Submandibular**
    Ref. Bailey and Love 25/e, p 755; Current Otoloryngology 2/e, p 299; CSDT 13/e pp 239-240; Mohan Bansal p 393

    Stone formation is *most common* in submaxillary (submandibular) gland (80–90% cases) followed by parotid gland (10–20%).

    It can occur at any age with a predilection for men.
    - **Predisposing factors for stone formation** are systemic disease (Hyperparathyroidism, hypercalcemia, gout, diabetes and hypertension) therefore submandibular calculi contain primarily calcium phosphate and hydroxyapatite and are radiopaque and visualized on X-ray
    - Parotid gland calculi are less radiopaque
    - M/C presentation – Recurrent swelling and pain in the submandibular gland exacerbated with eating.
    - **IOC** to detect stones – CT scan *(CSDT/13th/ed p 240)*
    - Sialography is not done routinely and is contraindicated in a patient of sialadenitis.^{Q}

    Management

    Depending on the size of stone and the site at which it is located, it can be removed by:
    - Intraoral extraction
    - Surgical excision
    - Endoscopic removal

24. **Ans. is d i.e. Pleomorphic adenoma**
    Ref. Devita 7/e, p 725; Bailey and Love 24/e, p 730; Scott's Brown 7/ed vol 2 p 2476; Mohan Bansal p 395
    "Pleomorphic adenoma is the commonest tumor found at any site and outnumbers all other tumors in major glands."
    —Scott's Brown 7/e, Vol 3/e, p 2476
    "Pleomorphic adenomas or benign mixed tumors are the M/C neoplasms of salivary gland" —Current Otolaryngology 3/e, p 329

Most common tumor of salivary gland	**Pleomorphic adenoma**
Most common benign tumor of salivary gland	**Pleomorphic adenoma**
Most common malignant tumor of major salivary gland	**Mucoepidermoid carcinoma**
Most common malignant tumor of minor salivary gland	**Adenoid cystic carcinoma**
Most common benign and overall tumor of parotid in children (specially < 1 yr)	**Hemangioma** (Current Otolaryngology 3rd/ed p 332; Maqbool 12th/ed p 209)
Most common malignant tumor in children	**Mucoepidermoid** (Maqbool 12th/ed p 209)
Most common radiation induced neoplasm of salivary gland	**Mucoepidermoid carcinoma.**

25. **Ans. is c i.e. Pleomorphic adenoma** *Ref. Scott Brown 7/e, Vol 1, p 1248*
    "The commonest benign tumor encountered is pleomorphic salivary adenoma accounting for approximately 30% of all pediatric salivary neoplasma. The majority occur within the parotid gland."

    Most common **malignant tumor of salivary gland in childhood:** *Mucoeidermoid carcinoma*, approximately 50% followed by acinic cell carcinoma (20%)— *Ref. Scott Brown 7/e, Vol 1 p 1248, Current otolaryngology 3/e, p 341*

26. **Ans. is d i.e. None**
    Ref. Current Otolaryngology 2/e, p 307-308; 3/e, p 329,330; Dhingra 5/e, p 247

    Pleomorphic Adenoma
    - It is the M/C benign tumor of salivary glands^Q
    - It can arise from the parotid^Q, submandibular^Q or other minor salivary glands of palate and pharynx^Q
        Ref. Dhingra 5/e, p 247; Scotts Brown 7/e, Vol 2, p 2475
    - They represent ~ 60–70% of all parotid tumors and 90% of submandibular benign tumors
    - M/C age group affected is fourth decade
    - M/C gland involved – parotid gland
    - M/C site affected in parotid gland is – tail of parotid gland
    - They are slow growing painless tumors
    - Histologically, they contain both epithelial and mesenchymal elements and are therefore called as mixed tumors.
    - It can rarely undergo malignant transformation (current otolaryngology 2/e, p 308, 3/e, p 330)

    TOC – Surgery – Complete surgical excision of the tumor with uninvolved margins is the recommended treatment, for example, if the tumor is in superficial lobe – superficial parotidectomy is the surgery of choice.
    Prognosis is excellent with a 95% non-recurrence rate.

27. **Ans. is a i.e. Superficial parotidectomy**
    Ref. Dhingra 5/e, p 247, 6/e, p 234; Current otolaryngology 2/e, p 308, 3/e, p 330 and; Short Cases of Surgery 3/e, p 77

    Treatment of choice for pleomorphic adenoma is superficial parotidectomy but, if the deep lobe of parotid is involved, total parotidectomy is done.

28. **Ans. is c i.e. Conservative total parotidectomy** *Ref. Schwartz 8/e, p 540*

    "For parotid tumors that arise in lateral lobe superficial parotidectomy with preservation of CN VII is indicated. If the tumor extends into deep lobe of parotid, a total parotidectomy with nerve preservation is performed."

    In this question tonsil is pushed medially i.e. deep lobe of parotid is also invovled, so conservative total parotidectomy will be done.

29. **Ans. is b i.e. 2nd histologically benign recurrence** *Ref. Devita 7/e, p 725*

    Radiotherapy is indicated for malignant recurrence not for benign recurrence.

Indications of Radiotherapy in Salivary Gland Tumor
• Low-grade neoplasm with close or positive margin
• Facial nerve involvement
• Multiple regional node metastasis
• High-grade histology
• Deep lobe involvement
• Perineural invasion
• Recurrence of malignant tumors.

30. **Ans. is c i.e. Most common in parotid gland**
    Ref. Bailey and Love 24/e, p 731; Robbins 7/e, p 791,792; Dhingra 5/e, p 247, 6/e, p 234; Mohan Bansal p 395

    Mixed tumors of salivary glands are pleomorphic adenomas (as they have both epithelial and mesenchymal elements)
    "80% of salivary gland tumor occur in parotid. Of these tumors approximately 75–80% are pleomorphic adenoma (mixed tumor)."

    Note:
    M/C site for all salivary gland tumors is parotid gland except for:
    - Adenoid cystic carcinoma = M/C site is minor salivary gland.
    - Squamous cell carcinoma = M/C site is submandibular gland.

31. **Ans. is b i.e. Adenoid cystic carcinoma**
    Ref. Schwartz 8/e, p 539; Bailey 24/e, p 685; Dhingra 5/e, p 248, 6/e, p 235; Current Otolaryngology 2/e, p 315; 3/e, p 338

    Perineural invasion is the most constant microscopic finding in adenoid cystc carcinoma.

Adenoid Cystic Carcinoma (Cylindroma)
• *Most common* malignant tumor of submandibular glands.
• *Most common* minor salivary glands tumor.
• *Most common* site minor salivary gland.
• ***Characterized*** by its tendency to invade perineural space and lymphatics and thus causes ***pain*** (which may be a prominent and early symptom) and ***VII nerve paralysis.***
• ***Skip lesions*** along nerves are common.
• It is a ***treacherous tumor*** as it appears benign even when it is malignant.
• It can metastasize to lymph nodes.

- They are highly recurrent.
- Local recurrence after surgical excision are common and can occur as late as 20 years after surgery. Distant metastases go to lung, brain and bone.
- Treatment of choice is *radical parotidectomy* irrespective of its benign appearance under the microscopy.
- Radical neck dissection is not done unless nodal metastases are present.
- Postoperative radiation is given if margins of resected specimen are not free of tumor.

> **Extra Edge**
>
> - The most common histologic subtype (44%) is the **cribriform type**, characterized by a **"Swiss - Cheese"** pattern of vacuolated area. It has intermediate prognosis
> - The **tubular subtype** has the best prognosis while **solid subtype** has the worst prognosis.

32. **Ans. is a i.e. Parotid salivary gland** *Ref. Schwartz 8/e, p 539; Robbin's 7/e, p 794; Current Otolaryngology 2/e, p 315*

    "80–90% occur in the parotid gland and most of the remaining occur in submandibular gland"   –*Current Otolaryngology 2/e, p 316.*

    > **Remember**
    >
    > All salivary gland tumor are *most common* in parotid gland except **adenoid cystic** carcinoma (*most common* in minor salivary gland) and **squamous cell carinoma** (*most common* is submandibular gland).

    > **Important Points about Acinic Cell Carcinoma**
    > - Affect exlusively *parotid gland*
    > - *Low-grade* malignancy
    > - *Hypercellular* tumor with **relative absence of stroma.** It is enclosed in a fibrous capsule
    > - Treatment is **radical excision.**

33. **Ans. is a i.e. An adenolymphoma of parotid gland.**
34. **Ans. is a i.e. More common in females**.
35. **Ans. is a i.e. Superficial parotidectomy**.

    Ref. CSDT 13/e, p 257; Current Otolaryngology 2/e, p 308; 3/e, 330; Dhingra 5/e, p 248, 6/e, p 234; Mohan Bansal p 396

    - Warthin's tumor or **papillary cystadenoma lymphomatosum or adenolymphoma** is 2nd most common benign tumor accounting for 5% of parotid gland tumors.
    - It arises **exclusively** from parotid gland.
    - It almost always occur in **older males** (in 5th to 7th decade).
    - There is increased risk in smokers.
    - *Most common* **site is tail of parotid.**
    - It is *bilateral* in **10%** cases.
    - It consists of papillary cystic pattern lined with cuboidal and columnar cells with core of lymphoid tissue.
    - Treatment of choice is superficial parotidectomy but because of its benign nature and since it can be easily diagnosed cytologically, *surgical removal is not always necessary especially in older or unhealthy persons.*

    > **Remember**
    > - It is only salivary gland tumor that produces **hot spot in 99Tcm** scan so *its preoperative diagnosis is made without biopsy.*
    > - *It never involves facial nerve* i.e. it never becomes malignant.
    > - It is the only salivary gland tumor which is more common in males.

36. **Ans. is a i.e. Mucus secreting and epidermal cells.**

    Ref. Robbin's 7/e, p 793; Dhingra 5/e, p 248; 6/e, p 235; Current Otolaryngology 3/e, p 337

    Mucoepidermoid carcinoma is the M/C type of malignant salivary gland tumor.

    Mucoepidermoid tumor consists of following cells:

    - Squamous cells
    - Intermediate hybrid cells (progenitor of other cells)
    - Mucus secreting cells
    - Clear or hydropic cells.
    - **No myoepithelial cells are seen**

    ### ALSO KNOW

    - Mucoepidermoid tumors similar to other tumors are more common in parotid and have a female predominance.
    - They are malignant tumors which are slow growing and can invade facial nerve.
    - Histologically, the greater is the ratio of epidermoid element, the more malignant is the behavior of the tumor.
    - They are more aggressive in minor salivary glands as compared to major salivary glands.
    - Low-grade tumors are more common in children.

Management

Low-grade Tumors	High-grade tumor
Total parotidectomy with preservation of facial nerve	• Total parotidectomy • Facial nerve may be sacrificed if it is invaded by tumor • Radical neck dissection may be done.

37. **Ans. is a, c and e i.e. Pleomorphic adenoma can arise in subhmandibular gland; Pleomorphic adenoma is the most common tumor of submandibular gland; and Frey's syndrome can occur after parotid surgery**

Ref. Scott Brown 7/e, Vol 1, p 1248; MB p 395-396

Lets Analyze Each Option Separately

- **Option a** – Pleomorphic adenoma can arise in submandibular gland.
  This is correct as *"Pleomorphic adenoma – It can arise from the parotid, submandibular or other minor salivary glands"*
  Ref. Dhingra 5/e, p 247, 6/e, p 234

- **Option b** – Warthin's tumor arises from submandibular gland.
  This is absolutely incorrect as *"Warthin's tumor is found almost exclusively in the parotid gland."*
  –Current Otolaryngology 2/e, p 308, 3/e, p 338

- **Option c** – Pleomorphic adenoma is the M/C tumor of submandibular gland
  This is correct as – *"Plemorphic adenoma – represent approximated 60–70% of all parotid tumors and 90% of submandibular benign tumors."*
  —Current Otolaryngology 3/e p 329

- **Option d** – Acinic cell Ca is most malignant
  This is wrong because – *"Acinic cells carcinomas are low-grade malignancies."*
  – Current otolaryngology 2/e, p 316; 3/e, p 338

- **Option e** - Frey's syndrome *(gustatory sweating)* is a universal sequelae following parotid surgery. *– Bailey and Love 25/e, p 763*

Frey's Syndrome (Gustatory sweating)

- Usually manifests several months after parotid operation.
- Characterized by sweating and flushing of the preauricular skin during mastication.
- Occurs due to aberrant innervation of sweat glands by parasympathetic secretomotor fibers of parotid gland, so instead of causing salivary secretions from parotid, they cause secretions from sweat glands.

Treatment
  - Mostly reassurance.
  - In some cases tympanic neurectomy is done which intercepts these parasympathetic fibers at the level of middle ear.

38. **Ans. is a, c and d i.e. Hypoglossal, Facial and Lingual nerve.**

Ref. Bailey and Love 25/e, p757; Scott Brown 7/e, Vol 2, p 2487,88

Submandibular Gland Surgery

- Unlike the parotid gland where only a part of the gland is removed, total resection of the submandibular gland is always indicated for tumors of submandibular gland.
- Before performing the surgery, the patient should be warned about the following serious or frequent complications
  - **Damage to marginal branch of facial nerve:**
  - This may result in temporary or permanent weakness of the angle of mouth.
  - **Lingual and hypoglossal nerve damage:**
    * This results more frequently, if gland is being removed for chronic sialadenitis rather than tumor
    * It leads to motor dysfunction of tongue which impairs articulation and mastication
  - **Cosmetic defects**

39. **Ans. is d i.e. Acute sialadenitis** *Ref. Sutton 7/e, p 535; Diseases of Salivary Gland by Rankow and Prolayes, p 55; Current Surgical Diagnosis and Treatment 3/e, p 240*

Sialography:

"Use of sialography during period of an acute inflammation of salivary system is contraindicated." *—Sutton 7/e, p 535*
"Sialography is no longer routinely used and is contraindicated in patients with acute sialadenitis." *—CSDT 13/e, p 240*

Chapter 21: Oral Cavity

Sialography

Main Indications of Sialography
- Salivary duct stones
- Stricture
- Fistula, penetrating injury
- Intraglandular and sometimes extraglandular mass lesions.

Contraindications
- Iodine allergy
- Acute sialadenitis

Contrast
- Water soluble media (Meglumine diatrizoate)

ALSO KNOW
- M/C organism leading to bacterial sialadenitis – *Staphylococcus*
- M/C site of sialadenitis – Parotid Gland
- M/C site of sialolithiasis – Submandibular Gland

40. Ans. is b i.e. Pleomorphic adenoma *Ref. CSDT 13/e, p 257; Dhingra 5/e, p 247*
- Pleomorphic adenoma or benign mixed tumor accounts for 80% of parotid tumors and 60% of all salivary gland tumors.
- Most common site is parotid gland though it can arise from submandibular gland, salivary gland of palate upper lip and buccal mucosa.

> **Remember**
> Though Warthin's tumor occurs most common in males, but most common tumor in males still is pleomorphic adenoma.

41. Ans. is a and b i.e. Involves both submandibular and sublingual spaces; and Most common cause is dental infection
See the text for explanation

42. Ans. a. Wait and watch for 4–5 days to allow spontaneous healing *Ref. Dhingra 5/e, p 179; Scott-Brown 7/e, p 1636-1639, Internet search*

"Early cases of post-traumatic CSF rhinorrhea are managed conservatively by placing the patient in the semisitting position, avoiding blowing of nose, sneezing and straining. Prophylactic antibiotics are also administered to prevent meningitis. Persistent cases of CSF rhinorrhea are treated surgically by nasal endoscopic or intracranial approach. Nasal endoscopic approach is useful for leaks from the frontal sinus, cribriform plate, ethmoid or sphenoid sinuses." — *Dhingra 5/e, p 179*

The most appropriate management of a conscious patient of head injury with clear nasal discharge through right nostril with non-operable injury to frontobasal area on NCCT head is to wait and watch for 4–5 days to allow spontaneous healing.

43. Ans is d i.e. Edema of uvula *Ref. Scott Browns 6/e, p 4,5,10*

Quincke's Disease
- Acute edema of the uvula is called as **Quincke's disease.**
- **Etiology** is unknown; but it is related to
  (a) Allergy
     Other causes include
  (b) Trauma (foreign body, iatrogenic)
  (c) Infection
     – Viral pharyngitis   – Candidiasis
     – Syphilis   – TB
  (d) Tumors = Squamous cell carcinoma
- **Clinical features:** Trickling or irritating sensation in the throat together with sensation of gagging.
- **Treatment:** *Edema usually settles down spontaneously. IV hydrocortisone may help.*

> - Collection of pus in the peritonsillar space is known as **Quinsy and not Quincke.**
> - Recurrent edema of uvula with occasional laryngeal edema is seen in hereditary angioneurotic edema (HANE).

44. **Ans is d i.e. Mandible** *Ref. Dhingra 5/e, p 198,199; 6/e, p 185; Mohan Bansal p 346*

> **Le Fort's Fractures Involve**
> - Nasal septum
> - Pterygoid plates
> - Superior orbital fissure
> - Zygomatic processes (frontozygomatic and temporozygomatic)
> - Maxilla
> - Floor of orbit
> - Lacrimal bone

45. **Ans. is c i.e. Le Fort 3 fracture** *Ref. Dhingra 5/e, p 199; 6/e, p 185; Scott's Brown 7/ed. Vol 2 Chapter 128, p 1623*
In Le Fort 3 fracture, there is complete separation of facial bones from the cranial bones i.e. craniofacial dissociation/dysjunction occurs.

46. **Ans. is b i.e. May cause CSF rhinorrhea** *Ref. Dhingra 6/e, p 185*
   - Leforts fracture is fracture of maxilla and not zygomatic bone (i.e. option a is incorrect)
   - It is classified into 3 types – Type 1, 2 and Type 3 (not 5, hence option d is correct)
   - Type 3 is associated with complete separation of facial bones from cranial bones (craniofacial dissociation option c is incorrect)
   - Lefort II and Lefort III fracture may cause CSF rhinorrhea (i.e. option b is correct)

47. **Ans. is a i.e. Fracture of floor of orbit** *Ref. Dhingra 5/e, p 198, 6/e, p 184*
As discussed in theory section–"Tear Drop" sign is a radiological sign seen in blow out fracture of orbit. It signifies entrapment and herniation of orbital content through a defect in floor of orbit into maxillary antrum.

48. **Ans. is a, b, c, d and e i.e. Cheek swelling; Trismus; Nose bleeding; Infraorbital numbness and Diplopia.**

49. **Ans. is b i.e. CSF rhinorrhea.**

50. **Ans is d i.e. Zygoma.** *Ref. Dhingra 5/e, p 197, 6/e, p 183; Mohan Bansal p 344*

Clinical Featuers of Zygoma Fracture: (also k/a Tripod Fracture)
- Flattening of malar prominence
- Swelling of cheeks
- Ecchymosis of lower eyelids
- **Unilateral epistaxis**
- Numbness over infraorbital part of face
- **Diplopia** and **restricted ocular movements**
- **Trismus due to depression** of zygoma on underlying coronoid process
- Periorbital emphysema due to escape of air from the maxillary sinus on nose blowing —*Dhingra, 6/e p, 183*
- Step deformity of infraorbital margin. —*Dhingra, 6/e p, 183*

> **Note:**
> - After nasal bones, zygoma is the second most frequently fractured bone
> - The fracture and displacement can best be viewed by water's view
> - T/t – only displaced fractures require open reduction and internal wire fixation.

51. **Ans. is d i.e. Surgical emphysema** *Ref. Dhingra 5/e, p 199, 6/e, p 185; Tuli 1/e, p 201; Mohan Bansal p 344*
Fracture of maxilla as we have already discussed is classified as Le Fort 1/Le Fort 2/Le Fort 3.

Clinical Features of Fracture of Maxilla—Common to All Types
- Malocclusion of teeth
- Undue mobility of maxilla
- Elongation of mid face

Specific Clinical Features
- CSF rhinorrhea is seen in Le Fort 2 and Le Fort 3 fracture as cribriform plate is injured.
- Injury to infraorbital nerve is seen in Le Fort 2 fracture. *–Tuli 1/e, p 201*
- So anesthesia will be seen in area of supply of infraorbital nerve injury viz. cheek and upper lip (area of supply of infraorbital nerve). *– BDC 4/e, p 118*

52. **Ans. is b i.e. Cribriform plate of ethmoid bone.** *Ref. Logan and Turner 10/e, p 28;*

53. **Ans. is a i.e. Ethmoid sinus** *Scott Brown 7/e, Vol 2 p 1636-1639*
Historically, most common cause of CSF rhinorrhea was head injury with involvement of cribriform plate of ethmoid bone however, now most common cause of CSF rhinorrhea is iatrogenic trauma/surgery.

> **Note:**
> **According to Logan and Turner 10th/ed p 28**
> - Most common area of fracture of CSF rhinorrhea is the cribriform plate of the ethmoid bone as it is extremely thin
> - Other possible areas are –
>   – Posterior wall of the frontal sinus
>   – Floor of anterior cranial fossa
>
> **In the previous edition of Scott Brown** – it was given most common site of leak in CSF rhinorrhea is – **roof of ethmoid sinus > cribriform plate > sphenoid sinus**
> But now in latest edition it is not given.

54. **Ans. is c and d i.e. Nasoethmoid fracture; and Frontozygomatic fracture.**
    Ref. Logan and Turner 10/e, p 28; Dhingra 5/e, p 199, 6/e, p 182; Mohan Bansal p 348

    CSF rhinorrhea occurs in fracture of maxilla in Le Fort type 2 and type 3 (as cribriform plate is injured here) and also in nasal fracture class III.

55. **Ans. is a, b and d i.e. Occurs due to break in cribriform plate; Contains glucose and; Contains less protein.**
    Ref. Turner 10/e, p 28; Dhingra 5/e, p 178; 6/e, p 163–165

    Let us see each option Separately
    - **Option a** – Occurs due to break in cribriform plate. **This is correct**
    - **Option b** – CSF contains glucose and **option d** It has less proteins
      In comparison to nasal secretions – CSF contains more of glucose and less of proteins *(Turner 10/e, p 28)* hence both options b and d are correct
    - **Option c** – Requires immediate surgery
      This is not absolutely correct as:
      – Early cases of post-traumatic CSF rhinorrhea are managed conservatively. Only those cases where CSF rhinorrhea occurs persistently
      – Surgical management should be done.

56. **Ans. is a i.e. Traumatic CSF leak**
    Ref. Dhingra 6/e, p 164

    This is one of the traditional test to detect CSF rhirorrhea, where the bloody nasal discharge is collected on handkerchief or paper towel and a clear ring is seen surrounding a central bloody spot.

    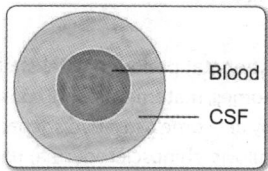

57. **Ans. is a i.e. Antibiotics and Observation**
    Ref. Dhingra 5/e, p 179, 6/e, p 164
    - **Early cases** of post-traumatic CSF rhinorrhea are managed conservatively (by placing the patient in propped up position, avoiding blowing of nose, sneezing and straining) and
    - Prophylactic antibiotics (to prevent meningitis).
    - **Persistent cases** are treated surgically by nasal endoscopy or by intracranial route.
      According to Scott-Brown's 7th/ed Vol 2 p 1641 –
      Endoscopic closure of CSF leak is now the treatment of choice in majority of patients but it should not be done immediately. First patient should be subjected to diagnostic evaluation and after site of leakage is confirmed, it should be closed endoscopically.

58. **Ans. is b i.e. Beta-2 transferrin.**
59. **Ans. is d i.e. Beta-2 transferrin.**
    Ref. Scott-Brown's Otolaryngology 7/e, Vol 2, Chapter 129 p 1638; Mohan Bansal p 348; Dhingra, 6/e, p 164 Table 29.1
    - The only test that should be used to determine if a sample is CSF or not, is **immunofixation of beta-2 transferrin**.
    - Beta-2 transferrin is a protein involved in ferrous ion transport and is found in CSF, perilymph and aqueous humor
    - The sensitivity of the test is 100% and specificity 95%

    > - There are certain conditions which can cause abnormal transferrin metabolism and thus β_2 formation in blood which could potentially lead to **false-positive result**:
    > These conditions are:
    > a. Chronic liver disease
    > b. Inborn errors of glycogen metabolism
    > c. Genetic variant form of transferrin
    > d. Neuropsychiatric disease
    > e. Rectal carcinoma

    For this reason, some authors recommend taking a simultaneous blood sample to exclude this possible source of error.

ALSO KNOW

- Imaging modality of choice to detect the site of leak in CSF rhinorrhea is **T2 weighted MRI**
- High resolution CT can detect CSF rhinorrhea in up to 84% cases but its result should be interpreted with caution, as if there is/has been a previous skull base surgery it will almost inevitably show a large defect in absence of a true leak.
- Historically, many dyes (methylene blue, indigocarmine) were used for diagnosis of CSF rhinorrhea but in recent time only fluorescein is being used. It is used in cases where site of leak is uncertain or there is the possibility of more than one defect.

60. **Ans. is c i.e. Surgical drainage**   *Ref. Tuli 1/e, p 148; Current Otolaryngology 2/e, p 252, 253*
    - The patient in the question had fall from bed following which there is a swelling in nose and slight difficulty in breathing.
    - This patient has probably had septal hematoma which should be drained immediately under LA.
    - For details of septal hematoma–Ref. to the Chapter-Diseases of Nasal Septum.

61. **Ans. is b i.e. After few days**   *Ref. Scott's Brown 7/e, chapter 127 Vol 2 p 1612; Dhingra 6/e, p 182; Tuli 2/e, p 208*

Management Protocol for Nasal Fractures/Injuries

- Most of the patients (~70–80%) do not require any active treatment, as many do not have a nasal fracture and those that do, the fracture is not displaced.
    - Soft tissue swelling can produce the misleading appearance of a deformity which disappears as the swelling subsides. Such patients require only reassurance and topical vasoconstrictors to alleviate congestion and obstructive symptoms. A re-examination should be carried out after 5 days, if there is uncertainty about the need for reduction.
- Immediate surgical intervention in acute phase is required in case of cosmetic deformity and nasal obstruction caused by septal hematoma.
- For rest of the cases the optimal time for clinical assessment is around 5 days, by which time the edema will have subsided and any underlying deformity apparent. Review at 5 days allows sensible planning for reduction of the fracture on an elective operating list within the next 2–3 days.
    - By 7 days the bony deformity will be easily palpable and still movable. Further delay makes effective reduction less likely and sometimes impossible without making osteotomies. Thus best time to reduce fracture of nasal bone is between 5 and 7 days. In children, healing can take place even more quickly and earlier intervention is indicated.

62. **Ans. is c and d i.e. Tertiary syphilis and Cocaine abuse**   *Ref. Internet search*

Causes of palatal perforation

- **Developmental:** During the sixth week of prenatal period, palatal shelve coalesce to form the hard palate. Failure to this integration results in cleft palate. Some syndromes, maternal alcohol consumption and cigarette smoking, folic acid deficiency, corticosteroid use and anticonvulsant therapy are some causative agents for this abnormality.
- **Infectious:** Leprosy, tertiary syphilis, tuberculosis, rhinoscleroderma, naso-oral blastomycosis, leishmaniasis, actinomycosis, histoplasmosis, coccidiomycosis and diphtheria.
- **Autoimmune:** Lupus erythematosus, sarcoidosis, Crohn's disease and Wegener's granulomatosis.
- **Neoplastic:** Different tumors can extend from maxillary sinus or nasal cavity and perforate the palate. Although these neoplasms usually form a mass, but in advanced cases perforation of palate may occur in course of disease or following treatment.
- **Drug related:** Palatal perforation due to *cocaine abuse* is a well-known situation. Other drugs (heroine, narcotics) can be responsible for palatal perforation.
- **Iatrogenic:** Sometimes following a tooth extraction an oro-antral fistula remains. Other procedures such as tumor surgery (maxillectomy), corrective surgeries (e.g. septoplasty) or intubation can cause palatal perforation.
- **Rare causes:** Rhinolith can result in palatal perforation. Patients with psychologic problems may present with a fictitious palatal perforation.

Note: Aphthous ulcers involve soft palate whereas spare the mucosa of hard palate and gingivae.

63. **Ans is a i.e. Lingual vein and e i.e. Cephalic vein**   *Ref. BD Chaurasia p 62-63; Maqbool 11/e, p 172*

Dangerous area of face

> Dangerous area of face includes upper lip and anteroinferior part of nose including the vestibule. This area freely communicates with the cavernous sinus through a set of valveless veins, anterior facial vein and superior ophthalmic vein. Any infection of this area can thus travel intracranially leading to meningitis and cavernous sinus thrombosis.

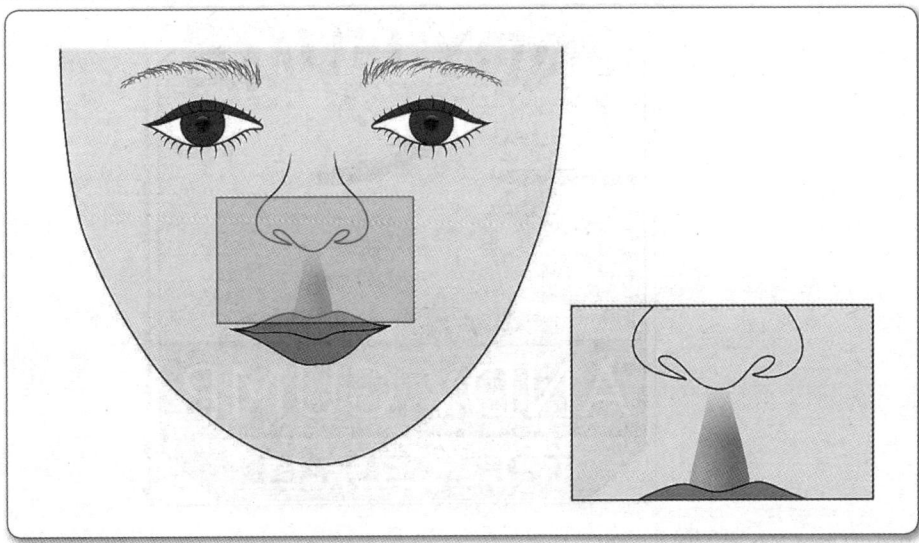

Vein draining dangerous area *M. Maqbool 11/e, p 172*

- Through facial veins communicating with ophthalmic veins (both having no valve)
- Through the pterygoid plexus of veins which communicate with facial vein on one hand and the cavernous sinus through emissary vein on the other hand.

According to B.D. Chaurasia Vol 3, 5/e, p 62

Deep connections of the facial vein include:
- A communication between the supraorbital and superior ophthalmic veins.
- Another with the pterygoid plexus through the *deep facial* vein which passes backwards over the buccinator.

The facial vein communicates with the cavernous sinus through these connections. Infections from the face can spread in a retrograde direction and cause *thrombosis* of the cavernous sinus. This is specially likely to occur in the presence of infection in the upper lip and in the lower part of the nose. This area is, therefore, called the *dangerous area of the face*.

64. **Ans. is a, c and d i.e. Occurs due to defects of the anterior mandibular arch, marginal mandibulectomy can cause it and treatment is adequate reconstruction of anterior mandibular arch with plate and graft** *Ref. Ballenger's Otorhinolaryngology 16/e, pgs962, 963f, 964, Journal of oral and maxillofacid surgery*

   Defects of the Anterior Mandibular Arch *Ballenger's 16th/962, 963f, 964*

   - **Defects of the anterior mandibular arch** cause severe problems that cannot be reversed without formal reconstruction. These problems combine to produce the classic **"Andy Gump" deformity**, named after the 1917 comic strip character whose appearance suggests loss of the anterior mandibular arch.
   - When the anterior mandibular arch is removed, there is usually an associated soft tissue deficit too large to close primarily. A **mandibular reconstruction plate** can be used to secure the remaining mandibular bodies and restore continuity to the arch.
   - As the plate and screws used for reconstruction of the anterior mandibular arch are subject to multiplanar shear, torsion, bending, and loading, the high failure rate of plates not secured to a continuous bony arch is not surprising.
   - Functionally, resection of the anterior arch of the mandible results in disabilities, including drooling and interference with eating, directly related to the amount of bone removed. Esthetically, this "Andy Gump" deformity results in an inferior cosmetic appearance.
   - For instance, **resection of the anterior mandibular arch produces the "Andy Gump" deformity,** which is a complete loss of anterior oromuscular support and oral competence. Because this is such a debilitating functional and esthetic problem, it is important to reconstruct this defect at the time of resection.
   - The " Andy Gump deformity" is a euphemism for an anterior mandibular defect that creates the appearance of an absent chin and lower lip and severly retrognathic lower jaw (Fig. 1). Most commonly, this defect is due to ablative head and neck cancer surgery; however, this deformity is also to describe bilateral body fractures of the edentulous and atrophic mandible or severely retrognathic mandible. 1 In all cases patients with this deformity are at risk for airway compromise cosmetic embarrassment, excessive drooling, mastication difficulties, and speech impairment. Reconstruction is difficult but has become more successful over with improved surgical technology.

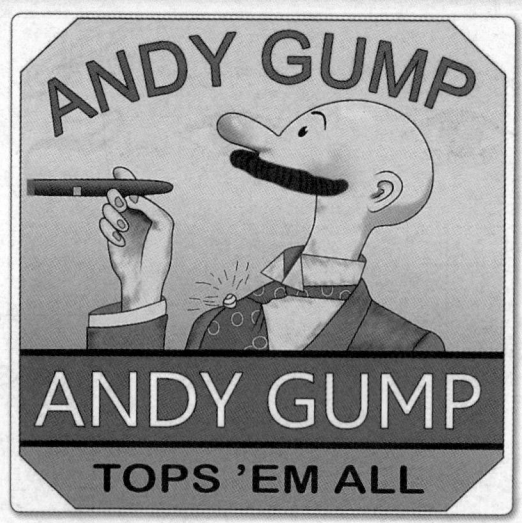

From Journal of Oral & Maxillofacial surgery.

65. **Ans. is a, b and e i.e. Inferior alveolar nerve damage may occur. Panorex radiograph is very useful in management and condylar fracture is the M/C site.** *Ref. P.L. Dhingra 5/e, pgs199-200; L & B 25/e, pgs331-32; CSDT 11/e, pgs1256; Washington Manual of Surgery 5/e, pgs481; Sabiston 18/e, pgs494-95, 2143*

> "The **condylar** neck is the **weakest part of** the **mandible** and is the most frequent site of fracture" Bailey & Love 25/e, pgs331 i.e. option e is correct

> "Many patients with mandibular fractures experience trauma to the **inferior** alveolar **nerve** (a branch of the trigeminal nerve), which runs through a canal within the body of the mandible and terminates in the lower lip as the mental nerve. These patients may experience permanent numbness of the lower lip and teeth on the affected side. Fractures of the coronoid process of the mandible can result in **trismus** (inability to open the mouth) because the coronoid process normally passes beneath the zygomatic arch with mouth opening"—Sabiston 18/e, pgs2143

Thus option 'a' is correct

Fracture of Mandible *Ref. Dhingra 5/e, pgs199-200;*
- Condylar fractures are the most common. They are followed in frequency, by fracture of angle, body & symphysis. Fractures of the ramus, coronoid & alveolar processes are uncommon
- In fracture of condyle, if fragments are not displaced, pain & trismus are the main features & tenderness is elicited at the site of fracture. If fragments are displaced, there is in addition, malocclusion of teeth & deviation of law to the opposite side on opening the mouth.
- X-ray useful in mandibular fractures are PA view of the skull (for condyle), right & left oblique view of mandible & panorex view (i.e. option b is correct).

SECTION 4

Pharynx

Section Outline

22. **Anatomy of Pharynx, Tonsils and Adenoids**

23. **Head and Neck Space Inflammation and Thornwaldt's Bursitis**

24. **Lesions of Nasopharynx and Hypopharynx including Tumors of Pharynx**

25. **Pharynx Hot Topics**

Chapter 22

Anatomy of Pharynx, Tonsils and Adenoids

PHARYNX

Pharynx extends from the base of skull to lower border of cricoid cartilage. Its length is 12–14 cm and width is 3.5 cm at base to 1.5 cm at pharyngoesophageal junction, which is the narrowest part of digestive tract (apart from appendix).

Anatomically pharynx is divided into 3 parts (Figs. 22.1 and 22.2):
- Nasopharynx
- Oropharynx
- Hypopharynx/Laryngopharynx

Nasopharynx

- It is the oval upper part of pharynx situated behind the nose and above the lower border of soft palate and passavant ridge (at C_1 level). It extends vertically from the base of skull to soft palate.
- Since it lies above oropharynx it is also called **epipharynx.**
- It communicates with nasal cavity anteriorly through posterior nasal apertures and posteriorly with oropharynx at nasopharyngeal isthmus.
- The lateral wall of nasopharynx has following structures from below upwards:
  - **Pharyngeal opening of Eustachian tube** (situated 1.25 cm behind the posterior end of inferior turbinate.[Q]) It is bounded above and behind by an elevation called **torus tubaris.**[Q]
  - Behind the tubal elevation lies a pharyngeal recess called **fossa of rosenmuller** (Fig. 22.3). This is not entirely visible even on nasopharyngoscopy.
  - 1 cm behind the middle turbinate is the **spheno palatine foramen**.

> **Point to Remember**
>
> ➤ **Fossa of Rossenmuller** (also called as pharyngeal recess or lateral recess) is the M/C site of origin of nasopharyngeal carcinoma.
> ➤ **Spheno palatine foramen** is the M/C site for origin of angiofibroma.

Contents of Nasopharynx

- **Adenoids/Nasopharyngeal tonsil:** Subepithelial collection of lymphoid tissue at the junction of roof and posterior wall of nasopharynx.
- **Nasopharyngeal Bursa:** Epithelial lined median recess extending from pharyngeal mucosa to the periosteum of basiocciput. Represents attachment of notochord to pharyngeal endoderm during embryonic life. Abscess of this bursa is called as Thornwald's disease.[Q]
- **Rathke pouch:** Reminiscent of buccal mucosal invagination to form the anterior lobe of pituitary. Represented by a dimple above adenoids. A craniopharyngioma may arise from Rathke pouch.

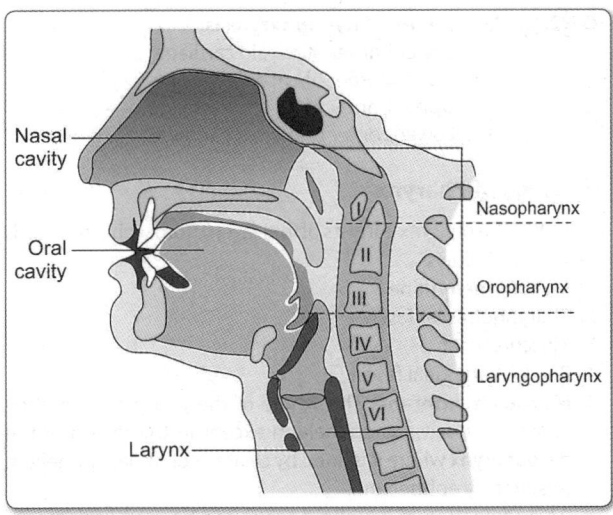

Fig. 22.1: Anatomy of pharynx

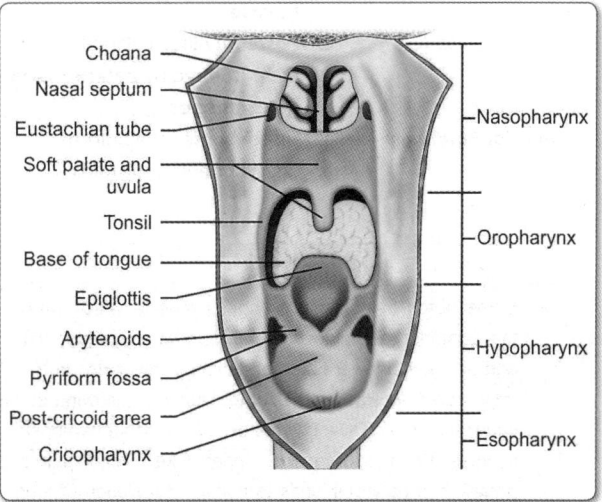

Fig. 22.2: Extent of the pharynx and its divisions

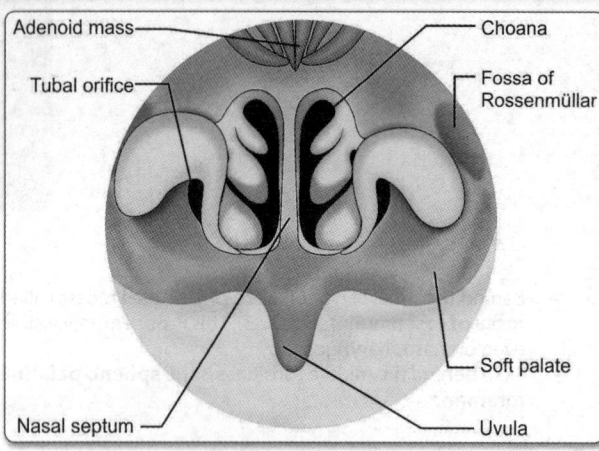

Fig. 22.3: Posterior rhinoscopic view showing the structures of the nasopharynx

Oropharynx

Extends from hard palate above to hyoid bone below:

Boundaries (Fig. 22.2)

Posterior Wall	— Posterior pharyngeal wall lying opposite C2 and C3
Anterior Wall	— a. Base of tongue—posterior to circumvallate papillae
	b. Lingual tonsils
	c. Valleculae—is a depression lying between base of tongue and anterior surface of epiglottis.
Lateral Wall	— a. Palatine (faucial) tonsil
	b. **Anterior pillar** (palatoglossal arch)^Q formed by **palatoglossus muscle**
	c. **Posterior pillar** (palatopharyngeal arch)^Q formed by **palatopharyngeus muscles**
Inferior Boundary	— a. Upper border of epiglottis
	b. Pharyngoepiglottic folds

> **Point to Remember**
>
> ➢ Some fibres of palato pharyngeus muscle which make the posterior pillar, go posteriorly in the posterior wall and along with lower fibres of superior constrictor form a ridge called as **Passavant ridge**. During swallowing and speaking the passavants ridge closes the nasopharyngeal isthmus. When this cannot happen (like in cleft palate, paralysis of palate) it leads to nasal regurgitation of food and nasal tone in speech (called as **rhinolalia aperta**)

Hypopharynx/Laryngopharynx (Lower part of Pharynx)

Lies between body of hyoid to lower border of cricoid cartilage, opposite 3, 4, 5, and 6 cervical vertebrae.

Subdivided into three regions (Fig. 22.3):

- **Pyriform sinus (fossa)**—*Bounded by*:
    - Superiorly — Pharyngoepiglottic folds
    - Inferiorly — Lower border of cricoid
    - Laterally — Thyrohyoid membrane and thyroid cartilage
    - Medially — Aryepiglottic fold.
    - — Posterolateral surface of arytenoids and cricoid cartilages
    - Importance — Forms lateral channel for food
    - — Foreign bodies may lodge here
    - — Internal laryngeal nerve runs submucosally here thus easily accessible for anesthesia and pain is referred to ear in carcinoma pyriform sinus via this nerve.
- **Postcricoid region:** — Lies between upper and lower border of cricoid lamina
    - — Commonest site of carcinoma in females suffering from Plummer-Vinson syndrome
- **Posterior pharyngeal wall:** — Extends from hyoid bone to cricoarytenoid joint.

NEW PATTERN QUESTIONS	
Q N1.	**True regarding nasopharynx are all *except*:**
	a. Fossa of rosenmuller corresponds to the internal carotid artery
	b. Lateral wall has pharyngeal opening of Eustachian tube
	c. Passavant's muscle is formed by Stylopharyngeus
	d. Also called as epipharynx
Q N2.	**Lower limit of hypopharynx is:**
	a. Lower border of cricoid cartilage
	b. Upper border of cricoid cartilage
	c. Upper border of thyroid cartilage
	d. Lower border of thyroid cartilage

Histology of Pharynx

The wall of the pharynx consists of four layers; from within outwards these are as follows:

1. Mucous membrane
2. Pharyngobasilar fascia
3. Muscular coat
4. Buccopharyngeal fascia

1. **Mucous membrane:** The whole of the pharynx is lined by stratified squamous epithelium except in the region of the nasopharynx where it is lined by ciliated columnar epithelium (respiratory epithelium).

An aggregation of lymphoid tissue can be seen underneath the eipthelial lining of pharynx, surrounding the commencement of food and air passage. These aggregation together are called as **waldeyer's ring** which is in the form of an interrupted circle.

2. **Pharyngobasilar fascia:** It is a fibrous sheet between the mucous membrane and pharyngeal muscles. It is thick near the base of skull where it fills the gap between the upper border of superior constrictor and base of skull.

Posteriorly, it is stengthened by a strong band (**median raphe**) which gives attachment to the constrictors.

Note:
- Pharyngobasilar fascia forms the capsule of tonsil.

3. **Muscular layer:**
It is arranged into inner longitudnal layer and outer circular layer.
   a. Inner muscle layer consists of consists of three pair of longitudinal muscles:
      - Stylopharyngeus
      - Palatopharyngeus
      - Salpingopharyngeus
   b. Outer layer muscles consists of three pair of circular muscles:
      - Superior constrictor
      - Middle constrictor
      - Inferior constrictor

Points to Remember

➢ Each constrictor muscle's lower end is surrounded by upper fibres of one below. All the constrictor muscles are inserted into median raphe (Fig. 22.4).
➢ **Gaps in pharyngeal wall:** Total 4 gaps exist in pharyngeal wall.
   1. There is a gap between the base of skull and upper edge of superior constrictor called as **sinus of morgagni**. This gap is closed by pharyngobasilar fascia.
   2 & 3. Two gaps exist between the constrictor muscles.
      - One between superior and middle constrictor and other between middle and inferior constrictor.
   4. Fourth gap lies below inferior constrictor.

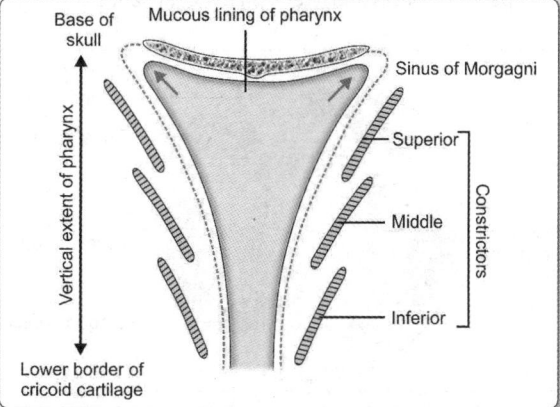

Fig. 22.4: Overlapping arrangement of the constrictor muscles of the pharynx

Table 22.1: Structures passing through the gaps in pharyngeal wall

Gap	Structures passing through
• **Sinus of Morgagni**	P = Palatine branch of ascending pharyngeal artery L = Levator palati muscle A = Ascending palatine artery T = Tensor vetli palatini E = Eustachian tube (Auditory tube)
• Between superior and middle constrictor	• Stylopharyngeus muscle • Glossopharyngeal nerve
• Between middle and inferior constrictor	• Internal laryngeal nerve • Superior laryngeal vessel
• Between lower border of inferior constrictor and esophagus	• Recurrent laryngeal nerve • Inferior laryngeal vessels

4. **Buccopharyngeal fascia:** It covers the outer surface of the constrictor muscles.

Extra Edge

Killian's Dehiscence:

The inferior constrictor consists of two parts:
a. Upper part, i.e. thyropharyngeus with oblique fibers arising from oblique line of thyroid cartilage.
b. Lower part, i.e. cricopharyngeus arises from lateral side of cricoid cartilage and transverse fibers from cricopharyngeal sphincter.

Killian's dehiscence is a gap between oblique and transverse fibers of inferior constrictor.

Significance:
i. A pharyngeal pouch (or **Zenkers diverticulum**) can be formed by outpouching of pharyngeal mucosa at this site.
ii. It is a common site for perforation during esophagoscopy hence called as **Gateway of Tears.**

Benign Hypopharyngeal lesions

ZENKER'S DIVERTICULUM (PHARYNGEAL POUCH) (FIG. 22.5)

- It is a **posterior pharyngeal pulsion diverticulum** through the Killian's dehiscence (area of weakness also called gateway of tears), **between the thyropharyngeus and circopharyngeus parts of inferior constrictor muscle**.
- There is incoordination between the descending peristaltic wave and circopharyngeus muscle at the upper esophageal sphincter leading to abnormally high intraluminal pressure and mucosal herniation through the weak area of Killian's dehiscence.
- Usually seen in elderly above 60 years.
- **M/c symptom is dysphagia**; initially intermittent which becomes progressive later on.
- It is associated with regurgitations of food and cough. Patient may experience **halitosis** and **regurgling sounds in neck**.
- The gurgling sensation palpation of neck is known as **Boyce sign**.
- Diagnosis is by **Barium swallow + videofluoroscopy**.
- Malignancy can develop in 0.5-1% cases.

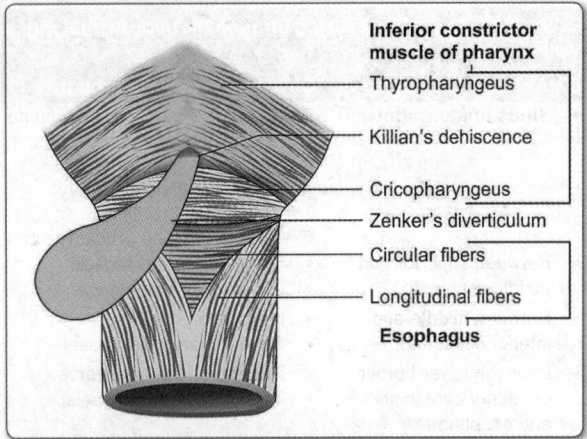

Fig. 22.5: Zenker's diverticulum of hypopharynx herniating through the Killian's dehiscence between the thyropharyngeal and cricopharyngeal parts of the inferior constrictor muscle

Courtesy: Textbook of Diseases of EAr, Nos and Throat, Mohan Bansal, Jaypee Brothers Medical Publishers Pvt. Ltd., p 463

Treatment

- Endoscopic stapling of the diverticulo esophageal septum (Earlier excision of diverticulum with circopharyngeal myotomy was considered to be the treatment of chocie
- In patient not fit for major procedures Dohlman's surgery diverticulotomy may suffice.

Note:
Zenker's Diverticulum is not a true diverticulum.

Points to Remember

- A true diverticulum contains all layers of the esophageal wall while Zenker's diverticula consists primarily of mucosa and submucosa only. It does not have a muscle layer, hence it is not a true diverticulum.
- Zenker's diverticula is a pulsion diverticula.

NEW PATTERN QUESTIONS

Q N3. Tonsils are lined by:
a. Ciliated columnar epithelium
b. Stratified squamous epithelium
c. Cuboidal epithelium
d. Transition at epithelium

Q N4. Which of the following is called as gateway of Tears?
a. Sinus of morgagni
b. Waldeyer's ring
c. Killian's dehiscence
d. Passavant ridge

Q N5. All of the following are true regarding zenkers diverticulum *except*:
a. It occurs in children
b. M/C site for diverticulum is killians dehiscence
c. It is a false diverticulum
d. M/C symptom is dysphagia
e. It is a posterior pharyngeal pulsion diverticulum

Q N6. Boyce sign is seen in:
a. Zenkers diverticulum
b. Barretts esophagus
c. Epiglottis
d. Plummer-Vinson syndrome

Q N7. Dohlmann procedure is done in:
a. Achlasia cardia   b. Zenkers diverticulum
c. Barretts oesophagus d. Schatzki ring

Q N8. A patient presents with regurgitation of food with foul smelling breath and intermittent dysphagia and diagnosis is:
a. Achalasia cardia
b. Tracheoesophageal fistula
c. Zenker's diverticulum
d. Diabetic gastropathy

Waldeyer's Ring (Fig. 22.6)

- It is a group of lymphoid tissue guarding the oropharynx and nasopharynx in the form of a ring.
- The ring is bounded above by pharyngeal tonsil (adenoids) and tubal tonsil, below by lingual tonsil and on left and right side by palatine tonsils and lateral pharyngeal bands.

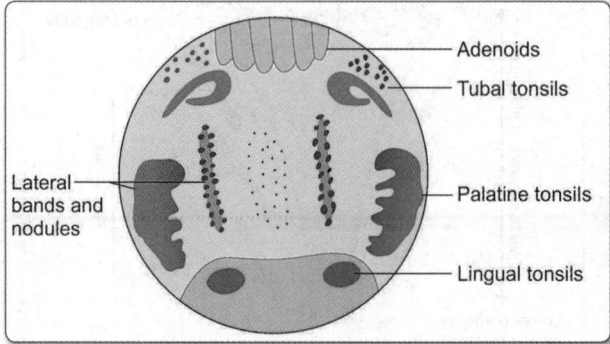

Fig. 22.6: Waldeyer's ring

Chapter 22: Anatomy of Pharynx, Tonsils and Adenoids

Points to Remember

Components of Waldeyer's ring
1. **Palatine tonsils:** Situated in between the anterior and posterior pillars of fauces on each side of oropharynx
2. **Adenoids or nasopharyngeal tonsil:** Lies at the junction of the roof and posterior wall of nasopharynx
3. **Tubal tonsils:** Lies in the fossa of Rosermuller behind the Eustachian tube opening in nasopharynx
4. **Lingual tonsils:** near the posterior 1/3rd, i.e. base of tongue
5. **Lateral pharyngeal bands and nodules:** Lies in posterior pharyngeal wall behind posterior facial pillar

NEW PATTERN QUESTIONS

Q N9. Gerlach tonsil is another name for:
a. Tubal tonsil
b. Palatine tonsil
c. Adenoids
d. Lingual tonsil

Q N10. Which of the following does not form the Waldeyer ring?
a. Palatine tonsil
b. Adenoids
c. Jugulodigastric node
d. Lateral pharyngeal band

Arterial Supply of Pharynx

- Ascending pharyngeal branch of external carotid artery. Ascending palatine branch of facial artery (branch of external carotid), greater palatine branch of maxillary artery.
- Venous drainage is through pharyngeal plexus into internal jugular vein.

Nerve Supply

It is by pharyngeal plexus of nerves which is formed by:
- Branch of vagus (Xth nerve)/Motor supply.
- Branches of glossopharyngeal (IXth nerve)/Sensory supply.
- Sympathetic plexus/Vasomotor supply.

NEW PATTERN QUESTIONS

Q N11. Stylopharyngeus is supplied by:
a. VIII cranial nerve
b. IX cranial nerve
c. X cranial nerve
d. None of the above

Q N12. Supply of inferior constructor is by:
a. Pharyngeal plexus
b. Recurrent laryngeal nerve
c. External laryngeal nerve
d. All of the above

Lymphatic Drainage of Pharynx

- **Nasopharynx**
  - Nasopharynx drains into upper deep cervical nodes either directly or indirectly through retropharyngeal.

Point to Remember

Rouviere's node
➢ This most superior node of the lateral group of retropharyngeal lymph nodes.

- **Oropharynx**
  - Lymphatics from the oropharynx drain into *upper jugular particularly the jugulodigastric (tonsillar) nodes.*
  - The soft palate, lateral and posterior pharyngeal walls and the base of tongue also drain into retropharyngeal and parapharyngeal nodes and from there to the jugulodigastric and posterior cervical group. Note: Lymphatics of base of tongue drain bilaterally.

- **Hypopharynx**
  - **Pyriform sinus drains into upper jugular chain and then to deep cervical group of lymph nodes.**
  - Note: Pyriform fossa have rich lymphatic network and carcinoma of this region has high frequency of nodal metastasis.
  - Postcricoid region drains into parapharyngeal and paratracheal group of lymph nodes.
  - Posterior pharyngeal wall drains into parapharyngeal lymph nodes and finally to deep cervical lymph nodes.

■ PALATINE TONSIL (COMMONLY CALLED AS TONSIL)

- *Palatine tonsil* is specialized subepithelial lymphoid tissue situated in *tonsillar fossa* on the lateral wall of oropharynx.
- **Tonsillar fossa** is bounded by palatoglossal fold in front and palatopharyngeal fold behind.
- Tonsils are almond shaped.
- **It develops from 2nd pharyngeal pouch.**
- **It achieves its maximum size by 6 or 7 years of age**
  (Ref. John Hopkins Manual of Medicine)
- **Tonsils are lined by:** Non-keratinized stratified squamous epithelium,[Q] which dips into the substance of tonsil forming crypts.
- Medial surface of each tonsil has 15–20 crypts, the largest of which is called Intratonsillar cleft or *crypta magna* (which represents the remnant of the second pharyngeal pouch).
- The lateral surface of tonsil is covered by capsule (formed by pharyngobasilar fascia).
- The deep part of tonsil is separated from the wall of oropharynx by loose areolar tissue. This provides for easy dissection of tonsil from tonsillar fossa. Suppuration of this tonsillar space can cause peritonsillar abscess.
- Laterally tonsil is related to tonsillar bed.

- **Tonsillar bed** (Fig. 22.7) is formed from within—outward by:
  - Pharyngobasilar fascia
  - *Superior constrictor (above)* and palatopharyngeus muscle *(below)*
  - *Buccopharyngeal fascia*
  - *Styloglossus*
  - *Glossopharyngeal nerve*

> **Points to Remember**
>
> **Important Relationships**
> - The styloid process lies is relation to lower part of tonsillar fossa, therefore, a hard elongated swelling felt in the posterior wall of tonsil may be on enlarged styloid also.
> - Glossopharyngeal nerve lies in relation to posterior pole of tonsil. This leads to earache in peritonsillar abscess and after tonsillectomy.
> - Since styloid process and glossopharyngeal nerve are related to bed of tonsil hence in styalgia/eagles syndrome (enlarged styloid process) and glossopharyngeal neuralgia these structures are approached by tonsillectomy.
> - Internal carotid artery lies lateral to tonsil so aneurysm of Internal cartoid artery can cause **pulsatile tonsil**.

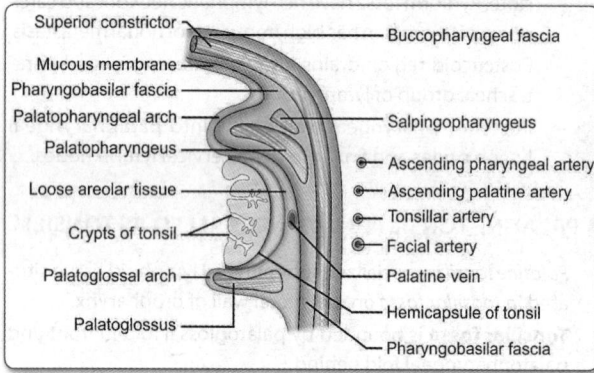

Fig. 22.7: Bed of tonsil

- In between the tonsil and superior constrictor muscle is a space called **peritonsillar space** in which runs the paratonsillar vein.

Nerve Supply

- By the tonsillar branch of the 9th nerve.
- Upper part of the tonsil is supplied by: Lesser palatine branch of maxillary division of trigeminal nerve.

Blood Supply

The entire tonsil is supplied by external carotid artery. The branches of external carotid artery which supply the tonsil are:

- *Tonsillar branch of facial artery (main source)* and is the **most common arterial cause of bleeding** during tonsillectomy.
- Ascending palatine artery another branch of facial artery.

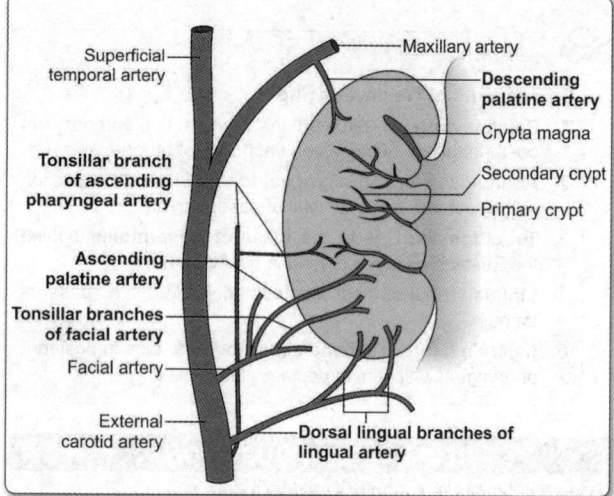

Fig. 22.8: Blood supply and crypts of tonsil

Courtesy: Textbook of Diseases of Ear, Nose and Throat, Mohan Bansal, Jaypee Brothers Medical Publishers Pvt. Ltd., p 55

- Dorsal lingual branch of lingual artery.
- Greater/descending palatine branch of maxillary artery.
- Tonsillar branch of ascending pharyngeal artery (Fig. 22.8).

Venous Drainage

Paratonsillar vein

Lymphatic Drainge

Jugulodigastric lymph nodes (upper deep cervical).

> **Point to Remember**
> - Tonsils have efferent lymphatic vessels but, no afferent vessels.

NEW PATTERN QUESTIONS	
Q N13.	**Crypta magna is seen in:**
	a. Nasopharyngeal tonsil
	b. Tubal tonsil
	c. Palatine tonsil
	d. Lingual tonsil
Q N14.	**Tonsils reach their maximum size by:**
	a. 1 year b. 3 years
	c. 5 years d. 12 years
Q N15.	**Arterial supply of tonsil is mainly by:**
	a. Maxillary artery
	b. Tonsillar branch of facial artery
	c. Middle meningeal artery
	d. Internal carotid artery

Q N16.	The palatine tonsil receives its arterial supply from all of the following except:
	a. Tonsillar branch of facial artery
	b. Ascending palatine artery
	c. Sphenopalatine artery
	d. Dorsal lingual artery
Q N17.	During tonsillitis, pain in ear is due to involvement of:
	a. Vagus N
	b. Chorda tympani N
	c. Glossopharyngeal N
	d. Hypoglossal N

DISEASES OF TONSIL

ACUTE TONSILLITIS

Most commonly seen in school going children but can be seen in adults.

Microbiology

- **M/C cause-viral infections:** Tonsilitis initially starts with viral infection followed by secondary bacterial infection
  - **Viral causes:** Adenovirus > Ebstein-Barr virus > Influenza virus
- In bacteria M/C cause is Group β-hemolytic streptococcus^Q (GABHS)
- **Others:** *Staphylococcus*, *Haemophilus*, and *Pneumococcus*.

Types of Tonsillitis

The components of a normal tonsil are:
- Surface epithelium or mucosa (continuous with oropharyngeal lining)
- Crypts
- Lymphoid tissue

Thus, tonsillitis is classified depending on the component involved:
- **Acute catarrhal or superficial tonsillitis:** It involves the mucosa of tonsils. Tonsillitis is a part of generalized pharyngitis and is mostly seen in viral infections.
- **Acute follicular tonsillitis:** Infection spreads into the crypts. They become filled with purulent material, presenting as yellowish spots.
- **Acute membranous tonsillitis:** It is a stage ahead of acute follicular tonsillitis. The exudation from the crypts coalesces to form a membrane on the surface of tonsil.
- **Acute parenchymatous tonsillitis:** Here, the substance of tonsil is affected. Tonsil appears swollen & uniformly enlarged.

Clinical Features

Symptoms
- Fever (high grade), headche, malaise, general bodyache
- *In acute phase*—sore throat
- Difficulty in swallowing
- Foul breath with coated tongue
- Ear ache

Signs
- Inflamed tonsils, pillars, soft palate, uvula
- Bilateral jugulodigastric lymph nodes are enlarged and tender.^{Q}

Diagnosis
- Pus can be squeezed from the crypts of tonsils
- Throat culture with blood agar plate

Treatment
- **Antibiotics:** Crystalline pencillin for 7–10 days.^{Q}
- Analgesics

[Extra Edge]

Grading of tonsillar hypertrophy: It is based on the percentage projection of tonsil medially from the anterior tonsillar pillar.
- **1+:** up to 25% projection
- **2+:** 25-50% projection
- **3+:** 50-75% projection
- **4+:** 75-100% projection such as kissing tonsils

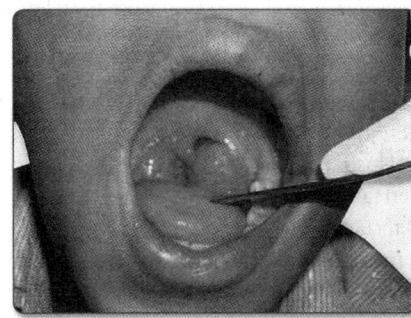

Fig. 22.9: Kissing tonsils

Complication

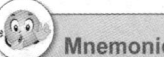 **Mnemonic**

ORA (N)TGE
- O – Acute **o**titis media
- R – **R**heumatic fever and scarlet fever
- A – **A**bscess:
  - Peritonsillar
  - Parapharyngeal
  - Cervical
- (N) T – Chronic **t**onsillitis/Chronic adenotonsillar hypertrophy
- G – **G**lomerulonephritis (Post streptococcal)
- E – Subacute bacterial **e**ndocarditis

Note: Recently, a temporal association between pharyngotonsillitis induced by group A, β-hemolytic streptococci and a new set of obsessive compulsive disorders (OCDs) and other tics has been recognized. This has been called as PANDAS (Pediatric Autoimmune Neuropsychiatric Disorder associated with Streptococcal infection).

Points to Remember

Differential Diagnosis of Membrane Over the Tonsil
- Trauma
- Tumors of tonsil and aphthous ulcer
- Infections: – Candidal Infection (monoliasis)
  – Diphtheria
  – Tonsillitis—membranous
- *For rest*
  VIAL – **V**incent angina (Caused by fusiform bacilli and *Borrelia vincentii*)
  – **I**nfectious mononucleosis
  – **A** – **A**granulocytosis
  – **L** – **L**eukemia.

Chronic Tonsillitis

- It is the chronic inflammation of palatine tonsils which occurs as a result of repeated attacks of acute tonsillitis or due to inadequately resolved acute tonsillitis.
  - **Symptoms**
    * Sore throat—recurrent attacks 3-4 times in a year
    * Cough
    * Halitosis (bad breath)
    * Bad taste in mouth
    * Difficulty in swallowing
  - **The four cardinal signs are**
    * Persistent congestion of arterior pillar
    * **Ervin Moore sign**—A tongue depressor is placed on the anterior pillar and pressed against the tonsil–a yellowish cheesy discharge escapes out from the crypts.
    * Non tender, enlarged ingulo digastric nodes
    * Enlarged tonsils

NEW PATTERN QUESTION

Q N18. Ervin Moore sign in positive in:
a. Acute tonsillitis
b. Chronic tonsillitis
c. Adenoid hypertrophy
d. Epiglottitis

■ TONSILLECTOMY (TABLE 22.2)

Indications

A. Tonsillar Indications (Table 22.2)

Table 22.2: Indications for tonsillectomy

Tonsillectomy	
Absolute Indications	**Relative Indications**
1. Recurrent tonsillitis (most important)	• Chronic Tonsillitis
2. Huge hypertrophic tonsil causing oropharyngeal obstruction leading to sleep apnea	• Tonsillitis in a cardiac valvular disease patient
3. Suspected malignancy of tonsil	• Diphtheria carrier
4. Peritonsillar abscess (after single episode in children and after 2 episodes in adult)	• Streptococcal carrier
5. Febrile seizures due to tonsillitis	• Long-term management of IgA nephropathy
	• Severe infectious mononucleosis with upper airway obstruction

Note:
Criteria for recurrent tonsillitis:
- 7 or more episodes in 1 year or
- 5 episodes year for 2 years or
- 3 episodes per year for 3 years.

B. Non-tonsillar Indications for Tonsillectomy

- As an approach for elongated styloid process (styalgia or eagle syndrome)
- Glossopharyngeal neuralgia
- As a part of uvulopalatopharyngoplasty in obstructive sleep apnea.

Contraindication

Contraindication of tonsillectomy

Mnemonic

- **A.** **A**ctive infection or acute tonsillitis within 2 weeks
- **B.** **B**leeding and clotting disorders
- **C.** **C**left palate, submucous cleft
- **D.** Uncontrolled systemic **d**iseases like HT, diabetes
- **E.** Polio **e**pidemic

Points to Remember on Tonsillectomy

- **Position of patient during tonsillectomy:** Rose position:
- **Position of patient after tonsillectomy:** Lateral position to avoid any aspiration
- **Method of performing tonsillectomy:** Dissection and snaring method
- **M/C complication of tonsillectomy:** Hemorrhage
- **Average blood loss during tonsillectomy:** 50 to 80 ml
- **Average blood loss during adenoidectomy:** 80 to 120 ml
- **M/C cause of bleeding during tonsillectomy:** Paratonsillar vein (Dennis Browne vein)
- **M/C arterial cause of bleeding during tonsillectomy** → Tonsillar branch of facial artery (called as artery of tonsillar hemorrhage)

Hemorrhage Following Tonsillectomy

- The M/C complication of tonsillectomy is haemorrhage
- Haemorrhage can be:
  - **Primary**-occuring at time of operation
  - **Reactionary**-occuring within 24 hours of surgery

  Reactionary haemorrhage is mainly due to slippage of ligature or blood clot formation.
  - **Secondary**-seen between 5th-10th postoperatively.

  The secondary haemorrhage is mainly due to infection.

Management of reactionary hemorrhage following tonsillectomy:
- Removal of clots
- Use of vasoconstrictors
- Ligation of blood vessel in OT under GA
- Applying a pressure pack.

Management of secondary hemorrhage:
- Systemic antibiotics
- Any blood clot removed
- Pressure pack

Instruments used during tonsillectomy

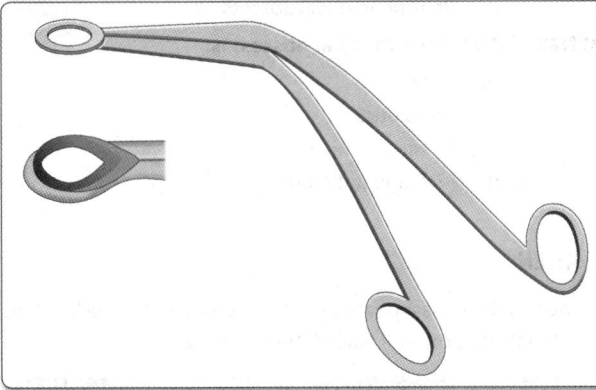

Fig. 22.10: Dennis Browne tonsil holding forceps

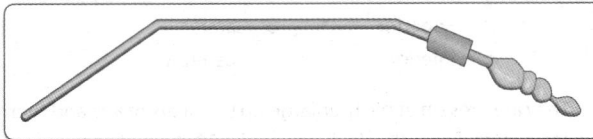

Fig. 22.11: Tonsillar suction

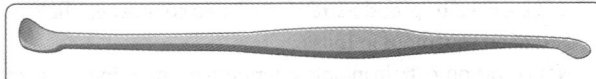

Fig. 22.12: Mollison's tonsil pillar retractor and dissector

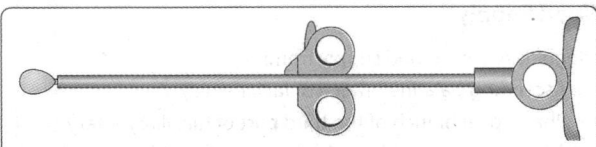

Fig. 22.13: Eve's tonsillar snare

NEW PATTERN QUESTIONS

Q N19. Torrential bleed during tonsillectomy is due to:
a. Facial artery
b. Tonsilar artery
c. Paratonsillar vein
d. None of the above

Q N20. M/C cause of hemorrhage during tonsillectomy:
a. Paratonsillar
b. Maxillary A
c. Lingual A
d. Middle meningeal A

Q N21. Identify the position of the patient during surgery and select the surgeries from the following list where it is used:

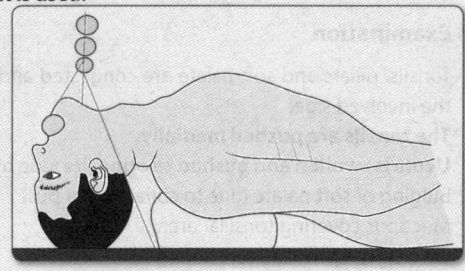

a. Submucous resection of nasel septum
b. Tonsillectomy
c. Myringoplasty
d. Adenoidectomy

Q N22. After tonsillectomy, secondary hemorrhage occurs:
a. Within 24 hours
b. After 2 weeks
c. 5–10 postoperative days
d. After 1 month

Q N23. Tonsillectomy is contraindicated in:
a. Small atrophic tonsils
b. Quinsy
c. Poliomyelitis epidemic
d. Tonsillolith

Q N24. Tonsillectomy is indicated in all except:
a. Quinsy
b. Atrophic tonsillitis
c. Polioepidemic
d. Recurrent acute tonsillitis

PERITONSILLAR ABSCESS (QUINSY)

It is collection of pus between the fibrous capsule of the tonsil, and the superior constrictor muscle of the pharynx.
- **Commonest site:** Upper pole of tonsil.
- **Etiology:** Generally occurs as a complication of acute tonsillitis, but may arise *de novo* without a preceding history of tonsillitis.

- It is generally unilateral.
- **Age group:** Young adults between 20 and 39 years of age. Children rarely affected.
- **Organisms:** Mixed flora (anaerobes and aerobes)/Group A beta-hemolytic streptococcus.

Clinical Features

- High-grade fever with chills and rigor
- **Unilateral throat pain**
- **Hot potato voice**
- Ipsilateral earache (referred pain via IXth cranial nerve)
- **Foul breath**
- Trismus (due to spasm of pterygoid muscles which are in close proximity to superior constrictor muscle)
- **Painful swallowing (odynophagia).**

On Examination

- Tonsils, pillars and soft palate are congested and swollen on the involved side.
- **The tonsils are pushed medially.**
- **Uvula is swollen and pushed to opposite side by the tonsil.**
- Bulging of soft palate (due to collection of pus)
- Mucopus covering tonsillar area
- Cervical lymph nodes are enlarged
- Torticollis: patient keeps neck tilted to side of abscess.

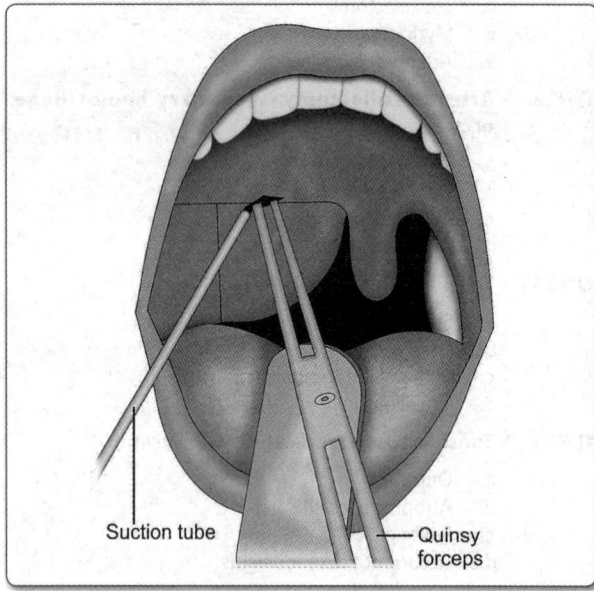

Fig. 22.14: Site of giving stab incision in quinsy

Treatment

Hospitalization

- IV fluids, antibiotics analgesics
- **I and D:** If there is bulging of soft palate or if adequate response is not seen within 24 hours of the antibiotic therapy.

For D and C a stab incision is given at one of the following sites:

1. Imaginary horizontal line drawn at the base of uvula which intersects at a vertical line drawn along the arterior pillar (Fig. 22.14).
2. At the point of maximum bulge.

- **Interval tonsillectomy:** Tonsillectomy done after 6 weeks of quinsy. In children tonsillectomy is done after 6 weeks of 1st attack of quinsy whereas in adults it is done after 2nd attack.
- **Hot tonsillectomy/abscess tonsillectomy:** Tonsillectomy performed in the acute stage. This is not preferred as it can lead to septicemia and hemorrhage.

NEW PATTERN QUESTIONS	
Q N25.	Swelling between tonsillar area and superior constrictor muscle is known as:
	a. Quinsy
	b. Dental abscess
	c. Parapharyngeal abscess
	d. Retropharyngeal abscess
Q N26.	T/t for peritonsillar abscess is:
	a. I & D
	b. Antibiotics
	c. Tonsillectomy
	d. I & D and antibiotics

ADENOIDS (LUSCHKA TONSIL)

- Adenoids are nasopharyngeal tonsils, situated at the junction of roof and posterior wall of the nasopharynx.

NEW PATTERN QUESTION		
Q N27.	Location of adenoids on pharyngeal wall is:	
	a. Superior	b. Lateral
	c. Inferior	d. Posterior

- They are present at birth, enlarge up to 6 years of age and then atrophy and completely disappear by 20 years of age.
- Unlike palatine tonsils, they have no crypts and no capsule and are lined by pseudo-stratified ciliated columar epithelium (stratified squamous in Tonsil).
- Not visible on X-ray in infants < 1 month of age. Clinically seen by the 4th month.

Blood Supply

Adenoids receive blood supply from:
- Ascending palatine branch of facial artery.
- Pharyngeal branch of the third part of maxillary artery
- Ascending cervical branch of inferior thyroid artery of thyrocervical trunk

Lymphatic Drainage

Is into upper jugular nodes directly or indirectly via retro pharyngeal and parapharyngeal nodes.

Nerve Supply

Through CN IX and X **(It is also responsible for referred pain to ear due to adenoiditis).**

Differences between Palatine Tonsils and Adenoids

	Adenoids	Palatine Tonsils
Number	Single	One on each side
Site	Nasopharynx	Tonsillar fossa in oropharynx
Crypts or Furrows	Only furrows	Only crypts
Capsule	Absent	Present
Epithelium	Ciliated columnar	Squamous stratified
In adults after 20 years of age	Absent	present

DISEASES OF ADENOID

ADENOID HYPERTROPHY

Etiology

Rhinits, Sinusitis, Allergy and tonsilitis

Clinical Symptoms (Table 22.3)

Table 22.3: Clinical symptom of adenoid hypertrophy		
Nasal Symptoms	**Aural Symptoms**	**General Symptoms/ Adenoid facies**
• B/L nasal obstruction (M/C symptom)	• Conductive hearing loss due to tubal obstruction	• Elongated dull face • Mouth breathing
• Wet bubbly nose		• Dull expression
• Sinusitis	• Recurrent attacks of acute	• Open mouth
• Epistaxis • Voice change	Otitis media • CSOM	• Crowded upper teeth • Hitched up upper lip
• Voice is toneless, loses nasal quality (Rhinolalia clausa)	• Serous OM	• Pinched appearance of nasal ala • High arched palate • Systemic symptoms – Pulmonary Hypertension

Diagnosis

- Diagnostic nasal endoscopy
- Soft tissue lateral radiograph reveals size of adenoid (CT has no role in diagnosis).

Treatment

Adenoidectomy

- *Traditional method* – Transoral curettage
- *Newer method* – Endoscopic adenoidectomy with forcep, suction diathermy and microdebrider

Point to Remember

> Endoscopic adenoidectomy was first described by Naik et al in 1998 for a case of schiele syndrome.

Indications	Contraindication
• Obstructive sleep apnea • Recurrent ear infections/ Glue ear • Snoaring/UARS • Recurrent sinusitis (Scott Brown's 7th/ed Vol 1 p 1084) • Dental malocclusion	• Submucous cleft of palate (as it can lead to postoperative **velopharyngeal insufficiency**) • Acute adenoiditis, age < 3 years • Bleeding disorders

Instrument used during Adenoidectomy

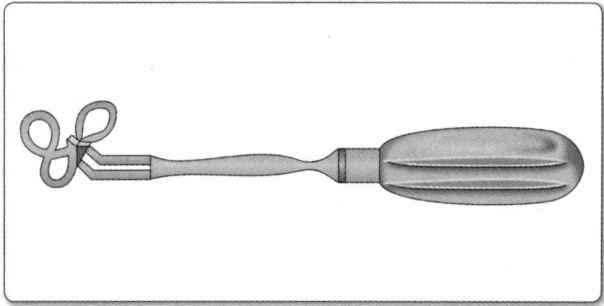

Fig. 22.15: St. Clair Thomson's adenoid curette with cage

Extra Edge

Rhinolalia clausa: It is toneless voice with no nasal component.
Causes:
> Adenoid hypertrophy
> B/L nasal polyp
> Hypertrophic turbinates
> Nasal allergy
> Nasopharyngeal angiofibroma.

NEW PATTERN QUESTIONS

Q N28. A 6-year-old boy presented to ENT OPD with recurrent URTI, mouth breathing and impaired hearing. The boy was diagnosed as having adenoid hypertrophy for which adenoidectomy was done and grommet inserted; 1 week after surgery the boy was again brought to the OPD with torticollis. Which of the following are true about above clinical scenario^Q?

a. Antlantoaxial subluxation is the cause for his torticollis
b. The condition is M/C in children with Down's syndrome
c. Torticollis is not a complication after adenoid surgery and it is a sheer coincidence
d. Adenoidectomy should not have been done in the patient as adenoids would have spontaneously regressed

Q N29. Hot potato voice is seen in all except:

a. Glottic cancer
b. Tonsillar malignancy
c. Posterior tongue malignancy
d. Peritonsillar abscess

Chapter 22: Anatomy of Pharynx, Tonsils and Adenoids

Explanations and References to New Pattern Questions

N1. Ans is c i.e Passavant's muscle is formed by Stylopharyngeus *Ref. Essentials of ENT, Mohan Bansal, p 290*
Passavant's ridge is formed by fibres of palatopharyngeus and not stylopharyngeus.

N2. Ans is a i.e. Lower border of cricoid cartilage
Divisions of pharynx

Division of pharynx	Superior border	Inferior border
Nasopharynx/epipharynx	Base of skull	Soft palate anteriorly, deficient posteriorly (nasopharyngeal isthmus)
Oropharynx	Hard palate	Plane of hyoid bone
Hypopharynx	Plane of hyoid bone	Lower border of cricoid cartilage opposite 3, 4, 5 & 6th in cervical vertebrae

N3. Ans is b i.e. Stratified squamous epithelium *Ref. Dhingra 6/e, p 257*
Tonsils are a part of oropharynx, hence they are lined by stratified squamous epithelium.
Also know: Adenoids are a part of nasopharynx, so they are lined by ciliated columnar epithelium.

N4. Ans is c. i.e. Killians dehiscence *Ref. Dhingra 6/e, p 238*
See the text for explanation.

N5. Ans is a. i.e. It occurs in children
Zenkers diverticulum is seen in elderly above 60 years.

N6. Ans is a. i.e. Zenkers diverticulum
See the text for explanation.

N7. Ans is b. i.e. Zenkers diverticulum
See the text for explanation.

N8. Ans. is c i.e. Zenker's diverticulum *Ref. Dhingra 5/e, p 289-90; 6/e, p 274*
- In Zenker's diverticulum patients present with intermittent dysphagia + regurgitation of food + foul smelling breath.
- Later on the dysphagia becomes progressive.
- In case of achalasia cardia patients present with dysphagia to liquids initially which later on progresses to involve solids also.
- In trachea esophageal fistula patients present with cough during meals causing difficulty in eating.

N9. Ans. is a. i.e. Tubal tonsil

Waldeyer's Ring component	Alternative name
Adenoids	Lushka's tonsil or Nasopharyngeal tonsil
Tubal tonsil	Gerlach tonsil
Palatine tonsil	Faucial tonsil

N10. Ans. is c i.e. Jugulodigastric node

See the text for explanation

N11. Ans is b. i.e. IX cranial nerve *Ref. BDC Anatomy, Vol. 3, p 235*
All the pharyngeal muscles are supplied by the cranial root of accessory nerve (via pharyngeal branch of vagus and pharyngeal plexus) except the stylopharyngeus which is supplied by the Glossopharyngeal nerve.

N12. Ans is d. i.e. All of the above *Ref. BDC Anatomy, Vol 3, p 235*
The superior and middle constructor are supplied by pharyngeal plexus.
The inferior constrictor receives an additional supply from the external and recurrent laryngeal nerves

N13. Ans. is c i.e. Palatine tonsil *Ref. Dhingra 6/e, p 257*
The medial surface of palatine tonsils is covered by non keratinizing stratified squamous epithelium which dips into the substance of tonsil in the form of crypts. One of these crypts is very large and deep and is called crypta magna or intratonsillar cleft.

N14. Ans. is c. i.e. 5 years   *Ref. John Hopkins Manual medicine*

Tonsils reach there maximum size by 6-7 years of age. But here the closest option is 5 years.

N15. Ans. is b. i.e. Tonsillar branch of facial artery   *Ref. Dhingra 6/e, p 257*

Main artery supplying tonsil is tonsillar branch of facial artery.

N16. Ans. is c i.e. Sphenopalatine artery   *Ref. Dhingra 6/e, p 257*

The tonsils are supplied by five arteries viz:
1. Tonsillar branch of facial artery
2. Ascending pharyngeal artery from external carotid artery
3. Ascending palatine, branch of facial atery
4. Dorsal lingual branches of lingual artery
5. Descending palatine branch of maxillary artery

N17. Ans. is c i.e. Glossopharyngeal N

The tympanic nerve (Jacobson nerve, a branch of cranial nerve IX) directly innervates the ear but also has pharyngeal, lingual and tonsillar branch to supply the posterior 1/3rd part of tongue, tonsillar pillar, pharynx and eustachian tube.

N18. Ans is b i.e. Chronic tonsillitis   *Ref. Textbook of ENT, Hazarika 3/e, p 480*

Irwin-Moore sign: Expression of cheesy material from the tonsil, on pressing anterior pillar in case of chronic tonsillitis.

N19. Ans. is b i.e. Tonsillar artery

N20. Ans. is a i.e. Paratonsillar vein

> - M/C cause of bleeding during tonsillectomy: Paratonsillar vein (Denis Browne vein)
> - M/C arterial cause of bleeding or M/C cause of torrential bleeding during tonsillectomy: Tonsillar branch of facial artery (called as artery of tonsillar haemorrhage).

N21. Ans. is b i.e. Tonsillectomy   *Ref. Dhingra 5/e, p 438,439–442; Mohan Bansal p 569*

The position drawn in figure is 'Rose position' where patient lies supine with head extended by placing a pillow under the shoulder—Rose position is used during.
  i. Tonsillectomy
  ii. Adenoidectomy
  iii. Tracheostomy

N22. Ans is c. i.e. 5–10 postoperative days   *Ref. Dhingra 6/e, p 430*

Haemorrhage following tonsillectomy can be:
- Primary – occuring at the time of surgery
- Reactionary – occuring within 24 hours of surgery
- Secondary – Seen between 5–10 postoperative days.

N23. Ans. is c i.e. Poliomyelitis epidemic   *Ref. Dhingra 6/e, p 257*

Already expalined.

N24. Ans. is c i.e. Polioepidemic

Tonsillectomy is contraindicated during polio epidemic.

N25. Ans is a i.e. Quinsy

Peritonsillar abscess or Quinsy is collection of pus between the fibrous capsule of the tonsil and superior constrictor muscle of pharynx.

N26. Ans. is d i.e. I & D and antibiotics

See the text for explanation.

N27. Ans. is d i.e. Posterior   *Ref. Dhingra 6/e, p 243*

See the text for explanation.

N28. Ans. is a and b i.e. Antlantoaxial subluxation is the cause for his torticollis and the condition is M/C in children with Down's syndrome.   *Ref. Current Otolaryngology 3/e, p 363*

Torticollis can occur as a complication of adenoidectomy due to ligamentous laxity secondary to inflammatory process following adenoidectomy. It is called as Grisel syndrome.

This is M/C in patients of Down syndrome as children with Down's already have asymptomatic atlantoaxial instability which manifests after surgery.

N29. Ans. is a i.e. Glottic cancer

Hot potato voice is a speech which has muffled quality.

Aetiology

- **Space occupying lesions of oropharynx**, e.g. lymphoid masses (Tonsillar lymphoma) Quinsy, Tumors of the vallecula between the epiglottis and base of tongue
- **In patients with supraglottic cancer** — Hot potato voice can be seen.
- **Post one-third/base of tongue malignancy** (SRB Manual of Surgery, pg 394).

Thus note: Hot potato voice is seen in supraglottic cancer, not glottic cancer.

QUESTIONS

1. Which of the following part is NOT included in hypopharynx is? [UP 01]
   a. Pyriform sinus
   b. Post cricoid region
   c. Anterior pharyngeal wall
   d. Posterior pharyngeal wall

2. Which of the following structures is seen in oropharynx? [TN 06]
   a. Pharyngotympanic tube
   b. Fossa of Rosenmuller
   c. Palatine tonsil
   d. Pyriform fossa

3. The lymphatic drainage of pyriform fossa is to: [Delhi 96]
   a. Upper deep cervical nodes
   b. Prelaryngeal node
   c. Parapharyngeal nodes
   d. Mediastinal nodes

4. Killian's dehisence is seen in: [MH 00]
   a. Oropharynx
   b. Nosophrynx
   c. Cricopharynx
   d. Vocal cords

5. 6-year-old child with recurrent URTI with mouth breathing and failure to grow with high arched palate and impaited hearing is: [AIIMS May 07, 2012]
   a. Tonsillectomy
   b. Grommet insertion
   c. Myringotomy with grommet insertion
   d. Adenoidectomy with grommet insertion

6. Regarding adenoids true is/are: [PGI 02]
   a. There is failure to thrive
   b. Mouth breathing is seen
   c. CT scan should be done to assess size
   d. High-arched palate is present
   e. Immediate surgery even for minor symptoms

7. Indication for Adenoidectomy in children include all except: [AP 00]
   a. Recurrent respiratory tract infections
   b. Recurrent middle ear infection with deafness
   c. Chronic serous otitis media
   d. Multiple adenoids

8. The inner Waldeyer's group of lymph nodes does not include: [AP 93 test I- General; TN 86, 00]
   a. Submandibular lymph node
   b. Tonsils
   c. Lingual tonsils
   d. Adenoids

9. The most common organism causing acute tosillitis is: [TN 95]
   a. Staph aureus
   b. Anaerobes
   c. Hemolytic streptococci
   d. Pneumococcus

10. All of the following cause a gray-white membrane on the tonsils, except: [AIIMS May 04]
    a. Infectious mononucleosis
    b. Ludwig's angina
    c. Streptococcal tonsillitis
    d. Diphtheria

11. Tonsillectomy is indicated in: [AI 94]
    a. Acute tonsillitis
    b. Aphthous ulcers in the pharynx
    c. Rheumatic tonsillitis
    d. Physiological enlargement

12. A 5-year-old patient is scheduled of for tonsillectomy. On the day of surgery he had running nose, temperature, 37.5°C and dry cough. Which of the following should be the most appropriate decision for surgery? [AI 06]
    a. Surgery should be canceled
    b. Can proceed for surgery, if chest is clear and there is no history of asthma
    c. Should get X-ray chest before proceeding for surgery
    d. Cancel surgery for 3 weeks and patient to be on antibiotic

13. Tonsillectomy: following peritonsillar abscess is done after weeks: [PGI 97, 98]
    a. 1–3 weeks
    b. 6–8 weeks
    c. 4–6 weeks
    d. 8–12 weeks

14. Most common postoperative complication of tonsilectomy is: [PGI 85]
    a. Palatal palsy
    b. Hemorrhage
    c. Injury to uvula
    d. Infection

15. Secondary hemorrhage after tonsillectomy develops:
    a. Within 12 hrs [AI 11]
    b. Within 24 hrs
    c. Within 6 days
    d. Within 1 months

16. Ramu, 15 years of age presents with hemorrhage 5 hours after tonsillectomy. Treatment of choice is: [AIIMS 99]
    a. External gauze packing
    b. Antibiotics and mouth wash
    c. Irrigation with saline
    d. Reopen immediately

17. Contraindication of adenotonsillectomy: [PGI 04]
    a. Age < 4 years
    b. Poliomyelitis
    c. Haemophilus infection
    d. Upper RTI

18. In which of the following locations, there is collection of pus in the quinsy: [AIIMS 04]
    a. Peritonsillar space
    b. Parapharyngeal space
    c. Retropnaryngeal space
    d. Within the tonsil

19. **Feature(s) of peritonsillar abscess:** *[PGI Nov 16]*
    a. Foul breath
    b. Hot potato voice
    c. Shifting of uvula in opposite side
    d. Difficulty in swallowing even own saliva
    e. Always present as B/L severe pain in threat
20. **True about quinsy is:** *[PGI 02]*
    a. Penicillin is used in treatment
    b. Abscess is located in capsule
    c. Commonly occurs bilaterally
    d. Immediate tonsillectomy should be done
    e. Patient presents with toxic features and drooling
21. **7-year-old child has peritonsillar abscess presents with trismus, the best treatment is:** *[AIIMS 96]*
    a. Immediate abscess drain orally
    b. Drainage externally
    c. Systemic antibiotics up to 48 hours then drainage
    d. Tracheostomy
22. **All of the following are ture about Zenker's diverticulum except:** *[PGI 02]*
    a. It is an acquired condition
    b. It is a false diverticulum
    c. Barium swallow, lateral view is the investigation of chioce
    d. Out poucing of anterior pharyngeal wall above circopharyngeus muscles
    e. Patient presents with toxic features and drooling
23. **Which of the following is not a complication of adenoidectomy?** *[AIIMS Nov 14]*
    a. Hyponasality of speech
    b. Retro pharyngeal abscess
    c. Velopharyngeal insufficiency
    d. Grisel syndrome

Explanations and References

1. **Ans. is c i.e. Anterior pharyngeal wall**   *Ref. Mohan Bansal p 56; Dhingra 6/e, p 241*
2. **Ans. is c i.e. Palatine tonsil**   *Ref. Scott Brown's 7/e, Vol 2, p 1944,1945; Mohan Bansal, p 52; Dhingra 6/e, p 240*

   Pharynx is divided into:

Nasopharynx	Hypopharynx/Laryngopharynx	Oropharynx
Important contents of nasopharynx	It is further divided into	Major structures included in it are:
• Adenoids	• Pyriform sinus	• Liagual tonsil
• Nasopharyngeal bursa	• Postcricoid region	• Palatine tonsil
• Rathke pouch	• Post pharyngeal wall	• Soft palate
• Sinus of Morgagni		• Tongue base
• Passavant ridge		

3. **Ans. is a i.e. Upper deep cervical nodes**   *Ref. Tuli 1/e, p 231, 232; Dhingra 5h/e p 257*
   - *Pyriform sinus* drains into upper jugular chain and then to deep cervical group of lymph nodes.
   - *Postcricoid region* drains into parapharyngeal and paratracheal group of lymph nodes.
   - *Posterior pharyngeal* wall drains into parapharyngeal lymph nodes and finally to deep cervical lymph nodes.
4. **Ans. is c i.e. Cricopharynx**   *Ref. Scott Brown's 7/e, Vol 2, Chapter 155, p 2045; Dhingra 5/e, p 253, 6/e, p 238*

   Killian's Dehiscence (Fig. 22.7)
   - It is an area of weakness between the two parts of inferior constrictor muscle—subthyropharyngeus and cricopharyngeus
   - Since it is an area of weakness it is one of the sites of esophageal perforation during instrumentation and scopy—hence also called **'Gateway of Tears'**.
   - It is lined by stratified squamous epithelium.

   Also Know:

   > - **Killian-Janieson's space** – It lies between cricopharyngeus and circular fibres of the esophagus.
   > - **Lamier Hackerman triangle** – It lies between circular and longitudinal fibers of esophagus.

5. **Ans. is d i.e. Adenoidectomy with grommet insertion**   *Ref. Scott Brown 7/e, Vol 1 p 896-906*
   The child is having recurrent URTI with high arched palate and failure to grow which indicates child is having adenoids and since there is impaired hearing it means child has developed otitis media as a complication.
   Hence logically the child should be treated with adenoidectomy with grommet insertion. This is further supported by following lines from Scott Brown.
   "Current practice is to perform adenoidectomy as an adjunct to the insertion of ventilation tubes."   *Ref: Scott Brown's 7/e, Vol 1, p 902*

6. **Ans. is a, b, d i.e. There is failure to thrive; Mouth breathing is seen, and High arched palate**
        Ref. Dhingra 5/e, p 258, 259, 6/e, p 243–244; Logan Turner 10/e, p 367; Mohan Bansal p 52
   - High arched palate and mouth breathing are features of hypertrophied adenoids which leads to adenoid facies
   - In adenoids as a consequence of recurrent nasal obstruction and URTI, child develops failure to thrive
   - Size of adenoids may well be assessed using lateral radiograph of nasopharynx, and CT scan is not necessary (Ruling out option c). Surgery is indicated only in hypertrophy causing severe symptoms. (Ruling out option e)
7. **Ans. is b i.e. Recurrent Middle ear infection with deafness**   *Ref. Dhingra 5/e, p 442, 6/e, p 131*
   There is growing evidence in literature for adenoidectomy as a first-line surgical intervention for chronic rhinosinusitis in children who have failed maximal medical treatment   *Ref. Scott Brown 7/e, Vol 1, p 1084*

   Indications for Adenoidectomy
   - Recurent otitis media with effusion (glue ear)
   - Recurrent sinusitis
   - Obstructive sleep apnea
   - Snoring UARS
   - Dental malocclusion

   Note: There is no term like multiple adenoids.

Chapter 22: Anatomy of Pharynx, Tonsils and Adenoids

8. **Ans. a i.e. Submandibular lymph nodes** *Ref. Current Otolaryngology 2/e, p 340, 341; Scott Brown 7/e, Vol 2, p 1793*
   Submandibular nodes do not form part of Waldeyer's lymphatic ring. They form part of the outer group of lymph nodes into which efferents from the constituents of the Waldeyer's lymphatic ring may drain.

   > Waldeyer ring consists of:
   > 1. Adenoids (nasopharyngeal tonsil)
   > 2. Tubal tonsil (Fossa of Rosenmuller)
   > 3. Lateral pharyngeal bands
   > 4. Palatine tonsils
   > 5. Nodules (postpharyngeal wall)
   > 6. Lingual tonsils

9. **Ans. is c i.e. Hemolytic streptococci** *Ref. Dhingra 5/e, p 341, 6/e, p 288; Current Otolaryngology 2/e, p 341*
   Group A beta-hemolytic streptococci is the M/C bacteria causing acute tonsillitis
   Other causes are:
   - *Staphytococci*
   - *Pneumococci*
   - *H. influenza*

10. **Ans b i.e. Ludwig angina** *Ref. Dhingra 5/e, p 274, 6/e, p 259–260*
    Ludwigs angina is cellulitis of submandibular space. It does not lead to membrane formation over tonsils.
    For causes of membrane over tonsil see the preceding text for explanation.

11. **Ans. is c i.e. Rheumatic tonsillitis**
    Ref. Scott Brown's 7/e, Vol 2, p 1989,1990, Vol 1 p 1232; Dhingra 5/e, p 438, 6/e, p 428; Mohan Bansal p 567
    Kindly see the preceding text for indications of tonsillectomy.

12. **Ans. is d i.e. Cancel surgery for 3 weeks and patient to be on antibiotic**
    Ref. Logan Turner's 10/e, p 365,366, Current Otolaryngology 2/e, p 178; Dhingra 6/e, p 428
    "There are no absolute contraindications to tonsillectomy. As such tonsillectomy is an elective operation and should not be undertaken in presence of respiratory tract infections or during the period of incubation of after contact with one of the infectious disease, if there is tonsillar inflammations. It is much safer to wait some 3 weeks after an acute inflammatory illness before operating because of the greatly increased risk of postoperative haemorrhage." *Ref. Turner 10/e, p 365,366*

    Tonsillectomy and Adenoidectomy
    "Patient may present with upper respiratory tract infections. Surgery for these patients should be postponed until the infection is resolved. Usually 7–14 days. These patients may develop a laryngospasm with airway manipulation. This complication carries the potential for significant morbidity and even mortality." *Ref. Current Otolaryngology 2/e, p 173*

13. **Ans. is b i.e. 6–8 weeks** *Ref. Turner 10/e, p 86; Head and Neck Surgery by Chris DeSouza Vol 2, p 1583*
    - Friends, Dhingra and Turner have a different opinions on this one.
    - According to Turner 10th/ed p 86—**"The tonsils should be removed 6–8 weeks following a Quinsy."**
    - According to Dhingra 6th/ed p 265—**"Tonsils are removed 4-6 weeks following an attack of Quinsy."**
    - According to Head and Neck Surgery-
    - Quinsy – **"Most people would practise interval tonsillectomy for these patients, deferring surgery for 6 weeks following resolution of an attack."** *Ref. Head and Neck Surgery by Chris de Souza Vol 2, p 1583*
    So, after reading all the above texts – I think 6–8 weeks is a better option.

14. **Ans. is b i.e. Hemorrhage**
    Ref. Dhingra 5/e, p 441; 6/e, p 430; Maqbool 11/e, p 288; Scott Brown's 7/e, Vol 2, p 1994; Mohan Bansal, p 571

15. **Ans. is c i.e. Within 6 days** *Ref. Mohan Bansal, p 571, Dhingra 6/e, p 430*
    "The main complication is hemorrhage which occurs in 3–5% patients" Ref. Head and Neck Surgery de Souza Vol 2, p 1588
    "Most common complication following tonsillectomy is hemorrhage." *Ref. Maqbool 11/e, p 288*
    "Reactionary hemorrhage is the most feared complication post tonsillectomy because of the risk of airway obstruction, shock and ultimately death." *Ref. Scott Brown's 7/e, Vol 2, p 1994*

    Hemorrhage can be

Primary	Reactionary	Secondary
Occurring at the time of surgery	Occurring within 24 hours of surgery	Seen between the 5th to 10th postoperative day

    Also know: Most common time of hemorrhage after tonsillectomy is within 4 hrs of surgery

16. **Ans. is d i.e. Reopen immediately** *Ref. Turner 10/e, p 366*
    "Reactionary hemorrhage occurs within a few hours of the operation and may be severe. It may occur after operation and is treated by a return to the theater when the vessle is ligated under anesthesia." *Ref. Turner 10/e, p 366*

Also Know
- Reactionary haemorrhage mostly occurs due to dislodgement of any clot or because BP of patient comes back to normal after hypotensive anaesthesia.
- Secondary haemorrhage mainly occurs due to infection.

Indications for blood transfusion in a case of Tonsillectomy
- End-stage renal disease
- Hypertension
- Reduced hemoglobin and hematocrit

In all these patients, if secondary hemorrhages occur – immediately return to OT to avoid severe complications

17. Ans. is b, c and d i.e. Poliomyelitis; Haemophilus infection; and Upper RTI *Ref. Turner 10/e, p 365,366; Mohan Bansal, p 568*
- As explained earlier, Tonsillectomy should not be performed during epidemics of poliomyelitis. This is because there are evidences that the virus may gain access to the exposed nerve sheaths and give rise to the fatal bulbar form of the disease.
- It should not be undertaken in the presence of respiratory tract infections or during the period of incubation of after contact with one of the infectious disease (i.e. Haemophilus) or if there is tonsillar inflammation.
- It is safer to wait for 3 weeks after an acute inflammatory disease, before performing tonsillectomy

According of Turner - Tonsillectomy can be performed at any age, if there are sufficient indications for their removal.
According to Dhingra - 6/e, p 428, Children < 3 years (Not < 4 years as given in the options) are poor candidates for surgery. So tonsillectomy should not be done in them.

According to Head and Neck Surgery de Souza –
"As tonsillar tissue has a role in the development of the immune system, it is advisable that surgery should be delayed until the age of 3 whenever possible." *Ref. Head and Neck Surgery Chris de Souza, Vol 2, p 1587*

18. Ans. is a i.e. Peritonsillar space *Ref. Dhingra 5/e, p 278, 279, 6/e, p 264*
Quinsy is collection of pus in the peritonsillar space which lies between the capsule of tonsil and superior constrictor muscle i.e. peritonsillar abscess.

19. Ans. is a, b, c and d i.e. foul breath, hot potato voice shifting of uvula in opposite side and difficulty in swallowing even own saliva

Quinsy/Paratonsillar abscess
- Collection of pus in peritonsillar space
- It leads to severe **unilateral throat pain (option e is incorrect)**
- Odynophagia–i.e. pain during swallowing is so much that patient has difficulty in swallowing his/her own salivas (i.e. option d is correct)
- Muffled and thick speech called as **hot potato voice (i.e. option b is correct)**
- Foul breath due to sepsis in oral **cavity (i.e. option a correct)**
- Ipsilateral ear ache (referred pain via CNIX)
- Trismus due to spasm of pterygoid muscles

O/E
- Uvula is swollen and pushed to opposite side
- Tonsils and soft pillar of involved side are congested and swollen
- Torticollis is seen

20. Ans. is a and e Penicillin is used in treatment and Patient presents with toxic features and drooling
Ref. Logan Turner 10/e, p 86; Dhingra 5/e, p 279, 6/e, p 248; Scott's Brown 7/e, Vol 2, p 1996,1997
- Quinsy is collection of pus outside the capsule (not in capsule) in peritonsillar area
- t is usually unilateral
- Patient present with toxic symptoms due to septicemia as well as local symptoms (e.g. dribbling of saliva from mouth)
- Antibiotics: High-dose panicillin. (IV benzipenicillin) is the DOC. In patients allergic to penicillin, erythromycin is the DOC. If antibiotics fail to relieve the condition within 48 hours, then the abscess must be opened and drained.

21. Ans. is c i.e. Systemic antibiotics up to 48 hours and then drainage
Ref. Harrison 17/e, p 211; Scott's brown 7/e, Vol 2, p 1997; Turner 10/e, p 86
Treatment of quinsy include IV antibiotics and if it fails to relieve the condition in 24–48 hours, the abscess must be opened and drained.

22. Ans. is d i.e. Outpouching of anterior pharyngeal wall above cricopharyngeus muscle *Ref. Dhingra 5/e, p 289-90, 6/e, p 274*
Zenker's diverticulum is an acquired **posterior pharyngeal pulsion diverticulum** in which only the mucosa and submucosa herniate through the Killian's dehiscence. It is a false diverticulum. IOC is barium study.

23. **Ans. a. Hyponasality of speech** *Ref. Dhingra 6/e, p 315, 5/e p 443, 335; Scott and Brown 7/e, p 1098, 1236*

Hyponasality of speech is not a complication of adenoidectomy. Adenoidectomy results in hypernasality.

Causes of Hyponasality (Rhinolalia clausa)	Causes of Hypernasality (Rhinolalia aperta)
• Common cold • Nasal allergy • **Nasal polyp**[Q] • **Nasal growth**[Q] • **Adenoids**[Q] • **Nasopharyngeal mass**[Q] • Familial speech pattern • Habitual	• Velopharyngeal insufficiency • **Congenitally short soft palate** • Submucous palate • **Large nasopharynx**[Q] • **Cleft of soft palate**[Q] • **Paralysis of soft palate**[Q] • **Post-adenoidectomy**[Q] • Oronasal fistula • Familial speech pattern • Habitual

Grisel Syndrome

- It is non-traumatic atlanto-axial subluxation which occurs secondary to any inflammatory process in the upper neck[Q]
  - The condition is described following tonsillectomy and adenoidectomy[Q]
- It may be associated with **overuse of diathermy** either for **removal of adenoid or following curettage**[Q], when used for hemostasis.
- Children with **Down syndrome**[Q] have atlanto-axial instability

Treatment:
- **Cervical immobilization**[Q]; **Analgesia**[Q]; **Antibiotics**[Q] to reduce the risk of neurological deficit

Chapter 23

Head and Neck Space Inflammation and Thornwaldt's Bursitis

SPACES OF PHARYNX

The posterior wall of the pharynx is lined by **bucco pharyngeal fascia**, behind which is another fascia called as **'Alar fascia'** (actually a layer of prevertebral fascia). Behind alar fascia lies the **prevertebral fascia** covering the cervical vertebra (Fig. 23.1).

The space between	Name
Buccopharyngeal fascia and alar fascia	Retro pharyngeal space
Alar fascia and prevertebral fascia	Danger space
Prevertebral fascia and cervical vertebra	Prevertebral space

Important Points

Retropharyngeal Space

- Extends from base of skull to bifurcation of trachea
- **Boundaries:**
  - **Anterior:** Buccopharyngeal fascia covering the pharyngeal constrictor muscle
  - **Posterior:** Alar fascia
  - **Laterally:** Carotid sheath
- **Contents:** Retropharyngeal nodes
- A midline fibrous raphe divides this space into two lateral compartments **(spaces of gillete)** one on each side. This is why an abscess of Retropharyngeal space causes unilateral bulge
- Space of Gillette contains lymphnodes called as **'Node of Rouvier'** (Into which drain nasopharynx and oropharynx).

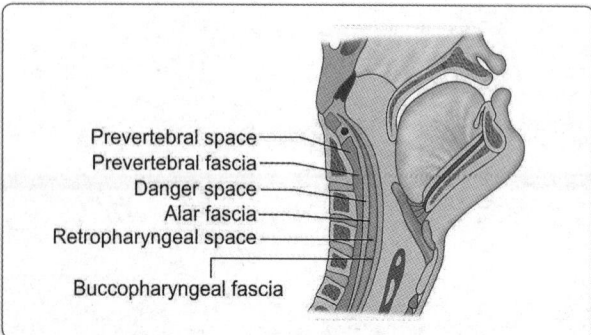

Fig. 23.1: Deep neck spaces for abscesses

Danger Space

- Lies between alar fascia anteriorly and prevertebral fascia posteriorly.
- The space doesnot have a midline raphe and so infection can spreads easily to either side.
- The space connects cervical spaces to mediastinum that is why it is called as **danger space** because infection can spread from here to mediastinum leading to mediastinitis.

Prevertebral Space

- Lies between the prevertebral fascia anteriorly and vertebral bodies posteriorly
- Extends from base of skull to coccyx
- Not divided in the midline; so abscess of this space presents as midline bulge.

NEW PATTERN QUESTIONS	
Q N1.	Gillette space is seen in:
	a. Parapharyngeal space
	b. Retropharyngeal space
	c. Peritonsillar space
	d. None of the above
Q N2.	Nodes of Rouviere are:
	a. Retropharyngeal nodes
	b. Parapharyngeal nodes
	c. Cervical nodes
	d. Adenoids
Q N3.	Danger space is bounded by:
	a. Buccopharyngeal fascia anteriorly and alar fascia posteriorly
	b. Alar fascia anteriorly and prevertebral fascia posteriorly
	c. Prevertebral fascia anteriorly and vertebral body posteriorly
	d. Tonsils anteriorly and superior constrictor muscle posteriorly

RETROPHARYNGEAL ABSCESS

Acute Retropharyngeal Abscess

- Most commonly seen in children below 6 years with a peak incidence between 3 and 5 years.

Causes

- **In children M/C cause** is suppuration of retropharyngeal lymph nodes due to infection at its draining sites—adenoids, nasopharynx, posterior nasal sinuses or nasal cavity.
- **In Adults M/C cause** is penetrating injuries to the posterior pharyngeal wall or the cervical esophagus.
- **Rarely:** Acute mastoiditis.

Point to Remember	
M/c organism	: *Streptococcus viridans* (46%)
	: *Staphylococcus aureus* (26%)

Clinical Features

- Fever
- Torticollis
- Difficulty in breathing—Stridor or Croupy cough
- Dysphagia

On Examination

Unilateral bulge in the posterior pharyngeal wall
(Friends, do not mug up these features—as their is abscess—obviously fever will be present.

Since it is situated in retropharynx it will—lead to a bulge in posterior pharyngeal wall and torticollis. It will press trachea and esophagus. so, it will cause difficulty in breathing and dysphagia.

Treatment

- I and D without general anesthesia (due to risk of rupture of abscess during intubation). The incision is given intraorally at the site of maximum bulge.
- Antibiotics
- **Tracheostomy: Done**, If abscess is large and causes mechanical obstruction of the airway.

NEW PATTERN QUESTIONS
Q N4. Which is the following is not true about acute retropharyngeal abscess? a. Dysphagia b. Swelling on posterolateral wall c. Torticollis d. Caries of cervical spine is usually a common cause
Q N5. Regarding retropharyngeal abscess all are true except: a. Lies only on one side b. Presents behind prevertebral fascia c. Surgical drainage is required d. Can be palpated by inserting finger in mouth

Chronic Retropharyngeal Abscess

- Mostly seen in adults

Cause

- Tuberculosis of the cervical spine (Potts spine)
- TB of the retropharyngeal lymph nodes secondary to tuberculosis of the deep cervical lymph nodes

Features

- Discomfort in the throat
- Pain
- Fever
- Progressive neurological signs and symptoms due to spinal cord compression
- Neck may show tubercular lymph nodes.

Investigation

X-ray

Radiological criteria to diagnose retropharyngeal abscess:
• Widening of retropharyngeal space (≥ 3/4th diameter of corresponding cervical vertebra) • Straightening of cervical space • Presence of gas shadow.

Treatment

- Antituberculous therapy (ATT)
- Anti gravity aspiration (if no relief then drainage done)
- **External drainage:**
  - Drainage through cervical incision
  - High abscess: vertical incision along the posterior border of sternocleidomastoid muscle[Q]
  - Low abscess: vertical incision along the anterior border of sternocleidomastoid muscle.[Q]

PARAPHARYNGEAL ABSCESS (ABSCESS OF LATERAL PHARYNGEAL SPACE, PTERYGOMAXILLARY SPACE, PHARYNGOMAXILLARY SPACE

Anatomy of Parapharyngeal Space (Pharyngomaxillary space)

Parapharynx lies on either side of the superior part of pharynx i.e. the nasopharynx and oropharynx.

- It is pyramidal in shape with base at the base of skull and apex at hyoid bone.
- It is the smallest space of pharynx but most commonly infected.
- Relations (Fig. 23.2):

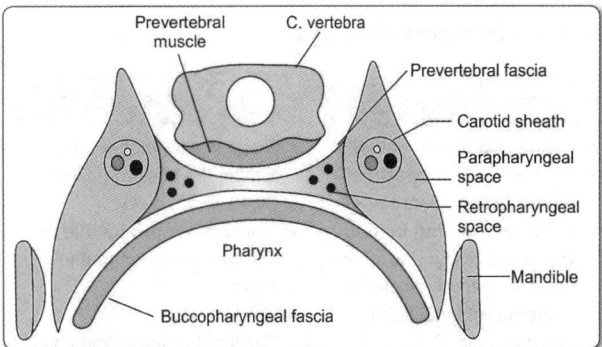

Fig. 23.2: Relation of parapharyngeal space

- **Laterally:** Medial ptyergoid muscle and mandible; deep lobe of the parotid
- **Medially:** Eustachian tube, Pharynx, and Palatine tonsil, medial pterygoid muscle
- **Posteriorly:** Vertebral and Prevertebral muscles
- **Anteriorly:** Pterygoid muscles and interpterygoid fascia (Fig. 23.2).

Note: Medial wall of the parapharyngeal space is the lateral wall of the peritonsillar space. It is formed by the superior constrictor muscle.

- Styloid process divides this space into 2 compartments.

Anterior compartment (related to tonsillar fossa medially and medial pterygoid muscle laterally)	Posterior compartment (related to posterior part of lateral pharyngeal wall medially and parotid gland laterally)
Contents	Contents
• Pterygoids	• Internal carotid artery
• Tensor villi palati	• Internal Jugallar vein
• Maxillary A	• IX, X, XI, XII cranial nerves
• Branches of mandibular N	• Sympathetic chain
	• Upper deep cervical nodes

Parapharyngeal Abscess

The parapharyngeal space communicates with the retropharyngeal, parotid, submandibular, carotid and visceral spaces.

Etiology

Infection in parapharyngeal space can occur through.

• Pharynx, tonsils, and adenoids infections		
• Teeth	:	Dental infections (Or extraction of lower third molar tooth) in 40% cases.
• Ear	:	Petrositis and Bezold's abscess
• External trauma	:	Penetrating injuries of the neck

Clinical Symptoms and Signs

Anterior compartment (lies lateral to tonsil)	Posterior compartment
• **Tonsil is pushed medially**	• Bulge in pharyngeal wall behind the posterior pillar
• **Trismus** (due to spasm of medial pterygoid muscles)	• IX, X, XI, XII palsy
• **External swelling behind the angle of the jaw** (at the posterior part of middle third of sternocleidomastoid)	• **Horners syndrome** due to involvement of sympathetic chain
• Odynophagia	• Parotid bulge
	• **Torticollis** (due to spasm of prevertebral muscles)

Note: Abscess of anterior compartment of Parapharyngeal space can be confused with quinsy as, trismus & tonsil pushed medially are seen in quinsy also. But in quinsy, there will not be a bulge at the angle of jaw or anterior 1/3rd of sternocleidomastoid.

Investigation of Choice: CT scan

Treatment

- Admission to hospital for intravenous (IV) antibiotics (penicillin/cefuroxime) is the baseline treatment
- Failure to respond to conservative treatment or clinical deterioration should prompt surgical abscess drainage
- *Abscess drainage* is done through a collar incision in the neck at the level of hyoidbone under general anaesthesia

NEW PATTERN QUESTIONS	
Q N6.	The medial bulging of pharynx is seen in:
	a. Parapharyngeal abscess
	b. Retropharyngeal abscess
	c. Peritonsillar abscess
	d. Paratonsillar abscess
Q N7.	Trismus in parapharyngeal abscess is due to spasm of:
	a. Medial pterygoid b. Lateral pterygoid
	c. Masseter d. Temporalis
Q N8.	Middle age diabetic with tooth extraction with ipsilateral swelling over middle one-third of sternocleidomastoid and displacement of tonsils towards contralateral side:
	a. Parapharyngeal abscess
	b. Retropharyngeal abscess
	c. Ludwig's angina
	d. None of the above

VINCENT'S ANGINA (TRENCH MOUTH/ULCERATIVE GINGIVITIS)

Organisms

- Spirochete
- *Borellia vincentii*
- Anaerobe
- *Bacillus fusiformis*

Predisposing Factor

- Very poor dental hygiene
- Debilitated patient
- Seen in young adults and middle-aged persons.

Features

Clinical

- Necrotizing gingivitis, i.e. gums are covered with necrotic membrane
- Bleeding of gums
- Ulceration of mucosa of tonsils, pharynx and mouth
- Patients parent with low-grade pyrexia and sore throat

On Examination

Greyish black membrane is present on one tonsil but may involve gums, soft and hard palate. The membrane bleeds when it is removed. It gives a characteristic foul smell to the breath.

Treatment

- Sodium bicarbonate gargles
- Penicillin + Metronidazole
- Dental care.

LUDWIG ANGINA

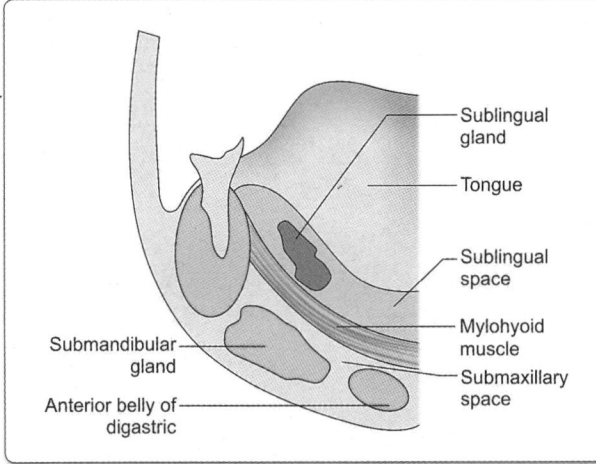

Fig. 23.3: Anatomy of submandibular space

Submandibular Space

- It lies between mucous membrane of floor of mouth and tongue on one side and superficial layer of deep cervical fascia extending between the hyoid bone and mandible on other side.
- It is divided into 2 compartments by mylohyoid muscle
  - **Sublingual space** – above the mylohyoid
  - **Submaxillary space** – below the mylohyoid

Ludwig Angina

- Infection of submandibular space is called *Ludwig angina*
- **Bacteriology:** Infections involved both aerobes and anaerobes. The M/c causative organism are hemolytic Streptococci, Staphylococci and bacteroides.
  For details see Flowchart 23.1.

NEW PATTERN QUESTION	
Q N9.	The spaces involved in Ludwig's angina are:
	a. Sublingual b. Submandibular
	c. Submaxillary d. All of the above

Extra Edge

KERATOSIS PHARYNGIS

Feature—Benign Condition:

- Horny excrescences on the tonsillar surface, pharyngeal wall or lingual tonsils which appear as white/yellow dots which cannot be wiped off.
- No constitutional symptoms
- *Treatment:* Reassurance.

THORNWALDLT'S BURSITIS (NASOPHARYNGEAL BURSITIS)

- It is infection of pharyngeal bursa (Lushka pouch) which is a remnant of notochord.

Flowchart 23.1: Ludwig angina

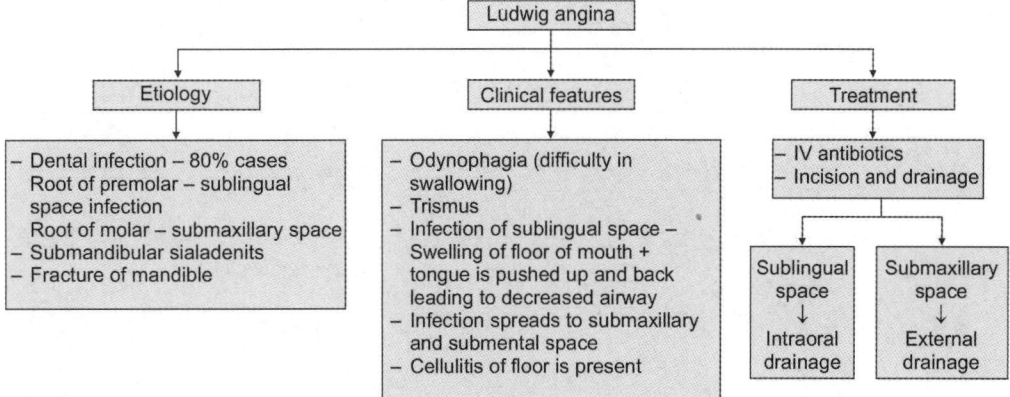

- Pharyngeal bursa is located in the midline of posterior wall of nasopharynx in the adenoid mass.
- The opening of the bursa may get closed leading to cyst or abscess.

Clinical Features
- Persistent postnasal discharge with crusting in the nasopharynx.
- Nasal obstruction due to swelling in the nasopharynx.
- Obstruction of eustachian tube leading to serous otitis media.
- Dull type of occipital headache.
- Recurrent sore throat
- Low-grade fever

Examination would reveal a cystic and fluctuant swelling in the posterior wall of nasopharynx.

Treatment
- Antibiotics are given to treat infection
- Marsupialization of the cystic swelling and adequate removal of its lining membrane by oral or palatine approach. These days diode laser is being used.

NEW PATTERN QUESTIONS

Q N10. **Thornwaldt cyst is also called:**
- a. Laryngeal cyst
- b. Nasopharyngeal cyst
- c. Ear cyst
- d. None

Q N11. **All of the following are true about Thornwaldt's abscess except:**
- a. Marsupialization is done
- b. Also called as nasopharyngeal bursa
- c. Presents as persistent postnasal drip
- d. Antitubercular treatment is given

Chapter 23: Head and Neck Space Inflammation and Thornwaldt's Bursitis

Explanations and References to New Pattern Questions

N1. Ans. is b i.e. Retropharyngeal space *Ref. Dhingra 6/e p 265*

Space of Gillette is seen in retropharyngeal space and contains nodes of rouviere.

N2. Ans. is a i.e. Retropharyngeal nodes *Ref. Dhingra 6/e p 265*

Nodes of Rouviere are retropharyngeal lymph nodes.

N3. Ans. is b i.e. Alar fascia anteriorly and prevertebral fascia posteriorly

Read the text for explanation.

N4. Ans. is d i.e. Caries of cervical spine is usually a common cause *Ref. Dhingra 6/e, p 266*

As discussed in the text M/C cause of acute retropharyngeal abscess in children is suppuration of retropharyngeal lymphnodes secondary to infection of adenoids, nasopharynx and nasal cavity.
The M/C cause of acute retropharyngeal abscess in adults is penetrating injury of posterior pharyngeal wall or cervical esophagus.
Rest all options are clinical features seen in acute retropharyngeal abscess. Rest all options are correct.

N5. Ans. is b i.e. Presents behind prevertebral fascia.

Retropharyngeal space lies between buccopharyngeal fascia and alar fascia.
For rest all options – see the text.

N6. Ans. is a i.e. Parapharyngeal abscess

Retropharyngeal abscess leads to bulge in posterior pharyngeal wall.
Parapharyngeal abscess leads to medial bulging of pharynx.

N7. Ans. is a i.e. Medial pterygoid

Trismus in parapharyngeal abscess is due to spasm of medial pterygoid muscle.

N8. Ans. is a i.e. Parapharyngeal abscess *Ref. Dhingra 6/e, p 267*

H/O tooth extraction
+
Ipsilateral swelling over middle/3 of sternocleidomastoid] Indicate parapharyngeal abscess
+
Displacement of tonsils

N9. Ans. is d i.e. All of the above *Ref. Dhingra 6/e, p 263*

See the text for explanation.

N10. Ans. is b i.e. Nasopharyngeal cyst

Thornwaldt's bursa is also called as **nasopharyngeal bursa**, hence thornwaldt's cyst is also called as nasopharyngeal cyst.

N11. Ans. is d i.e. Antitubercular treatment is given *Ref. Dhingra 6/e, p 245*

See the text for explanation.

QUESTIONS

1. **A male Shyam, age 30 years presented with trismus, fever, swelling pushing the tonsils medially and spreading laterally posterior to the middle sternocleidomastoid. He gives H/O excision of 3rd molar few days back for dental caries. The diagnosis is:** [AIIMS 01]
   a. Retropharyngeal abscess
   b. Ludwig's angina
   c. Submental abscess
   d. Parapharyngeal abscess

2. **A postdental extraction patient presents with swelling in posterior one third of the sternocleidomastoid, the tonsil is pushed medially. Most likely diagnosis is:**
   a. Retopharyngeal abscess b. Parapharyngeal abscess
   c. Ludwig angina   d. Vincent angina

3. **Parapharygeal space is also known as:** [PGI June 05]
   a. Retropharyngeal space
   b. Pyriform sinus
   c. Lateral pharyngeal space
   d. Pterygomaxillary space

4. **The medial bulging of pharynx is seen in:** [AI 91]
   a. Pharyngomaxillary abscess
   b. Retropharyngeal abscess
   c. Peritonsillar abscess
   d. Paratonsillar abscess

5. **Trismus in parapharyngeal abscess is due to spasm to:** [PGI 98]
   a. Masseter muscle   b. Medial pterygoid
   c. Lateral pterygoid   d. Temporalis

6. **Most common cause of chronic retropharyngeal abscess:** [Kolkata 01]
   a. Suppuration of retropharyngeal lymph node
   b. Caries of cervical spine
   c. Infective foreign body
   d. Caries teeth

7. **True statement about chronic retropharyngeal abscess:** [PGI 03]
   a. Associated with tuberculosis of spine
   b. Causes psoas spasm
   c. Suppuration of Rouviere lymph node
   d. Treatment by surgery

8. **Retropharyngeal abscess, false is** [AIIMS Nov 10]
   a. It lies lateral to midline
   b. Causes difficulty in swallowing and speech
   c. Can always be palpated by finger at the post pharyngeal wall
   d. It is present beneath the vertebral fascia.

9. **Infection of submandibular space is seen in:** [Manipal 08]
   a. Ludwig angina   b. Vincent angina
   c. Prinzmetal angina   d. Unstable angina

Explanations and References

1. **Ans. is d i.e. Parapharyngeal abscess**
2. **Ans. is b i.e. Parapharyngeal abscess** *Ref. Turner 10/e, p 106; Tuli 1/e, p 260, 2/e, p 268; Mohan Bansal p 542; Dhingra 6/e, p 267*

   History of dental caries
   +
   Trismus
   +
   Swelling pushing the tonsils medially ⎫
   +   ⎬ Indicate parapharyngeal abscess
   Swelling spreading posterior to the sternocleidomastoid or
   Presenting with a swelling in middle 1/3rd of sternocleidomastoid ⎭

3. **Ans. is c and d i.e. Lateral pharyngeal space; and Pterygomaxillary space**
   Ref. Dhingra 5/e, p 281, 6/e, p 267; Mohan Bansal p 538
4. **Ans. is a i.e. Pharyngomaxillary abscess**
   - Parapharyngeal space is also called *lateral pharyngeal space* and *pharyngomaxillary space.*
   - Pharyngomaxillary abscess is a synonym for parapharyngeal abscess *(which is also called **Lateral Pharyngeal abscess**).*
5. **Ans. is b i.e. Medial pterygoid** *Ref. Dhingra 5/e, p 282, 6/e, p 268*
   Trismus in parapharyngeal abscess is due to spasm of medial pterygoid muscle.

   Note:
   - Styloid process divides the pharynx into anterior and posterior compartment.
   - Trismus occurs in infection of anterior compartment whereas torticollis (due to spasm of paravertebral muscles) occurs in the infection of posterior compartment.

6. **Ans. is b i.e. Caries of cervical spine**
7. **Ans. is a, c and d i.e. Associated with tuberculosis of spine; and Suppuration of Rouviere lymph node; and Treatment by surgery** *Ref. Dhingra 5/e, p 281, 6/e, p 266-267*
   - Chronic retropharyngeal abscess is associated with caries of cervical spine or tuberculous infection of **retropharyngeal lymph nodes** secondary to tuberculosis of deep cervical nodes (i.e. suppuration of Rouviere nodes)
   - It leads to discomort in throat, dysphagia, fluctuant swelling of postpharyngeal wall.
   - Retropharyngeal abscess doesnot lead to psoas spasm.

   Treatment
   - Incison and drainage of abscess
   - Full course of **ATT**

   Also Know: Most common cause of acute retropharyngeal abscess:

Children	Adults
• Suppuration of retropharyngeal lymph nodes secondary to infection in the adenoids, nasopharynx, posterior nasal sinuses or nasal cavity	• Due to penetrating injury of posterior pharyngeal wall or cervical esophagus

8. **Ans. is d i.e. It is present beneath vertebral fascia** *Ref. Dhingra 5/e, p 280,281, 6/e, p 266–267; Mohan Bansal p 543*
   - Retropharyneal space lies behind the pharynx between the buccopharyngeal fascia covering pharyngeal constrictor muscles and the prevertebral facia (i.e. behind the pharynx and in front of prevertebral fascia)
     Thus **option d, i.e.** it lies beneath the vertebral fascia is incorrect.
   - On physical examination, may reveal bulging of the posterior pharyngeal wall, although this is present in <50% of infants with retropharyngeal abscess. Cervical lymphadenopathy may also be present. There will be as smooth swelling on one side of the posterior pharyngeal wall with airway impairment.
   - Dysphagia and difficulty in breathing are prominent symptoms as the abscess obstructs the air and food passages.
9. **Ans. is a i.e. Ludwig angina** *Ref. Dhingra 5/e, p 277, 6/e, p 263; Mohan Bansal p 543*
   See the preceding text for explanation.

Chapter 24

Lesions of Nasopharynx and Hypopharynx including Tumors of Pharynx

NASOPHARYNX (ALSO CALLED AS EPIPHARYNX)

NASOPHARYNGEAL FIBROMA/JUVENILE NASOPHARYNGEAL ANGIOFIBROMA

- Most common **benign tumor** of nasopharynx (but overall angiofibroma is rare).
- Most common site is *posterior part of nasal cavity* close to the margin of **sphenopalatine foramen**.
- Seen almost exclusively in males of *10–20 years* (*testosterone dependent* tumor seen in prepubertal to adolescent males).
- **Locally invasive vasoformative** tumor consisting *of endothelium lined vessels with no muscle coat.*
- The major blood supply is from **internal maxillary artery.**

Clinical Features

Symptoms

Symptoms depend on spread of tumor to nasal cavity, paranasal sinuses, pterygomaxillary fossa, infratemporal fossa, cheek, orbits (through inferior orbital fissure), cranial cavity (most common site is *middle cranial fossa*).

- Most common symptom - *Spontaneous profuse and recurrent epistaxis.*
- Progressive, unilateral nasal obstruction, denasal speech, hyposmia/anosmia, broadening of nasal bridge.
- Otalgia, conductive hearing loss and serous otitis media, due to eustachian tube obstruction.
- Initially it is unilateral and later becomes bilateral.
- *Pink or purplish mass* obstructing one or both choanae in nasopharynx.
- Tumor in the orbit causes proptosis and frog-face deformity; diplopia and diminished vision.
- Swelling of cheek.
- Tumor in infratemporal fossa can cause trismus and bulge of parotid.
- II, III, IV, V, VI cranial nerve can be involved.

> **Point to Remember**
>
> *Juvenile nasopharyngeal angiofibroma:* In an adolescent male, profuse recurrent episodes of nosebleed suggests juvenile nasopharyngeal angiofibroma until proven otherwise.

Signs

- Splaying of nasal bones
- Pink or purplish mass obstructing one or both choanae in nasopharynx
- Swelling of cheek and fullness of face.

Diagnosis

- Soft tissue lateral film of nasopharynx and X-ray of paranasal sinuses and base of skull.
- **CT scan of head** *with contrast enhancement* (CECT) is now the IOC. It shows extent, bony destruction or displacements and anterior bowing of the posterior wall of maxilla due to tumor enlarging in pterygopalatine fossa

> Antral sign or Holman Miller sign[Q]:
> - Pathognomic of angiofibroma.
> - Anterior bowing of the posterior wall of maxilla due to tumor enlarging in pterygopalatine fossa.

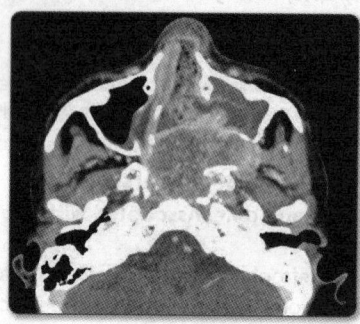

Fig. 24.1: Contrast CT scan juvenile nasopharyngeal angiofibroma. Note the pterygopalatine fossa and infratemporal fossa extension

Source: ENT, Essential of Mohan Bansal, Jypee Brothers Medical Publishers Pvt. Ltd.

- MRI is done to veiw the soft tissue extension and is complementary to CT scan.
- Carotid angiography: Shows extent of the tumor, its vascularity and feeding vessel.

> **Point to Remember**
>
> ➤ Biopsy is **contraindicated** as it contains only blood vessels and fibrous tissue with no muscular coat, so profuse bleeding can occur while taking biopsy.

Treatment

- **Surgical excision is** treatment of choice.
- **For decreasing blood loss during surgery:**
  (a) **Preoperative embolization**
  (b) **Estrogen therapy**
  (c) Cryotherapy
  (d) Radiotherapy

Chapter 24: Lesions of Nasopharynx and Hypopharynx including Tumors of Pharynx

Note: Preoperative embolization of the tumor reduces its blood supply and causes less bleeding, provided if tumor removal is performed within 24–48 hour of embolization before collaterals have time to develop. Preoperative angiography also helps to find any feeders from internal carotid system..

- **Surgical approaches** depend on the origin and extension of angiofibroma

Table 24.1: Radkowski classification of juvenile nasopharyngeal angiofibroma (JNA) and suggested surgical approach

Stage*	Tumor extent*	Surgical approach
IA	Tumor limited to nose and nasopharyngeal vault	Transpalatine or endoscopic (Wilson approach)
IB	Extension to paranasal sinuses	Medial maxillectomy by lateral rhinotomy or endoscopy
IIA	Minimal extenson to pterygomaxillary fissure (PMF)	Extended lateral rhinotomy or Le Forte 1
IIB	Full extension to PMF and/or erosion of orbital bones	Extended lateral rhinotomy and removing anterior wall of maxillary sinus and along with part of nasal pyriform aperture
IIC	Extension to infratemporal fossa and/or cheek or posterior to pterygoid plates	Infratemporal fossa approach or maxillary swing approach (facial translocation)
IIIA	Erosion of skull base: minimal intracranial	Combined intracranial and/or extracranial
IIIB	Extensive intracranial and/or cavernous sinus extension	Neurosurgery/radiation

*Radkowski D and others; Arch Otoalryngol Head and Neck 122:122, 1996

Point to Remember

- **Recurrence** is not uncommon after surgery (Recurrence rate 30–50%).
- **Recurrence rates** can be reduced by meticulous dissection of sphenopalatine foramen.
- Recurrences usually become evident within 2–3 years of initial resection.

Note: It is not a fast-growing tumor.

Also know

Other modalities of treatment in nasopharyngeal angiofibroma.

Radiotherapy	Hormonal	Chemotherapy
For intracranial extension of tumor when it derives its blood supply from Internal carotid artery	Since tumor occurs in young males testosterone has been implicated for its growth. Antitestosterone are being tried for management	Doxorubicin, vincristine and dacarbazine are used for residual with recurrent lesions

Radiotherapy	Hormonal	Chemotherapy
Recurrent angiofibromas are treated with intensity modulated radiotherapy	Diethylstilbestrol with Flutamide	

NEW PATTERN QUESTIONS

Q N1. Frog face deformity of nose is caused by:
a. Rhinoscleroma b. Angiofibroma
c. Antral polyp d. Ethmoidal polyp

Q N2. Which of the following is not true for juvenile angiofibroma?
a. Biopsy for diagnosis
b. Benign tumor
c. Surgical excision
d. Second decade

Q N3. Angiofibroma is classified as stage—if it extends to one or more paranasal sinuses:
a. Stage I b. Stage II
c. Stage III d. Stage IV

Q N4. Pharyngeal angiofibroma is treated with:
a. Surgery b. Radiotherapy
c. Chemotherapy d. None of the above

Q N5. Main arterial supply of nasopharyngeal fibroma is:
a. Facial artery
b. Internal maxillary artery
c. Internal carotid artery
d. Ascending pharyngeal artery

Q N6. Characteristic sign of nasopharyngeal fibroma on CT scan is:
a. Antral sign b. Furstenberg sign
c. Lhermitte's sign d. Ervin Moore sign

Q N7. IOC for angiofibroma:
a. MRI
b. CECT
c. Carotid angiography
d. Biopsy

NASOPHARYNGEAL CARCINOMA

Uncommon in India except in North-East region where people are predominantly of mongoloid origin.
- M/c in southern states of China, Taiwan and Indonesia.
- It is most common tumor of head and neck which gives rise to secondaries with occult primary.
- Most common **site** is *fossa of Rosenmuller* in the lateral wall of nasopharynx.
- Most common **histological type** of nasopharyngeal carcinoma squamous cell carcinoma.

Table 24.2: WHO classification of epithelial carcinoma based on histopathology	
Type 1 (25%)	Keratinizing squamous cell carcinoma, EBV –ve, 10% survival
Type 2 (12%)	Nonkeratinizing carcinoma, EBV +ve, 50% survival Without lymphoid stroma With lymphoid stroma
Type 3 (63%)	Undifferentiated carcinoma, EBV +ve, 50 survival Without lymphoid stroma With lymphoid stroma

%, % NPC; EBV, Epstein-Barr Virus, Survival, 5-year survival

Etiology

- **Genetic:** It is most common in Southern China.
- **Viral:** *Epstein-Barr virus* has identified in tumor epithelial cells of most undifferentiated and nonkeratinizing squamous cell carcinoma. IgA VC, i.e. IgA against viral capsid antigen of EBV is used as a serological marker for screening purpose.
- **Environmental:** Wood dust, smoking of tobacco and opium; air pollution; nitrosamines from dry salted fish along with vitamin C deficient diet, textile industry workers.

Clinical Features

- It usually affects males.
- It has a bimodal peak: 1st peak at 15-25 years and 2nd peak at 55-65 years of age.
- *Most common manifestation is upper neck swelling due to cervical lymphadenopathy since nasopharynx is richly supplied by lymphatics.*
- Unilateral neck swelling is more common than bilateral swelling
- *Most common* lymph node involved jugulodigastric (upper deep cervical) lymph node.
- *Earliest lymph node involved* is retropharyngeal lymph node. (Node of Rouviere)

Spread of Tumor	Findings
1. Nose and orbit	Unilateral nasal obstruction; epistaxis, rhinolalia clausa
2. Eustachian tube	– Serous/suppurative otitis media leading to U/L deafness and tinnitus
3. Parapharyngeal space	– Cranial nerve palsies IX, X, XI, XII; **Horner's syndrome;** trismus
4. Foramen lacerum and ovale	– Ophthalmic symptoms and facial pain (CN III, IV, V, VI) (Cavernous sinus thrombosis)
5. Retropharyngeal nodes	– Neck pain and stiffness
6. Krause's nodes	– These LNs are situated in the jugular foramen. Their enlargement compresses CN IX, X, and XI and produces **jugular foramen syndrome.**
7. Distant metastases	– Secondaries in bone (most common) lung, liver

- Most common **cranial nerve palsy** in nasopharyngeal carcinoma is *V cranial nerve* followed by VI nerve whereas M/C multiple cranial nerves involved are IX and X.

Extra Edge

Collet sicard syndrome Involvement of IX, X, XI and XII nerves.

Points to Remember

- Presence of **unilateral serous otitis media** in an adult should raise suspicion of nasopharyngeal growth.
- **Trotter's triad or sinus of Morgagni syndrome:** Seen in Nasopharyngeal cancer. Includes *conductive deafness; ipsilateral tempoparietal neuralgia due to involvement of CN V; palatal paralysis due to CN IX. Also called as sinus of Morgagni syndrome.*
- Unlike other squamous cell carcinoma, it can metastasize to posterior triangle (level V) in the absence of jugular lymph node involvement.
- **Neck is the M/C:** Site of clinically occult primary cancer of tonsillar fossa, tongue base, pyriform sinus and nasopharynx.

Diagnosis

- Most important is examination of postnasal space by nasopharyngeal mirror or nasopharyngoscope.
- Biopsy of nasopharynx is considered as the first necessary investigation for nasopharyngeal carcinoma if a suspected lesion is found.
- Imaging modality of choice—MRI with gadolinium and fat suppression.

Treatment

- *Irradiation* is treatment of choice. External beam radiotherapy of 6000 CGY is given

Intensity-modulated radiotherapy (IMRT) is now being preferred as it allows higher dose to be delivered with less damage to structures like brainstem and spinal cord.

- In stages I and II only radiotherapy is done. In stages III and IV chemoradiation is the treatment of choice.
- Radical neck dissection is required for persistent nodes when primary has been controlled and in postradiation cervical metastasis.

- **Prognosis**
- Poor

Complications of Radiotherapy

- Xerostomia of radiotherapy (M/c common complication because both major and minor salivary glands are well within the field of irradiation)
- Mucositis, altered taste sensation, dental caries
- Radiation otitis media with effusion, rhinosinusitis
- Radionecrosis of skull base
- Radiation myelitis
- Encephalomyelitic change
- Optic atrophy

 Note: Intensity-modulated radiation therapy (IMRT) have decreased the incidences of these complications.

Lhermitte's Sign

- Uncommon complication
- **Cause:** Due to radiation to the cervical spinal cord
- **Features:** Lightening - like electrical sensation spreading into both arms, down the dorsal spin, and into both legs on neck flexion.

Rhabdomyosarcoma

- It is the M/c malignant tumor of nasopharynx in children.
- Orbit is the M/c site of rhabdomyosarcoma in the head and neck region.

Nasopharyngeal Chordoma

- It originates from the notochord.
- After rearrange nasopharyngeal chordone give N5-N9, Then Hypopharynx
- Anatomy
- Benign hypopharyngeal lessons

- hypopharynx cases and last → Table 24.3

Characteristic histological feature includes **physaliferous cells**.

NEW PATTERN QUESTIONS

Q N8. Nasopharyngeal cancer occurs most commonly in:
   a. India
   b. Bangladesh
   c. Pakistan
   d. China

Q N9. Undifferentiated carcinoma of nasopharynx belongs to which category as per WHO classification?
   a. Type 1   b. Type 3
   c. Type 2   d. Type 4

Q N10. Most common presentation in nasopharyngeal carcinoma:
   a. Epistaxis
   b. Hoarseness of voice
   c. Nasal stuffiness
   d. Cervical lymphadenopathy

Q N11. Trotter's triad includes all *except*:
   a. Sensory disturbance over distribution of 5th cranial nerve
   b. Diplopia
   c. Conductive deafness
   d. Palatal palsy

Q N12. A 70-year-old man with cervical lymphadenopathy. What can be the cause?
   a. Nasopharyngeal carcinoma
   b. Angiofibroma
   c. Acoustic neuroma
   d. Otosclerosis

Q N13. Nasopharyngeal carcinoma is an occupational hazard of:

Table 24.3: Cancer of hypopharynx			
Feature	CA Pyriform Sinus	CA Postcricoid	CA Posterior Pharyngeal Wall
Incidence	Most common of all hypopharyngeal cancer (60%)	2nd most common hypopharyngeal cancer (30%)	Least common (10%)
Age and sex	Mostly males > 40 years	• Mostly females • May be seen as early as 20–30 years	Mostly males > 40
Clinical features Presenting symptoms Presenting sign	Generally symptomless and diagnosed late Pricking/sticking sensation in throat Enlarged lymph nodes	• Progressive dysphagia	Dysphagia, hemoptysis Enlarged lymph nodes
Lymphatic spread	Upper deep cervical nodes	• Paratracheal lymph nodes (Bilateral)	Retropharyngeal lymph nodes
Treatment of choice	Early growth-radiotherapy	• Poor prognosis with both surgery and radiotherapy	Early growths-radiotherapy Later surgery

a. Asbestos industry
b. Cement industry
c. Wood workers
d. Chimney workers

Q N14. Trotter's triad is seen in carcinoma of:
a. Maxilla
b. Larynx
c. Nasopharynx
d. Ethmoid sinus

Q N15. Following is true of carcinoma of nasopharynx:
a. Unknown etiology
b. Excellent prognosis
c. High incidence of nodal metastasis
d. Surgery offers good chances of cure

Q N16. TOC for nasopharyngeal carcinoma:
a. Surgery
b. Radiotherapy
c. RT + CT
d. Surgery + CT

HYPOPHARYNX

ANATOMY

- Hypopharynx extends from the floor of vallecula to the lower border of the cricoid.
- It has three parts:
  1. Pyriform sinus
  2. Posterior pharyngeal wall
  3. Postcricoid (see adjacent figure).

TUMORS OF HYPOPHARYNX

Hypopharynx Cancer

- Most common type of tumor of hypopharynx is – squamous cell carcinoma.^Q

Etiology
- Alcohol
- Tobacco
- Vitamin A deficiency
- Iron deficiency/Plummer-Vinson syndrome is an important etiology for carcinoma postcricoid.
- Low cholesterol levels.
  For details, *see* Table 24.3.

> **Points to Remember**
> ➤ **In cancer of pyriform fossa:** The referred ear pain is because of CN X as superior laryngeal nerve is a branch of vagus nerve.
> ➤ **Laryngeal crepitus:** Laryngeal crepitus is present in normal persons and absent in patients with postcricoid malignancy as larynx becomes fixed.

BENIGN HYPOPHARYNGEAL LESIONS

Plummer-Vinsion (Paterson-Brown-Kelly) Syndrome

- Mostly affects females more than 40 years.

Classical Features Include

- **Progressively increasing dysphagia for solids** (due to Webs in postcricoid region)
- Iron deficiency anemia
- Glossitis and stomatitis
- Koilonychia (spooning of nails)
- Achlorhydria

Signs
- Smooth tongue devoid of papillae.
- Craked lips and corners of mouth.
- Barium swallow shows web in the postcricoid region due to subepithelial fibrosis in the region.
- 2% cases develop postcricoid carcinoma.

Treatment
- Correction of anemia
- Dilatation of the webbed area by esophageal bougies.

Explanations and References to New Pattern Questions

N1. Ans. is b i.e. Angiofibroma *Ref. Dhingra 6/e, p 246*
Extension of angiofibroma to the orbit gives rise to proptosis and frog face deformity.

N2. Ans. is a i.e. Biopsy for diagnosis *Ref. Dhingra 6/e, p 247*
As discussed biopsy is never done for diagnosis of nasopharyngeal fibroma as it is extremely vascular tumor and taking a biopsy can lead to profuse bleeding.

N3. Ans. is a i.e Stage I *Ref. Esentials of ENT, Mohan Bansal, p 329*
Radkwoski classification of Juvenile nasopharyngeal carcinoma classifies JNA extending to paranasal sinuses as stage IB.

N4. Ans. is a. i.e. Surgery *Ref. Dhingra 6/e, p 248*
The mainstay of management of angiofibroma is surgery—in all stages except in stage 3 where the tumor spreads intracranially. Only in stage 3, Radiotherapy is the TOC.

N5. Ans. is b i.e. Internal maxillary artery
Major blood supply of nasopharyngeal angiofibroma is by internal maxillary artery.

N6. Ans. is a i.e. Antral sign
Antral sign (Holman-Muller sign): Anterior bowing of posterior wall of maxillary sinus (anterior wall of pterygopalatine fossa) is characteristic of juvenile nasopharyngeal angiofibroma.

N7. Ans. is b i.e. CECT
CECT is the Investigation of choice for nasopharyngeal angiofibroma.

N8. Ans. is d. i.e. China *Ref. Dhingra 6/e, p 250*
"Nasopharyngeal cancer is most common in China particularly in southern states and Taliwan" *Ref. Dhingra 6/e, p 250*

N9. Ans. is b i.e Type 3 *Ref. Dhingra 6/e, p 250*

WHO criteria for Nasopharyngeal carcinoma
Type I (25%)- Differentiated squamous cell CA
Type II (12%)- Non-keratinizing carcinoma
Type III (63%)- Undifferentiated carcinoma

N10. Ans. is d i.e. Cervical lymphadenopathy *Ref. Dhingra 6/e, p 252*
Cerivcal lymphadenopathy is the M/C presentation of nasopharyngeal carcinoma. It may be the only manifestation in some cases.

N11. Ans. is b i.e. Diplopia *Ref. Dhingra 6/e, p 251*
Nasopharyngeal can cause conductive deafness (eustachian tube blockage,) ipsilateral temporoparietal neuralgia (involvement of CN V) and palatal paralysis (CN X) collectively called Trotter's triad.

N12. Ans. is a i.e. Nasopharyngeal carcinoma *Ref. Dhingra, p 250-2*
A 70-year-male presenting with cervical lymphadenopathy should always raise the suspicion of nasopharyngeal carcinoma.

N13. Ans. is c i.e. Wood workers
Nasopharyngeal cancer is common in:
1. Epstein Barr virus infection
2. Environmental hazards: Wood dust exposure, Textile industry workers
3. Cigarette smokers
4. Netrosamine from dry salted fish
5. Diet deficient in vitamin C.

N14. Ans. is c i.e. Nasopharynx

> See the text for explanation

N15. Ans. is c i.e. High incidence of nodal metastasis

> See the text for explanation

N16. Ans. is b i.e. Radiotherapyc
Irradiation is the primary treatment of choice of nasopharyngeal cancers.

QUESTIONS

1. Most common site of origin of nasopharyngeal angiofibroma: [AI 00]
   a. Roof of nasopharynx
   b. At sphenopalatine foramen
   c. Vault of skull
   d. Lateral wall of nose
2. Nasopharyngeal angiofibroma is: [TN 91]
   a. Benign
   b. Malignant
   c. Benign but potentially malignant
   d. None of the above
3. A 14-year old boy presents with history of frequent nasal bleeding. His Hb was found to be 6.4 g/dL and peripheral smear showed normocytic hypochromic anemia. The most probable diagnosis is: [AIIMS May 2014]
   a. Juvenile nasopharyngeal angiofibroma
   b. Hemangioma
   c. Antrochonal polyp
   d. Carcinoma of nasopharynx
4. Chandu a 15-year-aged boy presents with unilateral nasal blockade mass in the cheek and epistaxis; likely diasnosis is: [AI 01]
   a. Nasopharyngeal Ca
   b. Angiofibroma
   c. Inverted papilloma
   d. None of the above
5. In angiofibroma of nasopharynx all are correct except: [Kolkata 00]
   a. Common in female
   b. Most common presentation is epistaxis
   c. Arises from roof of nasopharynx
   d. In late cases frog-face deformity occurs
6. The main vessel involved in bleeding from Juvenile nasopharyngeal angiofibroma: [AIIMS Nov 2015]
   a. Internal maxillary artery
   b. Ascending pharyngeal artery
   c. Facial artery
   d. Anterior Ethmoidal artery
7. All are true about nasopharyngeal fibroma except: [PGI Nov 2014]
   a. Most common age of presentation is 20-50 yr
   b. Radioresistant tumor
   c. Highly vascular
   d. Benign in nature
   e. Surgery is treatment of choice
8. Angiofibroma bleeds excessively because: [DNB 01]
   a. It lacks a capsule
   b. Vessels lack a contractile component
   c. It has multiple sites of origin
   d. All of the above
9. Clinical features of nasopharyngeal angiofibroma are:
   a. 3rd to 4th decades [PGI 02]
   b. Adolescent male
   c. Epistaxis and nasal obstruction is the cardinal symptom
   d. Radiotherapy is the management of choice
   e. Arises from posterior nasal cavity
10. A 14 years boy presented with repeated epistaxis, and a swelling in cheek. Which of these statements may be correct? [PGI 02]
    a. Diagnosis is nasopharyngeal angiofibroma
    b. Contrast CT scan should be done to see the extent
    c. High propensity to spread via lymphatics
    d. Arises from roof of nose
    e. Surgery is therapy of choice
11. True about juvenile nasopharyngeal angiofibroma:
    a. Surgery is treatment of choice [PGI June 06]
    b. It is malignant tumor
    c. Incidence in females
    d. Hormones not used in Rx
    e. Miller's sign positive
12. True about nasopharyngeal angiofibroma: [PGI Dec 03]
    a. Commonly seen in girls
    b. Hormonal etiology
    c. Surgery is treatment of choice
    d. Radiotherapy can be given
    e. Recurrence is common
13. Most appropriate investigation for angiofibroma is:
    a. Angiography
    b. CT scan [AIIMS 97]
    c. MRI scan
    d. Plain X-ray
14. A 2 years child presents with B/L nasal pink masses. Most important investigation prior to undertaking surgery is: [AI 97]
    a. CT scan
    b. FNAC
    c. Biopsy
    d. Ultrasound
15. A 10-year-old boy presents with nasal obstruction and intermittent profuse epistaxis. He has a firm pinkish mass in the nasopharynx. All of the following investigations are done in this case except: [UPSC 98]
    a. X-ray base of skull
    b. Carotid angiography
    c. CT scan
    d. Biopsy
16. IOC for angiofibroma is:
    a. CT scan
    b. MRI
    c. Angiography
    d. Plain X-ray
17. An 18-year-old boy presented with repeated epistaxis and there was a mass arising from the lateral wall of his nose extending into the nasopharynx. It was decided to operate him. All of the following are true regarding his management except: [AIIMS 02]
    a. Requires adequate amount of blood to be transfused
    b. A lateral rhinotomy approach may be used
    c. Transpalatal approach used
    d. Transmaxillary approach
18. Treatment of choice for angiofibroma: [RJ 02]
    a. Surgery
    b. Radiotherapy
    c. Both
    d. Chemotherapy

19. A 9 years boy presents with nasal obstruction, proptosis, recurrent epistaxis from 3 to 4 years. Management includes: [PGI Nov 10]
    a. Routine radiological investigations
    b. Embolization alone should be done
    c. Surgery is treatment of choice
    d. Embolization followed by surgery
    e. Conservative management is sufficient
20. Radiotherapy is used in treatment of angiofibroma when it involves: [MP 04]
    a. Cheek
    b. Orbit
    c. Middle cranial fossa
    d. Cavernous sinus
21. Most common site for nasopharyngeal carcinoma: [AIIMS 97; MP 02]
    a. Nasal septum
    b. Fossa of Rosenmuller
    c. Vault of nasopharynx
    d. Anterosuperior wall
22. Nasopharyngeal Ca involve: [PGI 02]
    a. Nasal cavity
    b. Orophaynx
    c. Oral cavity
    d. Tympanic cavity
    e. Orbit
23. Nasopharyngeal Ca is caused by: [AIIMS 98]
    a. EBV
    b. Papilloma virus
    c. Parvo virus
    d. Adeno virus
24. Most common presentation in nasopharyngeal carcinoma is with: [AI 97]
    a. Epistaxis
    b. Hoarseness of voice
    c. Nasal stuffiness
    d. Cervical lymphadenopathy
25. A 70-year-old male presents with Neck nodes. Examination reveals a Dull Tympanic Membrance, deafness and tinnitus and on evaluation Audiometry gives Curve B. The most probable diagnosis is: [AI 08]
    a. Nasopharyngeal carcinoma
    b. Fluid in maddle ear
    c. Tumor in interior ear
    d. Sensorineuronal hearing loss
26. A 70-year-old man presented with left sided conductive hearing loss, o/e TM intact and Type B curve on tympanogram. Next step is: [AIIMS May 2013]
    a. Myrinogotomy and grommet insertion
    b. Conservative management
    c. Type 3 tympanoplasty
    d. Endoscopic examination to look for nasopharyngeal causes
27. Nasopharyngeal Ca causes deafness by: [PGI Nov 05; PGI Dec 07]
    a. Temporal bone metastasis
    b. Middle ear infiltration
    c. Serous effusion
    d. Radiation therapy
28. Horner's syndrome is caused by: [PGI 97]
    a. Nasopharyngeal carcinoma metastasis
    b. Facial bone injury
    c. Maxillary sinusites
    d. Ethmoid polyp
29. Trotter's triad is seen in carcinoma of: [Comed 08]
    a. Maxilla
    b. Larynx
    c. Nasopharynx
    d. Ethmoid sinus
30. Trotter's triad includes all of the following except: [AI 09, PGI Dec 08]
    a. Mandibular Neuralgia
    b. Deafness
    c. Palatal palsy
    d. Seizures
    e. Associated with nasopharyngeal angiofibroma
31. Nasopharyngeal Ca: [PGI 02]
    a. M/c nerve involve is vagus
    b. Unilateral serous otitis media is seen
    c. Treatment of choice radiotherapy
    d. Metastasized to cervical lymph node
    e. EBV is responsible
32. Which among the following is not true regarding nasopharyngeal carcinoma? [PGI 01]
    a. Associated with EBV infection
    b. Starts in the fossa of Rosenmuller
    c. Radiotherapy is the treatment of choice
    d. Adenocarcinoma is usual
    e. If elderly patients present with unilateral otitis media, it is highly suggestive
33. Which of the following is not true about nasopharyngeal carcinoma? [AI 10]
    a. Bimodal age distribution
    b. EBV is implicated as etiological agent
    c. Squamous cell carcinoma is common
    d. Nasopharyngectomy and lymph node dissection is mainstay of treatment
34. Treatment of choice in nasopharyngeal carcinoma: [AI 98; PGI Dec 05 FMGE 2013]
    a. Radiotherapy
    b. Chemotherapy
    c. Surgery
    d. Surgery and radiotherapy
35. True about nasopharyngeal carcinoma: [PGI May 2016]
    a. Radiotherapy is treatment of choice
    b. Also k/a Guangdong tumour
    c. May associated with U/L otitis media
    d. Associated with EBV
36. True about Plummer-Vinson syndrome: [PGI 06]
    a. Web is M/C in lower esophagus
    b. Web is M/C in mid esophagus
    c. Web is M/C in postcricoid region
    d. It occurs due to abnormal vessels
    e. Reduced motility of esophagus

Explanations and References

1. **Ans. is b i.e. At sphenopalatine foramen**

2. **Ans. is a i.e. Benign**   *Ref. Dhingra 5/e, p 261, 6/e, p 246; Scott-Brown's 7/e, Vol 2, p 2437; TB of Ent Mohan Bansal, p 437*
   - Nasopharyngeal fibroma is the *most common* benign tumor of nasopharynx.
   - Most common site is posterior part of nasal cavity close to the margin of Sphenopalatine foramen.
   "Though it is a benign tumor, it is locally invasive and destroys the adjoining structures.
   Juvenile Angiofibroma is uncommon, benign and extremely vascular tumor that arises in the tissues within the sphenopalatine foramen."
       Ref. Scott-Brown's 7/e, Vol 2, p 2437

3. **Ans. is a i.e. Juvenile nasopharyngeal angiofibroma**
   A 14-year-old boy presents with history of frequent nasal bleeding. His Hb was found to be 6.4 g/dL and peripheral smear showed normocytic hypochromic anemia. The most probable diagnosis is juvenile nasopharyngeal angiofibroma.
   As the age of the patient (14 years), Sex: (male) and presentation (nasal bleeding) all favour it.
   In antrochoanal polyps, the presenting symptom is U/L nasal obstruction and not bleeding.
   Age of the patient goes against Nasopharyngeal cancer. As far as hematoma are concerned, a swelling is generally seen.

4. **Ans. is b i.e. Angiofibroma**   *Ref. Dhingra 5/e, p 261, 6/e, p 246; Scott-Brown's 7/e, Vol 2 p 2437; Mohan Bansal p 437*
   M/C presentation of angiofibroma is profuse and recurrent episodes of epistaxis and U/L nasal obstruction.
   It is seen in adolescent males

   > **Point to Remember**
   > So friends, remember—If the Question says a boy with age 10–20 years presents with swelling of cheek and recurrent epistaxis – Do not think of anything else but – 'Nasopharyngeal fibroma'

5. **Ans. is a i.e. Common in female**   *Ref. Read below*
   Let us see each option separately here:

Option	Correct/Incorrect	Reference	Explanation
Option a = Common in female	Incorrect	Dhingra 5th/ed p 261, 6th/ed, p 246; Scott-Brown's 7th/ed Vol 2 p 2437	It is seen almost exclusively in male
Option b = M/c presentation is epistaxis	Correct	Dhingra 5th/ed p 261, 6th/ed, p 246; Scott-Brown's 7th/ed Vol 2 p 2438	Profuse and recurrent epistaxis is the M/c presentation
Option c = Arises from roof of nasopharynx	Partly correct	Dhingra 5th/ed p 261, 6th/ed, p 246	This statement is partly correct as earlier it was thought to arise from roof of nasopharynx or anterior wall of sphenoid. But now it is believed to arise from posterior part of nasal cavity close to sphenopalatine foramen.
Option d In late cases frog-like deformity seen	Correct	Dhingra 5th/ed p 262, 6th/ed p 246	In later stages, it can lead to broadening of nasal bridge, proptosis, i.e. frog-like deformity.

   S/B = Scott-Brown 7th/ed
   Thus option a, i.e. Common in females is absolutely incorrect and the option of choice here.

6. **Ans. is a i.e. Internal maxillary artery**   *Ref. Tuli 2/e, p260*
   Major blood supply of Nasopharyngeal angiofibroma is through internal maxillary artery.
   Other arteries supplying Nasopahryngeal angiofibroma are:
   - Ascending pharyngeal artery
   - Vidian artery
   - Branches of internal carotid artery
   - Sphenopalatine artery

Chapter 24: Lesions of Nasopharynx and Hypopharynx including Tumors of Pharynx

7. **Ans. a and b i.e. M/c age of presentation 20-50 years; and radioresistant tumor**
   See the text for explanation
8. **Ans. is b i.e. Vessels lack a contractile component** *Ref. Dhingra 5/e, p 261*
   Angiofibroma as the name implies is made of vascular and fibrous tissues in varying ratios *"Mostly the vessels are just endothelium lined spaces with no muscle coat. This accounts for the severe bleeding as the vessels lose the ability to contract, and also, bleeding cannot be controlled by application of adrenaline."*
   – *Dhingra 5th/ed p 261, 6th/ed p 246*
9. **Ans. is b, c and e i.e. Adolescent male; Epistaxis and nasal obstruction is the cardinal symptom and arises from posterior nasal cavity** *Ref. Dhingra 5/e, p 261-3, 6/e, p 246; TB of ENT Mohan Bansal p 437-8*

   ### Nasopharyngeal Angiofibroma
   - Most commonly seen in adolescent males (i.e. option b is correct)
   - Most common age of presentation = second decade of life (option a incorrect)
   - Arises from posterior nasal cavity close to sphenopalatine foramen (option e is correct)
   - Epistaxis and nasal obstruction are the most common presentation. (correct)
   - Recurrent severe epistaxis accompanied by progressive nasal obstruction are the classical symptoms of juvenile angiofibromas at the time of presentation." – *Scott-Brown 7/e, Vol 2 p 2438*
   - TOC is surgical excision (i.e. option d is incorrect)

10. **Ans. is a, b and e i.e. Diagnosis is nasopharyngeal angiofibroma; Contrast CT scan should be done to see the extent; and Surgery is therapy of choice**
11. **Ans. is a and e i.e. Surgery is treatment of choice; and Miller's sign positive**
12. **Ans. b, c, d and e i.e. Hormonal etiology; Surgery is treatment of choice; Radiotherapy can be given; and Recurrence is common** *Ref. Dhingra 5/e, p 261-3, 6/e, p 246–9*
13. **Ans. is b i.e. CT scan**
    Ans. 8 is straightforward
    Ans. 9 also needs no explanation
    Ans. 10 lets see option 'e' recurrence is the most common complication
    "Recurrence is by far the most common complication encountered and is reported in 25% patients."
    [Scott-Brown's 7/e, Vol 2, p 2442]
    In Q13 the boy (14 years) is presenting with repeated epistaxis with swelling in cheek which points towards angio fibroma.
14. **Ans. is a i.e. CT scan**
15. **Ans. is d i.e. Biopsy**
16. **Ans. is a i.e. CT scan** *Ref. Dhingra 5/e, p 262, 6/e, p 252; Mohan Bansal p 437*

    ### Diagnosis of Nasopharyngeal Fibroma
    - **CT scan of head *with contrast enhancement* is now the IOC.** It shows the extent, bony destruction or displacements and anterior bowing of the posterior wall of maxillary sinus (called as *antral sign*) which is *pathognomic of angiofibroma*.
    - MRI is complimentary to CT and is done especially to see the soft tissue extension.
    - Carotid **angiography** shows the vascularity and feeding vessels. It is done when embolization is planned before operation.
    - Biopsy is **contraindicated**.

17. **Ans. is d i.e. Transmaxillary approach**
18. **Ans. is a i.e. Surgery**
19. **Ans. is a, c and e i.e. Routine radiological investigations; Surgery is the treatment of choice; and Conservative Management is sufficient** *Ref. Dhingra 5/e, p 262,263, 6/e, p 252*

    18 years male
    +
    Repeated epistaxis   ⎤
    +   ⎬ Indicates the patient has nasopharyngeal angiofibroma
    Mass arising from the lateral wall of
    nose and extending to nasopharynx ⎦

    ### Treatment
    - Surgical excision is the treatment of choice.
    - Before surgery at least 2–3 liters of blood should be given. —*Tuli 1/e, p 253*
    - Preoperative embolization and estrogen therapy or cryotherapy reduce blood loss in surgery. —*Dhingra 6/e, p 249*

Approach
- *Transpalatine approach*—done for tumor confined to nasopharynx.
- *Lateral rhinotomy approach*—done for large tumors involving, nasal cavity, paranasal sinuses and orbit. Nowadays, it is the best approach.

20. **Ans. is c i.e. Middle cranial fossa** *Ref. Dhingra 6/e, p 249*

    Radiotherapy is useful only for advanced cases of the tumor, when there is intracranial extension.

21. **Ans. is b i.e. Fossa of Rosenmuller** *Ref. Dhingra 5/e, p 264, 6/e, p 251; TB of ENT Mohan Bansal p 439*

    Nasopharyngeal carcinoma most commonly arises from **fossa of Rosenmuller in lateral wall of nasopharynx.**

22. **Ans. is a, d and e i.e. Nasal cavity; Tympanic cavity; and Orbit**

    ### Spread
    Ref. Dhingra 5/e, p 265, 6/e, p 250; Essential of ENT Mohan Bansal p 320

    Most common site of origin: Fossa of Rosenmuller
    Local spread:
    - **Anterior:** Choana, nasal cavity and orbit
    - **Posterior:** Retropharyngeal space
    - **Inferior:** Oropharynx and laryngopharynx
    - **Lateral:** Eustachian tube, parapharyngeal space, pterygoid muscles and infratemporal fossa (via sinus of Morgagani).
    - **Superior:** Middle cranial fossa (via foramen lacerum and ovale), jugular foramen, hypoglossal canal, posterior cranial fossa.

23. **Ans. is a i.e. EBV** *Ref. Dhingra 5/e, p 264, 6/e, p 250; TB of ENT Mohan Bansal p 439*

    ### Etiology of Nasopharyngeal Carcinoma
    - **Genetic:** It is *most common* in China.
    - **Viral:** Epstein-Barr virus is closely associated with nasopharyngeal cancer. Epstein-Barr virus has identified in tumor epithelial cells *(not lymphocytes)* of most undifferentiated and nonkeratinizing squamous cell carcinoma.
    - **Environmental:** Burning of incense or wood *(polycyclic hydrocarbon);* smoking of tobacco and opium; air pollution; nitrosamines from dry salted fish along with vitamin C deficient diet have been linked to the etiology of nasopharyngeal cancer.

24. **Ans. is d i.e. Cervical lymphadenopathy** *Ref. Dhingra 5/e, p 264, 6/e, p 252; Scott-Brown's 7/e, Vol 2, p 2451*

    "The most common complain at presentation is the presence of an upper neck swelling. Unilateral neck swelling is much more common although bilateral metastasis also occur." *Ref. Scott-Brown's 7th/ed Vol 2 p 2457*

25. **Ans. is a i.e. Nasopharyngeal carcinoma** *Ref. Dhingra 5/e, p 261,262, 6/e, p 251–2*

    Let us see the complains and examination findings one by one.
    - A 70 years male is presenting with neck nodes (which could either be due to infection or due to malignancy, but malignancy is more consistent with the age).
    - **On examination**—ear shows coincidental findings viz. Tympanic membrane appears dull and audiometry shows curve B which means fluid is present in middle ear (Ruling out **option "d"** i.e. SNHL).

    ### Fluid in Middle Ear can be Seen in

ASOM	CSOM	Serous otitis media
• Tympanic membrane appears red, bulging in early stages and later in the stage of resolution usually a small perforation is seen • Also here patient will have fever and excruciating earache (which is the chief complain) • So, ASOM ruled out	• On examination either cholesteatoma granulation or perforation will be seen • Neck nodes will not be the presenting So, CSOM ruled out	• Tympanic membrane appears dull and audiometry shows B type of curve. So, serous otitis media is a possibility

    Serous otitis media/Glue ear:
    It is mostly seen in school-going children. If serous otitis media is seen in adults (that too males) – always think of **Nasopharyngeal carcinoma.**

    "Presence of unilateral serous otitis media in an adult should raise the suspicion of a nasopharyngeal growth"
    Ref. Dhingra 5/e, p 264, 6/e, p 251

    The diagnosis is further consolidated by:
    - Age of patient = 70 years (*most common* age for nasopharyngeal carcinoma = 5th – 7th decade).
    - Sex of patient = male (nasopharyngeal carcinoma is *most common* in males).
    - Presenting symptom = Presence of neck nodes.
    - (It is the *most common* presenting symptom of nasopharyngeal carcinoma).

> **Point to Remember**
> Presence of unilateral serous otitis media in an adult should always raise suspicion of nasopharyngeal growth.

Chapter 24: Lesions of Nasopharynx and Hypopharynx including Tumors of Pharynx

26. **Ans is d i.e. Endoscopic examination to look for nasopharyngeal causes** *Ref. Dhingra 6/e, p 251*
    A 70-year-old man is presenting with U/L conductive deafness and on O/E—Tympanic membrane is intact (i.e. any otology cause for conductive deafness ruled out) and Type B tymparogram (i.e. serous otitis media is present which has to be due to a cause other than ear because tympanic membrane is intact).
    Always Remember—
    "Presence of a unilateral serous otitis media is an adult should raise suspicion of nasopharyngeal growth." *Dhingra 6/e, p 251*

27. **Ans. is c i.e Serous effusion** *Ref. Dhingra 5/e, p 264, 6/e, p 251; Scott-Brown's 7/e, Vol 2, p 2458*
    Nasopharyngeal carcinoma spreads to Eustachian tube, blocks it and causes Serous Otitis Media which in turn causes Conductive hearing loss.

28. **Ans. is a i.e. Nasopharyngeal carcinoma metastasis** *Ref. Dhingra 5/e, p 264, 6/e, p 251; TB of ENT Mohan Bansal p 439*
    Nasopharyngeal carcinoma can cause Horner's syndrome due to involvement of cervical sympathetic chain.

29. **Ans. is c i.e. Nasopharynx** *Ref. Dhingra 5/e, p 264; TB of ENT Mohan Bansal p 439*

30. **Ans. is d i.e. Seizures** *Ref. Dhingra 6/e, p 251; TB of ENT Mohan Bansal p 439*
    Trotter's triad – seen in nasopharyngeal carcinoma is characterised by (Fig. 24.2):

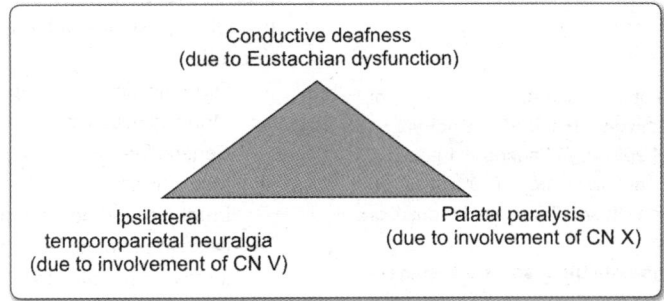

Fig. 24.2: Trotter's triad

31. **Ans. is b, c, d and e i.e. Unileteral serous otitis media is seen; Treatment of choice radiotherapy; Metastaised to cervical lymph node; and EBV is responsible**
    - *Most common* **nerve involved – VI nerve** *Ref. Current Otolaryngology 2/e, p 365; Textbook of ENT Mohan Bansal p 439*
    Rest all options are already discussed

32. **Ans. is d i.e. Adenocarcinoma is usual** *Ref. Dhingra 5/e, p 264,265, 6/e, p 250-251*
    Most common histological type of nasopharyngeal carcinoma – *Squamous cell carcinoma.*
    In squamous cell: It is the undifferentiated variety which is more common.
    Rest of the options have been explained earlier.

33. **Ans. is d i.e. Nasopharyngectomy and lymph node dissection is mainstay of treatment**
    Ref. Dhingra 5/e, p 264-6, 6/e, p 250-252
    In nasopharyngeal carcinoma, radiotherapy is the mainstay of treatment. Radical neck dissection is required for persistent nodes when primary has been controlled.
    For details on nasopharyngeal carcinoma, kindly see preceding text.

34. **Ans. is a i.e. Radiotherapy** *Ref. Dhingra 5/e, p 266, 6/e, p 252; Textbook of ENT Mohan Bansal p 439-40*
    TOC for nasopharyngeal fibroma – Surgery
    TOC for nasopharyngeal carcinoma – Radiaton
    TOC for advanced carcinoma – Chemotherapy + Radiation

35. **Ans is a. b. c and d. i.e. Radiotheraphy is the TOC also called Guangdong tumor associated with EBV and may be associated with U/L otitis media.**
    Nasopharyngeal carcinoma is M/C in Southern China hence it is also called Guangdong tumor.
    Rest all options have been discussed in the text

36. **Ans is c i.e. Web is M/C in postcricoid region** *Ref. Dhingra 5/e, p 351, 6/e, p 343; Text book of ENT Mohan Bansal p 461*
    In Plummer-Vinson syndrome patients present with dysphagia due to web in the postcricoid region and due to incoordinated swallowing secondary to esophageal spasm
    For more details see preceding text.

Chapter 25

Pharynx Hot Topics

SNORING

It is an undesirable disturbing sound that occurs during sleep. It is estimated that 25% of adult males and 15% of adult females snore. Its prevalence increases with ages.

Definition of Terms

- **Sleep apnea:** It is cessation of breathing that lasts for 10s or more during sleep. Less than five such episodes is normal
- **Apnea index:** It is number of episodes of apnea in 1 hour
- **Hypopnoea:** It is reduction of airflow i.e drop of 50% of airflow from the base line associated with an EFG defined arousal or 4% drop in oxygen saturation
- **Respiratory disturbance index (RDI):** Also called **apnea—hyponoea index.** It is the number of apnea and hypopnoea episodes per hour. Normally RDI is less than five. Based on RDI, severity of apnea has been classified as mild, 5–14; moderate, 15–29; and severe ≥ 30
- **Arousal index:** It is number of arousal events in 1 h. Less than four is normal.

Etiology

- In children most common cause is adenotonsillar hypertrophy
- In adults (Table 25.1).

Table 25.1: Causes of snoring in adults	
Site	Cause
Nose (nasopharynx)	• Septal deviation • Nasal hypertrophy • Nasal polyp • Nasal tumor
Oral cavity (oropharynx)	• Elongated self-palate/uvula • Large base of tongue • Tongue tumor
Larynx (laryngopharynx)	• Laryngeal stenosis • Omega-shaped epiglottis
Others	• Obesity • Use of alcohol, sedatives, hypnotics

Sites of Snoring

Site of snoring may be soft palate, tonsillar pillars or hypopharynx.

Symptomatology

- Excessive loud snoring is socially disruptive
- In addition, a snorer with obstructive sleep apnea may manifest with:
  - Excessive daytime sleepiness
  - Morning headaches
  - General fatigue
  - Memory loss
  - Irritability and depression
  - Decreased libido
  - Increased risk of road accidents.

Treatment

- Avoidance of alcohol, sedatives and hypnotics
- Reduction of weight
- Sleeping on the side rather than or the back
- Removal of obstructing lesion in nose, nasopharynx, oral cavity, hypopharynx and larynx. Radiofrequency has been used for volumetric reduction of tissues of turbinates, soft palate and base of tongue.
- **Performing uvulopalatoplasty (UPP) surgically with cold knife or assisted with radiofrequency (RAUP) or laser (LAUP).**

SLEEP APNEA

Apnea means no breathing at all. There is no movement of air at the level of nose and mouth. It is of three types:

1. **Obstructive** (M/C variety)**:** There is collapse of the upper airway resulting in cessation of airflow. Other factors may be obstructive conditions of nose, nasopharynx, oral cavity and oropharynx, base of tongue or larynx. An apnea—hypopnea index is ≥5.
2. **Central:** Airways are patent but brain fails to signal the muscles to breathe.
3. **Mixed:** It is combination of both types.

Chapter 25: Pharynx Hot Topics

Obstructive Sleep Apnea Hypopnea Syndrome (OSAHS)
- OSAHS is defined as the **coexistence of unexplained excessive daytime sleepiness with at least 5 obstructed breathing events (apnea or hypopnea) per hour of sleep.**[Q]
- Mild disease: apnea-hypopnea index (AHI): 5-15 moderate disease: 15-30, Severe disease ≥ 30

Mechanism of Obstruction:
- Apneas and hypopneas are caused by the airway being sucked closed on inspiration during sleep. This occurs as the **upper-airway dilating muscles like all striated muscles relax during sleep**[Q].
- In patients with **OSAHS**, the **dilating muscles fail to oppose negative pressure within the airway during inspiration**[Q].

Factors predisposing to OSAHS
- Obesity[Q]
- Shortening of the mandible and/or maxilla[Q]
- Hypothyroidism[Q]
- Acromegaly[Q]
- Male sex[Q]
- Middle age[Q] (40-65 years)
- Myotonic dystrophy[Q]
- Ehlers-Danlos syndrome[Q]
- Smoking[Q]

Epidemiology:
- OSAHS occurs in around **1-4% of middle-aged males and is about half as common in women**
- The syndrome also **occurs in childhood,** usually associated with **tonsil or adenoid enlargement;** and in the **elderly,** although the **frequency is slightly lower in old age**
- Irregular breathing during sleep *without* daytime sleepiness is much more common, occuring in perhaps a **quarter of the middle-aged male population.**

Clinical Features:
- OSAHS causes **daytime sleepiness; impaired vigilance, cognitive performance and driving; depression; disturbed sleep;** and **hypertension.**

Diagnosis:
- **OSAHS requires lifelong treatment,** and the diagnosis has to be made or excluded with certainly. This will hinge on obtaining a good sleep history from the patient and partner, with both completing sleep questionnaires, including the **Epworth Sleepiness Score.**
    - In those with **appropriate clinical features, the diagnostic test must demonstrate recurrent breathing pauses during sleep.**
    - This may be **full polysomnography with recording of multiple respiratory** and **neurophysiologic signals during sleep.**

Treatment:
- Change in lifestyle including **weight loss** and **alcohol reduction both to reduce weight** and because alcohol acutely decreases upper-airway dilating muscle tone, thus predisposing to obstructed beathing.

Positional Therapy:
- Positional therapy: Patient should sleep on the side as supine position may cause obstructive apnea. A rubber ball can be fixed to the back of shirt to prevent adopting supine position.

Continuous Positive Airway Pressure (CPAP)	Oral devices i.e. Mandibular Repositioning Splint (MRS)	Surgery	Drugs
• **CPAP therapy** works by **blowing the airway open during sleep**, usually with **pressures of 5-20 mm Hg** • The **main side effect of CPAP is airway drying** • It is the most commonly done treatment for obstructive sleep apnea	• **MRSs work by holding the lower jaw** and the **tongue forward.** thereby **widening the pharyngeal airway** • They help to improve or abolish smoking	• **Bariatric surgery can be curative** in the **morbidly obese** • *Tonsillectomy can be highly effective in children* but *rarely in adults* • **Uvulopalato - pharyngo- plasty**	• Unfortunately, **no drugs are clinically useful** in the prevention or reduction of apneas and hypopneas • A **marginal improvement in sleepiness in patients who remain sleepy despite CPAP** can be produced by **modafinil**, but the clinical value is debatable and the financial cost is significant

Contd...

Contd...

- **CPAP use is imperfect,** but around 94% of patients with **severe OSAHS** are still using their therapy after 5 years on objective monitoring
- MRS is also used in retrognathic patients
- **Tracheostomy is gold standard** but **rarely used** as it is socially unaccepted and has its own complications
- Jaw advancement surgery particularly "maxillomandibular osteotomy" is **effective in** those with **retrognathia** (posterior displacement of the mandible) and should be **considered particularly in young and thin patients**
- There is **no robust evidence** that **pharyngeal surgery, including uvulo palatopharyngoplasty** (whether by scalpel, laser, or thermal techniques) helps **OSAHS patients.**

Retrognathic patients: It is 80% effective in snoring but relieves OSA in 30% cases.

Treatment: Obstructive sleep apnea hypopnea syndrome

- **CPAP** and **MRS** are the **two most widely used** and **best evidence-based therapies**[Q].
- Direct comparisons in studies indicate better outcomes with CPAP in terms of apneas and hypopneas, nocturnal oxygenation, symptoms, quality of life, mood, and vigilance.
- **Adherence to CPAP is generally better than that to an MRS**[Q], and there is evidence that CPAP improves driving, whereas there are no such data on MRSs:
  - Thus, **CPAP is the current treatment of choice.**
  - However, **MRSs** are evidence-based **second-line therapy in those who fail CPAP.**[Q]
  - In **younger, thinner patients, maxillomandibular advancement** should be considered.[Q]

Note: Uvulopolatopharyngoplasty – here tonsils and uvula are removed along with the posterior edge of soft palate. The anterior and posterior faucial pillars are sutured together.
- UPPP is very effective in treating snoring but its role in OSA is doubtful.
- M/C complication – bleeding.
- Other complications
  - Temporary velopharyngeal incompetence and rarely nasopharyngeal stenosis.

OTHER IMPORTANT TOPICS

Point to Remember

Other important topics:
- Investigation of choice for dysphagia = Barium videofluoroscopy
- Dysphagia to solids is generally due to mechanical obstruction (e.g. tumors) → endoscopy should be done
- Dysphagia to liquids is generally due to motility disorders →

of arch of aorta, Recent MI, Trismus
In most of these cases new generations of flexible gastroscopes can be used successfully
- M/C complication of rigid esophagoscopy – Perforation
- M/C site for perforation – Just above cricopharyngeal.

Note: A rigid bronchoscope can be used for performing esophagoscopy but not vice versa.

RIGID ESOPHAGOSCOPY

- Anesthesia – General anaesthesia
- Position – **Boyce position** (Similar to direct laryngoscopy)
- C/I of rigid esophagoscopy—cervical spine injury, Aneurysm

ESOPHAGEAL PERFORATION

- **Features:** Fever after esophagoscopy
- **Diagnosis:** Swallow study confirms the diagnosis
- **Treatment:** Early intervention to repair is most desirable. Drain the perforation to prevent complications.

Chapter 25: Pharynx Hot Topics

QUESTIONS

1. **Gold standard test in evaluation of OSA is:**
   a. Polysomnography
   b. CT
   c. MRI
   d. EEG
2. **Muller's maneuver is done in:**
   a. Nasopharyngeal CA
   b. Tongue CA
   c. OSA
   d. Oropharyngeal CA
3. **All of the following are true about obstructive sleep apnea syndrome except:** [AIIMS Nov 14]
   a. Females affected more than males
   b. Commonly associated with hypertension
   c. Day time sleepiness is seen
   d. >5 episodes of apnea per hour
4. **A 36 years old obese man was suffering from hypertension and snoring. Patient was a known smoker. In Sleep test, there were 5 apnea/hyperapnoes episodes per hour. He was given antihypertensives and advised to quit smoking. Next line of management:** [AIIMS Nov 13]
   a. Uvulopalatopharyngeoplasty
   b. Weight reduction and diet plan
   c. Nasal CPAP
   d. Mandibular repositioning sling
5. **All are true about esophagoscopy except:**
   a. Compress the posterior part of tongue
   b. Tip of the esophagoscope lies in pyriform fossa
   c. Should be inserted from right side
   d. Epiglottis should be lifted up
   e. Incisiors must act as fulcrum

Explanations and References

1. **Ans. is a i.e. Polysomnography**   *Ref. Essentials of ENT, Mohan Bansal p 313*
   Polysomnography is the Gold standard test in evaluation of snoring and OSA.
   It differentiates snoring without OSA, with OSA and central sleep apnea. It also identifies the severity of the apnea.
2. **Ans. is c i.e. OSA**   *Ref. Essential of ENT, Mohan Bansal p 313*
   Muller's maneuver is a test to be done before the uvulopalatopharyngoplasty (UPPP) to know whether the patient will benefit from this surgery or not.
3. **Ans. is a i.e. Females affected more than males**   *Ref. Harrison 18/e p2186*
   OSAHS occurs in around 1-4% of middle aged males and is about half as common in women.
4. **Ans. is b i.e. Weight reduction and diet plan**   *Ref. Harrison 18/e p2186-2189*
   A 36 years old obese man was suffering from hypertension and snoring. Patient was a known smoker. In Sleep test, there were 5 apnea/hyperapnoes episodes per hour. He was given antihypertensives and advised to quit smoking. Next line of management is weight reduction and diet plan as patient is having mild sleep apnea (apnea-hypopnea index of 5-15 is mild).

   "All patients diagnosed with Obstructive sleep apnea/hypopnea syndrome (OSAHS) should have the condition and its significance explained to them and their partners. Rectifiable predispositions should be discussed; this often includes weight loss and alcohol reduction both to reduce weight and because alcohol acutely decreases upper-airway dilating muscle tone, thus predisposing to obstructed breathing."   *Ref. Harrison 18/e p2189*

   "The primary treatments of obstructive sleep apnea are: weight loss in those who are overweight, continuous positive airway pressure, and mandibular advancement devices. There is little evidence to support the use of medications or surgery."

   "Continuous positive airway pressure (CPAP) is effective for both moderate and severe disease. It is the most common treatment for obstructive sleep apnea."

   "Adherence to CPAP is generally better than that to an MRS, and there is evidence that CPAP improves driving, whereas there are no such data on MRSs. Thus, CPAP is the current treatment of choice (for both moderate and severe disease). However, MRSs are evidence-based second-line therapy in those who fail CPAP."   *Ref. Harrison 18/e p2189*

   "There is no robust evidence that pharyngel surgery, including uvulopalatopharyngoplasty (whether by scalpel, laser or thermal techniques) helps OSAHS patients."   *Ref. Harrison 18/e p2189*

5. **Ans. is e i.e. Incisors must act as fulcrum** *Ref. Dhingra 5/e p 436,437*
   Esophagoscopy Procedure
   - Hold the scope in a pen-like fashion and introduce it into the mouth from **the right side of tongue** and then toward the midline.
   - Never rotate the endoscope on the fulcrum of the upper teeth, rather it should be lifted up.
   - Lift up the epiglottis after passing through the tongue base to identify the arytenoids. Tip of the scope should be introduced into the pyriform sinuses on either to inspect them before passing behind the arytenoids.
   - Open up the cricopharyngeal sphincter by slow sustained pressure, never apply force on the sphincter for it can result in undue spasm and perforation.
   - Once the esophagus is entered keep the lumen in constant view.
   - Lower the head of the patient while negotiating the aortic and bronchial constriction.
   - Move the head slightly to the right while passing the cardia (Identified by redder and more velvety mucosa).

SECTION 5

Larynx

Section Outline

26. Anatomy of Larynx, Congenital Lesions of Larynx and Stridor
27. Acute and Chronic Inflammation of Larynx, Voice and Speech Disorders
28. Vocal Cord Paralysis
29. Tumors of Larynx

Chapter 26

Anatomy of Larynx, Congenital Lesions of Larynx and Stridor

- Larynx develops from tracheobronchial groove, a midline diverticulum of foregut.
- Development starts in the 4th week of embryonic life.
- Most of the anatomical characteristics of larynx develop by the 3rd month of fetal life.
- Angle of the thyroid cartilage at birth:
  - Males   : 110 degree
  - Females   : 120 degree
- The angle remains till puberty.
- Level of the larynx:
  - At birth   : till C3
  - Adults   : C3–C6
- Descent of the larynx continues throughout life.
- Vocal cord length:
  - Infants   : 6–8 mm
  - Adult males   : 17–23 mm
  - Adult females : 12–17 mm

EXTERNAL FEATURES OF LARYNX

Laryngeal Cartilages

- Laryngeal cartilages are 9 in number and derived from 4th, 5th and 6th arches.

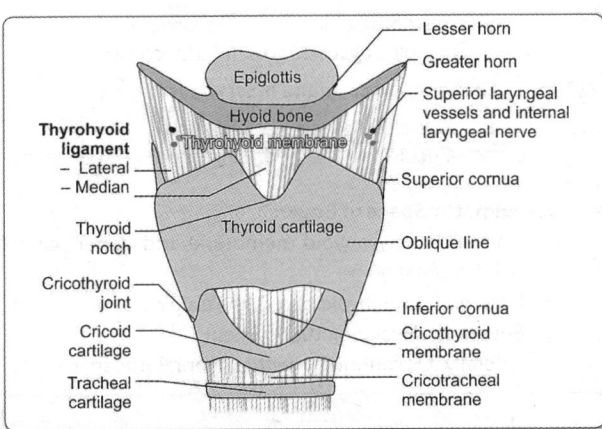

Fig. 26.1: Laryngeal framework—anterior view

Courtesy: Textbook of Diseases of Ear, Nose and Throat, Mohan Bansal, Jaypee Brothers Medical Publishers Pvt. Ltd., p 62.

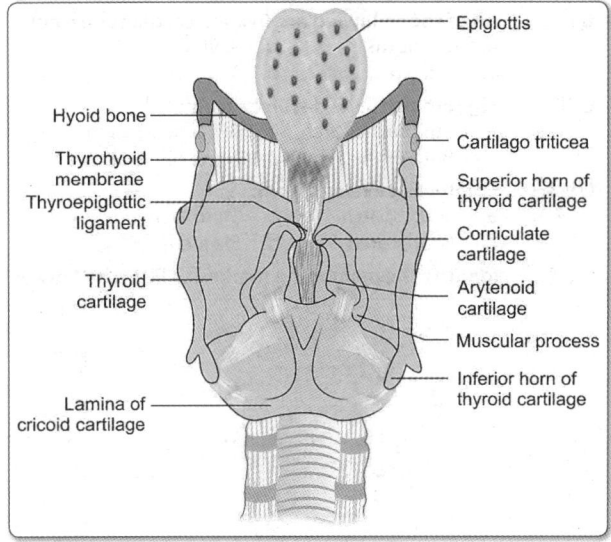

Fig. 26.2: Posterior view of larynx showing cartilages and ligaments

Courtesy: Textbook of Diseases of Ear, Nose and Throat, Mohan Bansal, Jaypee Brothers Medical Publishers Pvt. Ltd., p 62.

- Larynx has 9 cartilages of which 3 are paired and 3 are unpaired:

Paired	Unpaired
– Arytenoid	– Thyroid
– Corniculate	– Cricoid
– Cuneiform	– Epiglottis

- *Ossification of the various laryngeal cartilages:*

Thyroid and Cricoid	– Early 20s
Arytenoid	– Late 30s

 Points to Remember

➤ **Vocal process** Do Not ossify
➤ No ossification occurs in the cuneiform or the corniculate cartilage.

Histology of Laryngeal Cartilages

Hyaline cartilages (ossify)	Elastic cartilages (Do not ossify)
• Thyroid cartilages • Cricoid cartilages • Basal part of arytenoid cartilage	All the other cartilages

 Note: Other example of elastic cartilage is auricular cartilage

NEW PATTERN QUESTIONS

Q N1. All of the following are hyaline cartilages *except*:
  a. Epiglottis b. Arytenoid
  c. Cricoid d. Thyroid

Q N2. Thyroid cartilage develops from:
  a. 4th brachial arch b. 6th brachial arch
  c. Both of the above d. None of the above

Q N3. Epiglottis develops from:
  a. Second arch b. Third arch
  c. Fourth arch d. Six arch

Q N4. Identify the membrane marked as 'X' in the figure:

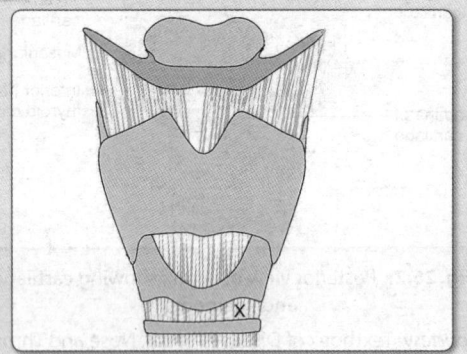

See Color Plate 19

  a. Thyrohyoid membrane
  b. Cricothyroid membrane
  c. Cricotracheal membrane
  d. None

Characteristics of Individual Laryngeal Cartilages

Thyroid Cartilage
The upper border of thyroid cartilage usually lies between the forth and fifth cervical vertebrae
- Largest cartilage, hyaline in nature.
- It is V-shaped and consists of right and left lamina. Which meet anteriorly in midline and form an angle (Adam's angle)
- Adam's angle:
  – Male : 90 degrees
  – Female : 120 degrees
- The outer surface of each lamina is marked by an **oblique line** which extends from superior thyroid tubercle to inferior thyroid tubercle.

> • Oblique line gives attachment to:
>   – Thyrohyoid   – Sternothyroid
>   – Inferior constrictor muscle.

- Vocal cords are attached to middle of thyroid cartilage.

Cricoid Cartilage
- It is hyaline cartilage and shaped like a ring (the only complete cartilaginous ring in the airway).
- It articulates with arytenoid cartilage. Cricoarytenoid joint is a **synovial joint**[Q]
- Cricothyroid joint is also a synovial joint.

Arytenoid Cartilage
- They are 2 small pyramid shaped cartilages. It articulates with cricoid lamina.

 Points to Remember
> ➤ It has a vocal process for: attachment of vocal folds.
> ➤ It has muscular process for: attachment of posterior crico-arytenoid and lateral cricothyroid

- Its apex articulates with corniculate cartilage.

Corniculate (Cartilage of Santorini) and Cuneiform (Cartilage of Wrisberg)
- Are fibroelastic cartilages. Corniculate cartilages are conical; cuneiform cartilages are rod shaped.
- Corniculate cartilage articulates through a synovial joint with apices of arytenoids cartilage.

Epiglottis
- It is Fibroelastic cartilage which is leaf shaped in adults and omega shaped in children.

NEW PATTERN QUESTIONS

Q N5. Which of the following is not attached at oblique line?
  a. Sternothyroid b. Thyrohyoid
  c. Middle constrictor d. Inferior constrictor

Q N6. Leaf-shaped cartilage of larynx is:
  a. Thyroid b. Epiglottis
  c. Cricoid d. Erythroid

- **Pre-epiglottic Space of Boyer:**
  – Anteriorly: Thyrohyoid membrane and upper part of thyroid cartilage
  – Posteriorly: Infrahyoid part of the epiglottis
  – Superiorly: Hyoepiglottic ligament
  – Laterally it is continuous with paraepiglottic space.

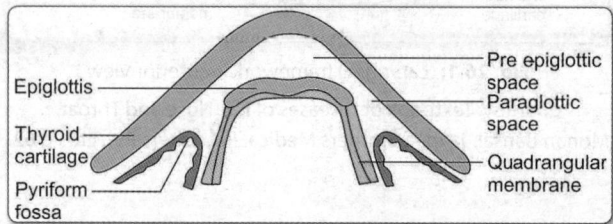

Fig. 26.3: Diagram to show pre-epiglottic and paraepiglottic space

- **Paraglottic Space** is continuous medially with the pre-epiglottic space.

  Boundaries:
  - Laterally — Thyroid cartilage
  - Medially — Quadrangular membrane and Conus elasticus
  - Posteriorly — Anterior reflection of pyriform fossa.

Joints of Larynx

Cricoarytenoid Joint
Cricothyroid Joint } Synovial Joints

Points to Remember

> *Larynx of infants differ from the adults as:*
> - It is situated high up (C3–C4) and funnel shaped/conical (Adults–Cylindrical in shape) with narrow epiglottis
> - Cartilages are soft and collapse easily on forced inspiration. Epiglottis is omaga shaped It has more of submucosal space
> - The narrowest part of infantile larynx is the junction of subglottic larynx with trachea.^Q

NEW PATTERN QUESTION

Q N7. All of the following spaces are seen in relation to larynx except:

a. Space of Boyer b. Space of Tucker
c. Reinke's space d. Space of Gillette

Membranes of Thyroid

A. External membranes

I. Thyrohyoid membrane: connects the thyroid cartilage to the hyoid bone. Its median and lateral parts are thickened to form the median and lateral thyrohyoid ligaments.

Point to Remember

Structures Piercing it are Superior Laryngeal Vessels and Internal Laryngeal Nerve.

II. Hypoepiglottic ligament: It connects the epiglottic cartilage to the body of hyoid bone.

III. Cricotracheal membrane: It connects cricoid cartilage to the first tracheal ring.

B. Internal membranes

- **Quadrangular membrane** is a fibroelastic membrane which extends between the border of the epiglottis and the arytenoid cartilage. It has upper border called the **aryepiglottic fold** and a lower margin called as **vestibular fold** (false cord).
- **Cricovocal membrane:** This triangular fibroelastic membrane has free upper border (true vocal cords), which stretches between middle of thyroid angle to the vocal process of arytenoids. The lower border is attached to the arch of cricoid cartilage.
  - **Conus elasticus:** The two sides of cricovocal membranes form conus elasticus.
  - **Cricothyroid membrane:** The anterior part of conus elasticus is thick and forms cricothyroid membrane, which connects thyroid cartilage to cricoid cartilage.

Point to Remember

> Any airway obstruction above the vocal cord due to tumor or foreign body can be quickly, easily and effectively bypassed by piercing the cricothyroid membrane (**cricothyrotomy**). Subglottic foreign bodies sometimes get impacted in the region of conus elasticus.

INTERIOR OF THE LARYNX

Inlet of the larynx

Anteriorly	Bounded on sides	Posteriorly
Free edge of the epiglottis	Aryepiglottic folds	Mucous membrane over the interarytenoid fold

- Cavity of larynx extends from inlet of larynx to the lower border of the cricoid cartilage.
- Within the cavity of larynx, there are 2-folds of mucous membrane on each side. The upper fold is called as **vestibular fold** (false vocal cords) and the lower fold is called as **vocal fold** (True vocal cords).

The space between the right and left vestibular fold is called as *Rima vestibuli* and the space between vocal fold is called as *Rima glottidis*. It is the narrowest part of larynx.

Point to Remember

Rima glottidis is the narrowest part of larynx in adults whereas in infants the narrowest part of larynx is subglottic region.

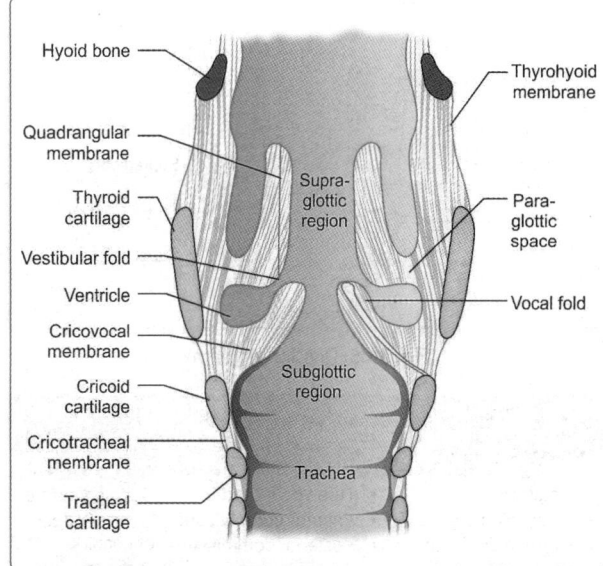

Fig. 26.4: Coronal section of larynx
Courtesy: Textbook of Diseases of Ear, Nose and Throat, Mohan Bansal, Jaypee Brothers Medical Publishers Pvt. Ltd., p 63.

Definition
Important Terminology
- The part above the vestibular fold – Vestibule of larynx
- The part between the vestibular and vocal fold – Sinus of Morgagni/ventricle of larynx
- The part below the vocal folds – Infraglottic part.

Point to Remember
> The anterior part of sinus of Morgagni is prolonged upward as a diverticulum between the vestibular fold and the lamina of thyroid cartilage, this extension is called as the Saccule of larynx. The secretion of mucus glands in the saccule provide lubrication for vocal cord region.

Clinical Correlation

Laryngocele: This abnormally enlarged and distended saccule contains air.

Retention cyst: The obstruction of duct of mucous gland in saccule can result in retention cyst.

Vocal Folds – True Vocal Cords

- Are twofold like structures which extend from the middle of the angle of the thyroid cartilage to the vocal process of the arytenoids posteriorly.
- True vocal cords — divide the larynx into 3 parts (Fig. 26.5):
    i. Part lying above the vocal cords — Supraglottis
    ii. At the level of true vocal cords — Glottis
    iii. Below the level of true vocal cords – Subglottis

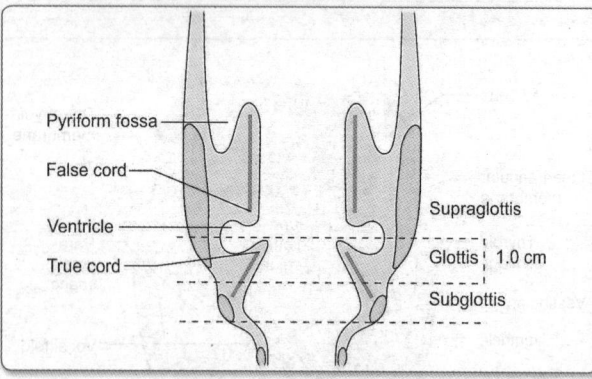

Fig. 26.5: Division of larynx

Table 26.1: Classification of sites and various subsites under each site in larynx (AJCC classification 2002)

Supraglottis	Glottis	Subglottis
• Epiglottis	• True vocal cord	Subglottis upto lower border of cricoid cartilage
• Aryepiglottic folds	• Anterior commissure	
• Drytenoids (laryngeal surface only)	• Posterior commissure	
• False vocal cords		
• Ventricle		
• Vestibule		

NEW PATTERN QUESTIONS

Q N8. Narrowest part in respiratory tract in adult is:
 a. Trachea   b. Glottis
 c. Supraglottis   d. Subglottis

Q N9. Narrowest part in an infant's respiratory tract is:
 a. Subglottis   b. Glottis
 c. Carina   d. None

Q N10. Which of the following is not true about Reinke's space?
 a. Potential space with scanty subepithelial connective tissue
 b. Lies under the epithelium of true vocal cords
 c. Lies superficial to elastic layer of vocal cords
 d. Lies under the epithelium of false vocal cords

Point to Remember
> *Mucous membrane of larynx:* The anterior surface and upper half of the posterior surface of epiglottis, the upper parts of aryepiglottic fold and the vocal folds are lined by nonkeratinizing stratified squamous epithelium. Rest of the laryngeal mucous membrane is covered with ciliated columnar epithelium.

Lymphatic drainage of the larynx

- Above the glottis : To upper deep cervical nodes
- Below the glottis : To lower deep cervical node chain through the prelaryngeal and pretracheal lymph nodes
- Glottis : Lymphatics in vocal cords are very scanty, hence glottic carcinoma rarely shows lymphatic metastasis.

Note: Delphian node – Prelaryngeal LNs in the region of thyroid isthmus are called Delphian nodes.

Nerve Supply

- **Superior laryngeal nerve:** Nerve of the 6th arch. It arises from the inferior ganglion of vagus and receives a branch from superior cervical sympathetic ganglion. It enters the larynx by piercing the thyrohyoid membrane.
- It divides at the level of greater cornu of hyoid into:
- **Internal laryngeal nerve:**
    - *Sensory (It supplies the larynx above the vocal cords i.e. supraglottic area)*
    - Secretomotor
- **External laryngeal nerve**—supplies cricothyroid muscle
    - The superior laryngeal nerve ends by piercing the inferior constrictor of pharynx and unites with ascending branch of recurrent laryngeal nerve. This branch is k/a Galen's anastomosis and is purely sensory.
- **Recurrent laryngeal nerve:**

Motor branch	Sensory branch
Supplies all the intrinsic muscles of the larynx except cricothyroid (which is supplied by external laryngeal nerve, a branch of superior laryngeal nerve).	Supplies larynx below the level of the vocal cords.

Chapter 26: Anatomy of Larynx, Congenital Lesions of Larynx and Stridor

- **Laryngeal muscles:** All muscles are paired except transverse arytenoid

Action	Muscle Responsible
Abductor:	• Posterior cricoarytenoid
Adductor:	• Lateral cricoarytenoid
	• Interarytenoid (transverse arytenoids)
	• Thyroarytenoid (external part)
Tensor:	• Cricothyroid^Q
Relax vocal cord:	• Thyroarytenoid (internal part)
	• Vocalis
Opener (of the laryngeal inlet):	• Thyroepiglotticus
Closure of the laryngeal inlet:	• Aryepiglotticus
	• Inter arytenoids (oblique part)

NEW PATTERN QUESTIONS

Q N11. Which of the following is the only intrinsic muscle of larynx that lies outside the laryngeal framework?
  a. Cricothyroid b. Superior constrictor
  c. Cricopharyngeus d. Lateral cricothyroid

Q N12. Abductor of vocal cord is:
  a. Posterior cricoarytenoid b. Lateral cricoarytenoid
  c. Cricothyroid d. None of the above

Q N13. A patient met with recurrent laryngeal nerve palsy while undergoing thyroid surgery. Which of the following muscles of larynx is/are affected?
  a. Posterior cricoarytenoid b. Lateral cricoarytenoid
  c. Thyroarytenoid d. Cricothyroid
  e. Vocalis

Arterial Supply

- **Up to vocal folds:** by superior laryngeal artery, a branch of superior thyroid artery.
- **Below vocal folds:** by inferior laryngeal artery, a branch of inferior thyroid artery.

The cricothyroid artery is a branch of superior thyroid artery and passes across the upper part of cricothyroid ligament to supply the larynx.

Venous Drainage

Superior laryngeal vein → Internal jugular vein
Inferior laryngeal vein → Inferior thyroid vein

EXAMINATION OF LARYNX

Indirect Laryngoscopy (IL)

Done using a laryngeal mirror

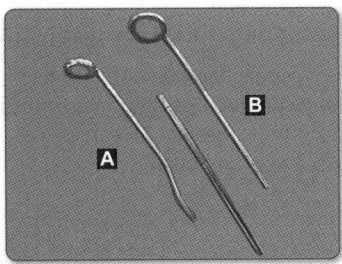

Fig. 26.6: Laryngoscopy (B) and rhinoscopy mirrors (A) with handle

Point to Remember

The posterior rhinoscopy mirror is smaller and its shaft is bayonet shaped, while the shaft of the laryngeal mirror is straight.

Structures which can be visualized by IL	Blind areas which cannot be visualized
• Larynx (with trachea rings)	• Laryngeal surface of epiglottis/infrahyoid epiglottis
• Parts of oropharynx (tongue base and vallecula)	• Ventricle of larynx
• Hypopharynx/laryngopharynx part viz.:	• Subglottis
– Pyriform sinus	• Anterior commissure
– Posterior wall of hypopharynx	• Apex of pyriform fossa
– Postcricoid region	

Points to Remember

- The movement of both the cords are observed when patient takes deep inspiration (abduction of cords) and says "Aa" (adduction cords) and "Eee" (for adduction and tension)
- To see the hidden areas—rigid or flexible endoscopy should be done.

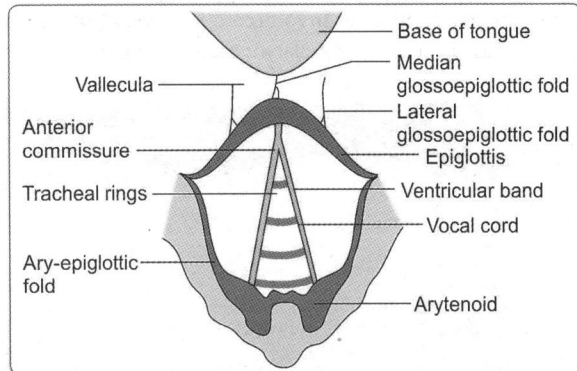

Fig. 26.7: Structures seen on indirect laryngoscopy

Direct Laryngoscopy (Fig. 26.8)

- Done using a rigid endoscope
- Position of patient – Boyce position/Barking-dog position.

Indications
1. To examine hidden areas of larynx
2. In infants and young children
3. To take biopsy
4. To perform microlaryngoscopic surgery.

Contraindications
- Cervical spine injury
- Aneurysm of arch of aorta
- Recent cardiac illness
- Stridor.

Note: In these condition and in voice disorders – Transnasal flexible laryngoscopy (TFL) is being done.

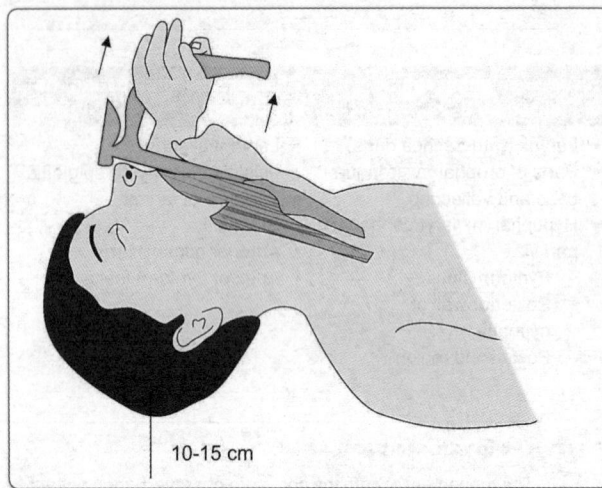

Fig. 26.8: Direct laryngoscopy

Microlaryngoscopy

- Combination of laryngoscope and operating microscopy done for precision in surgeries on vocal cord. Focal length of the lens of microscope used in microlaryngoscopy = 400 mm.

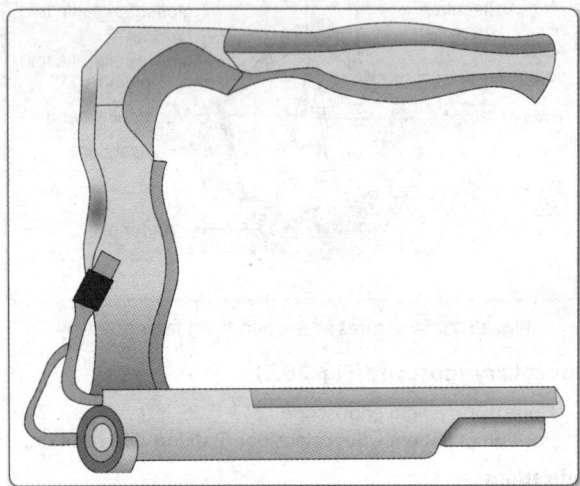

Fig. 26.9: Direct laryngoscope

NEW PATTERN QUESTION

Q N14. Laryngeal mirror is warmed before use by placing:
  a. Glass surface on flame
  b. Back of mirror on flame
  c. Whole mirror into flame
  d. Mirror in boiling water

CONGENITAL LESIONS OF LARYNX AND STRIDOR

Laryngocele

Definition

Laryngocele is an air-filled cystic swelling due to dilatation of saccule. The saccule is a diverticulum of mucous membrane which starts from the anterior part of ventricular cavity and extends upward between vestibular folds and lamina of thyroid cartilage. When it abnormally enlarges, it forms the air containing sac – *Laryngocele*.

Type

External 30%	Internal 20%	Mixed type 50%
Sac arises from the laryngeal ventricle and expands into the neck through the thyrohyoid membrane^Q	The dilatation remains confined to larynx	

Causes

Raised transglottic air pressure as in trumpet players, glass blowers or weight lifters.

Clinical Features

- Majority cases are asymptomatic.
- **The internal laryngocele** produces hoarseness of voice and may produce dyspnea due to pressure changes.
- **The external laryngocele** presents as a cystic swelling in neck which increases in size on coughing or performing Valsalva.
- It presents with hoarseness, cough and if large – obstruction to the airway.
- If neck of sac is blocked and it gets infected, pyocele is formed.

Investigation

- X-ray: Anteroposterior view with and without Valsalva maneuver.
- Indirect laryngoscopy helps to make the diagnosis.

Treatment

- Excision of the saccule at its neck together with removal of the upper half of thyroid lamina.
- Endoscopic marsupialization of internal laryngocele.

Note: In adults laryngocele may be associated with saccule carcinoma.

Laryngomalacia/Congenital Laryngeal Stridor

- *Most common* congenital anomaly of larynx.^Q
- *Most common* condition causing **inspiratory stridor** at or shortly afterbirth^Q (within first 2 weeks of life).
- In most cases, it is asymptomatic.
- M:F = 1:1
- There is abnormal flaccidity of laryngeal cartilage.^Q Stridor occurs as a result of sucking of supraglottic structures into the laryngeal inlet on inspiration.

- Manifests afterbirth (within first 2 weeks of life) and may persist throughout infancy.^Q (peak age – 6–9 months)
- Usually disappears by two years of age.^Q
- Inspiratory stridor is worse during exertion such as crying and feeding so stridor is intermittent.^Q
- *Strangely, stridor worsens during sleep, and positional variations occur—stridor is worse when patient is in supine position.*
- It decreases when child is placed in prone position and in hyperextension.
- Sometimes associated with cyanosis – (Dhingra 5th/ed, p 34)
- Cry is normal.
- Laryngoscopy finding—Omega shaped epiglottis.^Q Aryepiglottic folds are tall, thin and foreshortened.
- Treatment is conservative:
  - Reassure the patient.
  - Early antibiotic therapy for URI.
  - 10% patients need surgical intervention which includes supraglottoplasty (ary epiglottoplasty).
- In severe cases, tracheostomy may be needed.^Q

Point to Remember

Children with laryngomalacia have high prevalence of gastro-esophageal reflux disease (50–100%) and second synchronous airway lesion (17%).

Laryngeal Web/Atresia

- Mostly congenital but may be acquired.
- Congenital web is due to incomplete recanalization of larynx.
- *Most common* site: Anterior 2/3rd of the vocal cord.
- Webs have a concave posterior margin.

Symptom

The child presents with congenital airway obstruction (stridor), weak cry or aphomia.

Point to Remember

All patients need genetic screening and cardiovascular evaluation especially of aortic arch.

Treatment

- Tracheostomy - often required
- Thin web - cut with a knife or CO_2 laser
- Thick web - Excision via laryngofissure followed by placement of silicon keel (MC Naughter keel) and subsequent dilation.

Stridor

It is noisy respiration due to upper airways obstruction (i.e. from external naves up to trachea. Causes of stridor have been given in Flowchart 26.1.

Flowchart 26.1: Causes of stridor

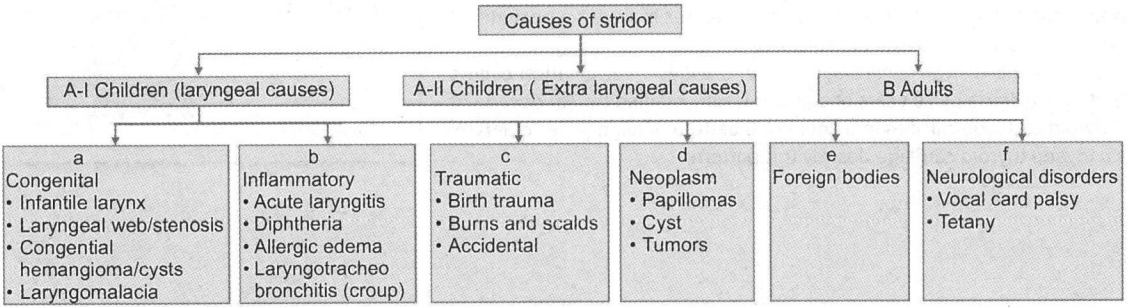

Extralaryngeal causes in children

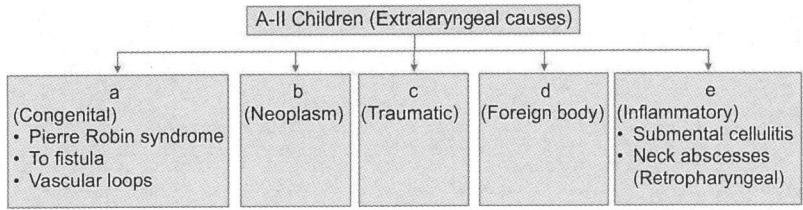

Causes in adults

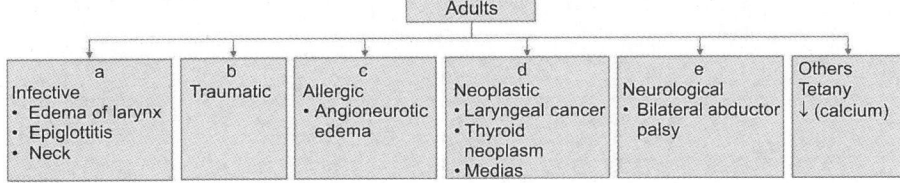

Section 5: Larynx

Points to Remember
- In children, chronic stridor is due to congenital lesions, mostly due to laryngomalacia.
- In children acute stridor is mostly due to acute upper respiratory tract infection.
- In adults stridor is uncommon chronic stridor may indicate laryngeal carcinoma.

NEW PATTERN QUESTION

Q N15. Palpatory thud or audible slap is seen in:
- a. Tracheal foreign body
- b. Bronchial foreign body
- c. Laryngeal foreign body
- d. None of the above

IMPORTANT CLINICAL CONCEPTS FOR NEET

- The only intrinsic muscle of the larynx which lies outside the laryngeal cartilages framework is cricothyroid.
- In thyroidectomy, the nerve commonly injured is external branch of superior laryngeal nerve.
- Posterior cricoarytenoid is the only abductor of vocal cord.
- Epiglottis is omega shaped in neonates and infants.
- Vocal cords have practically no lymphatics except for a small delphian node which lies on cricothyroid membrane (lymphatic watershed of larynx).
- Aryepiglottic fold has the richest lymphatic supply in larynx.
- Keyhole glottis is seen in thyroarytenoid weakness.
- Flag sign is seen in bilateral adductor palsy.
- In examination of neck, absence of laryngeal crepitus indicates a postcricoid growth or an abscess in the postcricoid area.
- Thyroid cartilage is hyaline cartilage and so calcifies – calcification occurs earliest in it. It starts by 20 years of age and is fully ossified by 7th decade of life. Thyroid cartilage calcifies in a figure of 8 pattern. Malignancies of larynx which invade thyroid cartilage destroy this pattern.

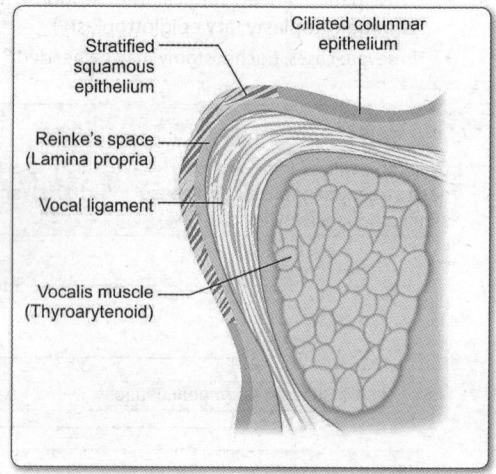

Explanations and References to New Pattern Questions

N1. Ans. is a i.e. Epiglottis   *Ref. Dhingra 6/e, p 282*

Epiglottis is elastic cartilage
Thyroid, cricoid and arytenoids are hyaline cartilage.

N2. Ans. is c i.e. Both of the above

N3. Ans. is c i.e. Fourth arch   *Ref. Dhingra 6/e, p 285*

Larynx develops from both 4th and 6th arch. The vocal cords are attached to middle of thyroid cartilage.
Part of larynx above the vocal cords, i.e. supraglottic part develops from 6th arch.
Part of larynx below the vocal cords (subglottis) and a glottis develop from 4th arch.
Therefore upper part of thyroid cartilage develops from 4th arch and lower part of thyroid cartilage develops from 6th arch.

Part of Larynx	Develops from
• Epiglottis	
• Upper part of thyroid	• Develop from 6th arch
• Lower part of thyroid	
• Cricoid cartilage	
• Corniculate cartilage	• Develop from 4th arch
• Cuneiform cartilage	

N4. Ans. is c i.e. Cricotracheal membrane

N5. Ans. is c i.e. Middle constrictor   *Ref. Essential of ENT, Mohan Bansal, p 286*

Attachments of oblique line:
- Sternothyroid
- Thyrohyoid
- Inferior constrictor

N6. Ans. is b i.e. Epiglottis   *Ref. Essential of ENT, Mohan Bansal, p 286*

Epiglottis is leaf-shaped fibrocartilage.

N7. Ans. is d i.e. Space of Gillette   *Ref. Dhingra 6/e, p 265*

Space of Gillette is seen in pharynx in relation to retropharyngeal space and not in larynx.
Also know
Spaces in relation to larynx
1. **Pre-epiglottic space (Space of Boyer)**
   Location: Between the thyroid and thyrohyoid membrane anteriorly and epiglottis posteriorly. Laterally it is continuous with paraglottic space.

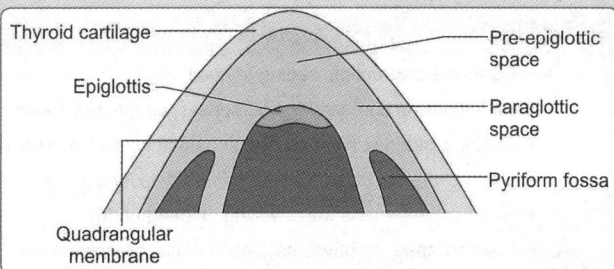

2. **Paraglottic space (space of Tucker):** It is bounded by the thyroid cartilage laterally conus elasticus inferomedially, the ventricle and quadrangular membrane medially, and mucosa of paraglottic with pre-epiglottic space. Growths which invade this space can present in the neck through cricothyroid space.
3. **Reinke's space:** Under the epithelium of vocal cords is a potential space with scanty subepithelial connective tissues. It is bounded above and below by the arcuate lines, in front by anterior commissure, and behind by vocal process of arytenoid. Oedema of this space causes fusiform swelling of the membranous cords (Reinke's oedema).

N8. Ans. is b i.e. Glottis

N9. Ans. is a i.e. Subglottis

- The narrowest part of larynx
- In adults – Glottis
- In children – Subglottis.

N10. Ans. is d i.e. Lies under the epithelium of false vocal cords *Ref. Dhingra 6/e, p 285*

Reinke's space
Reinke's space is a subepithelial space on the vocal cord
  Its bounded:
- Superiorly by mucous membrane of vocal cord
- Inferiorly by vocal cords
- Anteriorly by anterior commissure
- Posteriorly by vocal process of arytenoid cartilage
- Importance of this space is edema of the space leads to Reinke edema. Reinke's space also prevents spread of glottic carcinoma to deeper structures.

N11. Ans. is a i.e. Cricothyroid *Ref. Dhingra 6/e, p 284, Fig's 56.5, 56.6*

- Cricothyroid muscle is the only intrinsic muscle which is supplied by external laryngeal nerve and lies outside the laryngeal framework.

N12. Ans. is a i.e. Posterior cricoarytenoid *Ref. Dhingra 6/e, p 283*

Posterior cricoarytenoids are the only abductors of vocal cord.
Adductors of vocal cord can be memorized by mnemonic TALC as discussed in text.

N13. Ans. is a, b, c and e i.e. Posterior cricoarytenoid; Lateral cricoarytenoid; Thyroarytenoid; and Vocalis *Ref. Dhingra 6/e, p 298*

All muscles of larynx are supplied by the recurrent laryngeal nerve except the cricothyroid muscle which is supplied by external laryngeal nerve (a branch of superior laryngeal nerve); hence it will be spared.

N14. Ans. is a i.e. Glass surface on flame *Ref. Tuli 1/e, p 234*

Laryngeal mirror is warmed by:
- Dipping the mirror in warm water.
- Heating the glass surface against some heat such as bulb or spirit lamp.

N15. Ans. is a i.e. Tracheal foreign body *Ref. Dhingra 6/e, p 321*

A foreign body in trachea may move up and down the trachea between the carnia and the undersurface of vocal cords causing "audible slap" and "palpatory thud".

Symptoms and signs of foreign bodies at different levels

Site of foreign bodies	Symptoms and signs
Larynx	• Complete obstruction leading to death
	• Partial obstruction: stridor, hoarseness, cough, respiratory difficulty
Trachea	• Choking, striodor, wheeze, cough palpatory thud, audible slap
Bronchi	• Cough, wheeze and diminished air entry to lung forms a "triad"
	• Respiratory distress with swelling of foreign body
	• Lung collapse, emphysema, pneumonitis, bronchiectasis or lung abscess are late features

QUESTIONS

1. **All of the following are paired except:** [PGI Nov 05]
   a. Interarytenoids b. Corniculate
   c. Vocal cords d. Cricothyroids
   e. Thyroid
2. **Laryngeal cartilage forming complete circle:** [TN 08]
   a. Arytenoid b. Cricoid
   c. Thyroid d. Hyoid
3. **True about larynx in neonate:** [PGI 03]
   a. Epiglottis is large and omega shaped
   b. Cricoid narrowest part
   c. It extends C4,5,6 vertebrae
   d. Tongue is small in comparison to oral cavity
   e. Funnel shaped
4. **Narrowest part of infantile larynx is:** [Assam 95, RJ 05]
   a. Supraglottic b. Subglottic
   c. Glottic d. None of the above
5. **Abductor of vocal cord is:** [Kerala 95]
   a. Cricothyroid b. Posterior cricoarytenoid
   c. Lateral cricoarytenoid d. Cricohyoid
6. **All are elevators of larynx except:** [AP 04]
   a. Thyrohyoid b. Digastric
   c. Stylohyoid d. Sternohyoid
7. **Sensory nerve supply of larynx below the level of vocal cord is:** [AIIMS 98; AI 95]
   a. External branch of superior laryngeal nerve
   b. Internal branch of superior laryngeal nerve
   c. Recurrent laryngeal nerve
   d. Inferior pharyngeal
8. **Supraglottis includes all of the following except:**
   a. Aryepiglottic fold
   b. False cord
   c. Lingual surface of epiglottis
   d. Laryngeal surface of epiglottis
9. **Epilarynx include(s):** [PGI Nov 10]
   a. Suprahyoid epiglottis b. Infrahyoid epiglottis
   c. False cords d. Posterior commissure
10. **The water cane in the larynx (saccules) are present in:**
    a. Paraglottic space b. Pyriform fossa [UP 07]
    c. Reinke's space d. Laryngeal ventricles
11. **Vocal cord is lined by:** [Delhi 96]
    a. Stratified columnar epithelium
    b. Pseudostratified ciliated columnar epithelium
    c. Stratified squamous epithelium
    d. Cuboidal epithelium
12. **Inlet of larynx is formed by:** [Kolkata 03]
    a. Ventricular fold b. Aryepiglottic fold
    c. Glossoepiglottic fold d. Vocal cord
13. **A neonate while suckling milk can respire without difficulty due to:** [AIIMS Nov 10]
    a. Start soft palate b. Small tongue
    c. High larynx d. Small pharynx
14. **Laryngocele arises from:** [AIIMS May 05, 08]
    a. Anterior commissure b. Saccule of the ventricle
    c. True cords d. False cords
15. **Laryngocele arises as herniation of laryngeal mucosa through the following membrane:** [AI 06]
    a. Thyrohyoid b. Cricothyroid
    c. Cricotracheal d. Crisosternal
16. **Most common congenital anomaly of larynx:** [TN 99; Delhi-08]
    a. Laryngeal web b. Laryngomalacia
    c. Laryngeal stenosis d. Vocal and palsy
17. **Regarding laryngomalacia:** [PGI 02]
    a. Most common cause of stridor in newborn
    b. Omega-shaped epiglottis
    c. Inspiratory stridor
    d. Requires immediate surgery
    e. Stridor worsens on lying in prone position
18. **Which is not true about laryngomalacia?** [AI 12]
    a. Omega-shaped epiglottis
    b. Stridor increases on crying, but decreases on placing the child in prone position
    c. Most common congenital anomaly of the larynx
    d. Surgical management of the airway by tracheostomy is the preferred initial treatment
19. **About laryngomalacia, all are true except:** [PGI 08]
    a. MC neonatal respiratory lesion
    b. Decreased symptoms during prone position
    c. Self-limiting by 2–3 years of age
    d. Omega-shaped epiglottis seen
    e. Surgery is treatment of choice
20. **Most common mode of treatment for laryngomalacia is:** [UP 07]
    a. Reassurance b. Medical
    c. Surgery d. Wait and watch
21. **MC cause of intermittent stridor in a 10-day-old child shortly afterbirth is:** [AI 01; AIIMS 95]
    a. Laryngomalacia b. Foreign body
    c. Vocal nodule d. Hypertrophy of turbinate
22. **Most common cause of stridor in children is:** [UP 07]
    a. Laryngomalacia b. Congenital laryngeal paralysis
    c. Foreign body in larynx d. Congenital laryngeal tumors
23. **Causes of congenital laryngeal stridor is/are:** [PGI 00]
    a. Laryngomalacia b. Laryngeal papillomatosis
    c. Subglottic papilloma d. Laryngeal stenosis
    e. Hemangioma of larynx
24. **Main treatment of congenital laryngeal stridor is:**
    a. Tracheostomy [JIPMER 04]
    b. Steroid therapy
    c. Reassurance to the child's parents
    d. Amputating epiglottis

Section 5: Larynx

25. **Stridor is caused by all *except*:** [AP 96]
    a. Hypocalcemia   b. Asthma
    c. Epiglottis   d. Laryngeal tumor
26. **A 2-year-old boy presenting with sudden severe dyspnea, most common cause is:** [Bihar 06]
    a. Foreign body
    b. Bronchiolitis
    c. Asthmatic attack
    d. None
27. **Stridor in adults is most commonly caused by:** [Delhi 96]
    a. Reinke's edema
    b. Malignancy
    c. Acute severe asthma
    d. Toxic gas inhalation
28. **The most common cause of laryngeal stridor in a 60-year-old male is:** [JIPMER 91]
    a. Nasopharyngeal carcinoma
    b. Thyroid carcinoma
    c. Foreign body aspiration
    d. Carcinoma larynx
29. **Laryngofissure is:** [JIPMER 04]
    a. Opening the larynx in midline
    b. Making window in thyroid cartilage
    c. Removal of arytenoids
    d. Removal of epiglottis
30. **In an direct laryngoscopy which of the following can be visualized:** [PGI Dec 01]
    a. Cricothyroid   b. Lingual surface of epiglottis
    c. Arytenoids   d. Pyriform fossa
    e. Tracheal cartilage
31. **Which of the following is difficult to visualize or examine on indirect laryngoscopy?** [MH-PGM-CET 07; MH 08]
    a. True vocal cord   b. Anterior commmissure
    c. Epiglottis   d. False vocal cord
32. **Microlaryngoscopy was started by:** [MH 03]
    a. Bruce Benjamin   b. Kleinsasser
    c. Chevalier Jackson   d. None of the above
33. **The procedure that should precede microlaryngoscopy is:** [AI 91]
    a. Pharyngoscopy   b. Esophagoscopy
    c. Rhinoscopy   d. Laryngoendoscopy

Explanations and References

1. **Ans. is a and e i.e. Interarytenoid; and Thyroid**
   Ref. BDC, Vol. 3, 4/e, p 240,244; Scott-Brown's 7/e, Vol. 2 p 2133; Dhingra 5/e, p 299, 6/e, p 282; Mohan Bansal p 62

   - All intrinsic muscles of larynx are paired except transverse arytenoid/interarytenoid.
   - As far as cartilages of larynx are concerned 3 are paired and 3 are unpaired.

Unpaired cartilage	Paired cartilage
Thyroid cartilage	Arytenoid
Cricoid	Corniculate
Epiglottis	Cuneiform

   Vocal cords are also paired structures.

2. **Ans. is b i.e. Cricoid**
   Ref. BDC, Vol III, 4/e, p 240; Dhingra 5/e, p 299, 6/e, p 282; Mohan Bansal p 62

Cartilage	Shape
Thyroid cartilage	V shaped on cross section. Has 2 lamina right and left which are placed at an angle of 90° in males and 120° in females
Cricoid cartilage	Ring shaped (it is the only complete ring present in the air passages)
Epiglottic cartilage	Leaf shaped in adults, omega shaped in infants and neonates
Arytenoid cartilage	Pyramid shaped
Corniculate cartilage	Cone shaped
Cuneiform cartilage	Rod shaped

   Also know: The thyroid, cricoid and basal parts of arytenoid cartilages are made up of hyaline cartilage. They ossify after the age of 25 years. The other cartilages, e.g. epiglottis, corniculate, cuneiform and processes of the arytenoid are made of elastic cartilage and do not ossify.

3. **Ans. is a, b and e i.e. Epiglottis is large and omega shaped; Cricoid narrowest part; and Funnel shaped**
   Ref. Miller Anaesthesia 5/e, p 2090; Tuli 1/e, p 284; Scott-Brown's 7/e, Vol 2, p 2131; Mohan Bansal p 67; Dhingra 6/e, p 285

Chapter 26: Anatomy of Larynx, Congenital Lesions of Larynx and Stridor

Points to Remember

Infant's Larynx Differs from Adult in:
1. It is situated high up (C2 – C4).º (in adults = C3 – C6)
2. Of equal size in both sixes *(in adults it is larger in males)*
3. Larynx is funnel shaped
4. The narrowest part of the infantile larynx is the junction of subglottic larynx with trachea and this is because cricoid cartilage is very small
5. Cartilages:
   a. Epiglottis is *omega shaped, soft, large* and *patulous.*
   b. Laryngeal cartilages are soft and collapse easily
   c. Thyroid cartilage is flat
   d. Arytenoid cartilage is relatively large
6. The cricothyroid and thyrohyoid spaces are narrow
7. The submucosal tissue is thick and loose and becomes oedematous in response inflammation
8. Vocal cords are angled and lie at level of C8
9. Trachea bifurcates at level of T9

Note: Narrowest part of adult larynx is Rima Glottidis.

4. Ans. is b i.e. Subglottic   *Ref. Scott-Brown's 7/e, Vol 2, p 2131; Dhingra 5/e, p 303, 6/e, p 285*

The infantile larynx
" *The diameter of cricoid cartilage is smaller than the size of glottis, making subglottis the narrowest part.*"   *Ref. Dhingra 5/e, p 303*
"*Rima glottidis (Glottis) is the narrowest part of larynx in adults whereas in infants the narrowest part of larynx is subglottis region.*"
Ref. Mohan Bansal p 6

5. Ans. is b i.e. Posterior cricoarytenoid   *Ref. BDC, Vol 3, 4/e, p 245; Dhingra 5/e, p 300, 6/e, p 283*

Remember
Posterior cricoarytenoid is the only abductor of vocal cord.

Adductors of vocal cord are:
T = **T**hyroarytenoid
A = Transverse **a**rytenoid
L = **L**ateral cricoarytenoid
C = **C**ricothyroid

Mnemonic

Add TALC i.e. Adductors are TALC.

6. Ans. is a i.e. Thyrohyoid   *Ref. BDC 4/e, Vol 3 p 243 Table 16.2; Mohan Bansal p 66*
Elevation of larynx is carried out by – Thyrohyoid and mylohyoid   *Ref. BDC 4/e, Vol 3 p 243*

Movement	Muscles
1. Elevation of larynx	Thyrohyoid, mylohyoid
2. Depression of larynx	Sternohyoid, sternothyroid, omohyoid
3. Opening the inlet of larynx	Thyroepiglotticus
4. Closing of inlet of larynx	Aryepiglotticus
5. Abductor of vocal cord	Posterior cricoarytenoids
6. Adductor of vocal cord	T – Thyroarytenoid A – Transverse arytenoids L – Lateral cricoarytenoid C – Cricothyroid
7. Tensor of vocal cord	Cricothyroid
8. Relaxor of vocal cord	Thyroarytenoid

ALSO KNOW – According to Dhingra 5/e, p 301, 6/e, p 284

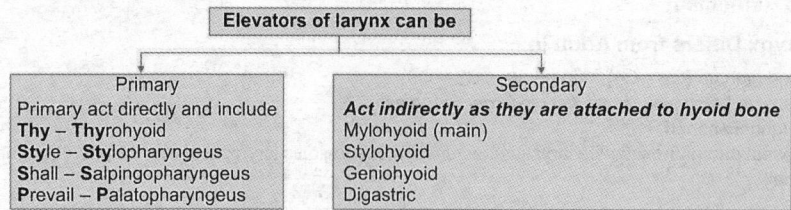

7. **Ans. is c i.e. Recurrent laryngeal nerve** *Ref. BDC, Vol 3, 4/e, p 246; Mohan Bansal p 66; Dhingra 6/e, p 298*

   Nerve supply of larynx
   - *Sensory:*
     - The internal laryngeal nerve supplies the mucous membrane up to the level of the vocal folds.
     - The recurrent laryngeal nerve supplies below the level of the vocal folds.
   - *Motor:*
     - All intrinsic muscles of the larynx are supplied by the recurrent laryngeal nerve except for the cricothyroid which is supplied by the external laryngeal nerve.

8. **Ans. is c i.e. Lingual surface of epiglottis** *Ref. Logan Turner 10/e, p 171*
   - The lingual surface of epiglottis and vallecula are a part of oropharynx according to *Logan Turner 10/e, p 171*
   - According to *Dhingra 6th/ed p 307*
     "Whole of epiglottis is included in supraglottic area."
   - According to Scott-Brown's 7th/ed Vol 3 p 2132 – whole of epiglottis is included in the supraglottic.
   - But since here we have to choose one option. Therefore, I am going with Turner.

9. **Ans. is a and c i.e. Suprahyoid epiglottis; and False cords** *Ref. Dhingra 6/e, p 307; Stell and Manran's Head and Neck Surgery 4/e, p 233*

   Classification of sites and various subsites under each site in larynx (AJCC classification, 2002)

Site	Subsite
Supraglottis	• Suprahyoid epiglottis (both lingual and laryngeal surfaces) • Infrahyoid epiglottis • Aryepiglottic folds (laryngeal aspect only) • Arytenoids • Ventricular bands (or false cords)
Glottis	True vocal cords including anterior and posterior commissure
Subglottis	Subglottis up to lower border of cricoid cartilage

    Note: Suprahyoid epiglottis, infrahyoid epiglottis, aryepiglottic folds and arytenoids together are called epilarynx.

10. **Ans. is d i.e. Laryngeal ventricles** *Ref. Dhingra 5/e, p 301, 6/e, p 284; BDC, Vol 3, 4/e, p 242; Mohan Bansal p 64,65*

    It is a diverticulum of mucous membrane which starts from the anterior part of laryngeal ventricle extending between the vestibular folds and lamina of thyroid cartilage. The saccule has plenty of mucous glands whose main purpose is to lubricate the vocal cords (vocal cord is devoid of mucous glands) and hence is known as water can of larynx.

     Note: When distended the saccule can protrude through the *thyrohyoid* membrane in the neck and is known as *Laryngocele*.

    ALSO KNOW

    Boyer's space – another name for the pre-epiglottic space which lies in front of epiglottic beneath the hyoid bone.

11. **Ans. is c i.e. Stratified squamous epithelium** *Ref. Dhingra 5/e, p 302, 6/e, p 285; Scott-Brown's 7/e, Vol 2, p 2137; Mohan Bansal p 65*

    Whole of larynx is lined by ciliated columnar epithelium except the vocal cords and upper part of vestibule which is lined by stratified squamous epithelium.

Chapter 26: Anatomy of Larynx, Congenital Lesions of Larynx and Stridor

ALSO KNOW

Mucous glands are distributed all over the larynx except the vocal cords, which is lubricated by mucus from glands within the saccule. The squamous epithelium of vocal fold is, therefore prone to desiccation if these glands cease to function as in radiotherapy.

12. **Ans. is b i.e. Aryepiglottic fold** *Ref. BDC 4/e, Vol 3, p 242; Dhingra 6/e p 284*

    Inlet of the larynx is bounded by:
    Anteriorly   – Epiglottis
    Posteriorily   – Interarytenoid fold of mucous membrane
    On each side by   – **Aryepiglottic fold**

13. **Ans. is c i.e. High larynx** *Ref. Dhingra 6/e, p 285*

    Infant's larynx is positioned high in the neck level of glottis being oppostie to C3 or C4 at rest and reaches C1 or C2 during swallowing. This high position allows the epiglottis to meet soft palate and make anasopharyngeal channel for nasal breathing during suckling. The milk feed passes separately over the dorsum of tongue and the side of epiglottis, thus allowing breathing and feeding to go on simultaneously.

14. **Ans. is b i.e. Saccule of the ventricle** *Ref. Dhingra 5/e, p 34, 6/e, p 295*

15. **Ans. is a i.e. Thyrohyoid** *Ref. Turner 10/e, p 168; Mohan Bansal 1st/ed p 487*

    Laryngocele is an air-filled cystic swelling which occurs due to dilatation of saccule.
    Saccule is a diverticulum arising from anterior part of ventricle/sinus of larynx.^{Q}
    External laryngocele is one in which distended saccule **herniates through the thyrohyoid membrane**^{Q} and presents as a reducible swelling in the neck, which increases in size on coughing or performing Valsalva.

16. **Ans. is b i.e. Laryngomalacia**

17. **Ans. is a, b and c i.e. Most common cause of stridor in newborn; Omega-shaped epiglottis; and Inspiratory stridor**

18. **Ans. is d i.e. Surgical management of the airway by tracheostomy is the preferred initial treatment**
    Ref. Dhingra 5/e, p 314, 6/e, p 285; Turner 10/e, p 385,386; Current Otolaryngology 2/e, p 462,463; Mohan Bansal p 514

Laryngomalacia

- It is the M/C congenital anomaly of the larynx
- It is the M/C condition causing inspiratory stridor afterbirth
- The stridor worsens during sleep and when baby is in supine position (not in prone position). Rather when the child is placed in prone position it is relieved
- On laryngoscopy – Epiglottis is omega shaped and aryepiglottis folds are floppy.

Treatment

Conservative Management

19. **Ans. is b and e i.e. Decreased symptoms during prone position; and Surgery is treatment of choice**
    Ref. Dhingra 5/e, p 314; Current Otolaryngology 2/e, p 462; Mohan p 514

Option	Correct/ Incorrect	Reference	Explanation
Option a M/C neonatal respiratory lesion	Not sure	Current 2nd/ed p 462	Laryngomalacia is the most common cause of stridor in infants and is also the most common congenital laryngeal abnormality but whether it is M/c neonatal respiratory lesion is not sure.
Option b Decreased symptoms during prone position	Incorrect	Current Otolaryngology 2nd/ed p 462; Dhingra 5th/ed p 314, 6th/ed p 295	– Stridor in laryngomalacia is intermittent and not constant. – It is worse during sleep or when patient is in supine position **It is improved in** – prone position
Option c Self-limiting by 2–3 years of age	Correct	Dhingra 5th/ed p 314; Current Otolaryngology 2nd/ed p 462	"It manifests at birth or soon after and usually disappears by 2 years of age" – Dhingra 5th/ed p 314, 6th/ed p 295

Contd...

Contd...

Option	Correct/ Incorrect	Reference	Explanation
Option d Omega-shaped epiglottis seen	Correct	Dhingra 5th/ed p 314, 6th/ed p 295; Current Otolaryngology 2nd/ed p 462	On direct laryngoscopy – Epiglottis is omega shaped – Aryepiglottic folds – floppy – Arytenoids – prominent
Option e Surgery is T/t of choice	Incorrect	Dhingra 5th/ed p 314, 6th/ed p 295; Current Otolaryngology 2nd/ed p 462	Treatment is mostly conservative Surgery is required in only 10% cases **Indications of surgery** – Severe stridor – Apnea – Failure to thrive – Pulmonary hypertension – Corpulmonale

20. **Ans. is a i.e. Reassurance** *Ref. Dhingra 5/e, p 314, 6/e, p 295; Turner 10/e, p 386; Current Otolaryngology 2/e, p 463*

    In most patients laryngomalacia is a self-limiting condition.
    Treatment of laryngomalacia is reassurance to the parents and early antibiotic therapy for upper respiratory tract infections.
    Tracheostomy is required only in severe respiratory obstruction.
    Surgical intervention (supraglottoplasty, i.e. reduction of redundant laryngeal mucosa) is indicated for 10% of patients. Main indications for surgery are:
    - Severe stridor
    - Apnea
    - Failure to thrive
    - Pulmonary hypertension
    - Cor pulmonale.

21. **Ans. is a i.e. Laryngomalacia** *Ref. Turner 10/e, p 385; Current Otolaryngology 2/e, p 462*

    Laryngomalacia is the most common cause of inspiratory stridor in neonates.
    The stridor in case of laryngomalacia is not constantly present, rather it is intermittent. So laryngomalacia is also the M/C cause of intermittent stridor in neonates.

22. **Ans. is c i.e. Foreign body in larynx** *Ref. Ghai 6/e, p 341*

    Read the question carefully.
    It says most common cause of stridor in **children**—which is not laryngomalacia, it usually resolves spontaneously by the age of 2 years and is rare after that.
    "Foreign body aspiration should always be considered as a potential cause of stridor and airway obstruction in children."
    Ref. Ghai 6/e, p 341

    ALSO KNOW

    > *Most common* causes of chronic stridor in children is long-term intubation causing laryngotracheal stenosis.

23. **Ans. is a, d and e i.e. Laryngomalacia; Laryngeal stenosis; and Hemangioma of larynx**
    Ref. Tuli 1/e, p 295; Current Otolaryngology 2/e, p 463; Mohan Bansal p 474

    Causes of congenital laryngeal stridor:

    - Infantile larynx
    - Laryngomalacia
    - Laryngeal web/stenosis
    - Laryngeal cyst
    - **Congenital hemangioma** (subglottic)
    - Posterior laryngeal cleft
    - Vocal cord paralysis
    - Cricoarytenoid joint fixation

24. **Ans. is c i.e. Reassurance to the child's parent** *Ref. Dhingra 5/e, p 314, 6/e, p 295*

    Congenital laryngeal stridor is synonymous with laryngomalacia. Hence, management remains the same i.e. reassurance to childs parent.

25. **Ans. is b i.e. Asthma** *Ref. Dhingra 5/e, p 315*
    - First you should know what exactly upper and lower airway means:
        i. **Upper airway:** The airway from the nares and lips to the lower border of larynx (includes nose, pharynx, larynx).
        ii. **Lower airway:** From the lower border of the terminal bronchioles (includes various level of bronchioles up to terminal bronchioles).

- **Stridor usually implies upper airway obstruction, so the level of obstruction is above the level of trachea (P)** (from nares to the larynx).
- *Wheezing and ronchi* are signs of lower airway obstruction.
  Epiglottitis and laryngeal tumors are common causes of stridor and do not need explanation.
  Hypocalcemia leads to tetany which causes stridor.
  Asthma leads to wheezing or ronchi (lower airway obstruction)
  Also know – Stridor is a harsh noise produced by turbulent air flow through a partially obstructed upper airway.
  It can be:
  - Inspiratory, i.e. originates from supraglottis glottis and pharynx
  - Expiratory, i.e. originates from thoracic trachea
  - Biphasic i.e. originates from subglottis and cervical trachea.
  Hence, stridor is mainly of laryngeal and tracheal origin.

26. **Ans. is a i.e. Foreign body**   *Ref. Scott-Brown's 7/e, Vol 1, p 1117; Dhingra 5/e, p 315, 6/e, p 295*
    In case of stridor with acute airway obstruction (i.e. dyspnea) always history of any foreign body ingestion should be taken.

27. **Ans. is b i.e. Malignancy**   *Ref. Read below*
    The answer to this question can be derived by exclusion.
    Reinke's edema leads to hoarseness of voice and not stridor. (Dhingra 5/e, p 311, 6/e, p 292) Ruling out **option 'a'.**
    - Acute severe asthma also does not lead of stridor.
    - Toxic gas inhalation does not lead to stridor. So we are left with one option i.e. malignancy.

28. **Ans. is d i.e. Carcinoma larynx**   *Ref. Dhingra 5/e, p 315-317, 6/e, p 296–297; Mohan Bansal p 474*
    Most common cause for stridor in 60 years old male will be carcinoma larynx as carcinoma larynx occurs in males (predominantly) at the age of 40–70 years.
    Most common and earliest symptom of subglottic cancer is stridor.

    Note:
    - Nasopharyngeal cancer does not lead to stridor
    - Thyroid cancer causes stridor rarely
    - Foreign body aspiration is a common cause of stridor in children and not adults.

29. **Ans. is a i.e. Opening the larynx in midline**   *Ref. Stedman Dictionary, p 937*
    Laryngofissure: Opening the larynx in midline.

30. **Ans. is a, b, c, d and e i.e. Cricothyroid; Lingual surface of the epiglottis; Arytenoids; Pyriform fossa; and Tracheal cartilage**
    Ref. Dhingra 5/e, p 432, 6/e, p 384; Tuli 1/e, p 527
    Structures seen on *Indirect laryngoscopy* are:
    - **Larynx:** Epiglottis, aryepiglottic folds, arytenoids, cuneiform and corniculate cartilage, ventricular ands, ventricles, true cords, anterior commissure, posterior commissure, subglottis and rings of trachea.
    - **Hypopharynx:** Both pyriform fossae, post-cricoid region, posterior wall of laryngopharynx.
    - **Oropharynx:** Base of tongue, lingual tonsils, valleculae, media and lateral glossoepiglottic folds.

    Note: *In indirect laryngoscopy* – The hidden ares of larynx viz. Anterior Commisure, Ventricle and Subglottic area are not seen properly.

31. **Ans. is b i.e. Anterior commissure**   *Ref. Dhingra 5/e, p 432, 6/e, p 384 p 70; Tuli 1/e, p 527; Mohan Bansal p 70*
    Hidden areas of larynx viz. infrahyoid epiglottis, anterior commissure, ventricles and subglottic region and apex of pyriform fossa are difficult to visualize by indirect laryngoscopy.

32. **Ans. is b i.e. Kleinsasser**   *Ref. Maqbool 11/e, p 323*
    "The present day microsurgical techniques of the larynx are a credit to **Kleinsasser.**"   *Ref. Maqbool 11/e, p 323*

33. **Ans. is d i.e. Laryngoendoscopy**   *Ref. Scott-Brown's 7/e, Vol 2, p 2236*
    The answer is not given directly but the following lines of *Scott-Brown's* leave no doubt about the answer—"Microlaryngoscopy concentrates mainly on the glottic area in cases where the diagnosis is already established and unlike direct laryngoscopy, is not primarily concerned with other areas of larynx which should have been assessed preoperatively."
    It is clear direct laryngoscopy (or laryngoendoscopy as given in the options) should always be done prior to microlaryngoscopy.

Chapter 27

Acute and Chronic Inflammation of Larynx, Voice and Speech Disorders

ACUTE LARYNGOTRACHEOBRONCHITIS (CROUP)

- It is a dangerous infection seen mostly in children which involves whole of tracheobronchial tree.

Organism

- Mostly viruses (parainfluenza type 1 and 2 and influenza A).
- In adults it can be caused by:
  - H. simplex
  - Cytomegalovirus
  - Influenza virus
  - Superimposed bacterial infection *[Hemolytic streptococci]* usually occurs.

Features

- Age group—*most common* in 6 months to 3 years although children < 7 years are susceptible
- Male > Female.

Pathology

- Mucosal swelling especially in subglottic area. Subglottic edema is most characteristic pathological feature^Q
- Production of thick tenacious mucus which can hardly be expectorated
- Pseudomembrane formation
- All these can lead to airway obstruction.

Clinical Features

- Onset is gradual with prodrome of upper respiratory symptoms
- Fever usually low grade
- Painful croupy cough (barking cough or seal barks cough)
- Hoarseness and stridor (initially inspiratory; then biphasic)
- Upper Airway obstruction which is visible in the form of suprasternal and intracostal recession.

> **Point to Remember**
> ➢ Acute laryngotracheo bronchitis is the M/C cause of infectious respiratory obstruction in children.

Investigation

- X-ray: "Steeple sign" i.e. symmetric steeple or funnel-shaped narrowing of subglottic region.

Treatment

- Broad-spectrum penicillin (for secondary bacterial infection)
- IV steroids, if child is in distress
- Humidified air
- IV fluids
- Nebulization with adrenaline.

In despite above measures respiratory obstruction increases intubation/tracheostomy is done.

> **Points to Remember**
> **Indications for Intubation**
> ➢ Rising CO_2 level
> ➢ Worsening neurologic status
> ➢ Decreasing respiratory rate.

NEW PATTERN QUESTION

Q N1. Steeple sign is seen in:
  a. Croup
  b. Acute epiglottis
  c. Laryngomalacia
  d. Quinsy

ACUTE EPIGLOTTITIS (SUPRAGLOTTIC LARYNGITIS)

- It is acute inflammatory condition of the supraglottic structures viz.
  - Epiglottis
  - Aryepiglottic fold and arytenoids.
- **Most common organism in children:** *H. influenza*—type B
- **In adults**—it can be caused by:
  - Group A streptococci, *S. pneumoniae, S. aureus, Klebsiella pneumoniae*
  - Recently, *Neisseria meningitidis* has been recognized as a cause of fulminant life-threatening supraglottitis.

Clinical Features

- Age group—mostly seen in 3–6 years but can occur in adults also
- There is usually a short history with rapid progression
- Starts with URI and fever (sometimes > 40°C)
- Sore throat and dysphagia are the most common presenting symptoms in adults.

- Dyspnea and stridor are the most common presenting symptoms in children. Stridor is inspiratory and increases on supine position
- Child prefers sitting position with hyperextended neck *(tripod sign)* which relieves stridor
- Drooling of saliva present as child has dysphagia
- Voice is not affected
- Stridor is uncommon in adults but tachycardia which is disproportionate to pyrexia is an important sign which preceedes airway obstruction.

Signs

- Epiglottis found cherry red and swollen on indiect laryngoscopy
- Care should be taken when depressing the tongue for examination as it can lead to the glottic spasm.

Investigations

Lateral soft tissue X-ray of neck shows:
- Swollen epitglottis **(Thumb sign)**[Q]

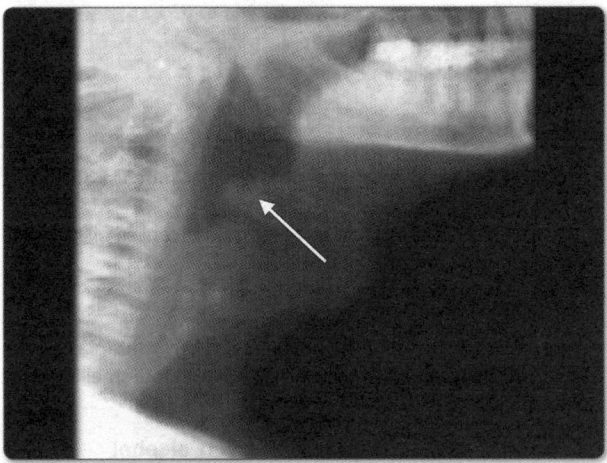

Fig. 27.1: X-ray showing thumb sign in acute epiglottitis
Courtesy: Textbook of ENT, BS Tuli, Jaypee Brothers Medical Publishers Pvt. Ltd., 2/e, p 296

- Absence of deep well-defined vallecula **(vallecula sign).**

Treatment

- Intubation/tracheostomy regardless of the severity of respiratory distress is the topmost priority
- Hospitalization
- Immediate IV antibiotics ampicillin/2nd and 3rd generation cephalosporins
- Ceftriaxone is the antibiotic of choice[Q]
- Steroid
- Adequate hydration to be maintained
- Humidification/O_2 inhalation
- If household contacts of the patient with *H. influenzae* epiglottitis include an unvaccinated child under the age of 4, all members of the household *(including the patient)* should receive prophylactic rifampin for 4 days to eradicate carriage of *H. influenzae*   *Ref. Harrison 17th/ed, p 213*
- *Main complication:* Death from respiratory arrest.

Table 27.1: Differential diagnosis of laryngotracheitis (croup) and epiglottitis

Feature	Croup	Epiglottitis
Age	Less than 3 years	Over 3 years
Onse	Gradual (d)	Rapid (h)
Cough	Barky	None
Posture	Supine	Sitting
Drooling	No	Yes
Radiograph	Steeple sign	Thumb sign
Etiology	Viral	Bacterial
Treatment	Supportive like corticosteroids	Airway management and antibiotics

NEW PATTERN QUESTION

Q N2. A 6-year-old girl complaining of high fever, hoarseness of voice and respiratory distress was bought to ENT OPD. The child gets some relief in the position shown in figure. The most probable diagnosis is:

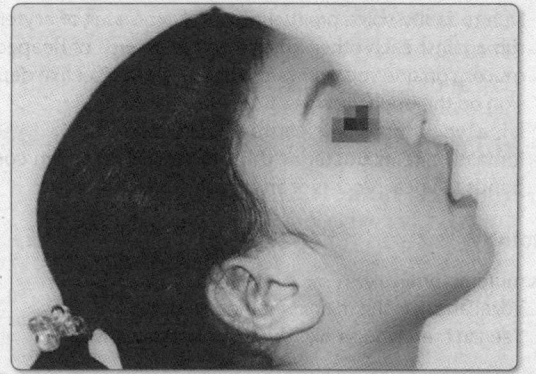

See Color Plate 20

Courtesy: Textbook of ENT, Mohan Bansal p 293, Jaypee Brothers Medical Publishers Pvt. Ltd.

a. Croup b. Laryngitis
c. Epiglottitis d. Pseudocroup

PSEUDOCROUP (SUBGLOTTIC LARYNGITIS)

Age: Children < 3 years

Pathology: Mucosal swelling is found on or near the undersurface of the vocal cords and in the subglottic region.

Clinical features:
- Starts abruptly
- No fever/mild fever

- Voice is raw resembling *barking of seals*
- Dry cough.

Treatment: Moist air.

CHRONIC LARYNGITIS

- Chronic inflammation of mucosa of larynx
- Exact cause is not known.

Can be due to:
- Repeated attacks of acute inflammation
- Smoking
- Voice abuse
- Pollution
- Chronic cough
- Chronic sinusitis.

Types of Chronic Laryngitis

- Hyperemic
- Hypertrophic
  The pseudostratified ciliated epithelium changes to squamous type. There may be hyperplasia and keratinization (**leukoplakia of squamous epithelium of the vocal cords**).

CONTACT ULCERS/PACHYDERMIA LARYNGITIS/CONTACT GRANULOMA

- Due to faulty voice production vocal processes of arytenoid rub against each other which leads to an area of heaped up mucosa on one vocal process which fits into ulcer like depression on the opposite side
- It is a type of chronic hypertrophic laryngitis
- It mainly affects **posterior third of vocal fold** which corresponds to vocal process of arytenoid cartilage.

Etiology

It is multifactorial:
- Vocal abuse is the main offending cause
- Seen in men who smoke/drink alcohol excessively.

Others

- Emotional stress
- Gastroesophageal reflux
- Chronic throat clearing and infections postural drip
- Allergy
- Idiopathic.

Lesions

- Saucer like lesions formed by heaping of granulation tissue
- **Site:** Medical edge of the vocal cord at the vocal process
- Lesion is B/L and symmetrical.

Points to Remember
- There is no epithelial defect (as is seen in true ulcers)
- It does not undergo malignant charge.

Clinical Features

- Seen exclusively in males > 30 years
- The only symptom is hoarseness of voice
- Diagnosis is made by biopsy which shows acanthosis and hyperkeratosis.

Treatment

- Voice rest for a long period of time and voice therapy, if required
- Management of psychological stress and GERD
- Microlaryngoscopic excision of granuloma

NEW PATTERN QUESTIONS	
Q N3.	All of the following are true about pachydermia laryngitis *except*:
	a. Hoarseness of voice
	b. Biopsy shows acanthosis and hyperkeratosis
	c. Premalignant condition
	d. Involves posterior part of larynx
Q N4.	The cause of contact ulcer in vocal cord is:
	a. Voice abuse
	b. Smoking
	c. TB
	d. Malignancy

ATROPHIC LARYNGITIS/LARYNGITIS SICCA

- Characterized by atrophy of laryngeal mucosa and crust formation
- Usually occurs as a part of atrophic rhinitis caused by *Klebsiella ozaenae* and atrophic pharyngitis.

Pathologically

- Respiratory epithelium shows squamous metaplasia with loss of cilia, mucous producing glands and foul smelling crust formation
- **Most common site:**
  - False cords
  - Posterior region and subglottic region.

Clinical Features

- ***Mostly seen in females:***
  - Hoarseness of voice which improves temporarily on coughing and on removing of crust
  - There may be dry irritating cough and dyspnea due to obstructing crusts
  - Patient may complain of blood stained thick mucoid discharge *Ref. Maqbool 11th/ed, p 335*
  - Crusts are foul smelling and mucosa bleeds when they are removed
  - Crusts may also be seen in trachea.

Treatment

- Treat the underlying cause (*poor nutrition, generalized infection rarely syphillis*)
- Laryngeal sprays with glucose in glycerine or oil of pine helps to loosen the crust

- Microlaryngoscopic removal of crust is new modality of treatment
- Expectorants containing ammonium chloride or iodide also help to loosen the crust.

TUBERCULAR LARYNGITIS

- Commonly associated with pulmonary TB
- *Rarely*: blood-borne infection.

> **Points to Remember**
>
> **Sites Affected**
> - All regions can be affected
> - Predilection for the posterior part of larynx (Interarytenoid region > vertricular bands > vocal cord > epiglottis).

Clinical Features

- Weakness of voice with periods of aphonia is earliest symptom
- Hoarseness, cough, dysphagia, odynophagia
- Referred otalgia.
  Laryngeal examination:
  - Hyperemia and ulceration of unilateral vocal cord with impairment of abduction—first sign
  - Vocal cords show shallow ulcers with undermined edges (*mouse nibbled appearance*)—Characteristic feature
  - Pseudoedema of the epiglottis called as **Turban epiglottis**
  - Swelling in *interarytenoid* region giving a *mammilated appearance.*

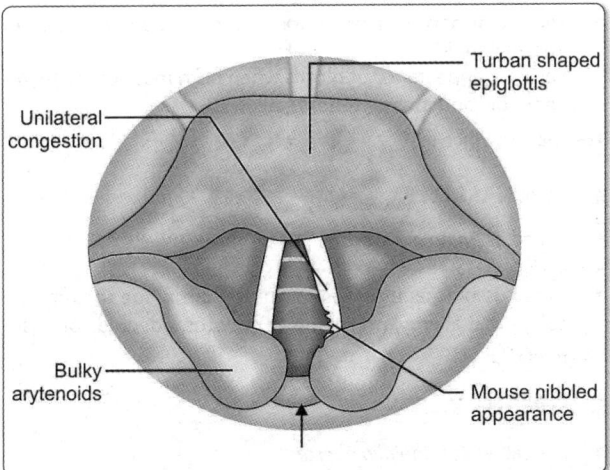

Fig. 27.2: Characteristic feature of tubercular laryngitis

Diagnosis

- Chest X-ray
- Sputum for AFB.

Treatment: ATT.

NEW PATTERN QUESTIONS

Q N5. Mouse nibbled appearance of vocal cord is seen in:
  a. Vocal cord palsy
  b. Vocal nodules
  c. Larynx Ca
  d. TB larynx

Q N6. Turban shaped epiglottis is seen in:
  a. Acute laryngitis
  b. Allergic laryngitis
  c. Laryngeal TB
  d. Carcinoma larynx

LUPUS OF THE LARYNX

It is an indolent tubercular infection associated with lupus of nose and pharynx.

> **Point to Remember**
>
> - **Site affected:** Anterior part of the larynx (Epiglottis > Aryepiglottic fold > ventricular bands).

Clinical Features

- It is a painless condition and the patient is asymptomatic
- No association with pulmonary tuberculosis.

Prognosis: Good

SYPHILIS OF THE LARYNX

- All stages of disease can be manifested
- *Primary stage:* Mucosal ulceration: Primary chancre
  Secondary stage: Multiple vesicles and papular lesions
  Tertiary stage: Gummatous lesion.

> **Point to Remember**
>
> - Sites affected: Anterior part of the larynx, i.e. epiglottis and aryepiglottic fold.

LEPROSY

- *Most commonly* affects the anterior part of larynx
- Supraglottic region affected first
- Lesions is appear dull grey in color epiglottis is destroyed gives appearance of hook over a buttonhole.

REINKE'S EDEMA

B/L symmetrical swelling of the **whole of the membranous part of vocal cord occurring** due to edema of the subepithelial space *(Reinke's space).*

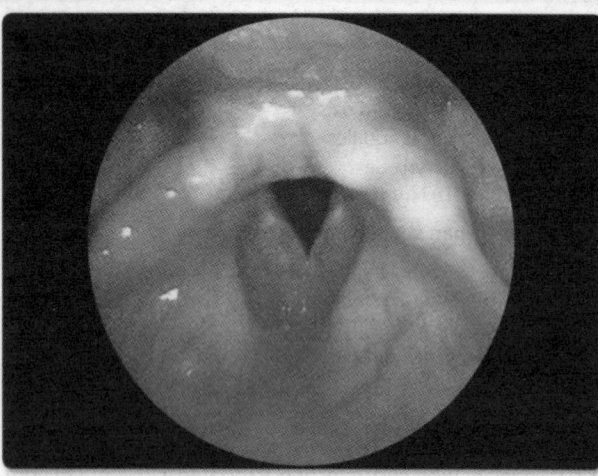

Fig. 27.3: Reinke's edema

Etiology

- *Chronic irritation of vocal cords due to:*
  Voice misuse, **Heavy smoking,** Chronic sinusitis, Laryngooesophageal reflex.
- Myxoedema.

Clinical Features

- Seen in middle age (40–60 years)
- **Most common symptom:** hoarseness of voice
- **Patient uses false vocal cords for voice production therefore voice is low pitched and rough.**

On examination: There is bilateral symmetrical swelling of the vocal cords.

Treatment

Decortication: A circumscribed strip of epithelium is removed from one side of vocal cord while preserving the vocal ligament. Other side to be operated after 3–4 weeks.
- **Voice rest and speech therapy.**

NEW PATTERN QUESTION

Q N7. Which of the following laryngeal condition involves posterior part of larynx?
  a. Pachyderma laryngis
  b. Intubation granuloma
  c. TB of larynx
  d. All of the above

VOICE AND SPEECH DISORDERS

DYSPHONIA PLICA VENTRICULARIS (VENTRICULAR DYSPHONIA)

Features : Voice production is by false cords (ventricular folds) rather than true vocal cord.
Cause can be functional (psychogenic) or organic eg in case of impaired function of true cords as in paralysis, fixation or tumors.

Quality of voice : Rough, low-pitched and unpleasant.
Diagnosis : On indirect laryngoscopy false cords approximate partially or completely and obscure the view of true cords on phonation Videotroboscopy is also helpful.
Treatment : Functional cases are dealt with voice therapy and psychological counseling. The condition is difficult to treat if, it is caused bylaryngeal disorders.

FUNCTIONAL APHONIA

- Mostly seen in emotionally labile females (in age group 15–30 years)
- Patient communicates with whisper but coughing is normal
- Aphonia is sudden and without any accompanying laryngeal symptoms/No vocal cord palsy^Q

On laryngoscopic examination: Vocal cords are seen in abducted position and fail to adduct on phonation; however, adduction of vocal cords is seen on coughing.

Treatment
Reassurance and psychotherapy.

PHONOSTHENIA

- Weakness of voice due to fatigue of phonatory muscles due to voice abuse or laryngitis
- Thyroarytenoid, interarytenoid or both may be affected.

Symptoms: Easy fatiguability of voice.

Signs: Indirect laryngoscopy:
- Elliptical space between cords in weakness of thyroarytenoid.
- Triangular gap near posterior commissure in weakness of interarytenoid.
- Key hole appearance of glottis when both muscles viz. thyroarytenoid and interarytenoids are involved.

Treatment: Voice rest

HYPONASALITY

- Called as *Rhinolalia clausa*
- Lack of nasal resonance
- Defect is blockage of nose or nasopharnx due to common cold, nasal allergy, polyps nasal growths, adenoids or nasopharyngeal mass.

HYPERNASALITY

- It is called as *rhinolalia aperta*
- Words with little nasal resonance are resonated through nose.
- **Defect:** failure of nasopharynx to cut off from oropharynx or abnormal communication between oral and nasal cavities.

PUBERPHONIA

- Presence of high pitched voice of childhood in adult males
- Seen in boys who are emotionally immature, feel insecure and show excessive attachment to their mothers.

Chapter 27: Acute and Chronic Inflammation of Larynx, Voice and Speech Disorders

Features
Adams apple prominent
Laryngeal contour-normal
Gutzmann Pressure test - positive
Secondary sexual characteristics - normal.

Treatment
- Training the boy to produce low-pitched voice.

SPASMODIC DYSPHONIA

Spasmodic dysphonia **is also called as laryngeal dysphonia**. The condition is characterised by spasm of phonatory muscles. It is a **neurological disorder** and is of following types:

(A) **Adductor spasm (M/C):** Adductor muscles go into spasm due to involuntary contraction of vocalis muscle leading to **strained and strangled voice** (scratchy creaky voice).

Management
Botulinum toxin injection in thyroarytenoid muscle. and voice therapy

(B) **Abductor spasm:** Abductor muscles i.e. Posterior cricoarytenoid go into spasm. Vocal cords are unable to abduct leading to leakage of air during speech. The voice is **breathy** or **whispery**.

Management
Botulinum toxin injection in posterior cricoarytenoid muscle. and patients who are not benefitted can be treated with thyroplasty type 1 or fat injection

(C) **Mixed type:**

NEW PATTERN QUESTIONS	
Q N8.	The muscle responsible for falsetto voice of puberphonia is: a. Vocalis b. Cricothyroid c. Thyroarytenoid d. Posterior cricoarytenoid
Q N9.	**Voice abnormality due to faulty use of false vocal cords is:** a. Dysphonia plica ventricularis b. Functional aphonia c. Puberphonia d. Mogiphonia

CONDITIONS CAUSING SPEECH DISORDERS

VOCAL CORD NODULE (SINGER'S/SCREAMER'S NODULES)

- It is localized epithelial hyperplasia and is a bilateral condition
- Seen symmetrically on the free edge of vocal cord, at the junction of anterior one third, with the posterior two thirds (i.e. area of maximum vibration of cord).

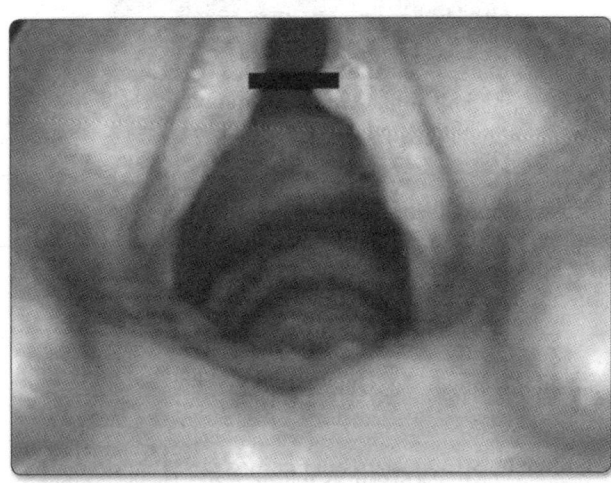

Fig. 27.4: Vocal nodule
Courtesy: Textbook of ENT, BS Tuli, Jaypee Brothers Medical Publishers Pvt. Ltd., 2/e, p 300

- Seen in singers, actors, teachers and hawkers
- Females > males in adults whereas in children it is more common in boys
- Most common age group = 20–30 years
- Main cause—Misuse or abuse of voice
- Patients complain of hoarseness of voice, which worsens by evening due to fatigue.
- Indirect laryngoscopy shows—pinkish white nodules at the junction of anterior one third and posterior two thrids.

Treatment
- Voice rest and speech therapy
- Microlaryngoscopic excision of nodules—Using microsurgical instruments or laser.

VOCAL CORD POLYP

- Usually unilateral at the junction of anterior and middle third of vocal cord.

Etiology

- Voice abuse, chronic irritation like smoking
- Sudden shouting results in hemorrhage and submucosal edema.

Management

- Microlaryngeal excision.

NEW PATTERN QUESTION

Q N10. Identify the condition shown in plate:

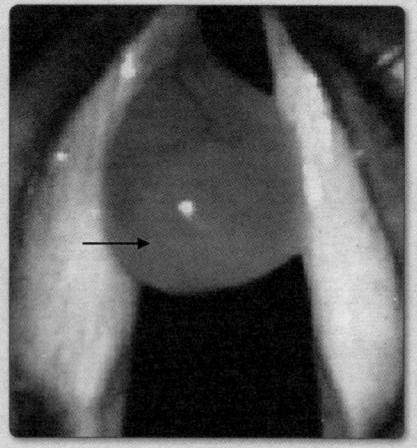

See Color Plate 21

Courtesy: Textbook of ENT, BS Tuli 2/e, p 300, Jaypee Brothers Medical Publishers Pvt. Ltd.

  a. Vocal nodule
  b. Vocal polyp
  c. Leucoplasia of vocal cords
  d. Vocal cord cyst

Extra Edge

- *Gutzmann's pressure test,* if positive confirms puberphonia. In this test, thyroid prominence is pressed backwards and downwards producing low tone voice.

- *Ortner's syndrome* consists of cardiomegaly and paralysis of recurrent layngeal nerve.
- *Mogiphonia:* It is a psychoneurotic disorder in which phonic spasm occurs in professional voice users, when they appear in public. Initially, the voice is normal but soon the vocal cords get adducted and person cannot speak.

NEW PATTERN QUESTIONS

Q N11. Following is not true about spasmodic dysphonia:
  a. Patient with the abductor type have strained and strangled voice
  b. Botulinum toxin is the standard treatment for it
  c. May be associated with other focal dysphonia
  d. Local laryngeal disorder

Q N12. Gutzman pressure test is done for:
  a. Laryngomalacia
  b. Puberphonia
  c. Laryngeal polyp
  d. Vocal cord polyp

VIVA VOCE

Differential diagnosis of stridor with fever in children:
1. Acute epiglottitis
2. Acute laryngotracheobronchitis
3. Laryngeal diphtheria
4. Angioneurotic edema
5. Laryngeal edema secondary to acute tonsillitis.

Chapter 27: Acute and Chronic Inflammation of Larynx, Voice and Speech Disorders

Explanations and References to New Pattern Questions

N1. Ans. is a i.e. Croup

See the text for explanation.

N2. Ans. is c i.e. Epiglottitis *Ref. Essentials of ENT, Mohan Bansal, p 362*

The position shown in the figure is—child is sitting upright with hyper extended neck called as **tripod position**. The child is presenting with fever, stridor and respiratory stress. All this points towards epiglottitis as the diagnosis.

N3. Ans. is c i.e. Premalignant condition *Ref. Dhingra 6/e, p 292*

See the text for explanation.

N4. Ans. is a i.e. Voice abuse *Ref. Dhingra 6/e, p 293*

See the text for explanation.

N5. Ans. is d i.e. TB larynx *Ref. Dhingra 6/e, p 293*

See the text for explanation.

N6. Ans. is c i.e. Laryngeal TB

Disease	Epiglottis
Normal epiglottis	Pink
Acute laryngitis	Bright red, swollen
Allergic laryngitis	Pale, swollen
TB larynx	Turban shaped

N7. Ans. is d i.e. All of the above *Ref. Dhingra 6/e, p 292, 293*

Conditions that commonly affect larynx.

	Condition	Part insoved
1	TB of larynx	Posterior half of larynx (Interarytenoid fold > verticular band > vocal cords > epiglottis)
2	Lupus	Anterior part of larynx (First to be involved-epiglottis)
3	Syphilis	Anterior part of larynx (Arterior commissure and anterior 1/3 vocal cord)
4	Leprosy	Anterior part of larynx (Epiglottis and aryepiglottic fold)
5	Scleroma	Subglottic area
6	Wegners granulomatosis	Subglottic area
7	Pachyderma laryngis (contact ulcer)	Posterior third of vocal cord and interarytenoid area
8	Intubation granuloma	Posterior third of vocal cord
9	Vocal nodule	Junction of anterior 1/3 and posterior 2/3 of vocal cord
10	Glottic cancer	Free edge and upper surface of anterior 1/3 of true vocal cord

N8. Ans. is b i.e. Cricothyroid *Ref. TB of ENT, Hazarika 3/e, p 636*

Cricothyroid is the main tensor responsible for the falsetto voice in puberphonia. There is hyperkinetic function and spasm of cricothyroid muscle.

N9. Ans. is a i.e. Dysphonia plica ventricularis

See the text for explanation.

N10. Ans. is b i.e. Vocal polyp

> The condition shown in the figure is vocal cord polyp.
> It is clear from the picture that it is not leucoplakia where by the whole of vocal cord appears white.
> Vocal nodule are sessile and bilaterally symmetrical lesions where as vocal polyp is pedunculated unilateral lesion. As seen in the figure, the lession is U/L hence it goes in favour of vocal polyp.

N11. Ans. is d i.e. Local laryngeal disorder *Ref. Dhingra 6/e, p 314*

Spasmodic dysphonia is not a local laryngeal disorder but a neurolgical disorder and is often associated with other dysphonia, e.g. blepharospasm, oromandibular dystonias.

N12. Ans. is b i.e. Puberphonia *Ref. Essentials of ENT, TB of Mohan Bansal, p 380*

> **Gutzman pressure test:** Done to confirm puberphonia. The thyroid prominence is pressed in a backward and downward direction. It relaxes the overstretched cords and low tone voice is produced. This can also be used therapeutically to train the patients of puberphonia to use low tone voice.

Chapter 27: Acute and Chronic Inflammation of Larynx, Voice and Speech Disorders

QUESTIONS

1. **Epiglottitis in a 2-year-old child occurs most commonly due to infection with:** *[AIIMS May 05, Nov 04]*
   a. Influenza virus
   b. *Staphylococcus aureus*
   c. *Haemophilus influenzae*
   d. Respiratory syncytial virus

2. **A child with features of upper respiratory infection, on investigations is found to have 'thumbprint sign' diagnosis is:**
   a. Acute larynagotracheobronchitis
   b. Acute epiglottitis
   c. Acute laryngeal diphtheria
   d. Laryngomalacia

3. **Thumb sign in lateral X-ray of neck seen in:** *[PGI Dec 04]*
   a. Epiglottitis   b. Internal hemorrhage
   c. Saccular cyst   d. Ca epiglottis
   e. Vallecular cyst

4. **In acute epiglottis, common cause of death is:** *[Delhi 96]*
   a. Acidosis   b. Respiratory obstruction
   c. Atelectasis   d. Laryngospasm

5. **The antibiotic of choice in acute epiglottitis pending culture sensitivity report is:** *[01]*
   a. Erythromycin   b. Rolitetracycline
   c. Doxycycline   d. Ampicillin

6. **An 1-year-old infant has biphasic stridor, barking cough and difficulty in breathing since 3–4 days. He has high-grade fever and leukocyte count is increased. Which of the following would not be a true statement regarding the clinical condition of the child?** *[AI 10]*
   a. It is more common in boys than in girls
   b. Subglotic area is the common site of involvement
   c. Antibiotics are mainstay of treatment
   d. Narrowing of subglottic space with ballooning of hypopharynx is seen

7. **Pachydermia laryngitis—M/C site of involvement:**
   a. Arytenoids cartilage
   b. Posterior 1/3 and anterior 1/3 commissure
   c. Anterior 1/3 commissure
   d. Vestibular fold

8. **The cause for contact ulcer in vocal cords is:** *[Kerala 94, 95]*
   a. Voice abuse   b. Smoking
   c. TB   d. Malignancy

9. **Which of the following statements is not true for contact ulcer?** *[AIIMS 03]*
   a. The commonest site is the junction of anterior 1/3rd and middle 1/3rd of vocal cord and gastroesophageal reflux is the causative factor
   b. Can be caused by intubation injury
   c. The vocal process is the site and is caused/aggravated by acid reflux
   d. Can be caused by adductor dysphonia

10. **In a patient hoarseness of voice was found to be having pachydermia laryngitis. All of the following are true except:** *[AIIMS 02]*
    a. It is a hyperkeratotic lesion present within the anterior 2/3rd of the vocal cords
    b. It is not premalignant lesion
    c. Diagnosis is made by biopsy
    d. On microscopy it shows acanthosis and hyperkeratosis

11. **A middle-aged male comes to the outpatient department (OPD) with the only complaint of hoarseness of voice for the past 2 years. He has been a chronic smoker for 30 years. On examination, a reddish area of mucosal irregularity overlying a portion of both cords was seen. Management would include all except:** *[AI 03]*
    a. Cessation of smoking
    b. Bilateral cordectomy
    c. Microlaryngeal surgery for biopsy
    d. Regular follow-up

12. **Steeple sign is seen in:** *[SGPGI 05; UP 05]*
    a. Croup   b. Acute epiglottitis
    c. Laryngomalacia   d. Quinsy

13. **True about laryngitis sicca:** *[PGI June 05]*
    a. Caused by *Klebsiella ozaena*
    b. Caused by *Klebsiella rhinoscleromatosis*
    c. Hemorrhagic crust formation seen
    d. Antifungal are effective
    e. Microlaryngoscopic surgery is a modality of treatment

14. **Wrong about laryngitis sicca:** *[PGI June 04]*
    a. Also known as laryngitis atrophica
    b. Caused by *Klebsiella ozaena*
    c. Caused by *Rhinosporodium*
    d. Common in women

15. **Reflux laryngitis produces:** *[PGI Dec 04]*
    a. Subglottic stenosis b. Ca larynx
    c. Cord fixation   d. Acute supraglottitis
    e. Laryngitis

16. **Tubercular laryngitis affects primarily:** *[TN 01]*
    a. Anterior commissure
    b. Posterior commissure of larynx
    c. Anywhere within the larynx
    d. Superior surface of larynx

17. **True about TB larynx:** *[PGI 02]*
    a. 'Turban' epiglottis   b. Odynophagia
    c. Cricoarytenoid fixation d. Ulceration of arytenoids
    e. Paralysis of vocal cord

18. **Mouse-nibbled apperance of vocal cord is seen in:**
    a. TB   b. Syphillis *[CUPGEE 01]*
    c. Cancer   d. Papilloma

19. **Patient following peanut consumption presented with laryngeal edema, stridor, hoarseness:** *[AIIMS Nov 2013]*
    a. Angioneurotic edema
    b. Pharyngeal abscess

c. Foreign body larynx
d. Foreign body bronches

20. **True about spasmodic dysphonia:** [PGI Nov 2016]
    a. A neurological problem
    b. Mostly psychogenic in origin
    c. Hyperadduction of vocal cord may be seen
    d. Botulinum toxin relieves spasm
    e. Speech therapy is beneficial

21. **Patient following peanut consumption presented with laryngeal edema, stridor, hoarseness of voice and swelling of tongue. Most likely diagnosis is:** [AIIMS Nov 13]
    a. Angioneurotic edema   b. Pharyngeal abscess
    c. Foreign body larynx   d. Foreign body bronchus

22. **Reinke's edema is seen in:** [JIPMER 98; Karn 01]
    a. Vestibular folds   b. Edges of vocal cords
    c. Between true and false vocal cords
    d. In pyriform fossa

23. **Reinke's layer seen in:** [CMC]
    a. Vocal cord   b. Tympanic membrane
    c. Cochlea   d. Reissner's membrane

24. **True about Reinke's oedema:** [PGI May 2016]
    a. Usually unilateral   b. Common in smoker
    c. Corticosteroid is mainstay of treatment
    d. Involve whole of membranous part of the vocal cords
    e. Patient has low pich voice

25. **Pharyngeal pseudosulcus is seen secondary to:** [AI 09]
    a. Vocal abuse   [AIIMS Nov 2012]
    b. Laryngopharyngeal reflux
    c. Tuberculosis
    d. Corticosteroid usage

26. **In dysphonia plica ventricularis, sound is produced by:**
    a. False vocal cords   b. True vocal cords [AIIMS 99]
    c. Ventricle of larynx   d. Tongue

27. **Features of functional aphonia:** [PGI June 06]
    a. Incidence in males
    b. Due to vocal cord paralysis
    c. Can cough
    d. On laryngoscopy vocal cord is abducted
    e. Speech therapy is the treatment of choice

28. **Habitual dysphonia is characterized by:** [PGI Dec 04]
    a. Poor voice in normal environment
    b. Related to stressful events
    c. Treatment is vocal exercise and reassurance
    d. Whispering voice
    e. Quality of voice is constant

29. **Rhinolalia clausa is associated with all of the following except:** [AI 07]
    a. Allergic rhinitis   b. Palatal paralysis
    c. Adenoids   d. Nasal polyps

30. **In a patient with hypertrophied adenoids, the voice abnormality that is seen is:** [JIPMER 00; Karn. 01]
    a. Rhinolalia clausa   b. Rhinolalia aperta
    c. Hot potato voice   d. Staccato voice

31. **Young man whose voice has not broken is called:**
    a. Puberphonia   b. Androphonia
    c. Plica ventricularis   d. Functional aphonia

32. **Androphonia can be corrected by doing:** [AI 05]
    a. Type 1 thyroplasty   b. Type 2 thyroplasty
    c. Type 3 thyroplasty   d. Type 4 thyroplasty

33. **Key nob appearance is seen in:** [MP 08]
    a. Functional aphonia   b. Puberphonia
    c. Phonasthenia   d. Vocal cord paralysis

34. **Most common location of vocal nodule:**
    a. Anterior 1/3 and posterior 2/3 junction
    b. Anterior commissure   [UP 04; PGI 00, PGI May 2013]
    c. Posterior 1/3 and anterior 2/3 junction
    d. Posterior commissure

35. **True about vocal nodule is/are:** [PGI 00]
    a. Also known as Screamer's node
    b. Occur at junction of ant. 1/3rd and post. 2/3rd of vocal cords
    c. Most common presentation is aphonia
    d. Microlaryngoscopic surgery is not useful

36. **All are true about vocal cord nodule except:** [PGI May 2014]
    a. Caused by phonotrauma
    b. Commonly occur at Junction of middle and posterior 1/3
    c. Common at junction of A 1/3 with P 2/3
    d. Common in teachers
    e. Treatment is speech therapy

37. **According to European Laryngeal Society, subligamentous cordectomy is classfied as:** [AIIMS May 11]
    a. Type I   b. Type II
    c. Type III   d. Type IV

38. **Change in pitch of sound is produced by which muscle?** [Jharkhand 04]
    a. Post cricoarytenoids   b. Lateral cricoarytenoids
    c. Cricothyroid   d. Vocalis

39. **True about croup:** [PGI Nov 2014]
    a. Caused by H. influenzae
    b. X-ray PA view shows steeple sign of subglottic narrowing
    c. Stridor is present
    d. Supraglottic edema is present
    e. Commonly present in 6 months to 3 years age group

Explanations and References

1. **Ans. is c i.e. *Haemophilus influenzae***
   Ref. Dhingra 5/e, p 307; Ghai 6/e, p 340; Harrison 17/e, p 212,213; Scott-Brown's 7/e, Vol 2, p 2250; TB of Mohan Bansal, p 479
   - **Most common organism causing epiglottitis in children is H. influenzae type B**
   - Though the introduction of Hib vaccine has reduced the annual incidence acute epiglottitis but still most of the pediatric cases seen today are due to haemophilus influenzae B   Ref. Harrison 17/e, p 212
   - In adults it can be caused by group A streptococcus, *S. pneumoniae*, *S. aureus* and *Klebsiella pneumoniae*.

2. **Ans. is b i.e. Acute epiglottis**

Chapter 27: Acute and Chronic Inflammation of Larynx, Voice and Speech Disorders

3. Ans. is a i.e. Epiglottitis *Ref. Dhingra 5/e, p 308; Scott-Brown's 7/e, Vol 2, p 2250; TB of Mohan Bansal, p 479*

In epiglottis: A plain lateral soft tissue radiograph of neck shows the following specific features:
- Thickening of the epiglottis—**the thumb sign**
- Absence of a deep well-defined vallecula—**the vallecula sign.**

ALSO KNOW

Steeple sign, i.e. narrowing of subglottic region is seen in chest X-ray of patients of laryngotracheobronchitis (i.e. croup).

4. Ans. is b i.e. Respiratory obstruction *Ref. Scott's Brown 7/e, Vol 2, p 2251; Turner 10/e, p 390; TB of Mohan Bansal, p 480*

Acute Epiglotlitis

"The main complication is death from respiratory arrest due to acute airway obstruction" *Ref. Scott's Brown 7/e, p 225*

- Respiratory arrest is more likely in patients with rapidly progressive disease and occurs within hours of onset of the illness
- Other complications are rare but include epiglottic abscess, pulmonary edema secondary to relieving airway obstruction and thrombosis of internal jugular vein (Lemierre's syndrome).

5. Ans. is d i.e. Ampicillin *Ref. Turner 10/e, p 390*

> Well friends, there is some controversy over this one.
> - Let's, first see what *Dhingra 5/e, p 308*, has to say:
> - *"Ampicillin or third generation cephalosporin are effective against H. influenzae and are given by parenteral route."*
>
> However, books like Turner and Harrison do not agree with Dhingra about ampicillin being the drug of choice.
>
> *Harrison 17/e, p 212* says:
>
> *"Once the airway has been secured and specimens of blood and epiglottis tissue have been obtained for cultrue, treatment with IV antibiotics should be given to cover the most likely organism particularly H. influenzae. Because rates of ampicillin resistance in this organism have risen significantly in recent years, therapy with a beta lactam / beta lactamase inhibitor combination or a second or third generation cephalosporin is recommended. Typically, ampicillin / sulbactam, cefuroxime, cefotaxime or ceftriaxone is given, with clindamycin and trimethoprim-sulfamethoxazole reserved for patients allergic to beta lactams."*
>
> So, according to *Harrison* **DOC are:**
> - Ampicillin + Sulbactam (Not ampicillin alone)
> - Cefuroxime
> - Cefotaxime
> - Ceftriaxone
>
> According to *Scott's Brown 7/ed Vol 2 p 2251*
>
> *"The antibiotics of choice are second and third generation cephalosporin. Ampicillin was often prescribed but resistant H. influenza are now emerging".*
>
> Now, lets read what *Turner 10/e, p 390* has to say:
>
> *"Treatment is to put the child in an atmosphere of moist oxygen. Sedation must be given cautiously, if at all, in case the respiratory centre is depressed. Chloramphenicol is the antibiotic of choice and it should be given intramuscularly or preferably intravenously. Amoxycillin or ampicillin is no longer advised as haemophilus organism are now sufficiently often resistant to make its use inappropirate."*
>
> Neither 2nd/3rd generation cephalosporins nor chloramphenicol is give in the option. Hence we will have to opt for ampicillin as no other opiton is correct.

Remember

DOC for epiglottitis—2nd/3rd generation cephalosporin. Treatment with ampicillin is not that effective due to b lactamase production by Hib. Prophylaxis with Rifampicin for 4 days is advocated in unimmunized household contacts < 4 years of age and in all immunocompromised contact.

6. Ans. is c i.e. Antibiotics are mainstay of treatment *Ref. Dhingra 5/e, p 308; TB of Mohan Bansal, p 478*

CROUP (laryngotracheitis and laryngotracheobronchitis)

Management

- Once the diagnosis of croup is made, mist therapy, corticosteroids and epinephrine are the usual treatments. Since croup is chiefly viral in etiology, **antibiotics play no role**. Mist therapy (warm or cool) is thought to reduce the severity of croup by moistening the mucosa and reducing the viscosity of exudates, making coughing more productive. For patients with mild symptoms, mist therapy may be all that is required and can be provided at home.
- For more severe cases, further intervention may be required like oxygen inhalation by mask, racemic epinephrine given by nebulizer, corticosteroids and intubation or tracheostomy.

Rest all options are correct for detail read the text.

7. Ans. is a i.e. Arytenoid cartilage *Ref. Scott's Brown 7/e, Vol 2, p 2196*

Pachyderma laryngitis affects the medial surface of arytenoid cartilage, in particular the vocal processes.

8. **Ans. is a i.e. Voice abuse** *Ref. Maqbool 11/e, p 334; TB of Mohan Bansal, p 486*
   Aetiology of contact ulcers is mutlifactorial but the most important cause is:
   - Voice abuse *(faulty production of voice rather than excess use).* — *Maqbool*
   - Smoking as a cause for contact ulcer is given only in Dhingra and is not supported by *Scotts Brown* or *Maqbool*.
9. **Ans. is a i.e. The commonest site is the junction of anterior 1/3rd and middle 1/3rd of vocal cord and gastroesophageal reflux is the causative factor** *Ref. Scotts Brown 7th/ed Vol 2, p 2196, 2197*
10. **Ans. is a i.e. It is a hyperkeratotic lesion present within the anterior 2/3rd of the vocal cords**
    Ref. Dhingra 5/e, p 311; Maqbool 11/e, p 334; Scotts Brown 7/e, Vol 2, p 2197
11. **Ans. is b i.e. Bilateral cordectomy** *Ref. Dhingra 6/e, p 292, 293, 309*
    Middle aged man + Chronic smoking + Hoarseness of voice + Bilateral reddish area of mucosal irregularity on cords
    All these indicate that either it is pachydermia laryngitis or it can be early carcinoma:
    - Both the conditions can be distinguished by biopsy only so **option "c"** is correct.
    - **In either conditions:** smoking is a causative factor and should be stopped.
    - Regular follow-up is a must in either of the conditions.
    - Bilateral cordectomy is not required even if it is glottic cancer because *early stages of glottic cancer are treated by radiotherapy*.
    - Management of pachydermia is microsurgical excision of hyperplastic epithelium *(cordectomy has no role)*.
12. **Ans. is a i.e. Croup** *Ref. Ghai Pediatric 6/e, p 339; Current Otolaryngology 2/e, p 472*
    Chest X-ray in croup *(Laryngotracheobronchitis)* reveals a characteristic narrowing of the subglottic region called steeple sign.
13. **Ans. is a, c and e i.e. Caused by *Klebsiella* ozaena; Hemorrhagic crust formation seen; and Microlaryngoscopic surgery is a modality of treatment** *Ref. Dhingra 5/e, p 312; Scott Brown 6/e, Vol. I, p 512, 513; TB of Mohan Bansal, p 481*
14. **Ans. is c i.e. Caused by *Rhinosporidium*** *Ref. Dhingra 6/e, p 293*
    For details see text
15. **Ans. is a, b and e i.e. Subglottic stenosis; Ca Larynx; and Laryngitis**
    - There are lots of controversies regarding the reflux laryngitis secondary to reflux gastrointestinal disease. But now some studies document that there is a clear relation between the two.
    - **Reflux laryngitis may have the following sequlae:**
      - Bronchospasm
      - Chemical pneumonitis
      - Refractory **subglottic stenosis**
      - Refractory contact ulcer
      - Peptic laryngeal granuloma
      - **A**cid laryngitis *(Heart burn, burning pharyngeal discomfort, nocturnal chocking due to interarytenoid pachydermia)*
      - **Laryngeal Carcinoma** *(According to recent reports laryngeal reflux is the cause of laryngeal carcinoma in patients who are life time non-smokers).*

Laryngopharyngeal Reflux

Here classical GERD symptoms are absent. Patients have more of daytime/upright reflux without the nocturnal/supine reflux of GERD. In laryngopharyngeal reflux esophageal motility and lower esophageal sphincter is normal, while upper esophageal sphincter is abnormal. The traditional diagnostic tests for GERD are not useful in LPR.
Symptom Chronic or Intermittent dysphonia, vocal strain, foreign body sensation, excessive throat mucus, Postnasal discharge and cough. *Laryngeal findings:* Interarytenoid bunching, Posterior laryngitis and subglottic edema (Pseudosulcus)

Sequelae of Laryngopharyngeal Reflux

- Subglottic stenosis
- Carcinoma larynx
- Contact ulcer/granuloma
- Cricoarytenoid joint fixity
- Vocal nodule/polyp
- Sudden infant deaths
- Laryngomalacia (Association)

Treatment is in similar lines as GERD, but we need to give proton pump inhibitors at a higher dose and for a longer duration (at least 6–8 months).

16. **Ans. is b i.e. Posterior commissure of larynx** *Ref. Dhingra 6/e, p 293*
    Tuberculosis affects posterior part of larynx more than anterior part.
    Parts affected are: Inter arytenoid fold > Ventricular bands > Vocal cords > Epiglottis

Chapter 27: Acute and Chronic Inflammation of Larynx, Voice and Speech Disorders

17. Ans. is a, b and d i.e. 'Turban' epiglottis; Odynophagia; and Ulceration of arytenoids

18. Ans. is a i.e. TB *Ref. Dhingra 6/e, p 293; TB of Mohan Bansal, p 481*

- Tuberculosis of larynx is always secondary to pulmonary TB.
- Tubercle bacilli reach the larynx by bronchogenic or haematogenous routes.
- Mostly affects males in middle age group.
- Affects posterior part of (Posterior Commissure) larynx more than anterior part.

Clinical Features

- Weakness of voice (earliest symptom), odynophagia, dysphagia.
- Pain radiates to the ears.
- **Laryngeal examination shows:**
  - *Vocal cord:* **Mouse nibbled ulceration**
  - *Arytenoids:* show ulceration.
  - **Interarytenoid region is swollen giving a mammillated appearance**[Q]
  - **Epiglottis shows:** Pseudoedema and is called as *'turban epiglottis'*.
  - Surrounding mucosa is pale.

 Note: Earliest sign = Adduction weakness

19. Ans. a i.e. Angioneurotic edema *Ref. Logan Turner 10/e p161*

Patient following peanut consumption presented with laryngeal edema, stridor, hoarseness of voice and swelling of tongue. Most likely diagnosis is angioneurotic edema.

> "**Allergic angioedema: Most common type** and usually affects those with some kind of **food allergy**. It can also be caused by **insect bites, contact with latex,** and some medications, such as **penicillin or aspirin**. In severe cases the **throat can swell,** making it hard for the patient to breath."

Angioneurotic Edema

- Angiodema, also known as Quincke's edema is the rapid edema (swelling) of the deep layers of skin[Q]- the dermis, subcutaneous tissue, mucosa and submucosal tissues.
- Due to the risk of suffocation, rapidly progressing angioedema is treated as a medical emergency[Q].
- When angioedema is the result of an allergic reaction the patient is usually injected with adrenaline (epinephrine)[Q].
- Adrenaline is not effective when the cause is hereditary.
- The edema, caused by an accumulation of fluid, can be severe and can affect any part of the body, including the hands, feet, genitals, lips and eyes[Q].

Four main kinds of angioedema:
- Allergic angioedema:
  - Most common type[Q] and usually affects those with some kind of food allergy[Q].
  - It can also be caused by insect bites, contact with latex, and some medications, such as penicillin or aspirin[Q].
  - In severe cases the throat can swell[Q], making it hard for the patient to breath.
  - There may also be a sudden drop in blood pressure.
- Drug-induced angioedema:
  - Certain medications can cause swelling in the deep layers of skin, such as angiotensin-converting enzyme (ACE) inhibitors which are used for treating hypertension (high blood pressure).
  - Symptoms may linger for a few months after the patient stops taking te medication.
  - Less commonly, this type of angioedema might be caused by bupropion, SSRI antidepressants, COX-II inhibitors, nonsteroidal anti-inflammatory drugs, statins, and proton pump inhibitors.
- Idiopathic angioedema:
  - Infection, fear, anxiety, stress, caffeine, overheating, wearing tight clothes, and alcohol may bring it on.
  - It may also be caused by a thyroid gland problem, iron (folic acid) and vitamin B_{12} deficiency.
- Hereditary angioedema:
  - Patient has inherited a faulty gene(s). Urticaria is very uncommon with this type of angioedema.
  - This is the rarest type. Blood levels of the protein C1-esterase inhibitor (C1-1NH protein) are low[Q].
  - C1-1NH protein plays a key role in regulating our immune system. In this type of angioedema symptoms develop gradually, rather than rapidly.
  - Patients usually start having symptoms after puberty[Q].
  - It can be triggered by pregnancy, contraceptive pills, infection, or trauma[Q].
  - Patients are usually effectively treated with medication.

20. Ans. is a, c, d and e. i.e. A neurological problem; hyper adduction of vocal cord may be seen, Botulinum toxin relieves the problem and speech therapy may be useful.

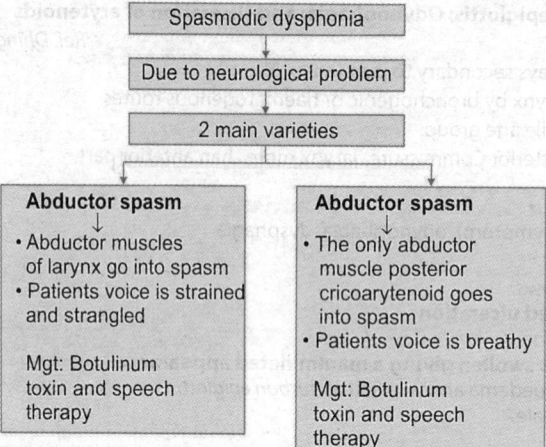

21. **Ans. a i.e. Angioneurotic edema**
    Ref. Logan Turner 10/e, p161
    Patient following peanut consumption presented with laryngeal edema, stridor, hoarseness of voice and swelling of tongue. Most likely diagnosis is angioneurotic edema.

22. **Ans. is b i.e. Edges of vocal cords**
    Ref. Dhirga 6/e, p 292; TB of Mohan Bansal 1/e, p 486

23. **Ans. is a i.e. Vocal cord**

Reinke's Edema
- It is diffuse edema of the Reinke's space (of vocal cords) leading to irreversible fusiform swelling of the vocal cord—usually bilateral.
- Commonest etiology is smoking though extra esophageal reflux, vocal strain and hypothyroidism has also been implicated.
- Patient has a *low-pitched hoarse voice*; may present as stridor in severe cases.
- *Treatment is superior cordotomy* (incising the superior surface of vocal cord preserving the medical vibrating edge) through microlaryngoscopy to decompress the edema fluid. The mucosal flap is then replaced after trimming off the excess epithelium.

24. **Ans. is b, d and e i.e. Common in smoker; involves whole of membranous part of vocal cord and patient has a low pitched voice**
    Ref. Dhingra 6/e p9
    See the text for explanation

25. **Ans. is b i.e. Laryngopharyngeal reflex**
    Ref. Ballenger's Otolaryngology 17/e, p 886; Scott Brown's 7/e, p 2238)

Vocal Sulcus/Laryngeal Sulcus
It is a groove along the mucosa and can be classified into three types:

Laryngeal sulcus

Laryngeal Pseudosulcus (Pseudosulcus Vocalis)	Laryngeal True Sulcus (Sulcus vergeture)	Sulcus Vocalis
Pseudosulcus arises due to swelling of the subglottic area secondary to **laryngotracheal reflux**. It refers to infraglottic edema extending from arterior commissure to posterior larynx	True sulcus is related **to scarring of the vocal fold in the phonatory strking zone**	Seen in deeper layers of ligament
The pseudosulcus is located between the true vocal folds and the subglottic swelling	This is located within the true vocal folds at the site of the adherence of vocal fold epithelium to the vocal ligament	

 Note: It is believed that vocal sulcus/laryngeal sulcus are more common in Indian subcontinent.
- They frequently present with persistent dysphonia following puberty.

Management
Phonosurgical treatment, i.e. either excising the sulcus, injecting collagen or fat to boost the underlying layer or giving a parallel incision in the mucosa running in cephalad to cordal direction to break up the linear scar and vocal fold.

Chapter 27: Acute and Chronic Inflammation of Larynx, Voice and Speech Disorders

26. **Ans. is a i.e False vocal cords**   *Ref. Dhingra 6/e, p 313; TB of Mohan Bansal, p 497*
    In dysphonia plica **ventricularis voice is produced by false vocal cords** *(ventricular folds)*.

27. **Ans. is c and d i.e. Can cough; and On laryngoscopy vocal cord is abducted**   *Ref. Dhingra 6/e, p 314; TB of Mohan Bansal, p 497*
    - *Functional aphonia or hysterical aphonia is a functional disorder mostly seen in emotionally labile females in the age group of 15-30 years.*
    - Laryngoscopy Examination shows vocal cord in abducted position and fails to adduct on phonation, *however* adduction is seen on *coughing, indicating normal adductor function.*
    - **Treatment :**
        - Reassurance of the patient of normal laryngeal function and psychotherapy.
        - Speech therapy has no role in it.

28. **Ans. is a, c, d and e i.e. Poor voice in normal environment; Treatment is vocal exercise and reassurance; Whispering voice; and Quality of voice is constant**
    - When a person always uses a poor voice in normal circumstances, is called habitual dysphonia. It is not related to stressful events and seems to be a habit.
    - The distinguishing characteristics of habitual and psychogenic functional dysphonia are:

Habitual dysphonia	Psychogenic functional dysphonia
Quality of voice is always poor	Previous good voice quality
Very gradual onset of voice problem	Abrupt change in voice quality.
Quality of voice is nearly constant changing with circumstances	Inconstant quality of voice
The voice fails repeatedly after prolonged speaking	Voice fails repeatedly in situations of emotional stress.

Some patients with habitual dysphonia need vocal excercises and very little counseling. Others are cured by a few counseling sessions and no voice practice at all.

29. **Ans. is b i.e. Palatal paralysis**   *Ref. Dhingra 6/e, p 315; TB of Mohan Bansal, p 497*

30. **Ans. is a i.e. Rhinolalia clausa**
    - Rhinolalia clausa is lack of nasal resonance (hyponasality).
    - It is seen in conditions which block the nose or nasopharynx. So will be see in case of allergic rhinitis, adenoids and nasal polyps.
    - Palatal paralysis will lead to hypernasality and not hyponasality.

31. **Ans. is a i.e. Puberphonia**   *Ref. Dhingra 6/e, p 315, TB of Mohan Bansal, p 497*
    - In males at the time of puberty, the voice normally drops by an octave and becomes low pitch.
    - It occurs because vocal cords lengthen
    - Failure of this change leads to persistence of childhood high pitched voice and is called as puberphonia
    - It is seen in boys who are emotionally insecure and show excessive attachment to their mothers. Their physical and sexual development is normal

32. **Ans. is d i.e. Type 4 thyroplasty**   *Ref. Dhingra 5/e, p 321*

    Thyroplasty

Type	Procedure	Indication
Type 1	Medialisation of vocal cord	Unilateral vocal cord paralysis, vocal cord atrophy and sulcus vocalis
Type 2	Lateralisation of vocal cord	Spasmodic dysphonia
Type 3	Shortening (relaxation) or cord	For lowering vocal pitch as in puberphonia
Type 4	Lengthening (stretching) of cord	For elevating the pitch as in androphonia

33. **Ans. is c i.e. Phoneasthenia**   *Ref. Dhingra 6/e, p 314*
    Phonasthemia is weakness of voice due to fatigue of phonatory muscles, i.e. either thyroarytenoids or intrarytenoids or both
    O/E – on Indirect laryngoscopy – 3 features may be seen

Elliptical space between the cords in case of weakness of thyroarytenoid	**Triangular gap** near posterior commissure in weakness of interarytenoid	**Keyhole** appearance of glottis when both thyroarytenoids are involved.

34. **Ans. is a i.e. Anterior 1/3 and posterior 2/3 junction**   *Ref. Dhingra 6/e, p 303; TB of Mohan Bansal, p 485*

35. **Ans. is a and b i.e. Also known as Screamer's node; and Occur at junction of ant. 1st/3rd and post. 2nd/3rd of vocal cords**
        Ref. Dhingra 6/e, p 303; Current Otolaryngology 2/e, p 432; TB of Mohan Bansal, p 485

36. **Ans. is b i.e. Commonly occur at junction of middle and posterior 1/3rd**
    Read the text for explanation.

37. **Ans. is b i.e. Type II**
    - The European Laryngological Society is proposing a classification of different layngeal endoscopic cordectomies in order to ensure better definitions of post-operative results.
    - The word "cordectomy" is used even for partial resections because is the term most often used in the surgical literature.
    - The classification comprises eight types of cordectomies.

    > - Tyepe I: A subepithelial cordectomy, which is resection of the epithelium
    > - Type II: A subligamental cordectomy, which is a resection of the epithelium, Reinke's space and vocal ligament.
    > - Type III: Transmuscular cordectomy, which proceeds through the vocalis muscle
    > - Type IV: Total cordectomy;
    > - Type Va: Extended cordectomy, which encompasses the contralateral vocal fold and the anterior commissure
    > - Type Vb: Extended cordectomy, which includes the arythnoid
    > - Type Vc: Extended cordectomy, which encompasses the subglottis
    > - Type Vd: Extended cordectomy, which includes the ventricle.

38. **Ans. is c i.e. Cricothyroid**   *Ref. PL Dhingra 3/e, p 337*
    The muscle responsible for charge in pitch of voice is cricothyroid.

39. **Ans. is a, b, c, and e i.e. Caused by H. influenza, X-ray PA view shows steeple sign of subglottic narrowing. Stridor is present; and Commonly presents in 6 months to 3 years age group**
    X-ray PA view shows steeple sign of subglottic narrowing, stridor is present and commonly presents in 6 month-3 years of age group.

    > See the text for explanation

Chapter 28

Vocal Cord Paralysis

NERVE SUPPLY OF LARYNX

The main cranial nerve innervating the larynx is the **vagus nerve** via its branches; **superior laryngeal nerve (SLN) and recurrent laryngeal nerve (RLN)**.

(A) **Superior laryngeal nerve:** arises from the inferior ganglion of vagus and receives a branch from superior cervical sympathetic ganglion. It enters the larynx by piercing the thyrohyoid membrane.
- It divides at the level of greater corner of hyoid into:
  (i) **Internal laryngeal nerve:**
    - Sensory (It supplies the larynx above the vocal cords)
    - Secretomotor
  (ii) **External laryngeal nerve**
    - Supplies cricothyroid muscle:
- The superior laryngeal nerve ends by piercing the inferior constrictor of pharynx and unites with ascending anastomosis of recurrent laryngeal nerve. This anastomosis is called as **Galen's anastomosis** and is purely sensory.

(B) **Recurrent laryngeal nerve:**

Motor branch	Sensory branch
Supplies all the intrinsic muscles of the larynx expect cricothyroid	Supplies below the level of the vocal folds

Note: On the right side recurrent laryngeal N originates from vagus and on left side it has a longer course since it originates in mediastinum at the level of arch of aorta and it is more vulnerable to injury.

Point to Remember
Muscle Actions
> In order to have a better understanding of the effects of nerve palsies: a summary of the nerve supply and actions of intrinsic muscles is given. In the table:

Muscle	Supplied by	Action
Cricothyroid	SLN	Tensor, Adductor
Posterior cricothyroid	RLN	Abductor
Lateral cricoarytenoid	RLN	Adductor
Interarytenoids	RLN	Adductor
Vocalis	RLN	Adductor

NEW PATTERN QUESTIONS

Q N1. All of the following are true about superior laryngeal nerve *except*:
a. Supplies cricothyroid
b. Internal laryngeal branch supplies larynx above vocal cord
c. External laryngeal nerve tenses vocal cord
d. Supplies all muscles except cricothyroid

Q N2. Galens anastomosis between SLN and RLN is:
a. Pure sensory
b. Pure motor
c. Secretomotor
d. Mixed

Q N3. Glottic chink, in cadaveric positions of vocal cords is:
a. 3.5 mm
b. 7 mm
c. 19 mm
d. 3 mm

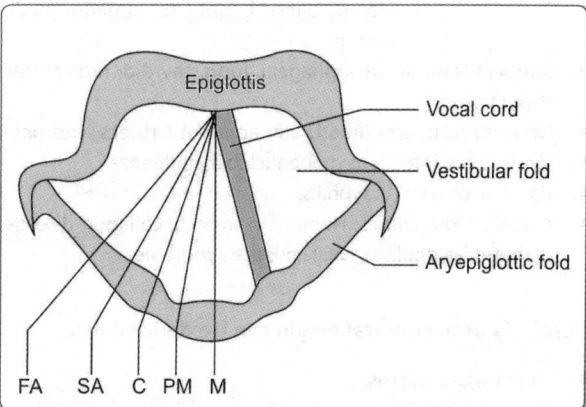
Fig. 28.1: Vocal cord positions
Abbreviations: **M,** Median; **PM,** Paramedian; **C,** Cadaveric (Intermediate); **SA,** Slight abduction; **FA,** Full abduction
Courtesy: Text book of Diseases of Ear, Nose and Throat, Mohan Bansal. Jaypee Brothers Medical Publishers Pvt. Ltd., p 491

Position of the Vocal Cord in Health and Disease

Position of the cord	Location of the cord from midline	Health	Situation in disease
Median	Midline	Phonation	RLN paralysis
Paramedian	1.5 mm	Strong whisper	RLN paralysis
Intermediate (cadaveric)	3.5 mm. This is neutral position of cricoarytenoid joint. Abduction and adduction take place from this position	–	Paralysis of both recurrent and superior laryngeal nerves
Gentle abduction	7 mm	Quiet respiration	Paralysis of adductors
Full abduction	9.5 mm	Deep inspiration	–

VOCAL CORD PARALYSIS

(a) Central causes (10% of all vocal cord paralyses).
   (i) Cortical causes: Rare, include–encephalitis, diffuse arterial sclerosis, etc.
   (ii) Corticobulbar causes: Basilar artery occlusion
   (iii) Bulbar causes: Vertebral artery occlusion bulbar poliomyelitis.
(b) Peripheral causes (90% of all vocal cord paralyses).

Causes of Vocal Cord Palsy

- Idiopathic
- *Malignancy:* – Bronchial (50%) – Oesophageal (20%)
  – Thyroid (10%) – Nasopharyngeal carcinoma/20%
  – Glomus tumor, lymphoma, superior mediastinum
- Surgical trauma (Oesophageal, lung, thyroid, radical neck dissection).
- Nonsurgical trauma (Road traffic accident, Ortner's syndrome).
- *Viral factors:* Infectious mononucleosis, Influenza.
- *Bacterial causes:* TB, syphilis.
- *Miscellaneous causes:* Hemolytic anemia, collagen disorder, diabetes, alcoholism. Guillain-Barré syndrome.

Paralysis of peripheral origin can be divided into:

- High vagal paralysis
- Low vagal paralysis.

High vagal paralysis: Is due to lesion at or proximal to the nodose ganglion. Therefore all the nerves supplying to half of the larynx are involved causing combined paralysis. Sometimes other cranial nerves may be involved due to tumor involvement at the base of the skull commonly due to nasopharyngeal carcinoma.

Low vagal paralysis: Here the nerve to cricothyroid is intact and the fibers to the recurrent laryngeal nerve are damaged. This is more common than the high vagal paralysis and occurs twice as frequently on the left side than the right because of its longer course. Neuritis is a common cause of isolated recurrent nerve paralysis following upper respiratory infection caused by influenza A or B virus.

> **Point to Remember**
>
> **Laws Related to Nerve Palsies**
> - **Semon's law:** States that in a gradually advancing organic lesion of recurrent laryngeal nerve or its fibres in the peripheral trunk, 3 stages can be observed.
>   - **1st stage**
>   - Only abductor paralyzed
>   - Vocal cord in the midline
>   - Adduction still possible
>   - **2nd stage**
>   - Additional contracture of the abductors. Cord immobilized in the median position.
>   - **3rd stage**
>   - Adductors paralyzed. Cords are present in the cadaveric position (Intermediate position).
> - **Wagner and Grossman theory:** It states that cricothyroid muscle innervated by superior laryngeal nerve keeps the cord in paramedian position due to its adductive function. In the absence of cricoarytenoid joint fixation, an immobile vocal fold lying in the paramedian position has a total Unilateral recurrent laryngeal nerve palsy, while an immobile vocal fold in the lateral (cadaveric) position has combined paralysis of superior and recurrent laryngeal nerves.

NEW PATTERN QUESTION

Q N4. Wagner and Grossman theory is related to:
   a. Palatal palsy
   b. Vocal cord palsy
   c. Facial palsy
   d. Hypoglossal palsy

SUPERIOR LARYNGEAL NERVE PALSY

Unilateral Paralysis

Muscle affected Cricothyroid-Adductor, Tensor
Features Voice not severely affected and recovers fast.
- Pitch of the voice cannot be raised
- Ipsilateral cord:
  - Bowed and floppy
  - Increased length
  - Cords sag down during inspiration and bulge up during expiration
- U/L anesthesia of larynx above the level of vocal cord.

Treatment: No treatment.

Bilateral Paralysis

- Features—voice is breathy and weak
- High chances of aspiration as there is bilateral anaesthesia of supraglottic part.

Treatment

- Tracheostomy may be required.
- Epiglottopexy to close the laryngeal inlet, to protect the lungs from repeated aspiration, may be done.

RECURRENT LARYNGEAL NERVE PALSY

U/L Abductor Paralysis

Recurrent laryngeal nerve palsy leads to ipsilateral paralysis of all intrinsic laryngeal muscles except cricothyroid.
- **Affected cord:** Paramedian position (vocal cord does not move laterally on deep inspiration)
- **Features:**
  - Slight hoarseness, which improves over the days.
  - Voice tires with use.

Treatment: Speech therapy.

Note:
Causes of Left Recurrent Laryngeal Nerve palsy:
- Pancoast tumor of lung
- Mitral stenoses—due to enlarged left atrium (k/a Ortner's syndrome)
- Aneurysm of arch of aorta
- Apical TB.

B/L Recurrent laryngeal nerve palsy–(B/L Abductor paralysis)

M/C cause = Thyroid surgery and neuritis.

Features

- Both cords lie either in the median or in the paramedian position due to unopposed action of cricothyroid muscle

- *Voice* is good
- **Dysponea/stridor:** May be present as airway is inadequate
- Stridor becomes worse on exertion or during an attack of acute laryngitis.

Treatment

- Emergency tracheostomy as an emergency procedure
- In long term cases choice is between a permanent tracheostomy with a speaking valve or a surgical procedure to lateralize the cord. The former relieves stridor, preserves good voice but has the disadvantage of a tracheostomy hole in the neck. The latter relieves airway obstruction but at the expense of a good voice, however, there is no tracheostomy hole in the neck.
- **Widening the respiratory airway without a permanent tracheostomy (endoscopic or through external cervical approach).** Aim is to widen the respiratory airway through larynx.

  This can be achieved by (i) arytenoidectomy with suture, woodman procedure, Dowine procedure, (ii) arytenoidopexy (fixing the arytenoid in lateral position), (iii) lateralization of vocal cord and (iv) laser cordectomy (removal of one cord).
- These operations have now been replaced by less invasive techniques such as:
  (i) Transverse cordotomy (kashima operation)
  (ii) Partial arytenoidectomy
  (iii) Reinnervation procedures. Aim to innervate paralyzed posterior cricoarytenoid muscle by implanting a nerve-muscle pedicle of sternohyoid or omohyoid muscle with its nerve supply from ansa hypoglossi. These procedures have not been very successful.
  (iv) Thyroplasty type II

COMBINED SUPERIOR AND RECURRENT LARYNGEAL NERVE PALSY

U/L Adductor Paralysis

(Both superior and recurrent laryngeal nerve gone).
There occurs unilateral paralysis of all laryngeal muscles except the inter arytenoid which receives innervation from both the sides.
- **Position of the cord:** U/L Cadaveric position (3.5 mm from midline)
- **Features:** – Voice produced is weak and husky
  – Chances of aspiration are present.
- *Treatment* – Cord medialization.
- **Surgery for medialization of the cord (Type I thyroplasty)**
  - **Intracordal injection:** Teflon and collagen
  - Arytenoid rotation
  - Nerve—muscle pedicle reinnervation.
  - Recurrent laryngeal nerve reinnervation
  - Muscle/cartilage implant

B/L Adductor Paralysis (M/C Cause = Functional → Flag sign is seen)

- **Position of the cord:** B/L cadaveric

- **Features:**
  - Aphonia
  - Inability of cough
  - Aspiration
  - Bronchopneumonia

There is also total anesthesia of the larynx.

Treatment

- Where recovery expected:
  - Tracheostomy with cuff
  - Epiglottopexy
  - Vocal cord plication.
- If neurological lesion is progressive and irreversible total laryngectomy to prevent aspiration and lung infection.

Points to Remember

Isshiki's thyroplasty: It is an innovative procedure developed to improve the laryngeal mechanics.

Types:
- Type 1: Medialization of the cord
- Type 2: Lateralization of the cord
- Type 3: Shortening the cord (lowers the vocal pitch)
- Type 4: Lengthening of the cord (to increase the pitch) to correct androphonia. The male character low pitch voice is converted to female pitch voice.

Note
Carcinoma bronchus is the most common cause of left RLN palsy, while thyroid surgery affects right RLN (as RLN is close to inferior thyroid artery, so increased chances of injury during thyroidectomy).

NEW PATTERN QUESTIONS

Q N5. Most common nerve injured in ligation of superior thyroid artery:
- a. Recurrent laryngeal nerve
- b. Facial nerve
- c. Mandibular nerve
- d. External laryngeal nerve

Q N6. The voice is not affected in:
- a. Unilateral abductor palsy
- b. Unilateral adductor palsy
- c. B/L superior laryngeal palsy
- d. Total adductor palsy

Q N7. Which of the following is life threatening?
- a. U/L abductor paralysis
- b. B/L abductor paralysis
- c. U/L adductor paralysis
- d. B/L adductor paralysis

Q N8. Muscular voice in females is treated by:
- a. Thyroplasty type 1
- b. Thyroplasty type 2
- c. Thyroplasty type 3
- d. Thyroplasty type 4

Q N9. Materials used for injection in thyroplasty are:
- a. Collagen
- b. A cellular micronized human debris
- c. Gelatin powder
- d. All of the above

Q N10. Voice in B/L abductor palsy:
- a. High pitch
- b. Aphonia
- c. Normal
- d. Hoarseness

Explanations and References to New Pattern Questions

N1. Ans. is d i.e. Supplies all muscles except cricothyroid *Ref. Dhingra 6/e, p 298*

See the text for explanation.

N2. Ans. is a i.e. Pure sensory *Ref. TB of ENT, Hazarika 3/e, p 623*

Galen's anastomosis is purely sensory.

N3. Ans. is b i.e. 7 mm *Ref. TB of Mohan Bansal 3/e, p 374*

Glottic chink: It is the distance between the vocal cords. In cadaveric position—the vocal cords are 3.5 mm away from midline so the distance between them, i.e glottic chink is 7 mm.
Similarly in full abduction it is about 19 mm^Q.

	Position of vocal cord	Distance from midline	Glottic chink
1.	Paramedian	1.5 mm	3 mm
2.	Intermediate (cadaver)	3.5 mm	7 mm
3.	Partial abduction	7 mm	14 mm
4.	Full abduction	9.5 mm	19 mm

N4. Ans. is b i.e. Vocal cord palsy *Ref. Dhingra 6/e, p 299*

Semon's law and **Wegner and Grossman hypothesis** are both related to vocal cord palsy.
Wagner and Grossman hypothesis states that in U/L recurrent laryngeal nerve palsy, cricothyroid muscle which receives innervation from superior laryngeal nerve keeps the cord in paramedian position due to its adduction action.

N5. Ans. is d i.e. External laryngeal nerve *Ref. Essentials of ENT, Mohan Bansal 3/e, p 350, 351*

- The external laryngeal nerve lies in relation to superior thyroid artery.
- The recurrent laryngeal nerve lies close to superior laryngeal artery.

N6. Ans. is a i.e. Unilateral abductor palsy

In U/L abductor palsy, the affected vocal cord assumes a median or paramedian position. The other is normal so one third patients are asymptomatic others may have some voice change.
"The voice in unilateral paralysis gradually, Improves due to compensation by the healthy cord which crosses the midline to meet the paralysed one." *Ref. Dhingra 6/e, p 299*

N7. Ans. is b i.e. B/L abductor paralysis *Ref. Dhingra 6/e, p 300*

In bilateral abductor paralysis (due to B/L recurrent laryngeal nerve palsy), both the cords assume a median position due to unopposed action of cricothyroid muscle. The airway is inadequate in this condition, causing dyspnea. The condition can be life-threatening.

N8. Ans. is d i.e. Thyroplasty type 4 *Ref. Dhingra 6/e, p 302*

Type 4 thyroplasty is used to lengthen the vocal cord and elevate the pitch. It converts male character of voice to female and is used in gender transformation.

N9. Ans. is d i.e. All of the above *Ref. Neurologic Disorder of Larynx by Andrew Bilitzer, p 152*

Materials used for medialization of the vocal cord include—fat, fascia, gelatin powder, collagen and micronized acellular human dermis.

N10. Ans. is c i.e. Normal
Voice remains normal in B/L abductor paralysis.

QUESTIONS

1. **Tensor of vocal cord includes:** [PGI May 2015]
   a. Arytenoid
   b. Thyroarytenoid
   c. Interarytenoid
   d. Posterior cricoarytenoid
   e. Cricothyroid

2. **Which of the following muscle is not supplied by recurrent laryngeal nerve?** [PGI Dec 08]
   a. Post cricoarytenoid
   b. Thyroarytenoid
   c. Lateral cricoarytenoid
   d. Cricothyroid
   e. Interarytenoids

3. **Cricothyroid muscle is supplied by:** [Jharkhand 2003]
   a. Superior laryngeal nerve
   b. External laryngeal nerve
   c. Vagus nerve
   d. Glossopharyngeal nerve

4. **Which of the following is true?** [PGI May 2014]
   a. Internal laryngeal nerve: supply cricothyroid muscle
   b. Internal laryngeal nerve–sensory supply below vocal cord
   c. Internal laryngeal nerve–tense vocal card
   d. External laryngeal nerve–tense vocal cord
   e. Internal laryngeal nerve–sensory supply above vocal cord

5. **Position of vocal cord in cadaver is:** [DNB 2000]
   a. Median
   b. Paramedian
   c. Intermediate
   d. Full abduction

6. **Why vocal cord looks pale?** [TN 2005]
   a. Vocal cord is muscle, lack of blood vessels network
   b. Absence of mucosa, no blood vessels
   c. Absence of submucosa, no blood vessels
   d. Absence of mucosa with blood vessels

7. **Right sided-vocal cord palsy seen in:** [AIIMS 99]
   a. Larynx carcinoma
   b. Aortic aneurysm
   c. Mediastinal lymphadenopathy
   d. Right vocal nodule

8. **The most common cause of vocal cord palsy is:** [UPSC 05]
   a. Total thyroidectomy
   b. Bronchogenic carcinoma
   c. Aneurysm of aorta
   d. Tubercular lymph nodes

9. **Left-sided vocal cord palsy is commonly due to:** [TN 2005]
   a. Left hilar bronchial carcinoma
   b. Mitral stenosis
   c. Thyroid malignancy
   d. Thyroid surgery

10. **Vocal cord palsy is not associated with:** [AP 2003]
    a. Vertebral secondaries
    b. Left atrial enlargement
    c. Bronchogenic carcinoma
    d. Secondaries in mediastinum

11. **Bilateral (B/l) recurrent laryngeal nerve palsy is/are caused by:** [PGI 00]
    a. Thyroid surgery
    b. Thyroid malignancy
    c. Aneurysm of arch of aorta
    d. Viral infection
    e. Mitral valve surgery

12. **Cause of B/L recurrent laryngeal nerve palsy is/are:**
    a. Thyroid Ca [PGI Nov 09]
    b. Thyroid surgery
    c. Bronchogenic Ca
    d. Aortic aneurysm
    e. Cervical lymphadenopathy

13. **Bilateral recurrent laryngeal nerve palsy is seen in:**
    a. Thyroidectomy [Delhi 2008]
    b. Carcinoma thyroid
    c. Cancer cervical oesophagus
    d. All of the above

14. **Most common cause of B/L recurrent laryngeal paralysis:**
    a. Thyroid surgery
    b. Cancer cervical oesophagus
    c. Blow from nasal cavity
    d. Thyroid cancer
    e. Bronchogenic carcinoma

15. **Which one of the following lesions of vocal cord is dangerous to life?** [UPSC 01, 02]
    a. Bilateral adductor paralysis
    b. Bilateral abductor paralysis
    c. Combined paralysis of left side superior and recurrent laryngeal nerve
    d. Superior laryngeal nerve paralysis

16. **In complete bilateral palsy of recurrent laryngeal nerves, there is:** [AIIMS Nov 03]
    a. Complete loss of speech with stridor and dyspnea
    b. Complete loss of speech but not difficulty in breathing
    c. Preservation of speech with severe stridor and dyspnea
    d. Preservation of speech and not difficulty in breathing

17. **In bilateral abductor paralysis which of the following is seen?**
    a. Vocal cord in paramedian position
    b. Voice is affected early
    c. Stridor and dyspnoea occurs
    d. Vocal cord lateralization done
    e. Hoarseness occurs

18. **The voice in a patient with bilateral abductor paralysis of larynx is:** [AP 2005]
    a. Puberphonia
    b. Phonasthenia
    c. Dysphonia plicae ventricularis
    d. Normal or good voice

19. **In B/L, abductor palsy of vocal cords following is done except:** [PGI 98]
    a. Teflon paste
    b. Cordectomy
    c. Nerve muscle implant
    d. Arytenoidectomy

Chapter 28: Vocal Cord Paralysis

20. Injury to superior laryngeal nerve causes: [AIIMS]
    a. Hoarseness
    b. Paralysis of vocal cords
    c. No effect
    d. Loss of timbre of voice
21. Paralysis of recurrent laryngeal nerve true is: [Bihar 05]
    a. Common in left side
    b. 50% idiopathic
    c. Cord will be laterally
    d. Speech therapy given
22. Partial recurrent laryngeal nerve palsy produces vocal cord in which position: [UP 96]
    a. Cadaveric
    b. Abducted
    c. Adducted
    d. Paramedian
23. U/L vocal cord palsy treatment includes: [PGI Nov 09]
    a. Isshiki type I thyroplasty
    b. Isshiki type II thyroplasty
    c. Woodman operation
    d. Laser arytenoidectomy
    e. Teflon injection
24. Type I thyroplasty is for: [AI 03]
    a. Vocal cord medialization
    b. Vocal cord lateralization
    c. Vocal cord shortening
    d. Vocal cord lengthening
25. In thyroplasty type 2, vocal cord is: [AP 2004]
    a. Lateralized
    b. Medialized
    c. Shorterned
    d. Lengthened
26. A 10-year-old boy developed hoarseness of voice following an attack of diphtheria. On examination, his right vocal cord was paralyzed. The treatment of choice for paralyzed vocal cord will be: [AIIMS Nov 05]
    a. Gel foam injection of right vocal cord
    b. Fat injection of right vocal cord
    c. Thyroplasty type–I
    d. Wait for spontaneous recovery of vocal cord
27. A patient presented with stridor and dyspnea which he developed after an attack of upper respiratory tract infection. On examination he was found to have a 3 mm glottic opening. All of the following are used in the management *except*: [AIIMS 02]
    a. Tracheostomy
    b. Arytenoidectomy
    c. Teflon injection
    d. Cordectomy
28. Which of the following is the most common cause of vocal cord palsy? [AIIMS Nov 2014]
    a. Trauma
    b. Malignancy
    c. Inflammatory
    d. Surgical

Explanations and References

1. **Ans. is e. i.e. Cricothyroid** *Ref. Dhingra 6/e, p 283; Logan Turner 10/e, p 146*
   The only tensor of vocal cord is cricothyroid.

2. **Ans. is d i.e. Cricothyroid**

3. **Ans. is a i.e. Superior laryngeal nerve** *Ref. Dhingra 6/e, p 298; Scotts Brown 7/e, p 2139*
   All the muscles which play any role in movement of vocal cord are supplied by recurrent laryngeal nerve except the **cricothyroid muscle** which receives its innervation from the external laryngeal nerve—a branch of **superior laryngeal nerve.**

4. **Ans. is d and e i.e. External laryngeal nerve–tense vocal cord; Internal laryngeal nerve–sensory supply above vocal cord**
   Ref. Dhingra 6/e, p 298;

> **Nerve Supply of Larynx**
> **Motor**
> - All the muscle which move the vocal cords (abductors, adductors or tensor) are supplied by **Recurrent Laryngeal nerve**[Q] except the cricothyroid muscle. The latter receive its innervation from External Laryngeal nerve[Q]–a branch of superior Laryngeal nerve
>
> **Sensory**
> - Above vocal cords-Internal Laryngeal nerve a branch of **Superior Laryngeal** nerve[Q]
> - **Below vocal cords–Recurrent Laryngeal** nerve[Q]
>
> RT Recurrent Laryngeal Nerve–It arises from the vagus[Q] **in the mediastinum at the level of arch of aorta**

5. **Ans. is c i.e. Intermediate** *Ref. Dhingra 6/e, p 299; Table 60.2*
   In cadaveric state – the position of vocal cord is intermediate (i.e. equal amount of adduction and abduction)

6. **Ans. is c i.e. Absence of submucosa, no blood vessels** *Ref. Maqbool 11/e, p 310*
   - Vocal cord are fibro elastic bands
   - They are formed by reflection of the mucosa over vocal ligaments
   - They have stratified squamous epithelium with no submucous layer
   - **Their blood supply is poor and are almost devoid of lymphatics. Hence vocal cords look pale in appearance.**

7. Ans. is a i.e. Larynx carcinoma *Ref. Dhingra 6/e, p 298*

This question can be solved easily, if you know the course of Left and Right recurrent laryngeal nerve.

As discussed in detail in text:
- *Lt. RLN:* Arises from vagus in the mediastinum at the level of arch of aorta loops around it and then ascends into the neck.
- *Rt. RLN:* Arises from vagus at the level of subclavian artery, hooks around it and then ascends up.

So, any mediastinal causes viz mediastinal lymphadenopathy and aortic aneurysm would paralyse Lt. RLN only (ruling out **options "b"** and **"d"**) Vocal nodule does not cause vocal cord palsy.

Laryngeal carcinoma especially glottic can cause U/L or B/L Vocal Cord paralysis—Conn's Current Theory

8. Ans. is a i.e. Total thyroidectomy

9. Ans. is a i.e. Left hilar bronchial carcinoma

10. Ans. is a i.e. Vertebral secondaries *Ref Schwartz Surgery 8/e, p 509; Dhingra 6/e, p 299*

Vocal cord paralysis is *most commonly* iatrogenic in origin following surgery to thyroid, parathyroid, carotid or cardiothoracic structures.

Right	Left	Both
• Neck trauma • Benign or malignant thyroid disease • Thyroid surgery • Carcinoma cervical oesophagus • Cervical lymphadenopathy • Aneurysm of subclavian artery • Carcinoma apex right lung • Tuberculosis of cervical pleura • Idiopathic	i. *Neck* • Accidental trauma • Thyroid disease (benign or malignant) • Thyroid surgery • Carcinoma cervical oesophagus • Cervical lymphadenopathy ii. *Mediastinum* • Bronchogenic cancer (M/C) • Carcinoma thoracic oesophagus • Aortic aneurysm • Enlarged left atrium • Intrathoracic surgery • Idiopathic	• Thyroid surgery • Carcinoma thyroid • Cancer cervical esophagus • Cervical lymphadenopathy

11. Ans. is a, b and d i.e. Thyroid surgery; Thyroid malignancy; and Viral infection

12. Ans. is a, b and e i.e. Thyroid Ca, Thyroid surgery and Cervical lymphadenopathy

13. Ans. is d i.e. All of the above *Ref. Dhingra 6/e, p 299; Turner 10/e, p 181; Current Otolaryngology 2/e, p 457*

Causes of bilateral recurrent laryngeal nerve palsy are:
- Idiopathic
- Post thyroid surgery
- Thyroid malignancy
- Carcinoma of cervical part of esophagus
- Cervical lymphadenopathy.

 Note: Peripheral neuritis causes high vagal palsy which leads to both superior as well as recurrent laryngeal nerve palsy, i.e. bilateral complete palsy. *Turner 10/e, p 181; Dhingra 5/e, p 318; 6/e, p301*

14. Ans. is a i.e. Thyroid surgery *Ref. Dhingra 6/e, p 300*

Bilateral Recurrent Laryngeal Paralysis:

"Neuritis or surgical trauma (thyroidectomy) are the most important causes of bilateral abductor paralysis or recurrent laryngeal nerve paralysis.." *Dhingra 6/e, p 300*

Other causes of B/L Recurrent Laryngeal Nerve:
- Carcinoma thyroid
- Cancer cervical oesophagus
- Cervical lymphadenopathy.

15. Ans. is b i.e. Bilateral abductor paralysis *Ref. Dhingra 6/e, p 300*
- Most dangerous lesion of vocal cords is bilateral abductor paralysis (Bilateral RLN palsy).
- This is because recurrent laryngeal nerve palsy will lead to paralysis of all laryngeal muscles except the cricothyroid muscle (as it is supplied by superior laryngeal nerve). The cricothyroid muscle is an adductor and therefore this will leave both the cords in median or paramedian position thus endangering proper airway, leading to stridor and dyspnoea.

16. **Ans. is c i.e. Preservation of speech with severe stridor and dyspnea**
17. **Ans. is a, c and d i.e. Vocal cord in paramedian position; Stridor and dyspnoea occurs; and Vocal cord lateralization done**
18. **Ans. is d i.e. Normal or good voice** *Ref. Dhingra 6/e, p 300; Current Otolaryngology, p 459,460*

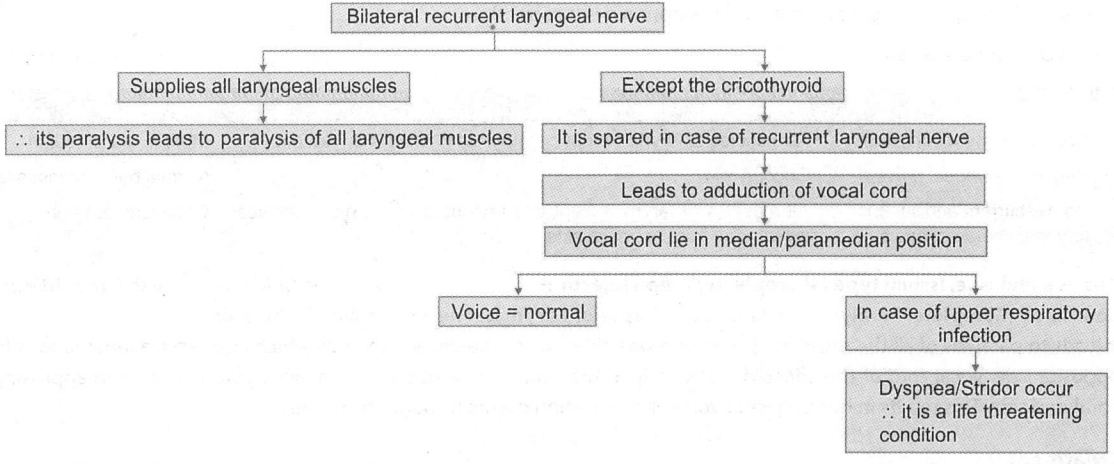

Management
- Lateralization of cord by arytenoidectomy, endoscopic surgery, thyroplasty type II, cordectomy
- In emergency cases—Tracheostomy may be required.

Also know
> - Generally patients with bilateral recurrent laryngeal nerve palsy have a recent history of thyroid surgery or rarely an advanced malignant thyroid tumor
> - Most common presentation—Development of stridor following URI
> - Since the voice of the patient is normal it is diagnosed very late.

19. **Ans. is a i.e Teflon paste** *Ref. Dhingra 6/e, p 300*
    - In bilateral abductor paralysis (i.e. bilateral paralysis of RLN), the cords lie in median or paramedian position due to unopposed action of cricothyroid muscle
    - Since, both the cords lie in median or paramedian position, the airway is inadequate causing dyspnea and stridor
    - Principle for managing such cases is: lateralisation of the cord and not further medialization of cord by injection of Teflon. For more details see the proceeding text.

20. **Ans. is d i. e. Loss of timbre of voice** *Ref Dhingra 6/e, p 300*

    Paralysis of Superior Laryngeal Nerve—causes paralysis of cricothyroid muscle which is a tensor of vocal cord.

Clinical Features
- Voice is weak and pitch cannot be raised.
- U/L Anaesthesia of larynx above the level of vocal cords causing occasional aspiration.

21. **Ans. is a i.e. Common in (left) side** *Ref. Dhingra 6/e, p 299; Current Otolaryngology 2/e, p 457*

Unilateral Recurrent Laryngeal Nerve Palsy
- More common on left side than right side because of the longer and more convoluted course of the left recurrent laryngeal nerve (Right side is involved only in 3-30% cases) (i.e. option a is correct)
- Most unilateral vocal cord paralysis are secondary to surgery (i.e. option b is incorrect)
- Unilateral injury to recurrent laryngeal nerve leads to ipsilateral paralysis of all intrinsic muscles except cricothyroid (which is an adductor of vocal cord). The vocal cord thus assumes a median or paramedian position which does not move laterally on deep inspiration (i.e. option c is incorrect).

Clinical Features
- Asymptomatic in 1/3rd cases
- In rest of the patients there may be some voice problem, i.e. dysphonia—the voice is hoarse and becomes weak with use. This gradually improves with time due to compensation by the healthy cord which crosses the midline to meet the paralysed one. Generally no speech therapy is required (i.e. option d is incorrect).

22. **Ans. is d i.e. Paramedian** *Ref. Dhingra 6/e, p 297*

Nerve paralysed	Muscles affected	Position of vocal cord
• Recurrent laryngeal nerve	All muscles of larynx except cricothyroid (Which is an adductor)	Median, paramedian
• Superior laryngeal nerve	Cricothyroid	Normal but cord loses tension
• Both recurrent and superior laryngeal nerve of one side	All muscles of larynx except interarytenoid which also receives innervation from opposite side	Cadaveric position

23. **Ans. is a and e i.e. Isshiki type I thyroplasty; Teflon injection** *Ref: Dhingra 6/e, p 300; Turner 10/e, p 182,183*

Combined (Complete) Paralysis (Recurrent and Superior Laryngeal nerve paralysis): Unilateral

It leads to paralysis of all the muscles of larynx on one side except the cricoarytenoid[Q] which also receive innervations from the opposite side. Vocal cord of the affected side will lie in the cadaveric position.[Q] The healthy cord is unable to approximate the paralysed side. This results in hoarseness of voice and aspiration occurs through the glottis.

Treatment
- **Speech therapy**—With proper speech therapy the healthy cord may approximate the paralysed cord
- Procedures to medialise the cord:
  - Injection of Teflon paste, lateral to the paralysed cord[Q]
  - Thyroplasty type I[Q]
  - Muscle or cartilage implant[Q]
  - Arthrodesis of cricoarytenoid joint (Also known as reversed Woodman's operation – Logan and Turner 10th/182)

> **Note: Woodman's operation**[Q] (external arytenoidectomy) is done in bilateral abductor paralysis—Logan and Turner 10th/183
> **Endoscopic laser arytenoidectomy and Isshiki type II thyroplasty**[Q] is done for lateralization of cord (in bilateral abductor paralysis)— *Dhingra 5/e p 318,319, 362*

24. **Ans. is a i.e. Vocal cord medialization** *Ref. Dhingra 5/e, p 321*

25. **Ans. is a i.e. Lateralized**

Isshiki divided thyroplasty procedures into 4 categories to produce functional alteration of vocal cords:
- **Type 1 :** Medial displacement of vocal cord (done by injection of gel foam/Teflon paste)
- **Type 2 :** Lateral displacement of cord (done to improve the airway)
- **Type 3 :** Shortening (relax) the cord, to lower the pitch (gender transformation from female to male)
- **Type 4 :** Lengthening (tightening) the cord, to elevate the pitch (gender transformation from male to female)

26. **Ans. is d i.e. Wait for spontaneous recovery of vocal cord** *Ref. Dhingra 6/e, p 300; Nelson 17/e, p 888, 889*

Unilateral paralysis of cord due to neuritis (as in diphtheria) does not require any treatment as it recovers spontaneously.
The characteristic features of diphtherial neuropathy is that it recovers completely.

27. **Ans. is c i.e. Teflon injection** *Ref. Dhingra 6/e, p 300*
- Glottic diameter of 3 mm indicates that the patient is having laryngeal paralysis (due to URTI)
- Because of the narrowness of the opening, the patient is having stridor and dyspnea
- Stridor and dyspnea can be managed by:
  - Tracheostomy
  - Fixing the cord in the lateral position by:
- Arytenoidectomy

- Arytenoidopexy
    - Vocal cord lateralisation through endoscope
    - Laser cordectomy
    - Thyroplasty type II
- Teflon injection is a method to medialise the cord and is therefore of no use in this patient. It would rather aggravate the condition.

Note: For a quiet respiration the glottic diameter should be 14 mm wide.

28. Ans. is d i.e. Surgical   *Ref. Dhingra 6/e, 299; 5/e, 320; Schwartz 8/e, p 509*

Surgical trauma is the most common cause of vocal cord palsy.

"Vocal cord paralysis is most commonly iatrogenic in nature following surgery to thyroid, parathyroid, carotid or cardiothoracic structures." (Schwartz 8/e, p501)

Vocal cord palsy
Vocal cord palsy can be attributed to the following causes:
• Surgical trauma (44%)[Q]
• Malignancy (17%)[Q]: Bronchial>Esophageal>Nasopharyngeal>thyroid
• Endotracheal intubation (15%)[Q]
• Neurologic disease (12%)
• Idiopathic causes (12%)

Chapter 29

Tumors of Larynx

Flowchart 29.1: Classification of laryngeal neoplasms

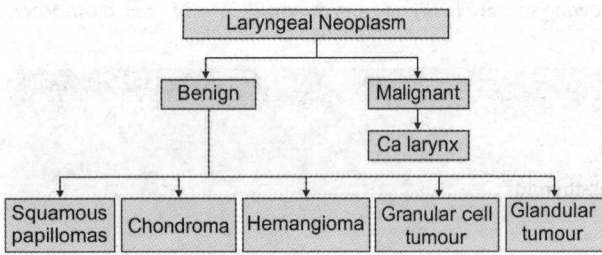

SQUAMOUS PAPILLOMAS

Most common **benign tumour**.

It is of two types:
1. **Juvenile onset/Recurrent respiratory papillomatosis (JORRP)/Multiple papillomatosis.**
   - Viral in origin, caused by **HPV types 6 and 11 and less commonly by subtypes 16 and 18**
   - **Multiple** sessile/pedunculated, friable papillomas which bleed on touch.
   - Occurs in infants and young children – peak age 2 to 5 years.

> **Point to Remember**
> ➤ **Most common site** – Vocal fold (first and predominant site)   *Ref. CSDT 12/e, p 971*

Other sites = other parts of larynx, nose, pharynx and trachea.
- Patient presents with **hoarseness** - Later as the lesion progresses **inspiratory dyspnea** with **stridor develops**.

Note: Vertical transmission also occurs.

Treatment
- **Microendoscopic CO_2 laser excision** of papillomas at fixed interval (2, 4 and 6 months) according to individual need is the treatment of choice.
- **Interferon alfa** can also be used as an adjuvant therapy in patients with severe disease but has several side effects like fever, chills, myalgia, arthralgia, headache, weight loss and bone marrow suppression.
- **Recurrence** after removal is common.

Adult Onset Papilloma
- Single, smaller in size, less aggressive and **do not recur** after surgery.
- Most common age affected is **30-50 years** and is more common in **males**.
- It arises from **anterior half of vocal cord or** anterior commissure.
- Hoarseness is the presenting symptom.
- Treatment is same as of juvenile papillomas.

NEW PATTERN QUESTIONS	
Q N1.	M/C benign tumor of larynx in a child from 2-5 years is:
	a. Chondroma
	b. Juvenile laryngeal papilloma
	c. Infantile hemangioma
	d. Scleroma
Q N2.	Juvenile papillomatosis is caused by:
	a. HPV b. EBV
	c. CMV d. HSV

CHONDROMA

- Most of them arise from **cricoid cartilage** (hyaline cartilage) and cause dyspnea, lump in throat, dysphagia.
- May also arise from thyroid, arytenoid or epiglottic cartilage (fibroelastic).
- Mostly affect **men** in age group 40-60.
- Diagnosis is by via endoscopy or external approach to endoscopic wedge biopsy and on CT of neck (calcification seen).
- Management is: excision of tumor.

NEW PATTERN QUESTIONS	
Q N3.	M/C site for laryngeal cartilaginous tumors is:
	a. Arytenoid cartilage
	b. Thyroid cartilage
	c. Cricoid cartilage
	d. Corniculate cartilage
Q N4.	Chondromas are most commonly seen in which cartilage?
	a. Cricoid
	b. Thyroid
	c. Arytenoid
	d. Epiglottis

Chapter 29: Tumors of Larynx

Q N5. Benign juvenile papilloma in children is:
   a. Solitary and senile
   b. Has tendency to develop into papillary carcinoma
   c. Multiple and friable
   d. Has familial inheritance

HEMANGIOMA

Infantile hemangioma involves the *subglottic area* and presents with stridor in first 6 months of life.
- Tends to **involute spontaneously** but a tracheostomy may be needed to relieve respiratory obstruction.
- **Treated** by CO_2 laser.

Adult hemangioma involves *vocal cord* or supraglottic larynx:
- Most are **cavernous type** and can't be treated with laser.
- *No treatment is required for asymptomatic cases, larger ones are treated by steroids or radiation therapy.*

GRANULAR CELL TUMOR

- Arise from **Schwann cells** and is often submucosal.
- Overlying epithelium shows pseudoepitheliomatous hyperplasia which *resemble well-differentiated cancer.*

CANCER LARYNX

- More prevalent in India.
- **Age:** Most common in age group 40-70 years.
- Males > **females:** M/C in lower socioeconomic class.
- **Occurrence:** Glottis (55-75%) > supraglottis (24-42%) > Subglottis (1-2%).

Etiology

Point to Remember
> Tobacco smoking and alcohol are most important. Combination of alcohol and smoking increase the risk 15 fold.

- Previous neck irradiation.
- *Occupational exposure* to **asbestos, mustard gas** and petroleum products.
- HPV–16 and 18 are also implicated.
- Premalignant conditions = Solitary papilloma, leukoplakia and keratosis.

Histopathology

- 90-95% of Ca larynx are **squamous cell ca.**
- Cordal lesions are **well-differentiated** while supraglottic ones are anaplastic.

Site of Laryngeal Tumors

As discussed previously, larynx is divided into supraglottic, glottic and subglottic regions for the purpose of anatomical classification of carcinoma of larynx. It is an important division and is based on lymphatic drainage. The area above the vocal cords, i.e., supraglottis drains upwards via the superior lymphatic to upper deep cervical group of lymph nodes. Vocal cords, i.e., glottis has practically no lymphatics, so it acts as a watershed. The area below the glottis (subglottis) drains to prelaryngeal and paratracheal glands and then to lower deep cervical nodes. Incidence of larynx cancer by site:

Point to Remember
> Supraglottis cancer = 40%
> Glottic cancer = 59%
> Subglottic cancer = 1%

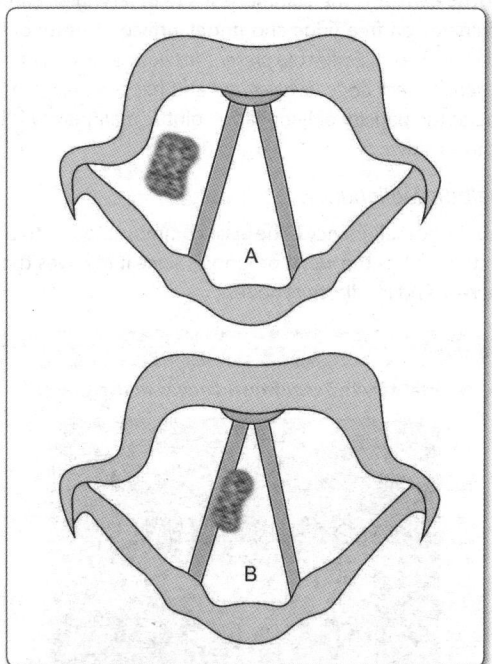

Fig. 29.1: Carcinoma larynx. (A) Supraglottic; and (B) Glottic
Courtesy: Text book of Diseases of Ear, Nose and Throat, Mohan Bansal. Jaypee Brothers Medical Publishers Pvt. Ltd., p 504

Classification

According to site Ca larynx is divided into:

a. Supraglottic Cancer: Less Common

- Majority of lesion is on epiglottis, false cords or ventricular bands followed by aryepiglottic folds (laryngeal aspect only); arytenoids.
- **Symptoms:** Pain on swallowing is the most frequent initial symptom. *Ref. Devita 7/e, p 698*
- Mass in neck may be the **first sign**.
- **Hoarseness** *is a late symptom.*
- *Pain may referred to ear by* **vagus nerve** *and* **auricular nerve of Arnold**.

- Late symptoms include foul breath, dysphagia and aspiration.
- Large tumors can cause hot potato voice/muffled voice.
- Hemoptysis, stridor, dyspnea, aspiration pneumonia may also occur.

Spread:
- *Locally* to invade vallecula, base of tongue and pyriform fossa.
- *Lymphatic*: Greatest incidence of nodal spread, nodal metastases *occurs* early and is bilateral *Upper* and **middle jugular nodes** are often involved.

b. Glottic Cancer (M/C)
- **Glottic cancer** is the commonest site of laryngeal cancers. It originates on free edge and undersurface of Anterior 1/3 of true vocal cord. Earliest *to present (as hoarseness[Q]), least predilection for neck node involvement* and has the best prognosis. Due to the paucity of lymphatics, glottic malignancy is highly radiosensitive.

c. Subglottic Malignancy
- Subglottic malignancy is the least common site, last to present as stridor[Q], has the worst prognosis since it involves the paratracheal and mediastinal nodes.

NEW PATTERN QUESTION

Q N6. Identify the condition shown in the plate:

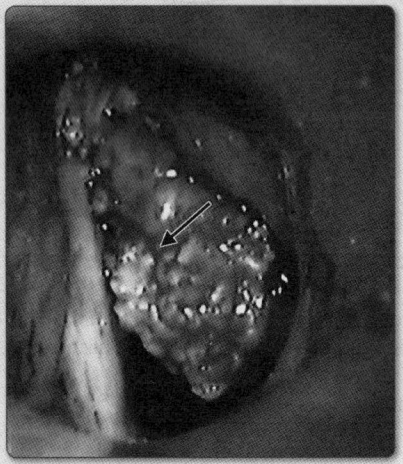

See Color Plate 22

a. Supraglottic CA   b. Glottic CA
c. Subglottic CA   d. None

Diagnosis

IOC = Direct laryngoscopy is used to assess the extent of tumor and for obtaining biopsy of the cancer.
- **CT:** Very useful investigation to find the extent of tumor and invasion of pre-epiglottic or paraepiglottic space.
- **MRI:** It is less suitable than CT due to motion artifacts associated with longer scanning time.

- **Supravital staining and biopsy:** *Toluidine* blue is applied to laryngeal lesion and then washed with saline. Carcinoma *in situ* and superficial carcinoma *take dye while leukoplakia does not.*

Staging
—*Devita 7/e, p 698*

Table 29.1: TNM classification of cancer larynx (AJCC 2002)	
Primary	Tumor (T)
Supraglottis	
T1	Tumor limited to one subsite of supraglottis with normal vocal cord mobility
T2	Tumor invades mucosa of more than one adjacent sub-site of supraglottis or region outside the supraglottis, without fixation of larynx.
T3	Tumor limited to larynx with vocal cord fixation and/or invades any of the following: postcoricoid area preepiglottic tissues, paraglottic space, and/or minor thyroid cartilage erosion (e.g. inner cortex).
T4a	Tumor invades through the thyroid cartilage and/or invades tissues beyond the larynx.
T4b	Tumor invades prevertebral space, encases carotid artery or invades mediastinal structures
Glottis	
T1	Tumor limited to one (T1a) or both (T1b) vocal cord(s) (may involve anterior or posterior commissure) with normal mobility
T2	Tumor extends to supraglottis and/or subglottis, or with impaired vocal cord mobility
T3	Tumor limited to the larynx with vocal cord fixation, and/or invades paraglottic space, and/or minor thyroid cartilage erosion (e.g. inner cortex)
T4	Same as supraglottis
Subglottis	
T1	Tumor limited to subglottis
T2	Tumor extends to vocal cords with normal or impaired mobility
T3	Tumor limited to larynx with vocal cord fixation
T4	Same as supraglottis

Regional Lymph Nodes (N)

 Note: Cancer larynx first spreads to the cervical nodes. The next M/C site of spread is lungs for this reason chest X-ray should be a part of the routine metastatic evaluation (in all head and neck cancers).

N_x Regional lymph nodes cannot be assessed.
N_0 No regional lymph node metastasis
N_1 Metastasis in a single ipsilateral lymph node, 3 cm or less in greatest dimension.
N_2 Metastatis in a single ipsilateral lymph node, more than 3 cm but not more than 6 cm in greatest dimension, or multiple ipsilateral lymph nodes, none more than 6 cm in greatest dimension, or bilateral or contralateral lymph nodes, nodes, not more than 6 cm in greatest dimension.
N_{2a} Metastasis in a single ipsilateral lymph node more than 3 cm but not more than 6 cm in greatest dimension.

N_{2b}	Metastases in multiple ipsilateral lymph nodes, none > 6 cm.
N_{2c}	Metastases in bilateral or contralateral lymph nodes, none > 6 cm.
N_3	Metastasis in a lymph node > 6 cm.

Modalities of Treatment

A. Endoscopic Resection with CO_2 Laser

Transoral endoscopic laser microsurgery (TLS): It is the TOC these days for early glottic cancer. It is less expensive and more convenient than traditional external beam radiotherapy. The drawback is that a relatively large number of laser-treated patients require radiotherapy for treating the residual disease as complete removal of tumor by laser is not possible in every case. This increases the treatment load on the patient, as well as increases the cost of treatment. Thus laser treatment is reserved for small, mid cord tumors at one vocal cord without impaired mobility (T_{1a}).

B. Radiotherapy

- Curative radiotherapy is given for early lesions $T_{1,2}$. The cords are mobile, and there is no involvement of cartilage and cervical nodes. The main advantage is preservation of voice.
- In cases of vocal cord cancer, radiotherapy gives 90% cure rate.
- In cases of superficial exophytic lesions of the tip of epiglottis and aryepiglottic folds, it gives 70-90% cure rate.
- The results are not good in cases of fixed cords, subglottic extension, cartilage invasion, and nodal metastases. These cases are candidates for surgery.

Other Indications of Radiotherapy
1. Recurrence after one or more prior vocal fold stripping
2. Recurrence in a short period after stripping
3. Inability for follow-up after treatment
4. In patients in whom voice quality is critical like in professional singers
5. Overall poor operative risks
6. Anterior commissure lesion which is inaccessible for complete endoscopic ablation

> **Point to Remember**
> - *Carcinoma glottis:* In comparison to supraglottis, nasopharynx and subglottic cancers, carcinoma glottis is the most radiosensitive tumor.

C. Surgery

- **Conservation surgery:** It preserves voice and avoids a permanent tracheal opening. Cases should be carefully selected:
  - *Cordectomy:* Excision of vocal cord via laryngofissure or endoscopy.
  - *Partial frontolateral laryngectomy (vertical laryngectomy):* Excision of vocal cord and anterior commissure.
  - *Partial horizontal laryngectomy (supraglottic laryngectomy):* Excision of supraglottis, which include epiglottis, aryepiglottic folds, false cords and ventricle used as TOC for supraglottic cancers not involving vocal cord.
- **Supracricoid partial laryngectomy (SCPL):** A SCPL is a suitable conservative procedure, which can be used as an alternative to total laryngectomy for advanced supraglottic and glottic cancers.

Ref: Otolaryngology Clinics Sep-Dec 2010;2(3):201-205.

There are 2 types of SCPL depending on the primary site of tumor and type of reconstruction:

1. The entire hyroid cartilage + true and false vocal cords + paraglottic space are resected.
   Leaving behind entire epiglottis, hyoid bone, minimum one side cricoarytenoid joint along with recurrent laryngeal nerve and entire cricoid cartilage. During reconstruction the cricoid is sutured to the hyoid and epiglottis, so it is called cricohyoid epiglottopexy (CHEP) and hence the term SCPL + CHEP.
2. In selected cases of supraglottic and transglottic cancers - In addition to structures removed in SCPL + CHEP, the entire pre-epiglottic space and epiglottis are resected and a pexy is made between cricoid and hyoid bone i.e. Cricohyoidopexy (CHP). Thus the term SCPL + CHP.

Table 29.2: Indications and contraindications of supracricoid partial laryngectomy

Indications	Contraindications
- Impaired mobility or even fixity of vocal cords but with mobile arytenoids in supraglottic or glottic cancer - T_{1b} glottic cancer where more than one-third of contralateral cord is involved - Supraglottic cancer with spread to anterior commissure - Thyroid cartilage involvement but without invasion of the outer perichondrum - Recurrent laryngeal cancer after failed laryngeal radiotherapy	- Cord fixity due to cricoarytenoid joint involvement - Pre-epiglottic space involvement in glottic cancer - In supraglottic cancer - if base of tongue, vallecula are involved or if there is massive involvement of pre-epiglottic space such that hyoid bone cannot be spared - Subglottic extension - Prior tracheostomy - Poor pulmonary reserve

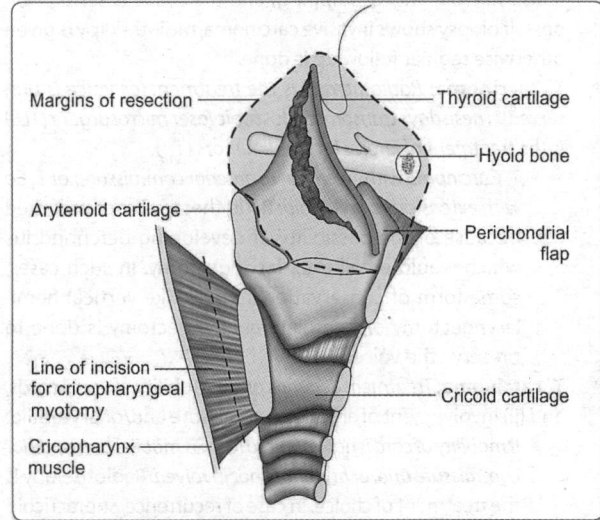

Fig. 29.2: Supraglottic laryngectomy
Courtesy: Disease of ENT, Tuli Jaypee Brothers Medical Publishers Pvt. Ltd., 2/e, p 326

- **Total laryngectomy:** The entire larynx is removed (upto 1 cm below the cord) along with hyoid bone, pre-epiglottic space, strap muscles and one or more rings of trachea. A tracheostome is formed above the suprasternal notch. The indications include T_{3-4} lesions and failure after radiotherapy or conservation surgery. It is combined with block dissection when nodal metastasis is present. It is not done in patients with distant metastasis. This procedure has low patient compliance.
- **Hemithyroidectomy or subtotal thyroidectomy:** The associated hemithyroidectomy or subtotal thyroidectomy is indicated in following conditions:
  - Palpable thyroid abnormality
  - Subglottic extension and tumors
  - T_4 glottic tumors
  - T_4 pyriform sinus tumors
  - Positive delphian nodes
  - Thyroid-cricoid cartilage destruction

D. Combined Therapy
- Earlier surgery was combined with pre- or postoperative radiation in a planned way to decrease the incidence of recurrence. These days chemoradiation is also being done.

> **Point to Remember**
> - **Verrucous carcinoma of larynx:** The treatment of choice is surgery.

Glottic/Vocal Cord Carcinoma
Stage dependent treatment include:
- **Carcinoma in situ (CIN):** *Best treated by transoral endoscopic CO_2 laser.* If laser is not available stripping of vocal cord is done (Endo/microlaryngeal stripping) and the tissue is sent for biopsy. If biopsy shows invasive carcinoma, radiotherapy is given otherwise regular follow up is done.
- **T_1 carcinoma:** *Radiotherapy is the treatment (as voice is preserved). These days transoral endoscopic laser microsurgery (TLS) is the treatment of choice for small tumors (T_{1a}).*
  - T_1 *Carcinoma with extension to anterior commissure: or T_1 Ca with extension to arytenoid:* Radiotherapy is not preferred because of the possibility of developing perchondritis which would entail total laryingectomy. In such cases, some form of conservation surgery like vertical hemilaryngectomy or frontolateral laryngectomy is done to preserve the voice.
- **T_2 carcinoma:** *Treatment depends on:* (i) Mobility of vocal cords, and (ii) Involvement of anterior commissure and/or arytenoid:
  - *If mobility of cord is not impaired (cord is mobile) and anterior commissure and/or arytenoid not involved:* Radiotherapy is the treatment of choice. In case of recurrence, supracricoid partial laryngectomy (SCPL) or total laryngectomy is done.
  - *If mobility of cord is impaired or anterior commissure and/or arytenoid involved:* Voice preserving conservative surgery such as SCPL is done. Total laryngectomy is done if there is recurrence on follow up.
- **T_3, T_4 carcinoma:** In T3 lesions – TOC is primary chemoradiation with total laryngectomy as salvage surgery in residual lesion.

NEW PATTERN QUESTIONS

Q N7. Ackerman's tumor is best treated by:
a. Surgery   b. Chemotherapy
c. Radiotherapy   d. Combined T/t

Q N8. Structures preserved in radical neck dissection is:
a. Vagus nerve
b. Submandibular gland
c. Sternocleidomastoid
d. Internal Jugular Vein

Q N9. Which structure is preserved during modified radical neck dissection?
a. Phrenic nerve
b. Submandibular gland
c. Sternocleidomastoid
d. Thoracic duct

Q N10. Level V cervical nodes includes:
a. Upper jugular nodes
b. Middle jugular nodes
c. Lower jugular nodes
d. Posterior triangle nodes

Q N11. Maintenance of airway during laryngectomy in a patient with carcinoma of larynx is best done by:
a. Tracheostomy
b. Laryngeal mask airway
c. Laryngeal tube
d. Combi tube

Q N12. IOC to detect involvement of laryngeal cartilage, laryngeal tumors
a. CT   b. MRI
c. Biopsy   d. Toluidine blue staining

Q N13. Bloom singer prosthesis for voice rehabilitation is used in:
a. Total laryngectomy
b. Near laryngectomy
c. Hemi laryngectomy
d. None

Q N14. Staging of glottic carcinoma of larynx with fixation of vocal cord is:
a. T_1 b. T_2
c. T_3 d. T_4

Q N15. Structures preserved in supracricoid partial laryngectomy are all except:
a. Hyoid bone   b. Cricoid cartilage
c. Thyroid cartilage   d. Recurrent laryngeal N

Vocal Rehabilitation after Laryngectomy

- Oesophageal speech:
  - Patient is taught to swallow air and hold it in inner oesophagus and then slowly burp out the into pharynx. Patient can speak 6-10 word before swallowing.
  - Rough voice but loud and understandable.
- Artificial larynx:
  - Electrolarynx and trans oral pneumatic device.
- Tracheoesophageal speech:
  - Here a fistula is created between the trachea and esophagus. This opening is called as tracheoesophageal puncture. A voice prosthesis is placed in this opening. Then it becomes possible to speak by occluding the stoma and blowing the air from the lungs through the inside of voice prosthesis and through the throat called tracheoesophageal speech.

Complications of Treatment

- **Surgery** — Speech loss after laryngectomy.
- **Radiation** — Laryngeal edema and odynophagia are *most common* complication after radiation for glottic or supraglottic lesion.

> **Points to Remember**
> **Also know**
> ➢ Glottic Ca carcinoma carries the best prognosis because of the early diagnosis and relatively few lymphatics.
> ➢ Most frequent site of recurrence in glottic Ca is around tracheal stoma in the base of tongue and in neck nodes.
> ➢ CT scan is the best investigation to find out the nature and extent of growth besides direct laryngoscopy examination.

Explanations and References to New Pattern Questions

N1. Ans. is b i.e. Juvenile laryngeal papilloma *Ref. Dhingra 6/e, p 305*

Juvenile Papillomatosis is the most common benign neoplasm of the larynx in children.

N2. Ans. is a i.e. HPV *Ref. Dhingra 6/e, p 305*

See the text for explanation.

N3. Ans. is c i.e. Cricoid cartilage *Ref. Essentials of ENT, Mohan Bansal, p 372*

N4. Ans. is a i.e. Cricoid cartilage

Laryngeal cartilaginous tumor i.e. Chondroma cricoid cartilage is the most common site of laryngeal cartilaginous tumor.

N5. Ans. is c i.e. Multiple and friable

See the text for explanation

> **Remember**
> Malignant change is uncommon or rare in multiple juvenile papillomatosis. Hence, it can be kept in +/– status in this question since option c is absolutely incorrect. ∴ it is be taken as the answer.

N6. Ans. is b i.e. Glottic cancer

The growth is seen in between the vocal cords in the plate, hence it is glottic cancer.

N7. Ans. is a i.e. Surgery *Ref. TB of ENT, Tuli 2/e, p 327*

Verrucous carcinoma is also called **Ackerman's tumor**.
Management of verrucous carcinoma of larynx is always surgery (partial or total laryngectomy).
These days endoscopic removal of tumor is the preferred method.

N8. Ans. is a i.e. Vagus nerve

N9. Ans. is c i.e. Sternocleidomastoid *Ref. Sabiston 19/e, p 796-797*

Structures Removed in Radical Neck Dissection	Modified Radical Neck Dissection
• Lymph nodes I-V + • Spinal accessory nerve + • Internal jugular vein + • Sternocleidomastoid muscle	Removal of Lymph nodes I-V Type I—Spinal accessory nerve preserved Rest removed Type II—Spinal accessory N + internal jugular vein preserved Type III—Spinal accessory N + internal jugular vein + sternocleidomastoid muscle preserved

N10. Ans. is d i.e. Posterior triangle nodes *Ref. Sabiston 19/e, p 796-797*

Cervical lymph nodes are divided into 7 levels:

Level	Lymph node
I A	Submental
IB	Submandibular
II	Upper Jugular
III	Middle Jugular
IV	Lower Jugular
V	Posterior triangle
VI	Central
VII	Superior mediastinal

Note: Virchow or left supraclavicular are included in level IV.

N11. Ans. is a i.e. Tracheostomy *Ref. Logan Turner 10/e, p 178*
During laryngectomy, airway of a patient is maintained by tracheostomy.

N12. Ans. is b i.e. MRI

N13. Ans. is a i.e. Total laryngectomy
Any type of voice prosthesis is needed after total laryngectomy.

There are several manufacturers that make voice prosthesis like Adeva, Eska, Medi Top, Hermomed. In 1980, the first commercially available prosthesis was introduced by Singer and Blom. The **Blom-singer Duckbill prosthesis**. All the voice prosthesis are used after total laryngectomy.

There are 2 main categories of voice prosthesis:
 a. Non-dwelling prosthesis: These prosthesis can be replaced by the patient themselves.
 b. Indwelling prosthesis: Those which have to be replaced by a medical professional.

N14. Ans. is c i.e. T_3
See the text for explanation.

N15. Ans. is c i.e. Thyroid cartilage
See the text for explanation.

QUESTIONS

1. **Premalignant conditions for carcinoma larynx would include:** [PGI 01]
   a. Leukoplakia
   b. Lichen planus
   c. Papillomas
   d. Smoking
   e. Chronic laryngitis

2. **Which of the following is precancerous lesion:** [UP 00]
   a. Pachydermia of larynx
   b. Laryngitis sicca
   c. Keratosis of larynx
   d. Scleroma larynx

3. **Of the following statements about Recurrent Laryngeal papillomatosis are true, except:** [AI-09]
   a. Caused by human papilloma virus (HPV)
   b. HPV6 and HPV11 are most commonly implicated
   c. HPV6 is more virulent than HPV11
   d. Transmission to neonate occurs through contact with mother during vaginal delivery

4. **True about juvenile respiratory papillomatosis:** [PGI 00]
   a. Affects children commonly
   b. Lower respiratory tract can be involved
   c. May resolve spontaneously
   d. Microlaryngoscopic surgery is treatment of choice

5. **True about multiple papillomatosis:** [PGI Dec. 05]
   a. HSV is causative agent
   b. Radiotherapy treatment of choice
   c. It is premalignant
   d. It is more common in 15 to 33 yrs
   e. It recurs due to parturition

6. **True about Juvenile laryngeal papillomatosis:**
   a. Caused by HPV [PGI May 2011]
   b. No risk of recurrence after surgical removal
   c. Tends to disappear after puberty
   d. Interferon therapy is useful

7. **Kamla 4 yrs of age presented in emergency with mild respiratory distress. On laryngoscopy she was diagnosed to have multiple juvenile papillomatosis of the larynx. Next line of management is:** [AIIMS 01]
   a. Tracheostomy
   b. Microlaryngoscopy
   c. Steroid
   d. Antibiotics

8. **Topical treatment for recurrent respiratory papillomatosis includes:** [AIIMS May 2015]
   a. Acyclovir
   b. Cidofovir
   c. Ranitidine
   d. Zinc

9. **All the following are true about Laryngeal carcinoma except:** [AI 94]
   a. More common in females
   b. Common in patients over 40 years of age
   c. After laryngectomy, esophageal voice can be used
   d. Poor prognosis

10. **Features of laryngeal Ca:** [PGI June 05]
    a. Glottis is the MC site
    b. Commonly metastasizes to cervical lymph node
    c. Lesions seen at the edge of the vocal cord
    d. Laryngeal compartments acts as barrier

11. **Supraglottic Ca present with:** [PGI June 03]
    a. Hot potato voice
    b. Aspiration
    c. Smoking is common risk factor
    d. Pain is MC manifestation
    e. Lymph node metastasis is uncommon

12. **The most common and earliest manifestation of carcinoma of the glottis is:** [AI 05, RJ-2006]
    a. Hoarseness
    b. Hemoptysis
    c. Cervical lymph nodes
    d. Stridor

13. **Lymph mode metastasis in neck is almost never seen with:** [AI 96]
    a. Carcinoma vocal cords
    b. Supraglottic carcinoma
    c. Carcinoma of tonsil
    d. Papillary carcinoma thyroids

14. **Which of the following carcinomas commonly presents with neck nodes:** [AI 95]
    a. Cricoid
    b. Glottic
    c. Epiglottis
    d. Anterior commissure

15. **True statement about infraglottic carcinoma larynx:** [PGI 96]
    a. Commonly spreads to mediastinal nodes
    b. Second most common carcinoma
    c. Most common carcinoma
    d. Spreads to submental nodes

16. **The treatment of choice for stage I cancer larynx is:**
    a. Radical surgery [AIIMS 03, PGI 98]
    b. Chemotherapy
    c. Radiotherapy
    d. Surgery followed by radiotherapy

17. **In laryngeal cancer if anterior commissure is involved best management would be:**
    a. Laryngectomy
    b. Conservative surgery
    c. RT
    d. Chemotherapy

18. **For a mobile tumor on vocal cord, treatment is:**
    a. Surgery [AIIMS 92, AP 96]
    b. Chemotherapy
    c. Radiotherapy
    d. None of the above

19. **For carcinoma larynx stage III treatment of choice:**
    a. Radiotherapy and surgery [AIIMS 96]
    b. Chemotherapy with cisplatin
    c. Partial laryngectomy with chemotherapy
    d. Radiotherapy with chemotherapy
20. **An elderly male presents with T3N0 laryngeal carcinoma. What would be the management?** [AIIMS Nov. 14]
    a. Neoadjuvant chemotherapy followed by radiotherapy
    b. Concurrent chemoradiotherapy
    c. Radial radiotherapy followed by chemotherapy
    d. Radical radiotherapy without chemotherapy
21. **Radiotherapy is the TOC for:** [AIIMS Nov. 09]
    a. Nasopharyngeal Ca $T_3 N_1$
    b. Supraglottic Ca $T_3 N_0$
    c. Glottic Ca $T_3 N_1$
    d. Subglottic Ca $T_3 N_0$
22. **A patient of carcinoma larynx with stridor presents in casualty, immediate management is:** [AIIMS 91]
    a. Planned tracheostomy
    b. Immediate tracheostomy
    c. High dose steroid
    d. Intubate, give bronchodilator and wait for 12 hours, if no response, proceed to tracheostomy
    e. None of the above
23. **Which of the following is not the indication of near total Laryngectomy?** [AP 2007]
    a. T3 stage
    b. Anterior commissure involvement
    c. Supraglotic involvement
    d. Both arytenoids involved
24. **A patient presents with carcinoma of the larynx involving the left false cord, left arytenoids and the left aryepiglottic folds with bilateral mobile true cords. Treatment of choice is:** [AIIMS Nov 07]
    a. Vertical hemilaryngectomy
    b. Horizontal hemilaryngectomy
    c. Radiotherapy followed by chemotherapy
    d. Total laryngectomy
25. **A case of carcinoma larynx with the involvement of anterior commissure and right vocal cord, developed perichondritis of thyroid cartilage. Which of the following statements is true for the management of this case?** [AIIMS May 06]
    a. He should be given radical radiotherapy as this can cure early tumors
    b. He should be treated with combination of chemotherapy and radiotherapy
    c. He should first receive radiotherapy and if residual tumor is present then should under go laryngectomy
    d. He should first undergo laryngectomy and then postoperative radiotherapy
26. **Treatment of choice for carcinoma larynx T1N0M0 stage:** [AI 02]
    a. External beam radiotherapy
    b. Radioactive implants
    c. Surgery
    d. Surgery and radiotherapy
27. **Select correct statements about Ca larynx:** [PGI 02]
    a. Glottic Ca is the most common
    b. Supraglottic ca has best prognosis
    c. Lymphatic spread is the most common in subglottic Ca
    d. T1 tumor is best treated by radiotherapy
    e. Smoking predisposes
28. **The preferred treatment of verrucous carcinoma of the larynx is:** [UP 07]
    a. Pulmonary surgery
    b. Electron beam therapy
    c. Total laryngectomy
    d. Endoscopic removal
29. **Laryngofissure is:** [JIPMER 04]
    a. Opening the larynx in midline
    b. Making window in thyroid cartilage
    c. Removal of arytenoids
    d. Removal of epiglottis
30. **About total laryngectomy all is correct except:**
    a. Loss of smell [Bihar 2005]
    b. Loss of taste
    c. Speech difficulty
    d. Difficult swallowing
31. **Laser used in laryngeal work?** [AI 2010]
    a. Argon   b. CO_2
    c. Holmium   d. Nd Yag
32. **Contraindication of supracricoid laryngectomy is/are:**
    a. Poor pulmonary reserve [PGI Nov 09]
    b. Tumor involving pyriform sinus
    c. Tumor involving preepiglottic space
    d. Vocal cord fixation
    e. Cricoid cartilage extension
33. **A 5-year-old male with worsening hoarseness for 3 months and stridor for 2 weeks. What is the likely diagnosis?** [AIIMS May 2016]

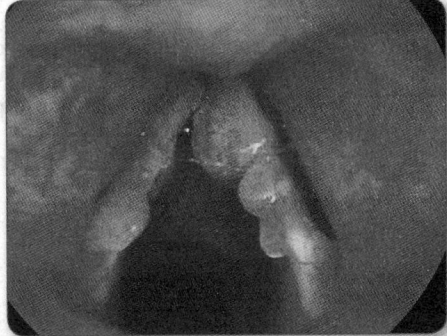

See Color Plate 23

    a. Vocal nodule
    b. Acute epiglottis
    c. Respiratory papillomatosis
    d. Carcinoma larynx

Explanations and References

1. **Ans. is a, c, and e i.e. Leukoplakia; Papillomas; and Chronic laryngitis**
   Ref. Read below
2. **Ans. is c i.e. Keratosis of larynx**
   Ref. Scotts Brown 7th/ed vol-2 pg-2221; Dhingra 5th/ed pg-323, 6th/ed p 304; Mohan Bansal p 487
   - Lichen planus has no malignant potential. *.... Turner 10/e, p 126*
   - Papilloma– "The malignant transformation from benign non keratinizing squamous papilloma to squamous cell carcinoma can occur in children, but is rarely seen" *– Current Otolaryngology 2/e, p 471*
   - Leukoplakia is a white patch, in which there is epithelial hyperplasia along with atypical cells. It is a premalignant condition. Another name for leukoplakia is hyperkeratosis dyskeratosis *– Scott's Brown 7/e, vol-2 p 2221*
   - Smoking is a predisposing factor, not a premalignant condition.
   - In some cases of chronic laryngitis, the laryngeal mucosa becomes dysplastic particularly over true vocal folds and is a premalignant condition. *... Bailey 24/e, p 765*
   - Chronic inflammatory conditions of larynx like chronic laryngitis may develop into malignancy. *... Maqbool 11/e, p 359*

   Keratosis of larynx/leukoplakia:-
   It is epithelial hyperplasia of the upper surface of one or both vocal cords.
   - Appears as a white plaque or warty growth on cord without affecting its mobility
   - Regarded as a precancerous condition as Ca in situ develops frequently
   - T/t = stripping of cords

3. **Ans. is c i.e. HPV6 is more virulent than HPV 11**
   Ref. Nelson's pediatrics 18/1772; Current Otorhinology 2/e, p 435/471 'Pediatric ENT' by Graham. Scadding and Bull (2008)/258

   ### Recurrent Laryngeal Papillomatosis/Recurrent Respiratory Papillomatosis
   Etiology
   - Associated with Human Papilloma Virus infection (HPV)
   - HPV6 and HPV 11 are most commonly associated with laryngeal disease whereas HPV 16 and HPV 18 are less commonly associated
   - HPV11 is associated with a more aggressive disease and makes the patient more prone to malignant change
   - Thus HPV 11 is more virulent.

4. **Ans. is a, b, c, and d i.e. Affects children commonly; Lower respiratory tract can be involved; May resolve spontaneously; and Microlaryngoscopic surgery is treatment of choice**
   Ref. Dhingra 5/e, p 324,325; Current Otolaryngology 2/e, p 471; Mohan Bansal p 488

   Juvenile respiratory papillomatosis:
   a. Affects children commonly, (option a is correct)
   b. Lower respiratory tract can be involved – though larynx is the M/C site affected – Mouth, pharynx, tracheobronchial tree and oesophagus can all be affected
      Hence option b is correct
   c. May resolve spontaneously (Hence option c is correct)
   d. Microlaryngoscopic surgery is the treatment of choice

   CO_2 laser surgery, which is a form of microlaryngoscopic surgery is the treatment of choice
   Hence option d is also correct.

5. **Ans. is c i.e. It is premalignant**
   Ref. Current Otolaryngology 2/e, p 471, 3/e, p 453-454

Option	Correct / Incorrect	Reference	Explanation
HSV is the causative Agent (**Option a**)	Incorrect	Current 2/e pg-471	It is caused by infection with human papilloma virus (HPV) subtype 6 and 11 not by Herpes simplex virus i.e. HSV is not the causative agent
Radiotherapy is the TOC (**Option b**)	Correct	Current 2/e pg-471	The primary treatment modality for respiratory papillomatosis is surgery" Current Otolaryngology 2/e pg-471
It is premalignant (**Option c**)	Incorrect	Current 2/e pg-471	Juvenile papillomatosis due to subtype 11,16,18 can undergo malignant transformations, though it is rare.

Contd...

Contd...

Option	Correct / Incorrect	Reference	Explanation
It is M/C in 15 to 33 yrs (**Option d**)	Incorrect	*Current 2/e pg-471* *Dhingra 6/e, p 305*	Respiratory papillomatosis m/c seen in children between the ages 2 to 5 years although it can be seen in adults in third decade also.
It recurs cause is due to parturition (**Option e**)	In correct	*Current 2/e pg-471* *Dhingra 5/e pg-324* *6/e, p 305-306*	These are 2 different statements – 1. Papilloma has a tendency to recur 2. Vertical transmission can occur from mother to child at the time of parturition. Both these statements are correct individually. **But** – It recurs and cause of recurrence is parturition is not correct

Point to Remember

- **Adult onset papilloma** – seen in adults in the third decade
- It is less aggressive, less chances of malignant transformation and less chances of recurrence.

6. **Ans. is a, c and d i.e. Caused by HPV; Tends to disappear after puberty; and Interferon therapy is useful** *(Ref. Read below)*
   See the text for explanation
7. **Ans. is b i.e. Microlaryngoscopy** *Ref. Current Otolaryngology 2/e, p 471, 3/e, p 454-455*
   - The patient (a 4 years girl) in the question is presenting with mild respiratory distress due to multiple Juvenile papillomatosis of larynx.
   - The management in such a case is microlaryngoscopic surgery using CO_2 laser to ablate the lesion.
   - Steroids and antibiotics have no role.
   - Tracheostomy is reserved for those patients who have severe respiratory distress.
8. **Ans is b. i.e Cidofovir** *Ref. Review therapy for recurrent respiratory papellometus- Karen J Auborn*
   Cidoflovir- is very effective in treatment of Recurrent Respiratory Papellonatos. It is a neucleoside analogue, and has broad spectrum activity against a wide variety of DNA viruses, interfering with viral DNA synthesis. It can be used systemically, intralesionally and topically.
   Adverse effects- Renal toxicity
9. **Ans. is a i.e. More common in females and d i.e. Poor prognosis**
   Ref. Current Otolaryngology 2/e, p 437 onwards; Mohan Bansal p 502,503

Cancer Larynx

- *Most common* histological type of laryngeal Ca - Squamous cell carcinoma (seen in 90% cases)
- It is more common in males
- Male: Female ratio is 4: 1) (option a is incorrect)
- *Most common* age = 60-70 years.

Mnemonic

Aetiology: Risk factors:- Mnemonic **"CA LARGES"**
- **C** – Chronic laryngitis
- **A** – Alcohol
- **L** – Leukoplakia
- **A** – Asbestosis
- **R** – Radiation
- **G** – Mustard Gas
- **E** – Exposure to petroleum products
- **S** – Smoking

Prognosis of Laryngeal Cancer

- Cure for larynx cancer, defined as 5 year disease free survival is generally better than for other primary site tumors of the aerodigestive tract. This reflects the prevalence of primary glottic tumors over supraglottic tumors and the early age at which glottic tumours are diagnosed (Hence option d is incorrect)
- So option a and d are both incorrect but if one option is to be chosen, go for option 'a'.

10. **Ans. is a, b, c and d i.e. All options are correct** Ref. Dhingra 5/e, p 302, 327; 6/e, p 308, 309; Tuli 1/e, p 310; Mohan Bansal p 502,503
    - As discussed previously, larynx is divided into supraglottic, glottic and subglottic regions for the purpose of anatomical classification of carcinoma of larynx.
    - It is an important division and is based on lymphatic drainage.
    - The area above the vocal cords i.e. supraglottis drains upwards via the superior lymphatics to upper deep cervical group of lymph nodes.
    - Vocal cords, i.e. glottis has practically no lymphatics. So, it acts as a watershed.
    - The area below the glottis, (subglottis) drain to prelaryngeal and paratracheal glands and then to lower deep cervical nodes. Hence option b and d are both correct

11. **Ans. is a, c and d i.e. Hot potato voice; Smoking is common risk factor; Pain is the most common manifestation**
    Ref. Devita 7/e, p 698; Scott's Brown 7/e, vol-2 p 2608; Mohan Bansal p 506

    ## Supraglottic Cancer
    - It is the second *most common* laryngeal cancer (most common is glottic cancer)
    - *Most common* initial symptom – pain on swallowing. (option d is correct)
    - *Most common* / first sign – mass is neck
    - Small supraglottic lesions not extending to glottis – may present with globus or foreign body sensation and parasthesia
    - If exophytic they may cause hemoptysis
    - Large tumors can cause "hot potato voice" (Option 'a' is correct)
    - Hoarseness is a late symptom
    - Smoking is a risk for all laryngeal carcinomas. (option c is correct)
    - Lymphatic spread occurs early in case of supraglottic cancer. (as it has rich supply of lymphatics).

    Note: Hoarseness of voice is the presenting symptom in glottic carcinoma.

12. **Ans. is a i.e. Hoarseness** Ref. Dhingra 5/e, p 327, 6/e, p 309; Current Otolaryngology 2/e, p 441, 3/e, p 460.
    In glottic cancer.
    "Hoarseness of voice is an early sign because lesion of cord affects its vibratory capacity."
    For details see the text.

13. **Ans. is a i.e. Carcinoma of vocal cords** Ref. Dhingra 5/e, p 327, 6/e, p 309
    "There are very few lymphatics in vocal cords and nodal metastasis are practically never seen in cordal lesions unless it has spread beyond the region of membranous cord."

14. **Ans. is c i.e. Epiglottis** Ref. Dhingra 5/e, p 326-327, 6/e, p 308-309.
    Supraglottic cancers: • Have earliest neck nodes involvement..
    • Presenting features is - pain on swallowing or neck mass.
    Glottic cancers: • No nodes involved presenting features is hoarseness.
    Subglottic cancers: • Nodal metastasis occurs to pretracheal, prelaryngeal nodes.
    • Presenting feature is stridor.
    In the options given–*epiglottis belongs to supraglottis so it will present with neck nodes.*

    Point to Remember
    - **Adult onset papilloma** – seen in adults in the third decade
    - Ca which presents with neck nodes = supraglottis Ca
    - Highest lymph node involvement occurs in – supraglottic Ca
    - Hoarseness is the presenting symptom – Glottic Ca
    - Stridor is the presenting symptom in Subglottic Ca.
    - Laryngeal cancer with worst prognosis = subglottic Ca
    - Ca with best prognosis = Glottic Ca

15. **Ans. is a i.e. Commonly spreads to mediastinal nodes** Ref. Dhingra 5/e, p 327, 6/e, p 309
    - Subglottic cancer is the rarest of laryngeal cancer.
    - Earliest presentation is a globus or foreign body sensation in throat followed by *stridor* or *laryngeal obstruction*.
    - Hoarseness is a *late feature* and occurs due to involvement of glottis or recurrent laryngeal nerve.
    - Lymphatic spread occurs to prelaryngeal, pretracheal, paratracheal and lower jugular nodes *(i.e. mediastinal nodes)*.

16. Ans. is c i.e. Radiotherapy *Ref. Dhingra 5/e, p 329-330; Mohan Bansal p 504*

Friends remember 2 very important concepts regarding laryngeal Ca:
- If the site of larynx caner viz supra glottis, glottis or subglottis is not mentioned, the cancer should be considered glottic (since it is the M/C variety)
- Generally stage I, II, III, IV means stage T_1, T_2, T_3, T_4 respectively.

According to Dhingra
- **Radiotherapy is the treatment of choice for all stage I cancers of larynx, which neither impair mobility nor invade cartilage or cervical nodes.**
- The greatest advantage of radiotherapy over surgery in Ca larynx glottic cancer is - preservation of voice.

It does not give good results:
- If cords are fixed
- In subglottic extension
- In cartilage invasion
- If nodal metastasis is present

– i.e. stages T_3 and T_4

But according to *Current otolaryngology 2/e pg-445*. Current Recommendations by the American Society of Clinical Oncology are that all patients with stage T_1 or T_2 laryngeal cancer, should be treated initially with the intent to preserve the larynx.

Microlaryngeal Surgery
i.e. endoscopic removal of selected larynx by operating microscope and microlaryngeal dissection instruments is used for treating early stages of glottic cancer.

17. Ans. is b i.e. conservative surgery *Ref. Read below*

The tumor is involving anterior commissure hence best management would be conservative surgery.

18. Ans. is c i.e. Radiotherapy *Ref. Dhingra 5/e, p 230-331*

According to Dhingra
- Radiotherpy is the treatment of choice for vocal cord cancer with normal mobility.
- Normal mobility of cord suggests that growth is only limited to the surface and belongs to either stage T1 or T2.
- TOC for stage T1 of glottic carcinoma - radiotherapy.
- TOC for stage T2 of glottic carcinoma - depends on mobility of the cord

If vocal cords are mobile (i.e. growth is limited to surface) Radiotherapy/microlaryngeal surgery is TOC	If local cords mobility is impaired (i.e. deeper invasion) Conservative surgery like vertical hemilaryngectomy or frontolateral hemilaryngectomy is TOC.

Note:
- If cord mobility is impaired radiotherapy is not preferred because of the possibility of developing perichondritis which would entail total laryngectomy.

19. Ans. is d i.e. Radiotherapy with chemotherapy

20. Ans. is b i.e. Concurrent chemoradiation *Ref. Harrison 18/e, p 734-735*

Management of stage 3 tumors days in concurrent chemoradiation earlier it was surgery followed by radiotherapy.

21. Ans. is a i.e., Nasopharyngeal Ca T_3N_1

Ref: Dhingra 5/e, p 263-266, 6/e, p 252 Cummings Otoloryngology: Head and Neck Surgery, 5/e, vol-2, Chapter-99

Treatment of nasopharyngeal carcinoma
- State I and II radiotherapy
- Stage III and IV radiotherapy + chemotherapy (preferred) or radiotherapy alone in some cases.

Now let's see about treatment of other options.
- Supraglottic T_3N_0 — Total laryngectomy with neck dissection followed by radiotherapy.
- Glottic T_3N_1 — Total laryngectomy $\pm$ neck dissection $\pm$ radiotherapy (In some centers organ preserving. surgery followed by chemoradiation is preferred).
- Sublottic Ca T_3N_0 — Total laryngectomy followed by post-operative radiation.

22. Ans. is b i.e. Immediate tracheostomy *Ref: Turner 10/e, p 178*

Carcinoma larynx presenting with stridor means it is subglottic laryngeal carcinoma .Ideally in such cases emergency laryngectomy should be performed.

"In the case of a large subglottic tumour presenting with respiratory obstruction a case could be made for doing an emergency laryngectomy."

But it is not given in the options:
- Intubation can not be done as growth is seen in subglottic area therefore tube can not be put.
- Planned tracheostomy can not be done as patient is suffering from stridor, which is an emergency. Therefore we will have to do emergency tracheostomy. With the precaution that the area of cancer should be removed within 72 hours.

23. **Ans. is d i.e. Both arytenoid involved**
Ref: Current otolaryngology 2/e, p 448-449

Type of Laryngectomy	Parts Removed	Indications	Comment
Hemilaryngectomy	Removal of one vertical half of larynx.	Tumor with: • Subglottic extension < 1 cm below the true vocal cord • A mobile affected cord • Unilateral involvement • No cartilage invasion • No extra laryngeal soft tissue involvement • For tumors with a T stage of T_1, T_2 or T_3 by pre epiglottic involvement only Vocal cords are mobile	Vocal cord reconstruction is done in this case by transposing a flap of strap muscle or microvascular free flap to provide bulk against which the remaining unaffected of cord can vibrate.
Near total laryngectomy	It is more extended partial laryngectomy procedure in which only one arytenoid is preserved and a tracheo-esophageal conduit is constructed for speech.	It should not- be offered to patients whose radiation treatment has failed, those with poor pulmonary reserve or those with tumor involvement below the cricoid ring. Patients with large T3 and T4 lesion with one uninvolved arytenoid or with U/L transglottic tumors with cord fixation are candidates for this surgery.	• Aspiration can occur • Pt is dependent on tracheostomy for breathing
Total laryngectomy	Entire larynx + thyroid + cricoid cartilages are removed along with some upper tracheal rings and hyoid bone, if possible.	Indications: • T4 malignancy • As a salvage surgery in recurrences following chemoradiation for T_3 esion • It is TOC in perichondritis larynx	Most important constraint is speech problem which can be obtained by tracheoesophageal speech

24. **Ans. is a i.e. Vertical hemilaryngectomy**
Ref. Essential of ENT, Mohan Bansal p 385

In the Patient
- Involvement of unilateral false cord, aryepiglottic folds and arytenoids with mobile cord suggest supraglottic cancer in T2 stage (more than one subsites of supraglottis are involved).
- For T2 stage radiotherapy is best. But it is not given in options. Hence, we will go for voice conserving surgery-vertical hemilaryngectomy.
- Vertical hemilaryngectomy means excision of one half of larynx, one half of supraglottis, glottis and subglottis.

25. **Ans. is d i.e. He should first undergo laryngectomy and then post-operative radiotherapy**
Ref. Dhingra 5/e, p 328,330,331; 6/e, 310-311

Perichondritis of thyroid cartilage in a patient of Ca larynx suggests invasion of thyroid cartilage, i.e. stage T4.
Stage T4 lesions glottic cancer earlier were managed by total laryngectomy with neck dissection for clinically positive nodes and post operative radiotherapy if nodes are not palpable.
These days chemoradiation is preferred.

26. **Ans. is a i.e. External beam radiotherapy**
Ref: Current otolaryngology 2/e, p 445, 450, 3/e, p 469-470

As I have said earlier–Treatment for stage I of cancer larynx (glottic cancer) is either microlaryngoscopic surgery or radiotherapy. Since microlaryngoscopic surgery is not given we will go for radiotherapy. Now the question arises which type of radiotherapy is used.

Chapter 29: Tumors of Larynx

External Bean Radiation or Brachytherapy

"External bean radiation is most often used to treat laryngeal and hypopharyngeal cancer."
"Brachytherapy is rarely used to treat laryngeal or hypopharyngeal cancer." —Oxford Basic reference
"Radiation given as the primary treatment for larynx cancer or as an adjuvant treatment after surgery is most often done using an external beam technique, a dose of 6000-7000 cGy is administered to the primary site." —Current otolaryngology 3/e, p 469-470

27. **Ans. is a, d and e i.e. Glottic Ca is the most common; T_1 tumor is best treated by radiotherapy; Smoking predisposes**
 Ref: Current otolaryngology 2/e, p 440,441, Dhingra 5/e, p 326, 327, 329-330; 6/e, p 308 onwards

Lets see each Option Separately

- **Option a** – Glottic CA is most common is correct

Correct –
Incidence of larynx cancer by site –

Supraglottic	–	40%
Glottic	–	59%
Subglottic	–	1%

- **Option b** – Supraglottic Ca has best prognosis *Incorrect* ....
- Supraglottic cancers are often silent and their only manifestation is presence of neck nodes which is a very late feature. Hence it does not have a good prognosis. (Best prognosis is with glottic cancer)
- **Option c** – Lymphatic spread is the M/C in subglottic CA
 Incorrect
- Lymphatic spread is more common in supraglottic CA as it has a rich lymphatic supply.
- **Option d** – T_1 tumor are best treated by radiotherapy
 Correct
 T_1 tumors are best treated by micro laryngoscopic surgery/radiotherapy
- **Option e** – Smoking predisposes - correct
 Cigarette smoking and alcohol are 2 main predisposing factors for CA larynx

28. **Ans. is d i.e. Endoscopic removal**
 Ref: Current otolaryngology 2/e, p 444, 3/e, p 463 Ref: Scotts Brown 7/e, vol-2 p 2604 – Table – 194.3 Turner 10/e, p 169

Verrucous Carcinoma

- Verrcous carcinoma makes up only 1-2% of laryngeal carcinomas.
- The larynx is the second most common site of occurance in the head and neck after the oral cavity.
- Most common site of involvement is vocal cord.
- Grossly, verrucous carcinoma appears as a fungating, papillomatous, grayish white neoplasm.
- Microscopically, it is *well differentiated squamous cell carcinoma* with minimal cytological atypis.
- It has low metastatic potential
- Hoarseness is the most common presented symptom. Pain and dysphagia may occur but are less common.
- Treatment of most verrucous tumors is primary surgery. Endoscopic laser surgery is appropriate as the tumor is less aggressive than usual squamous cell carcinoma.

29. **Ans. is a i.e. Opening the larynx in midline** *Ref. Stedman dictionary, p 937*
 Laryngofissure: Opening the larynx midline.

30. **Ans. All are correct** *Ref: Scott-Brown's Otolaryngology 7/e, vol-2 p 2617, 2618*
 Loss of functioning larynx causes problems in speech, swallowing, coughing, altered appearance, lifting, weight, laughing, crying, smelling, tasting and even kissing.

31. **Ans. is b i.e. CO_2 Laser** *Ref. Dhingra 5th/e, p 362, 6/e, p 357*
 CO_2 laser is used in laryngeal surgery to excise vocal nodules, polyps, cysts, granulomas or juvenile laryngeal papilloma. Also used in case of leukoplakia, T_1 lesion of vocal cord or localized lesions of supraepiglottis and infraglottis.

ALSO KNOW

- CO_2 laser has wavelength 10,400 nm
- It is the work horse laser and has been used widely in ENT
- It can cut precisely (0.3 mm precision), coagulate bleeders and vaporize tissues
- Besides laryngeal surgery it is used in oropharyngeal surgery to excise benign or malignant lesions and in plastic surgery

Extra Edge

Laser	Use in ENT	Comment
Argon laser	• Used to treat port wine stain, hemangioma and telangiectasia • Used to create hole in stapes footplate	• Lies in the visible spectrum of light • Wavelength 485-514 nm (blue green colour) • Easily transmitted through clear fluid e.g. cornea, lens, vitreous humor • Absorbed by Hemoglobin
KTP laser	• Stapes surgery • Endoscopic sinus surgery to remove polys or inverted papillomas and vascular lesions • Microlaryngeal surgery • To remove tracheobronchial lesions through bronchoscope	• Lies in the visible spectrum of light • Wavelength 532 nm
Nd yad laser	For debulking tracheobronchial and esophageal lesions for palliation, hereditary hemorrhagic telangiectasia and turbinectomy	Wavelength 1064 nm (lies in infra red zone of electro magnetic spectrum)
Diode laser	Turbinate reduction, laser assisted stapedectomy and mucosa intact tonsillar ablation	Wavelength 600-1000 nm

Laser	Use in ENT	Comment
Argon laser	• Used to treat port wine stain, hemangioma and telangiectasia • Used to create hole in stapes footplate	• Lies in the visible spectrum of light • Wavelength 485-514 nm (blue green colour) • Easily transmitted through clear fluid e.g. cornea, lens, vitreous humor • Absorbed by Hemoglobin
KTP laser	• Stapes surgery • Endoscopic sinus surgery to remove polys or inverted papillomas and vascular lesions • Microlaryngeal surgery • To remove tracheobronchial lesions through bronchoscope	• Lies in the visible spectrum of light • Wavelength 532 nm
Nd yad laser	For debulking tracheobronchial and esophageal lesions for palliation, hereditary hemorrhagic telangiectasia and turbinectomy	Wavelength 1064 nm (lies in infra red zone of electro magnetic spectrum)
Diode laser	Turbinate reduction, laser assisted stapedectomy and mucosa intact tonsillar ablation	Wavelength 600-1000 nm

Note: Gas preferred in laser surgery is enflurane[Q].

O_2 concentration in inhaled gases should not be more than 40%.

Do not use N_2O

32. Ans. is a, c and e i.e. Poor pulmonary reserve; Tumor involving preepiglottic space and cricoid cartilage extension

As explained in the text—Contraindications of supracricoid laryngectomy are:
- Poor pulmonary reserve (option a)
- Tumor involving preepiglottic space (option c)
  As far as involvement of cricoid cartilage is concerned.
  In SCPL—thyroid cartilage is removed and hyoid bone and cricoid cartilage are sutured together. If cricoid is involved it becomes a contraindication.
- Vocal cord fixity as such is not a contraindication; only if fixity is due to involvement of cricoarytenoid joint, then it becomes a contraindication.

33. Ans. is c i.e. Respiratory papillomatosis

A 5 year old child presenting with hoarseness and stridor and the lesion showing multiple small papillomas on vocal cords leaves no doubt that it is (Juvenile respiratory papillomatosis).

SECTION 6

Operative Procedures

Section Outline

30. Important Operative Procedures

Chapter 30

Important Operative Procedures

UPPER AIRWAY OBSTRUCTION AND TRACHEOSTOMY

Diagnostic sign of upper airway obstruction is stridor
- Other symptoms can be restlessness, Hoarseness (as in laryngeal pathology), Nostril flaring, suprasternal/intercostal retraction, Coughing or wheezing (as in trachea bronchial pathology)
- Investigation of choice in upper airway obstruction – Fiberoptic endoscopy

Management of Upper Airway Obstruction

See Table 30.1

 Note: Most definitive management of upper airway obstruction = Tracheostomy

Table 30.1: Management of upper airway obstruction

Immediate maneuvers	Medical management	Alternate airway
– Heimlich maneuver – Jaw Thrust	– O_2 inhalation through laryngeal – Mask/Nasal cannula – Heliox (80% helium and – 20% oxygen – Principle – It converts the turbulent – flow at the site of obstruction into – laminar pattern	– **Oral airway** – **Nasopharyngeal airway** – **Endotracheal intubation** (C/I in fracture of cervical spine, facial/oral – trauma, laryngeal trauma) – **Laryngeal mask ventilation** C/I = Large retropharyngeal tumors, – Retropharyngeal abscess – Hiatus hernia Pregnancy – **Cricothyrotomy** (Figure 1B) – Emergency procedure done by piercing the cricothyroid membrane called as minitracheostomy

TRACHEOSTOMY

- Site—2nd, 3rd and 4th tracheal rings which lie under the isthmus of thyroid gland.
- If tracheostomy is done above this, it is called as **high tracheostomy**; it can lead to perichondritis of cricoids cartilage and subglottic stenosis. If it is made below isthmus, it is called **low tracheostomy** and may injure great vessels of neck and the apical pleura especially in children.
- **Elective high tracheostomy** is done in malignancy of larynx presenting with stridor where a laryngectomy has to be done later. This is because after laryngectomy, a new tracheostoma has to be created lower down.
- **Elective low tracheostomy** is done in patients with laryngeal trauma to prevent aggravation of the laryngeal injury and in laryngeal papillomatoses to avoid implantation.

Features of Tracheostomy Tubes

- **Material:** Silicon is the preferred material especially in children since it is flexible and it reduces risk of mucosal trauma and skin injury around the stoma.
  Metal tubes (made of German silver) and Portex tube also available. Portex tube (PVC tube/Nonmetallic tubes) is the best tube during radiotherapy
- **Cuff:** Inflatable cuffs prevent aspiration of blood or saliva and form a seal to prevent leakage of ventilating gases during anesthesia or prolonged mechanical ventilation. But cuffs can be associated with the risk of subglottic stenosis. For this reason Low Pressure Cuffs are preferred. **In children, cuffed tracheotomy tube should not be used.**
- **Inner tube:** It projects 2–3 mm beyond the main outer tube and helps in periodic cleaning without disturbing the patency of the main tracheostomy. So they are the best for home tracheostomy care.

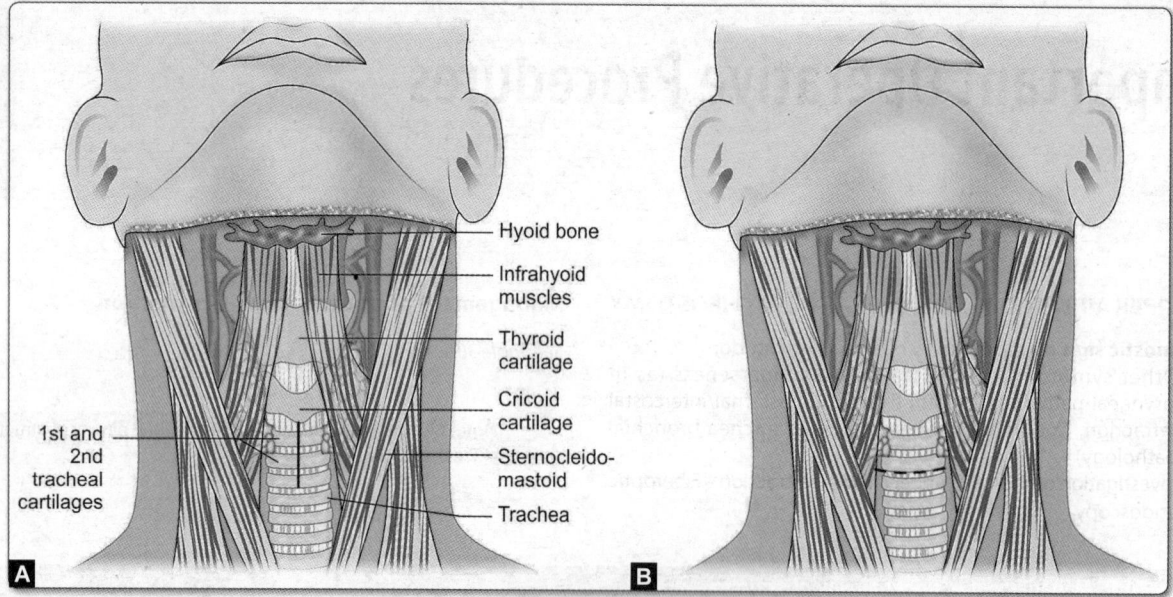

Figs. 30.1A and B: Incisions for tracheostomy. (A) Surface landmarks for the midline skin vertical incision for tracheostomy; (B) Horizontal skin incision for cricothyrotomy

Courtesy: Textbook of Diseases of Ear, Nose and Throat, Mohan Bansal. Jaypee Brothers Medical Publishers (p) Ltd., p 511.

- **Fenestration**: Allows air to pass through the tube and aids phonation, it is the tube of choice in children. Drawback—Oral contents and stomach contents can enter the lungs through these fenestrations.

   Disadvantage: Patient who are at risk of aspiration and are on IPPV should not be given fenestrated tube.

Structures Damaged in Emergency Tracheostomy

1. Isthmus
2. Left bracheocephalic vein, Jugular vein
3. Pleura
4. Thymus
5. Inferior mesenteric artery
6. Esophagus

Drawbacks

1. Post tracheostomy apnea–it is due to wash out of CO with rapid improvement in oxygenation after tracheostomy. Treatment is Carbogen inhalation which is a mixture of 95% oxygen and 5% CO_2.
2. Emphysema—In Immediate postoperative period surgical emphysema is either due to tight skin closure or large opening on the trachea. Immediate management is to release the skin sutures.
3. Bleeding—Anterior jugular vein and inferior thyroid veins are the commonest sites of bleeding.
4. Difficult decannulation- Patients who are on tracheostomy for long time, develop psychological dependence. This is the commonest long term complication in children.

Types of Tracheostomy Tube

See Table 30.2 for details

Table 30.2: Classification of tracheostomy tube
• On the basis of cuff
– Uncuffed
– Cuffed tubes
▪ Single cuff tube
▪ Double cuff tube
▪ Low pressure cuff tube
• On the basis of fenestra at the upper curvature of the tube
– Tubes without fenestra
– Single fenestrated tube
– Multiple fenestrated tube
• On the basis of length of the tube
– Standard length
– Extra length tracheostomy tube
▪ Adjustable flange long tub
• On the basis of number of lumens (cannula)
– Single lumen (cannula) tube – Nonmetallic
– Double lumen (cannula) tube – Jackson and Fuller
• Suction-aided tracheostomy tubes – metallic
• On the basis of the material
– Metallic
▪ Jackson
▪ Fuller
– Nonmetallic
▪ Polyvinyl chloride (PVC)
▪ Silicone
▪ Siliconized pVc
▪ Silastic
▪ Rubber tube
– Mixed
▪ Armored tubes

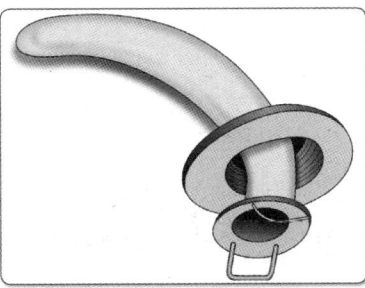

Fig. 30.2: Fuller's tracheostomy tube

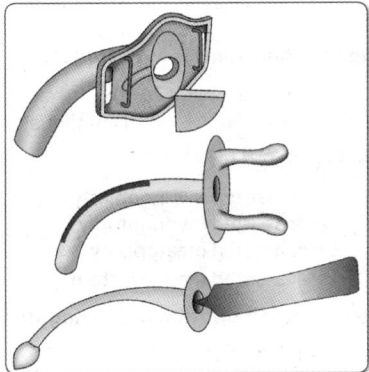

Fig. 30.3: Jackson's tracheostomy tube

FOREIGN BODIES OF UPPER AERODIGESTIVE TRACT

- Foreign body aspiration is more common in children in <4 yrs (vegetable foreign bodies even peanuts are the M/C foreign body)
- M/C Site for lodging of foreign body of upper digestive tract—Cricopharynx—since it is the narrowest part.
- Other sites of foreign body impaction are— Tonsil, Vallecula and Pyriform sinus.

Presentation

- In foreign body in cricopharynx - B/L pooling of saliva
- In foreign body in pyriform sinus - U/L pooling of saliva

FOREIGN BODY OF LARYNX

1. A smaller foreign body may present as hoarseness, stridor and cough.
2. But a large laryngeal foreign body is an emergency since it leads to total airway obstruction and patient may asphyxiate to death, if first-aid measures are not taken.

Management

- Emergency measure is Heimlich's maneuver. In children pounding the back after turning the patient head down can be tried.
- When these measures fail, cricothyrotomy (Laryngotomy) is done to gain rapid entry to airway and is converted into a normal Tracheostomy once the patient is shifted to a primary care set-up since it can lead to laryngeal stenosis later on.

FOREIGN BODY OF BRONCHUS

Presentation

- Initial choking, cyanosis followed by cough and wheeze.
  Other **Features Which Point Towards Foreign Body in Bronchus** are—unexplained or unilateral wheeze, or unexplained cough or hemoptysis or obstructive emphysema (if it leads to partial obstruction), or to atelectasis which in turn can cause pneumonitis (if it leads to complete obstruction)

 Note: Foreign bodies are more common on right side as right bronchus is short, wide and more in line with the trachea.

Management

Bronchoscopy	
Rigid bronchoscopy	**Flexible fiberoptic bronchoscopy**
Done via mouth	Done through nose
Structures seen—Uvula, Epiglottis, vocal cords, tracheal rings, carina and segmental bronchi	Structures seen—Posterior choana, pharynx, larynx, tracheal rings, carina, segmental bronchi and subsegmental bronchi
Advantage—in removal of foreign body and in children due to problem of ventilation and in establishing emergency airway	*Advantage*—Better magnification and better vision, can be used in conditions where rigid bronchoscopy is C/I like in cervical spine instability, trismus, micrognathia, recent MI, and it is useful in bedside examination of the critically ill patients. It can be passed easily through endotracheal tube or tracheostomy opening.

 Note: Flexible fiberoptic bronchoscopy is replacing rigid bronchoscopy but its utility limited in children because of the problems of ventilation.

Named Incisions used in Nasal Surgeries

Incision	Surgery
• Killian's incision	• Submucous resection
• Weber Ferguson incision	• Total maxillectomy
• Freer's incision	• Septoplasty
• Moure's incision	• Lateral rhinotomy

Pituitary Surgeries

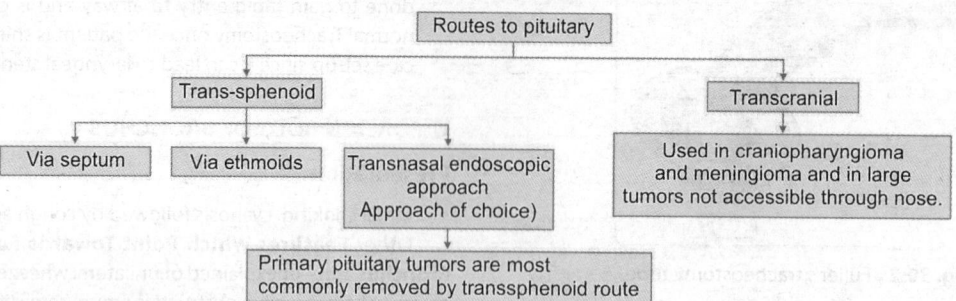

NEW PATTERN QUESTIONS

Q N1. Which of the following anesthetics should be avoided in middle ear surgery?

- a. Halothane
- b. N_2O
- c. Ether
- d. Isoflurane

Q N2. Brewer-Luckhardt reflex includes the following except:

- a. Associated with ear surgeries
- b. Associated with tonsillectomy
- c. Causes laryngospasm
- d. Causes cardiac arrhythmias/tachypnea

Q N3. High tracheostomy is indicated in:

- a. Carcinoma
- b. TB
- c. Tetanus
- d. Diphtheria

Q N4. LAM is related to:

- a. Laser assisted myringoplasty
- b. Laser assisted myringotomy
- c. Laser assisted meatoplasty
- d. Laser assisted mastoidectomy

Q N5. Commonest indication for myringotomy is:

- a. Myringitis bullosa
- b. Serous otitis media
- c. Middle ear defect
- d. Mastoiditis

Explanations and References to New Pattern Questions

N1. Ans. is b i.e. Nitrous oxide

Nitrous oxide should not be used in ear surgeries as it can enter middle ear from bloodstream and lead to expansion of air cavity. This may cause displacement of graft or prosthesis.

N2. Ans. is a i.e. Associated with ear surgeries *Ref. Lees Synopsis of Anesthesia, 11/e, p 448*

- **Brewer Luckhardt Reflex** is reflex inspiratory closure of glottis and tracheal inlet by adduction of vocal cords which is unresponsive to airway manoeuvres
- Afferent arc: Superior laryngeal nerve (vagus)
  Efferent arc: Recurrent laryngeal nerve (vagus)
- M/c seen in children and neonates, URTI, smoking, asthma, during tonsillectomy or adenoidectomy
- It is characterized by intense pain, reflex body movements, sudden stridor, bradycardia and laryngeal spasm.

N3. Ans. is a i.e. Carcinoma

See text for explanation.

N4. Ans. is b i.e. Laser assisted myringotomy

LAM stands for laser assisted myringotomy. CO_2 laser can be used for doing myringotomy, which is an OPD procedure and is done under topical anesthesia.

N5. Ans. is b i.e. Serous otitis media

Myringotomy is a surgical procedure in which a tiny incision is created in the eardrum to relieve pressure due to collection of fluid and pus. Its M/C indication is serous otitis media.

Chapter 30: Important Operative Procedures

QUESTIONS

1. **Tracheostomy is indicated in all except:** *[AI 91]*
   a. Tracheal stenosis
   b. Bilateral vocal cord palsy
   c. Foreign body larynx
   d. Uncomplicated bronchial asthma
2. **Tracheostomy is indicated in all except:** *[MP 97]*
   a. Carcinoma larynx
   b. Uncomplicated bronchial asthma
   c. Diphtheria
   d. Comatose patient
3. **The most common indication for tracheostomy is:** *[JIPMER 91]*
   a. Laryngeal diphtheria   b. Foreign body aspiration
   c. Carcinoma   d. Asthma
4. **Tracheostomy is not indicated in:** *[Rajasthan 97; TN 04]*
   a. Emphysema   b. Bronchiectasis
   c. Atelectasis   d. Pneumothorax
5. **A high tracheostomy may be indicated in:** *[SGPGI 05]*
   a. Scleroma of the larynx
   b. Multiple papillomatosis of larynx
   c. Bilateral vocal cord paralysis
   d. Carcinoma of larynx
6. **True about tracheostomy tube are all except:** *[AI 99]*
   a. Double tube
   b. Made of titanium silver alloy
   c. Cuffed tube for IPPV
   d. Has to be changed ideally in every 2 to 3 days
7. **All are true about tracheostomy tube except:** *[MP 2001]*
   a. Jackson's tube has 2 lumens
   b. Removal of metallic tube in every 2–3 days
   c. Cuffed tube is used to prevent aspiration of pharyngeal secretion
   d. Made up of titanium-silver alloy
8. **Montgomery tube used in ENT procedure is a:**
   a Double barrel tub   b. Lobster tail tube
   c. Airway tube   d. Silicone tube
9. **In emergency tracheostomy following structures are damaged except:** *[AIIMS Nov 07]*
   a. Isthmus of thyroid
   b. Inferior thyroid vein
   c. Inferior thyroid artery
   d. Thyoid IMA
10. **Most common complication of tracheostomy is:** *[PGI 97]*
    a. Tracheoesophageal fistula
    b. Tracheocutaeneous fistula
    c. Surgical emphysema
    d. Tracheal stenosis
11. **A 30-year-old Ravi presented with gradually increasing respiratory distress since 4 days. She gives history of hospitalization and mechanical ventilation with orotracheal intubation for 2 weeks. Now she is diagnosed as having severe laryngotracheal stenosis. Next step in the management is:**
    a. Laser excision and stent insertion
    b. Steroid
    c. Tracheal dilation
    d. Resection and end-to-end anastomosis
12. **Topical Mitomycin C is useful in treatment of?** *[AI 09, 10,12]*
    a. Angiofibroma   b. Tracheal stenosis
    c. Skull base osteomyelitis   d. Laryngeal carcinoma
13. **Which of the following statements regarding Heliox are correct:** *[AI 09]*
    a. It is inert
    b. Has low viscosity
    c. Decreases airway resistance
    d. Safe in pulmonary HT
14. **Foreign body in trachea & bronchus can cause:** *[PGI May 2015]*
    a. Bronchiectasis
    b. Atelectasis
    c. Subcutaneous emphysema
    d. Pneumothorax
15. **The commonest site of aspiration of a foreign body in the supine position is into the:** *[PGI 99]*
    a. Right upper lobe apical   b. Right lower lobe apical
    c. Left basal   d. Right medial
16. **"Gold standard" surgical procedure for prevention of aspiration is:** *[AIIMS Nov 03]*
    a. Thyroplasty
    b. Tracheostomy
    c. Tracheal division and permanent tracheostomy
    d. Feeding gastrostomy/jejunostomy
17. **Best management for inhaled foreign body in an infant is:**
    a. Bronchoscopy   b. IPPV and intubation *[AI 97]*
    c. Steroid   d. Tracheostomy
18. **Openings of the tube of bronchoscope are known as:**
    a. Holes   b. Apertures *[MH 03]*
    c. Vents   d. Any of the above
19. **In a one-year-old child intubation is done using:**
    a. Straight blade with uncuffed tube *[MP 2002]*
    b. Curved blade with uncuffed tube
    c. Straight blade with cuffed tube
    d. Straight curved blade with cuffed tube
20. **A 2-year-old child with intercostal retraction and increasing cyanosis was brought with a history of foreign body aspiration which might be a lifesaving in this situation:**
    a. Oxygen through face mask *[AIIMS 99]*
    b. Heimlich's manoeuvre
    c. Extracardiac massage
    d. Intracaridiac adrenaline
21. **Bronchoscopy visualizes all except:** *[AI 2010]*
    a. Trachea
    b. Vocal cords
    c. First segmental subdivision of bronchi
    d. Subcarinal lymph nodes

22. Which of the following is not a contraindication for bronchoscopy: [JIPMER 79, Delhi 83]
    a. Lesions of cervical spine
    b. Cardiac failure
    c. Active bleeding
    d. Trismus

23. A 2-year-old child develops acute respiratory distress. O/E breath sounds are decreased with wheeze on right side. Chest X-ray shows diffuse opacity on right side—Most probable diagnosis:
    a. Pneumothorax
    b. Foreign body aspiration
    c. Pleural effusion
    d. U/L emphysema.

24. A 5-year-old boy having dinner suddenly becomes aphonic and is brought to causality for the complaint of respiratory difficulty. What is the most appropriate management?
    a. Cricothyroidotomy   b. Tracheostomy
    c. Humidified O_2 d. Heimlich maneuver

25. Rigid esophagoscopy is not done in: [PGI 01]
    a. Cervical spine rigidity   b. Aortic aneurysm
    c. Carcinoma esophagus   d. Esophageal web
    e. Lung abscess

26. Route of approach of glossopharyngeal neurectomy:
    a. Tonsillectomy approach   [Kolkata 00]
    b. Transpalatal approach
    c. Transmandibular approach
    d. Transpharyngeal approach

27. All are true statement about tracheostomy and larynx in children except: [PGI May 2012]
    a. Omega shaped epiglottis
    b. Laryngeal cartilages are soft and collapsable
    c. Larynx is high in children
    d. Trachea can be easily palpated
    e. Avoid too much extension of neck during positioning

28. Kashima operation is done for: [AIIMS May 2015]
    a. Vocal cord palsy
    b. Recurrent cholesteatoma
    c. Atrophic rhinitis
    d. Choanal atresia

29. Structures preserved in radical neck dissection
    a. Internal jugular vein   [PGI May 2015]
    b. Carotid artery
    c. Accessory nerve
    d. Brachial plexus
    e. Sternocleidomastiod muscle

30. In right-handed person, direct laryngoscope is held by which hand? [AIIMS May 2012]
    a. Left   b. Right
    c. Both   d. Either of these

31. Laser uvulopharyngopalatoplasty is the surgery done for which of the following?
    a. Snoring of diseases of ear
    b. Recurrent pharyngotonsillitis
    c. Cleft palate
    d. Stammering

32. A construction worker met with an accident and presented to the trauma centre when a heavy concrete block fell over his face. He was found to have severe maxillofacial and laryngeal injury. He was not able to open his mouth and, on examination, he is found to have multiple fractures and obstruction in nasopharynx as well as oropharynx. In order to maintain a patent airway, the following procedure was done for him. Which of the following options correct define the procedure?
    [AIIMS 2016]

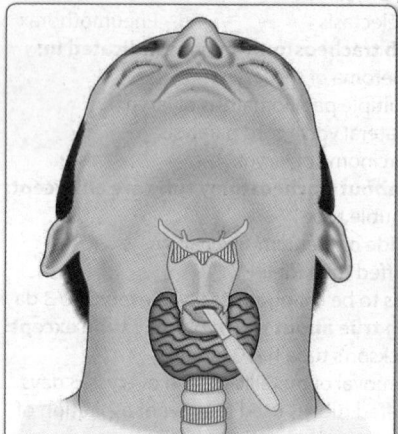

See Color Plate 24

    a. Submental endotracheal intubation
    b. Emergency tracheostomy
    c. Cricothyroidotomy
    d. Subcutaneous tracheostomy

33. True about foreign bodies of air passage in children except: [PGI May 2017]
    a. Vegetable foreign bodies are not common
    b. Tracheal obstruction can causes sudden death
    c. More common in right bronchus
    d. More common in children of less than 4 year of age
    e. CT scan of chest is done in all cases

Chapter 30: Important Operative Procedures

Explanations and References

1. **Ans. is d i.e. Uncomplicated bronchial asthma**
2. **Ans. is b i.e. Uncomplicated bronchial asthma**

Ref. Maqbool 11/e, p 351-352; Dhingra 5/e, p 337, 6/e, p 317; Head and Neck Chris deSouza Vol 2 p 1643

Indications for Tracheostomy

a. **Respiratory obstruction:**
   - Infections :
     - Acute laryngotracheobronchitis, acute epiglottitis, diphtheria
     - Ludwig's angina, peritonsillar, retropharyngeal or parapharyngeal abscess, tongue abscess.
   - **Trauma:**
     - External injury to larynx and trachea
     - Trauma due to endoscopies especially in infants and children
     - Fractures of mandible or maxillofacial injuries
   - **Neoplasms:** Benign and malignant neoplasms of larynx, pharynx, upper trachea, tongue and thyroid.
   - Foreign body in larynx
   - Edema larynx due to steam, irritant fumes or gases, allergy (angioneurotic or drug sensitivity), radiation.
   - Bilateral abductor paralysis
   - Congenital anomalies:
     - Laryngeal web, cysts, tracheooesophageal fistula
     - Bilateral choanal atresia.

b. **Retained secretions:**
   - Inability to cough:
     - Coma of any cause, e.g. head injuries, cerebrovascular accidents, narcotic overdose.
     - Paralysis of respiratory muscles, e.g. spinal injuries, polio, Guillain-Barre syndrome.
     - Spasm of respiratory muscles, tetanus, eclampsia, strychnine poisoning.
   - Painful cough : Chest injuries, multiple rib fractures, pneumonia.
   - Aspiration of pharyngeal secretions : Bulbar polio polyneuritis, bilateral laryngeal paralysis.

c. Prolonged ventilation/For assisted ventilation (m/c indication these days)
   Note: If IPPR is expected to prolong beyond 12 hours, tracheostomy is preferred over endotracheal intubation.

d. Respiratory insufficiency – chronic lung conditions – viz emphysema, chronic Bronchitis, bronchiectasis, atelectasis

e. As a part of other surgeries

3. **Ans. is b i.e. Foreign body aspiration / none**

Ref. Head and Neck Surgery – Chris deSouza vol 2 p. 1643; Mohan Bansal p 510; Scotts Brown 7th e, vol 2 p 2293

Friends – earlier – when this Question was framed – the answer was Foreign body aspiration but now in to days scenario – the answer is … (Read for yourself)

> "Historically, the main indication for a tracheostomy was to bypass upper airway obstruction caused by a foreign body or infection, particularly diphtheria. Nowadays upper airway obstruction is the least common indicator for tracheostomy. Almost two thirds of tracheostomies are currently performed on intubated intensive care patients, mainly to aid removal of secretions from the distal tracheobronchial tree and to facilitate weaning from distal tracheobronchial tree in acute respiratory failure and prolonged ventilation"
> – Head and Neck Surgery Chris De Souza 2/e, p 1643

"Today, prolonged intubation usually with mechanical ventilation is the most common indication for tracheostomy formerly it was upper respiratory obstruction."
—Mohan Bansal p 510

4. **Ans. is d i.e. Pneumothorax** *Ref. Dhingra 5/e, p 36, 339*

Friends, it is quite obvious that pneumothorax can be a complication of tracheostomy (if not performed properly) rather than an indication.

5. **Ans. is d i.e. Carcinoma of larynx** *Ref. Dhingra 5/e, p 337; Scott Brown 7/e, vol 2 p 2295; Mohan Bansal p 510*

"It is important (in tracheostomy) to refrain from causing any damage in the region of cricoid cartilage.
An exception to this rule is when a patient has laryngeal malignancy and under these circumstances tracheostomy should be placed high so as to allow resection of tracheostomy site at the time of laryngectomy". – Scott Brown 7/e, vol 2 p 2295

"The high tracheostomy is generally avoided because of the postoperative risk of perichondritis of the cricoid cartilage and subglottic stenosis. In cases of carcinoma larynx with stridor when total laryngectomy would be done, high tracheostomy is indicated."
—Mohan Bansal p 510

6. **Ans. is d i.e. Has to be changed ideally in every 2 to 3 days**
7. **Ans. is b i.e. Removal of metallic tube in every 2-3 days**

   Ref. Mohan Bansal p 592, 593; Maqbool 11/e, p 354; Turner 10/e, 195; Head and Neck Surgery Chris dSouzavol 2 p 1647

   A tracheostomy tube may be metallic or nonmetallic

Metallic Tracheostomy Tube

Metallic tubes are formed from the alloy of silver, copper phosphorus (option b in Q6 and option d in Q7).
Has an inner and an outer tube. The inner tube is longer than the outer one so that secretions and crusts formed in it can be removed and the tube reinserted after cleaning without difficulty. However, they do not have a cuff and cannot produce an airtight seal.

Nonmetallic Tracheostomy Tube

- Can be of cuffed or noncuffed variety, e.g. rubber and PVC tubes.

Cuffed Tracheostomy Tubes

- A cuff is a balloon-like device around the distal end of the tracheostomy tube. Most cuffed tubes now available have low pressure cuffs with a high volume. This significantly reduces the possibility of pressure necrosis and potential stenosis formation. Pediatric tubes do not have a cuff^Q. Cuffed tubes are used in situation where positive pressure ventilation is required, or when the airway is at risk from aspiration. (In unconscious patient or when patient is on respiration).
  The cuff should be deflated every 2 hours for 5 mins to present pressure damage to the trachea.

Uncuffed Tracheostomy Tubes

As the name suggest, this tube does not have a cuff that can be inflated inside the trachea. It is suitable for a patient who has returned to the ward from a prolonged stay in intensive care and requires physiotherapy and suction via trachea. This type of tube is not suitable for patients who are unable to swallow due to incompetent laryngeal reflexes, and aspiration of oral or gastric contents is likely to occur. An uncuffed tube is advantageous in that it allows the patient to breathe around it in the event of the tube becoming blocked. Patients can also speak with an uncuffed tube.

"Jackson and Fuller tracheostomy tube have two lumens (see the box given in the text)."s   —Mohan Bansal p 592

"Tracheostomy tubes should not be disturbed for the first 48-72 hours, but thereafter the tube is changed daily and cleaned at regular intervals."   ... Turner 10/e, p 195

According to S/B 7 e, vol 2 p 2298

"The frequency with which the inner tube needs to be cleaned will vary. In the early postoperative period. It may need cleaning every couple of hours".

8. **Ans. is d i.e. Silicone tube**   *Ref. Internet Search*

   Montgomery tracheal tube is designed to give the surgeon a complete program for creating a secondary airway - from initial incision through long-term tracheostomy care. It is a tracheal cannula system used in place of tracheostomy tubes. The system provides long-term access to the tracheal airway in situations that require an artificial airway or where access is needed for pulmonary hygiene.
   - It is so designed that the thin inner flange of the cannula is shaped to fit snugly against the contour of the inner anterior tracheal wall. No tube projects into the tracheal lumen.
   - All tracheal cannulas are made of flexible implant grade silicone to assure patient comfort and safety while reducing complications.

9. **Ans. is. c i.e. Inferior thyroid artery**   *Ref. Keith L Moore 5/e, p 1100*

   Structures which lie below the midline viz. isthmus of thyroid and thyroid IMA artery can be damaged in emergency tracheostomy. Inferior thyroid veins emerge at the lower border of the isthmus form a plexus in front of the trachea and drains into brachiocephalic vein can be damaged during tracheostomy but inferior thyroid artery, a branch of thyrocervical trunk of subclavian artery lies laterally away from midline and can thus escape injury.

10. **Ans. is a, b and c i.e. Tracheoesophageal fistula; Tracheocutaneous fistula; and Surgical emphysema**
    Ref. Dhingra 5/e, p 339-340; Scotts Brown 7/e, vol 2 p 2300-2301; Current Otolaryngology 3/e, p 542

Complications of Tracheostomy

Immediate

Most common complication of tracheostomy is hemorrhage. The commonest cause of bleeding during tracheostomy is Anterior jugular vein.

Chapter 30: Important Operative Procedures

Other Immediate Complication of tracheostomy
- Air embolism
- Cardiac arrest
- Pneumothorax (d/t injury to apical pleura)
- Apnea (due to sudden release of retained CO2)
- Local damage to structures

Intermediate

During first few hours or days
- Dislodgement/Displacement of the tube
- Surgical emphysema:
  - May occur as the air may leak into the cervical tissues.
  - This is occasionally found in the immediate postoperative period.
  - Presents as a swollen area around the root of the neck and upper chest, which displays crepitus on palpation. It is due to overtight suturing of the wound and is not dangerous unless it leads to mediastinal emphysema and cardiac tamponade.
- Pneumothorax/pneumomediastinum
- Tubal obstruction by Scabs/crusts
- Infection (tracheitis and tracheobronchitis, local wound infection).
- Dysphagia:
  - This is fairly common in the first few days after tracheostomy.
  - In normal swallowing a positive subglottic pressure is created by the closing of the vocal cords - which is why one cannot speak during swallowing. This is not possible with a tracheostomy tube in place, and thus swallowing is incoordinate.
  - Another reason for dysphagia is that if an inflatable cuff is blown up it will press on and obstruct the oesophagus.
- Tracheal necrosis
- Tracheoarterial (Tracheal innominate artery fistula) / Tracheoeshophageal fistula
- Recurrent laryngeal nerve injury.

Late
- Hemorrhage due to erosion of major vessels
- Stenosis of the trachea (at the level of stoma)
- Laryngeal stenosis due to perichondritis of cricoid cartilage.
- Difficulty with decannulation
- Tracheocutaneous fistula/scars.

 Note: According to Scott-Brown's 7th vol 2 p. 2301 - Tracheoarterial fistula / Tracheoesophageal fistula are intermediate complications and not late complications like tracheocutaneous fistula.

11. **Ans. is d i.e. Resection and end-to-end anastomosis.**

Laryngeal Stenosis	
M/C cause	– Endotracheal intubation followed by in tracheostomy
M/C site	– Subglottis at the level of cricoid cartilage
Management	
Mild stenosis (No cartilage involved)	– Repeated dilatation, removal of stenosis with CO_2 laser or intralesional steroid injection
Moderate stenosis	– Laryngotracheal reconstruction/self-expanding stents
Severe stenosis	– Partial cricotracheal resection + anastomosis

12. **Ans. is b i.e. Tracheal stenosis** *Ref. Internet search: www.bcm.edu/oto/grand.htm*
    - Laryngotracheal stenosis treated by (serial dilatation using Jackson bronchoscopes/laser have tendency to recur and hence adjuvant methods are done to decrease the rate of restenosis.
    - Mitomycin C is an example of one of these adjunctive agents. It is a chemical derived from the Streptomyces caespitosus bacterium. It is an alkylating agent which has both antineoplastic and antiproliferative properties and inhibits fibroblast production and thus prevents restenosis.

13. **Ans. is a, b and d i.e. It is inert; Has low viscosity; Safe in pulmonary HT**
    Ref. Current Otolaryngology 3/e, p 538
    - Heliox is a mixture of 80% helium and 20% oxygen
    - It has low density and high viscosity which decreases airway resistance

- It converts turbulent flow at the site of obstruction to a regular flow, which ensures better oxygen delivery to tissues and thus serves as a temporary method to improve ventilation until definitive control of airway can be achieved.

14. **Ans. is a. i.e. Bronchiectasis, b. Atelectasis, c. Subcutaneous emphysema & d. (Pneumothorax)** *Ref. TB of ENT, B.S. Tuli 2/e*

Sudden onset of cough or a unilateral wheezing should give rise to suspicion of foreign body in tracheobronchial tree.

Clinical Features of foreign body in trachea and bronchus.
- There may be no symptoms at all.
- At the onset, there may be bout of coughing, dyspnea and wheeze. Cyanosis and death may occur.
- Once these symptoms settle down, again there may be no symptoms, although signs may be present depending upon the nature of foreign body. Vegetable foreign bodies initiate chemical reaction, while metallic foreign bodies may remain silent for a sufficiently long time.
- Ultimately, later on, it may produce atelectasis of the lung segment leading to lung abscess. Obstructive emphysema occurs if bronchus is partially obstructed by foreign body due to check value obstruction.
- Symptoms of tracheobronchitis occur more in cases of vegetable foreign bodies.
- Tracheal flutter is felt as a click or flap by finger palpation of trachea.
- Examination of chest may show rales, evidence of emphysema, atelectasis or lung abscess.

15. **Ans. is b i.e. Apical lobe of right lung**

Foreign Body Aspiration

Supine position	Erect or sitting position
• Right upper lobe posterior segment • Right lower lobe superior segment • Left lower lobe superior segment	• Right posterior basilar segment of lower lobe

Site of aspiration and foreign body in lung depends upon position of patient due to anatomical elation of lung:
- If the patient has aspirated in upright or sitting position basilar segment of lower lobe is most likely to be involved
- In supine position either the posterior segment of upper (apical) lobe or superior segment of lower lobe is likely to be involved.
- In both cases right side is more likely to be involved due to straight and shorter course of right bronchi.

16. **Ans. is c i.e. Tracheal division and permanent tracheostomy**
    Ref. Scotts Brown 7/e, vol 1 p 1278; Internet search – www.bcn.edu/oto/grad

Aspiration is the passage of foreign material beyond the vocal cords:
- Larynx has 3 distinct functions – respiration, phonation and airway protection. Dysfunction of larynx can lead to aspiration.
- The primary goal of treatment of aspiration is to separate the upper digestive tract from the upper respiratory tract for a short period of time or in some cases, permanently.
  There are 3 broad categories of treatment.

1. *Temporary/Adjunct Treatments*
- Medical Therapy – in the form of antibiotics is important to prevent aspiration pneumonia.
- It is important to make the patient nil orally, to avoid further aspiration and to find an alternate feeding route to maintain the patients nutritional status. A nasogastric tube (feeding gastrostomy/jejunostomy) is commonly placed, but this may actually increase the aspiration reflux by making the lower esophageal and upper esophageal sphincters incompetent.

But Still

"Tubal feeding (either by nasogastric tube or gastrostomy) however is often unavoidable." – *Scotts Brown 7/e, vol 1 p 1278*
- Here it is important to note that feeding gastrostomy/jejunostomy are not the gold standard methods of preventing aspiration but rather are done to maintain the nutritional status of patient and prevent further aspiration. In fact according to most texts – they are a common cause of aspiration.
- Vocal cord medialization (by injecting Gel foam) is useful in unilateral paralysis. This is helpful but is rarely curative, if there is a serious aspiration problem.
- Tracheostomy will often make aspiration worse by preventing laryngeal elevation on swallowing. It does however, allow easy access to the chest for suctioning. Even a cuffed tube doesn't prevent aspiration as secretions pool above the cuff and the seal is never perfect" – *Scotts Brown 7/e, vol 1 p 1278*

2. Definite – Reversible Procedures
- **Endolaryngeal stents**: They function like a cork in the bottle. There job is to seal the glottis and therefore they need to be used in conjunction with a tracheostomy tube. But they are not often used as they are effective only as a short-term solution, plus there is risk of glottic stenosis.

- **Laryngotracheal separation:** The procedure involves transecting the cervical trachea and bringing out the lower end as a permanent end stoma

  According to Scotts Brown and Internet sites: It is the procedure of choice as it is reversible. But it has disadvantage of sacrificing voice.
- Alternative procedure is **Tracheoesophageal diversion** but has higher complication rates.

3. Definite – Irreversible Procedure

It includes: Narrow field laryngectomy: it was considered as a gold standard prior to 1970s, when the irreversible procedures like laryngo tracheal separation were not done.

Also Know

- Investigation of choice for diagnosing aspiration = Fiberoptic endoscopic evaluation of swallow (FESS)

17. **Ans. is a i.e. Bronchoscopy** *Ref. Scotts Brown 7/e, vol 1 p 1188-1190; Dhingra 5/e, p 344*
    - The peak incidence of inhaled foreign bodies is between the ages of one and three years with a male to female ratio of 2:1
    - Only 12% of the inhaled bodies impact in the larynx while most pass through the cords into the tracheobronchial tree.
    - In contrast to adults, where objects tend to lodge in the distal bronchi or right main bronchus, in children they tend to lie more centrally within the trachea (53%) or just distal to the carina (47%)
    - The treatment of choice for airway foreign bodies is prompt endoscopic removal with a Bronchoscope.
    - "In children – The choice of either using a rigid or flexible endoscope remains controversial. Otolaryngologists traditionally believe rigid endoscopes to be the optimal instrument for tracheobronchial foreign bodies. However, there are certain objects that may be more suitably removed with flexible fiberoptic instruments or a combination of rigid and flexible techniques."

    "The treatment of choice for airway foreign bodies is endoscopic removal with a rigid instrument"–Nelson 18/ed pp 169,170

18. **Ans. is c i.e. Vents** *Ref. Bronchology by Lukomsky, 40*

    Bronchoscope is similar to esophagoscope, but has openings at the distal part of the tube, called Vents which help in aeration of the side bronchi.

19. **Ans. is a i.e. Straight blade with uncuffed tube** *Ref. Scotts Brown 7/e vol 1 p 511*

    Pediatric Airway Management – Equipment
    - Tracheal intubation remains the standard for airway maintenance during many procedures.
    - Generally, a tracheal tube of the largest possible internal diameter should be chosen to minimize resistance to gas flow and avoid an excessive leak around the tube. It is important, however, to avoid inserting too large tube, which may cause mucosal damage.

    The length of the tube is calculated as:

Length = + 12 cm	For orotracheal intubation
Length = + 15 cm	For nasotracheal intubation

    - Uncuffed tubes are used in children – as there is potential for mucosal damage with the cuffed tubes (with high volume, low pressure cuffs)
    - In older children approaching puberty – Cuffed endotracheal tubes are used, reflecting the anatomical development of the airway.
    - Endotracheal tubes are available in a variety of materials although the use of PVC and silicone rubber is now almost universal.
    - As far as blades are concerned – A huge range of laryngoscopes blades are available. Anatomical considerations and to some extent personal choice, determine the most appropriate blade to use. In general position of the infant larynx and the long epiglottis makes intubation easier with a straight blade and are often used in children under 6 months of age.

    So from above description, it is clear that in children straight blade with uncuffed tube is the best for intubation.

20. **Ans. is b i.e. Heimlich's maneuver** *Ref. Dhingra 5/e, p 344, Scotts Brown 7/e vol 1 p 1188*
    - The child is presenting with cyanosis and intercostal retraction which indicates that the foreign body is lodged in the larynx.
    - Initial management for a foreign body lodged in trachea/larynx is Heimlich's maneuver where a person stands behind the child and places his arms around his lower chest and gives four abdominal thrust.
    - In infants, lying the child on its back on the adults knee and pressing firmly on the upper abdomen is the preferred maneuver.
    - If Heimlich's maneuvre fails, cricothyrotomy or emergency tracheostomy should be done.
    - Once acute respiratory emergency is over foreign body can be removed by direct laryngoscopy or by laryngofissure, if it is impacted.

Note:
- Tracheal and bronchial foreign bodies are removed by bronchoscopy with full preparation and under GA.
- Emergency removal of bronchial foreign bodies is not indicated.

21. **Ans. is d i.e. Subcarinal lymph nodes** *Ref. Read below*
    - Carina – midline partition between the two bronchi is the first endobronchial landmark during bronchoscopy. Subcarinal lymph nodes cannot be visualized on bronchoscopy but widening of carina is suggestive of subcarnial lymphadenopathy, and pulsations of the carina may be seen in aneurysm of arch of aorta
    - Rest all structures viz. vocal cord, trachea and first segmental subdivision of bronchi can be visualized.

    Note: Rigid bronchoscope visualises only up to segmental bronchus while it is possible to inspect the 2nd to 5th order subsegmental bronchi or beyond using the flexible bronchoscope.

22. **Ans. is c i.e. Active bleeding** *Ref. Tuli 1/e, p 529*
    Bronchoscopy is a procedure used for endoscopic examination of tracheobronchial tree.

    ### Contraindications of Bronchoscopy
    - Emergency bronchoscopy has no contraindication as it may be a lifesaving procedure.
    - Elective bronchoscopy may have the following contraindications:
      – General contraindications such as HT, DM, bleeding disorders, active infections.
      – Trismus
      – Aortic aneurysm
      – Cervical spine problems
      – Active recent massive hemoptysis
      – Metastatic involvement of cervical spine
      – Pulmonary hypertension.
    Although, cardiac arrest has not been mentioned as one of the contraindication but it is a very important complication of bronchoscopy. Hence, in patients of cardiac arrest bronchoscopy should not be performed.

    Note: Bronchoscopy should always be preceded by laryngoscopy during which the subglottis should be examined.

23. **Ans. is b i.e. Foreign body aspiration**
    Foreign body aspiration is a very common problem in pediatric age group (< 4 years). In the question, child is presenting with sudden onset respiratory distress and there is U/L decreased breath sounds + U/L wheezing and on chest X-ray a diffuse opacity is seen on right side i.e. there is clinical and radiological evidence of bronchospasm and collapse suggestive of a foreign body in bronchus

24. **Ans. is d i.e. Heimlich's maneuver**
    Ref. Scotts Broun 7/e, p 1188-1191, Emergency medicine 6/e, p 68, 69; Dhingra 5th/ed p344; Emergency medicine (American college of Emergency Physicians) 6th/ed pp 68, 69
    - Aphonia (inability to speak) and sudden respiratory distress in a young boy while having food, suggests obstruction of the airway with a large bolus of food. Heimlich's maneuver is the recommended, initial procedure of choice for relieving airway obstruction due to solid objects.
    - Cricothyroidotomy or tracheostomy should be performed if the Heimlich's maneuver fails

25. **Ans. is a and b i.e. Cervical spine rigidity; and Aortic aneurysm** *Ref. Dhingra 5/e, p 436*
    Contraindications of esophagoscopy (rigid type):
    - Trismus
    - Aneurysm of aorta
    - Receding mandible
    - Advanced heart, liver, kidney diseases (relative contraindication).
    - Diseases of cervical spine, e.g. cervical trauma, spondylitis, TB, osteophytes, kyphosis, etc.

26. **Ans. is a i.e. Tonsillectomy approach** *Ref. Dhingra 5/e, p 438*
    Tonsillecotmy is done as a part of the following operations:
    - Palatopharyngoplasty which is done for sleep apnea syndrome
    - Glossopharyngal neurectomy—tonsil is removed first and then IX nerve is severed in the bed of tonsil
    - Removal of styloid process.

27. **Ans is d i.e. Trachea can be easily palpated** *Ref. Dhingra 6/e, p285; Logan and Turner 10/e, p 396*
    Infant's larynx differs from adult in:
    - It is situated high up (C2 – C4).^{Q} (in adults = C3 – C6)

- Of equal size in both sixes *(in adults it is larger in males)*
- Larynx is funnel shaped
- The narrowest part of the infantile larynx is the junction of subglottic larynx with trachea and this is because cricoid cartilage is very small
- Epiglottis is *omega shaped, soft, large* and *patulous.*
- Laryngeal cartilages are soft and collapse easily
- Short trachea and short neck.
- Vocal cords are angled and lie at level of C4
- Trachea bifurcates at level of T2
- Thyroid cartilage is flat. The cricothyroid and thyrohyoid spaces are narrow.

Tracheostomy in Infants and Children
Dhingra 5/e, p338

"*Trachea of infants and children is soft and compressible and its identification may become difficult* and the surgeon may easily displace it and go deep or lateral to *it injuring recurrent laryngeal nerve or even the carotid.*"

"*During positioning, do not extend too much* as this pulls structures from chest into the neck and thus injury may occur to pleura, innominate vessels and thymus or the tracheostomy opening may be made two low near suprasternal notch."

Tracheostomy in Infants and Children
Logan and Turner 10/e, p 396

"*The incision is a short transverse one, midway b/w lower border of thyroid cartilage and the suprasternal notch. The neck must be well extended*"

"*A incision is made through two tracheal rings, preferably the third or fourth.*"

28. **Ans. is a i.e. Vocal cord palsy** *Ref Dhingra 6/e p300*

    Kashima Operation is another name for cordotomy surgery done in case of the B/L vocal cord paralysis (B/L abductor paralysis) Laser cordotomy was first described by Kashima in 1989. In 1999, Friedman described the application of cordotomy in Children from 14 months to 13 years.

    Now Endoscopic laser cordotomy is being considered as an alternate procedure to tracheostomy for managing vocal cord palsy.

29. **Ans. is b Carotid Artery & d. Brachial plexus** *Ref. P.L. Dhingra 6/e, pgs 388-89; Bailey and Love 25/e, pgs 733; CSDT 11/e, pgs 1301*

    Classical radical neck dissection

Structures removed are:	Structures saved are: *Dhingra ENT*
1. Internal jugular vein	1. Carotid artery
2. **Accessory nerve**^Q	2. Brachial plexus
3. **Submandibular gland**^Q	3. Phrenic nerve
4. **Tail of parotid**	4. Vagus nerve
5. Sternocleidomastoid muscle	5. Cervical sympathetic chain
6. Omohyoid muscle	6. Marginal mandibular br. of facial, lingual and hypoglossal nerves
7. Cervical lymphatics and lymph node	

    > "RND does not remove nodes of **postauricular, suboccipital, parotid** (except those in tail), facial retropharyngeal & pretracheal regions"—*Dhingra 5/e, pgs 396*

    Modified radical neck dissection *L & B 25th/733*
    Structures preserved are one or more of the following:
    1. **Accessory nerve**
    2. **Sternocleidomastiod muscle**
    3. **Internal jugular vein**

30. **Ans. is a i.e. Left** *Ref. Dhingra 5/e, p 432*

    "*Laryngoscope is held by the handle in the left hand. Right hand is used to retract the lips and guide the laryngoscope and to handle suction and instruments.*" —*Dhingra*

31. **Ans. is a i.e. Snoring of Diseases of Ear** *Ref: Mohan Bansal Textbook of Diseases of Ear, Nose and Throat 1/e, p 435*

    Snoring : Noisy breathing, a rough, rattling inspiratory noise produced by vibration of pendulous soft palate or occasionally of vocal cords during sleep.
    - Snoring indicates some obstruction in upper airway and represents a continum of the similar pathology as of Obstructive Sleep Apnea (OSA), where snoring is on one end and OSA on the other.

- **Management of Snoring without Obstructive Sleep Apnea.**

- **Uvulopalatoplasty–Laser Assisted Uvulopalatoplasty (LAUP) or Bovie-Assisted Uvulopalatoplasty (BAUP)**. It can be performed under Local Anesthesia in OPD. In this procedure, uvula is amputated and 1 cm trenches are created in the soft palate on either side of uvula. The soft palate elevates and stiffens after healing.
- **Uvulopalatopharyngoplasty** – It is the M/C surgery performed for Obstructive Sleep Apnea. It is also very effective in treating snoring.

Also Know
- **OSA** – Obstructive sleep apnea is a disorder characterized by loud, habitual snoring and repetitive obstruction of the upper airway during sleep, resulting in prolonged intervals of hypoxia and fragmented sleep.
- Gold standard test in evaluation of OSA – Polysomnography. It differentiates snoring without OSA from snoring with OSA and also identifies the severity of apnea.
- Muller's maneuver – This test is done before uvulopalatopharyngoplasty to know whether the patient will benefit from the surgery or not.

32. **Ans. is c i.e. Cricothyroidotomy** *Ref: Scott-Brown's Otorhinolaryngology: Head and Neck Surgery, 7ed, pg 476*

    The procedure being done is Cricothyroidotomy. A **cricothyrotomy (or cricothyroidotomy)** is an incision made through the skin and cricothyroid membrane to establish a patent airway during certain life-threatening situations, such as airway obstruction by a foreign body, angioedema, or massive facial trauma. Cricothyrotomy is easier and quicker to perform than tracheotomy, does not require manipulation of the cervical spine, and is associated with fewer complications.

33. **Ans. is a, b and e. i.e. vegetative foreign bodies are not common, tracheal obstruction can cause sudden death & CT scan of chest is done in all cases.**

    ### Foreign body of air passages
    - A foreign body aspirated into air passage can lodge in larynx, trachea or bronchi
    - M/C in children in < 4 years of age
    - M/C foreign body is vegetative foreign body e.g. peanuts, almost seed, pieces of carrot etc.

    ### Symptoms of foreign body aspiration
    1. Initial period of choking, gagging and wheezing
    2. Then the respiratory mucosa adapts to the presence of foreign body and there is symptomless interval
    3. Later symptoms

Laryngeal foreign body	Tracheal foreign body	Bronchial foreign body
• A large foreign body may obstrcut the airway leading to sudden death • Partially obstructive foreign body can cause discomfort or pain in throat • Diagnosis is by X-ray	• Causes cough and hemoptysis • A loose foreign body may move up and down leading to palpatory mud	• Most foreign body enter the **Right Bronchus** as it is wider and more in line with the tracheal lumen • A foreign body in bronchus can lead to complete obstruction of segmental bonchus causing atelectasis son obstructive emphysema